# Applied Echocardiography in Coronary Artery Disease

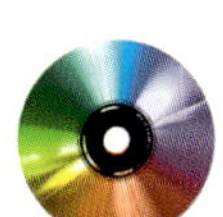

**System requirements:**

- Operating System—Windows Vista or above
- Web Browser—Internet Explorer 8 or above, Google Chrome and Mozilla Firefox
- Essential plugins—Java and PDF Reader
  - Facing problems in viewing content—it may be, your system does not have java enabled
  - You can test Java and download PDF reader by using the links from the help section of the **CD**

Accompanying **CD-ROM** is playable only in Computer and not in DVD player. CD has autorun function—it may take few seconds to load on your computer. If it does not work for you, then follow the steps below to access the contents manually:

- Click on my computer
- Select the CD/DVD drive and click open/explore—this will show list of files in the CD
- Find and double click file—"launch.html"

# Applied Echocardiography in Coronary Artery Disease

*Editor-in-Chief*

**Ravi R Kasliwal**
MD DM
Chairman
Clinical and Preventive Cardiology
Medanta Heart Institute
Medanta—The Medicity
Gurgaon, Haryana, India

*Co-editor*

**Manish Bansal**
MD DNB (Cardiology) FACC FASE FISCU
Senior Consultant Cardiology
Medanta—The Medicity
Gurgaon, Haryana, India

*Forewords*

**Naresh Trehan**
**Gilbert Habib**

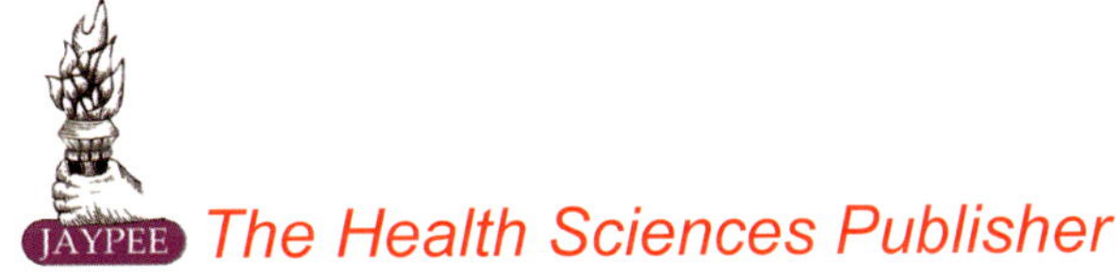


New Delhi | London | Philadelphia | Panama

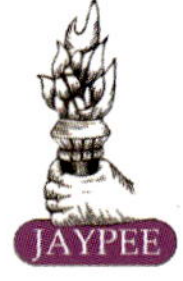


**Jaypee Brothers Medical Publishers (P) Ltd.**

**Headquarters**

Jaypee Brothers Medical Publishers (P) Ltd.
4838/24, Ansari Road, Daryaganj
New Delhi 110 002, India
Phone: +91-11-43574357
Fax: +91-11-43574314
E-mail: jaypee@jaypeebrothers.com

**Overseas Offices**

J.P. Medical Ltd.
83, Victoria Street, London
SW1H 0HW (UK)
Phone: +44 20 3170 8910
Fax: +44 (0) 20 3008 6180
E-mail: info@jpmedpub.com

Jaypee-Highlights Medical Publishers Inc.
City of Knowledge, Building 235, 2nd Floor
Panama City, Panama
Phone: +1 507-301-0496
Fax: +1 507-301-0499
E-mail: cservice@jphmedical.com

Jaypee Medical Inc.
325, Chestnut Street
Suite 412, Philadelphia, PA 19106, USA
Phone: +1 267-519-9789
E-mail: support@jpmedus.com

Jaypee Brothers Medical Publishers (P) Ltd.
17/1-B, Babar Road, Block-B, Shaymali
Mohammadpur, Dhaka-1207
Bangladesh
Mobile: +08801912003485
E-mail: jaypeedhaka@gmail.com

Jaypee Brothers Medical Publishers (P) Ltd.
Bhotahity, Kathmandu, Nepal
Phone: +977-9741283608
E-mail: kathmandu@jaypeebrothers.com

Website: www.jaypeebrothers.com
Website: www.jaypeedigital.com

© 2017, Jaypee Brothers Medical Publishers

The views and opinions expressed in this book are solely those of the original contributor(s)/author(s) and do not necessarily represent those of editor(s) of the book.

All rights reserved. No part of this publication and CD-ROM may be reproduced, stored or transmitted in any form or by any means, electronic, mechanical, photocopying, recording or otherwise, without the prior permission in writing of the publishers.

All brand names and product names used in this book are trade names, service marks, trademarks or registered trademarks of their respective owners. The publisher is not associated with any product or vendor mentioned in this book.

Medical knowledge and practice change constantly. This book is designed to provide accurate, authoritative information about the subject matter in question. However, readers are advised to check the most current information available on procedures included and check information from the manufacturer of each product to be administered, to verify the recommended dose, formula, method and duration of administration, adverse effects and contraindications. It is the responsibility of the practitioner to take all appropriate safety precautions. Neither the publisher nor the author(s)/editor(s) assume any liability for any injury and/or damage to persons or property arising from or related to use of material in this book.

This book is sold on the understanding that the publisher is not engaged in providing professional medical services. If such advice or services are required, the services of a competent medical professional should be sought.

Every effort has been made where necessary to contact holders of copyright to obtain permission to reproduce copyright material. If any have been inadvertently overlooked, the publisher will be pleased to make the necessary arrangements at the first opportunity.

**Inquiries for bulk sales may be solicited at:** jaypee@jaypeebrothers.com

***Applied Echocardiography in Coronary Artery Disease***

*First Edition :* **2017**

ISBN : 978-93-5152-972-9

*Printed at* Replika Press Pvt. Ltd.

**Dedicated to**

*The 'fab four' who would have truly appreciated this work and given a warm hug:*
*Prayag and Rajkumari Kasliwal*
*RamRatan and Rajmal Kasliwal*

# Contributors

**Adrian Chong** MBBS (Hons) BPharm FRACP FASE FCSANZ
Cardiologist
Department of Cardiology
Princess Alexandra Hospital
Mater Health Services
University of Queensland
Brisbane, Queensland, Australia

**Alina Nicoara** MD FASE
Assistant Professor of Anesthesiology
Director, Perioperative Echo Service
Duke University Health System
Durham, North Carolina, USA

**Amrita Kushal** MD
Cardiovascular Fellow
Lenox Hill Heart and Vascular Institute of New York
New York, USA

**Anuj Mediratta** MD
Advanced Cardiovascular Imaging Fellow
Section of Cardiology
Department of Medicine
University of Chicago
Chicago, Illinois, USA

**Asrar Ahmed** MD DM MRCP
Clinical Research Fellow
Department of Cardiovascular Medicine, Northwick Park Hospital
Harrow, London, UK

**Ayman A Farag** MD
Instructor/Fellow
Medicine-Cardiovascular Disease
Department of Medicine
Division of Cardiovascular Disease
University of Alabama
Birmingham, Alabama, USA

**Bijoy K Khandheria** MD FACP FESC FASE FACC
Clinical Adjunct Professor of Medicine
University of Wisconsin
School of Medicine and Public Health
Milwaukee, Wisconsin
Medical Director, Echocardiography
Aurora Cardiovascular Services-Aurora Medical Group, Milwaukee, Wisconsin
Co-Director
Aurora Center for Cardio-Oncology Research and Innovation
Milwaukee, Wisconsin, USA

**Brian Mott** MD
Fellow in Cardiology
Knight Cardiovascular Institute,
Oregon Health and Science University
Portland, Oregon, USA

**Cheuk-Man Yu** MD FACC FRCP
Professor of Medicine and Therapeutics
Division of Cardiology, Department of Medicine and Therapeutics
Honorary Consultant
Prince of Wales Hospital
Director (Clinical Sciences)
Institute of Vascular Medicine
Director of Heart Education and Research Training (HEART) Center
Faculty of Medicine
Division of Cardiology and HEART Center
The Chinese University of Hong Kong
Hong Kong

**Divya Malhotra** MD Diplomate American Board of Cardiovascular Disease Diplomate American Society of Echocardiography FACC FASE
Head and Senior Consultant
Department of Noninvasive Cardiology
Max Superspecialty Hospital
Saket, New Delhi, India

**Francesco Maffessanti** PhD
Postdoctoral Research Fellow
Department of Medicine
Section of Cardiology
University of Chicago
Chicago, Illinois, USA

**G Vijayaraghavan** MD DM (Cardiology) FRCP (Lon) FRCP (Edin) FACC FAHA
Vice Chairman and Director
Dean Academics
President SOCOMER
Senior Consultant Cardiologist
Department of Cardiology
Kerala Institute of Medical Sciences
Thiruvananthapuram, Kerala, India

**Itzhak Kronzon** MD FASE FACC FACP FESC FAHA
Chief, Cardiac Imaging
Professor of Cardiology
Lenox Hill Heart and Vascular Institute of New York
Hofstra University—NSLIJ School of Medicine
New York, USA

**Jagdish C Mohan** MD DM FASE
Director of Cardiac Sciences
Department of Cardiac Sciences
Fortis Hospital
Shalimar Bagh, New Delhi, India

**Karima Addetia** MD FRCPC
Clinical Associate of Medicine
Department of Medicine
Section of Cardiology
University of Chicago
Chicago, Illinois, USA

**Madhav Swaminathan** MD FASE FAHA
Associate Professor of Anesthesiology
Clinical Director, Cardiothoracic Anesthesiology and Critical Care Medicine
Duke University Health System
Durham, North Carolina, USA

**Manish Bansal** MD DNB (Cardiology) FACC FASE FISCU
Senior Consultant Cardiology
Medanta—The Medicity
Gurgaon, Haryana, India

**M Sonia Jain** MD MRCP (UK)
Cardiologist
Olmsted Medical Center
Rochester, Minnesota, USA

**Munesh Tomar** MBBS MD FNB
Associate Director
Department of Pediatric Cardiology and Congenital Heart diseases
Medanta—The Medicity
Gurgaon, Haryana, India

**Navin C Nanda** MD DSc (Med) (Hon) DSc (Hon) FACC FAHA FISCU (D)
Distinguished Professor of Medicine and Cardiovascular Disease
University of Alabama
Birmingham, Alabama, USA

**Nitin J Burkule** MD DM DNB FASE FACC
Consultant Cardiologist
Jupiter Hospital
Thane, Maharashtra, India

**Patrizio Lancellotti** MD PhD FESC FACC
Head
Intensive Care Cardiology Unit
University of Liege
Hospital Center
Professor
Clinical Medicine
University of Liege
Liege, Belgium

**Qing Zhang** MD PhD
Professor
Department of Cardiology
West China Hospital
Sichuan University
Chengdu, Sichuan, China

**Rahul Mehrotra** MBBS MD DNB (Cardiology)
Senior Consultant Cardiology
Medanta Heart Institute
Medanta—The Medicity
Gurgaon, Haryana, India

**Raj Kumar** MD (Physician) PG Diploma in Clinical Cardiology FNIC
Consultant
Department of Noninvasive Cardiology
Max Superspecialty Hospital
Saket, New Delhi, India

**Raluca Dulgheru** MD
Cardiologist
Department of Cardiology
Heart Valve Clinic
University Hospital Sart Tilman
University of Liege
Liege, Belgium

**Ram Bedi** PhD MBA
Affiliate Assistant Professor
Department of Bioengineering
University of Washington
Seattle, Washington, USA

**Ravi R Kasliwal** MD DM
Chairman
Clinical and Preventive Cardiology
Medanta Heart Institute
Medanta—The Medicity
Gurgaon, Haryana, India

**Roberto M Lang** MD FASE
Professor
Department of Medicine and Radiology
Director
Noninvasive Cardiac Imaging Laboratories
Section of Cardiology
Department of Medicine
University of Chicago
Chicago, Illinois, USA

**Roxy Senior** MD DM FRCP FESC FACC
Professor of Clinical Cardiology
Consultant Cardiologist and Director of Echocardiography
National Heart and Lung Institute
Imperial College, London
Royal Brompton Hospital, London
Consultant Cardiologist and Director of Cardiac Research
Northwick Park Hospital
Harrow, London, UK

**Sanjay Mittal** MD DM (Cardiology)
Senior Director
Clinical Cardiology and Research
Medanta—The Medicity
Gurgaon, Haryana, India

**Sanjiv Kaul** MD FACC FASE FAHA FESC FRCP (London)
Ernest C Swigert Endowed Chair in Cardiovascular Medicine
Professor of Medicine and Radiology
CEO, Knight Cardiovascular Institute
Oregon Health and Science University
Portland, Oregon, USA

**S Baskaran** MBBS DNB (Medicine) DNB (Cardiology)
Senior Registrar
Deparment of Cardiology
Kerala Institute of Medical Sciences
Thiruvananthapuram, Kerala, India

**Shantanu P Sengupta** MD DNB FACC FASE FCCP
Director
Sengupta Hospital and Research Institute
Nagpur, Maharashtra, India

**SK Parashar** MD FACC
Senior Consultant Cardiologist
Metro Heart Institute
New Delhi, India

**Srikanth Sola** MD
Additional Senior Consultant
Department of Cardiology
Sri Sathya Sai Institute of Higher Medical Sciences
Bengaluru, Karnataka, India

**Sudhir Wahi** MBBS MD FRACP FCSANZ
Associate Professor
Department of Cardiology
Director of Echocardiography
Princess Alexandra Hospital
University of Queensland
Brisbane, Queensland, Australia

**Sunil Mankad** MD FACC FCCP FASE
Associate Professor of Medicine
Mayo Clinic College of Medicine
Associate Director, Cardiology Fellowship
Director, Transesophageal Echocardiography
Board of Directors, American Society of Echocardiography
ACC Governor, Minnesota, USA

**Ty Whitfield** MD
Cardiovascular Diseases Fellow
Department of Medicine
Division of Cardiovascular Diseases
University of Alabama
Birmingham, Alabama, USA

**Vinayak Agrawal** MD DNB (Cardiology) FACC FASE
Senior Consultant
Department of Cardiology
Medanta—The Medicity
Gurgaon, Haryana, India

**Vishwas Mohan** MBBS Dip Card (UK)
Attending Cardiologist
Primus Hospital
Chanakyapuri, New Delhi, India

**Vivek Jain** MD Physican PGDCC
Senior Resident
Medanta—The Medicity
Gurgaon, Haryana, India

**Yu-Jia Liang** PhD MD
Associate Professor
Department of Cardiology
West China Hospital of Sichuan University
Chengdu, Sichuan, China

# Foreword

It gives me immense pleasure to write the foreword for the book *Applied Echocardiography in Coronary Artery Disease*. Having known Dr Kasliwal for over three decades now, I should say a work like this, with internationally renowned faculty and some of the best known Indian authors, was long overdue! This book fulfills a hiatus that existed in our practical understanding of patients of coronary artery disease: from the outpatient clinics to the emergency room and from the critically ill patients in the ICU to the cardiac operation theater.

As a cardiac surgeon, I have been witness, as well as a part, of the stupendous growth echocardiography has achieved during the past decades. I remember vividly the pioneering work of Drs Kronzon and Kasliwal in evaluation of protruding atheromas of the aortic arch not so far back and here we are, in an era wherein the use of 3D technology for mitral valve repair has become commonplace in the operation theaters across the globe.

As coronary artery disease constitutes the largest number of patients in any cardiac department, echocardiography has emerged as a key investigation, something that is truly indispensable. However, echocardiography needs to be viewed in clinical context and therein lies the true significance of this book—from scientific thinking to practical demonstration for clinical decision making for the patients.

I unhesitatingly recommend this text to everyone who is interested in learning the nuance of echocardiography. My colleague Ravi Kasliwal and the "who's-who" of the world of echocardiography who have contributed to this book, deserve my appreciation.

**Naresh Trehan**
Diplomate American Board of Cardiothoracic Surgery
Chairman and Managing Director, and
Chief Cardiac Surgeon
Medanta—The Medicity
Gurgaon, Haryana, India

# Foreword

It is my pleasure and honor to write a few words about my Indian colleagues and the current edition of the *Applied Echocardiography in Coronary Artery Disease*. Indian cardiologists have always been an example for the rest of the world in the field of echocardiography, with dynamic pioneers and innovative specialists of this fantastic technique. More important, facing such an important clinical problem as ischemic heart disease, we need to be not only echocardiographists, but also clinicians, that means doctors able to integrate the echocardiographic results in their clinical context, and to use these results to give the best therapy to the patient. Several echocardiographic techniques, including 2D, 3D echocardiography, stress echocardiography, contrast echocardiography and other more recent techniques such as tissue Doppler imaging and deformation imaging, are perfectly described in this book, and their use in ischemic heart disease is clearly depicted.

In that way, *Applied Echocardiography in Coronary Artery Disease* is the perfect example of what we can expect from a medical book: to be complete, exhaustive, comprehensive, but also easy to use in clinical practice by all practicing physicians. The result is here: this book will be an easy and fantastic tool for all Indian cardiologists, and probably around the world.

This foreword is also the opportunity for me to underline the strong and friendly relationship between Indian and European echocardiographists. As a specialist of echocardiography, but also President of the European Association of Cardiovascular Imaging, I am happy to see that in this book, the patient is at the center, and all the efforts are done to use echocardiography to find the best way to treat him/her.

The next step will be multimodality imaging. Other imaging techniques are also useful for the assessment of coronary artery disease. I am sure that the next objective of the authors will be to teach us how and when to use echocardiography and other imaging techniques in different clinical scenarios.

At the moment, we are learning echocardiography. Enjoy the *Applied Echocardiography in Coronary Artery Disease*!

**Gilbert Habib**
President
European Association of
Cardiovascular Imaging (EACVI)
Head
Department of Cardiology
University Hospital of Timone
Marseille, France

# Preface

Coronary artery disease (CAD) is one of the leading causes of death worldwide, and its prevalence continues to increase in many parts of the world. The patients of CAD thus constitute a major chunk of the patients seen by cardiologists today. For optimal management of these patients, the cardiologists rely on a thorough clinical evaluation supplemented by appropriate investigations. Echocardiography is one of the most useful imaging modalities available for this purpose in these patients.

Echocardiography is noninvasive, versatile, and safe and provides a vast amount of information about cardiac structure and function almost instantly. With its various modalities encompassing the entire spectrum of CAD—from visualization of early evidence of atherosclerosis to assessment of myocardial ischemia and viability to guiding therapeutic interventions—echocardiography assists at every step in critical decision making in these patients. For example, in a patient with CAD slated to undergo percutaneous coronary intervention, detection of significant mitral regurgitation will alter the entire course of treatment. Hence, a clinician dealing with the patients of CAD today cannot afford to be ignorant of the various aspects of echocardiography and the implications thereof.

Elaborate texts have been written and a huge amount of information is available about various aspects of echocardiography, both in the print form and on the internet. These are mainly textbooks of echocardiography describing the techniques and the role of echocardiography in all forms of cardiovascular diseases. However, the vastness of the available literature means that very often the interested reader has to sift through volumes of material on the subject and is left bewildered at the end of it all. This is the very need that the book aims to fulfill by compiling the state-of-the-art and updated knowledge about the role of echocardiography in the evaluation and management of patients with the various facets of CAD. When confronted with a patient of CAD and assailed with doubts regarding any aspect, the practicing physician needs to just pick-up this book and find the solution!

The book is divided into two sections—the first section deals with the technical aspects of the commonly used echocardiographic modalities while the second section discusses the clinical application of these modalities in the evaluation of patients with CAD. The contributors are the respected and renowned names in the field of echocardiography with years of experience behind them. They have graciously spent time and energy to give their best for this book. My grateful thanks to all of them for having responded to my numerous emails and conceding to my demands elegantly.

I hope the book will be widely read and will satisfy the needs of the discerning physicians!

**Ravi R Kasliwal**

# Acknowledgments

I am extremely thankful to Shri Jitendar P Vij (Group Chairman), Mr Ankit Vij (Group President), Mr Tarun Duneja (Director-Publishing), Mr KK Raman (Production Manager), as well as the editorial team of Mr Sarvesh Singh, Mr Mohit Bhargava, Mr Pramod Rout (Typesetter), Mr Amit Mathur (Graphic Designer) and Ms Monika Arora of M/s Jaypee Brothers Medical Publishers (P) Ltd, New Delhi, India, for all their efforts and support in bringing out our ideas in print form.

# Contents

## SECTION 1

## Echocardiographic Techniques Used in the Evaluation of Patients with Coronary Artery Disease

## SECTION 2

# Clinical Applications

# CD Contents

## Chapter 1: Assessment of Left Ventricular Systolic Function

*Shantanu P Sengupta, Bijoy K Khandheria*

**Video 1.1** Apical 4-chamber view in a patient with previous myocardial infarction. Left ventricular apex and distal parts of mid-inferoseptal and mid-anterolateral segments are akinetic, consistent with involvement of the left anterior descending coronary artery. Left ventricular apical thrombus is also present.

**Video 1.2** Apical 2-chamber view in a patient with inferior wall myocardial infarction demonstrating akinesia of basal and mid-inferior wall.

**Video 1.3** Typical septal bounce in a patient with chronic constrictive pericarditis. Marked thickening of the pericardium in the posterior region can also be easily appreciated.

**Video 1.4** Apical 4-chamber view in a patient with nonischemic dilated cardiomyopathy. Although there is global left ventricular hypokinesia, basal and mid-inferoseptal segments are almost akinetic, giving an impression of regional involvement.

## Chapter 3: Echocardiographic Evaluation of the Right Atrium and Right Ventricle

*Anuj Mediratta, Francesco Maffessanti, Karima Addetia, Roberto M Lang*

**Video 3.1** Three-dimensional echocardiographic imaging of tricuspid valve. All the three valve leaflets are visualized simultaneously.

**Video 3.2** Parasternal right ventricular inflow view.

**Video 3.3** Parasternal right ventricular outflow view.

**Video 3.4** Parasternal short axis view showing both right ventricular inflow and outflow.

**Video 3.5** Right ventricular focused apical four-chamber view.

## Chapter 5: Nonpharmacologic Stress Echocardiography

*Asrar Ahmed, Roxy Senior*

**Video 5.1** (A) Contrast-enhanced images showing parasternal long-axis (upper left), parasternal short-axis (upper right), apical four-chamber (lower left) and apical two-chamber (lower right) views at rest. There is no regional wall motion abnormality at rest. (B) Same views obtained immediately after exercise stress demonstrating akinesia of mid-anteroseptum, apex and mid-anterior wall indicative of a significant stenosis in the left anterior descending coronary artery.

## Chapter 6: Contrast Echocardiography

*Adrian Chong, Sudhir Wahi*

**Video 6.1** (A) Standard 2D apical 4-chamber view demonstrating an aneurysmal left ventricular apex with near-field clutter and a possible apical thrombus. (B) Contrast enhancement confirming the presence of an intraluminal filling defect in the apical lateral region consistent with an intracavitary thrombus.

**Video 6.2** (A) 2D transesophageal echocardiographic assessment of the left atrial appendage demonstrating an echodensity suspicious for a thrombus. (B) Off-label use of Definity contrast confirms the presence of an intraluminal filling defect at the base of the left atrial appendage consistent with a thrombus with a layered extension to the opening of the appendage.

**Video 6.3** (A) 2D transesophageal echocardiographic assessment demonstrating an echodensity in the left atrial appendage suspicious for a potential thrombus in the setting of suboptimal anticoagulation. (B) Definity contrast was administered resulting in full opacification of the left atrial appendage with no evidence of a filling defect to suggest thrombus. The patient was successfully cardioverted with no adverse outcome.

**Video 6.4** (A) Standard 2D apical 4-chamber view with suboptimal endocardial definition and poor delineation of the left ventricular apex. (B) Contrast enhancement demonstrating hypertrophy of the apical myocardium with the classic end-diastolic spade-shaped appearance of apical hypertrophic cardiomyopathy.

**Video 6.5** (A) Standard 2D apical 4-chamber view demonstrating an ill-defined echodensity at the left ventricular apex. (B) Contrast enhanced focused apical view revealing the prominent trabeculae and deep intertrabecular recesses typical of noncompaction cardiomyopathy.

**Video 6.6** (A) Standard 2D apical 4-chamber view with color Doppler demonstrating a communication between the left ventricular cavity and an echo-free extracardiac collection through the anterolateral wall. (B) Contrast extravasation through a narrow neck consistent with a left ventricular free wall rupture or pseudoaneurysm.

## Chapter 8: Echocardiographic Workup of Chest Pain in the Emergency Department

*Brian Mott, Sanjiv Kaul*

**Video 8.1** Right ventricular outflow view in a patient with pulmonary embolism. The arrow denotes thrombus in the right pulmonary artery.

**Video 8.2** Using direct color comparison, the right ventricular outflow into the main pulmonary artery and its right and left branches can be seen. There is trace pulmonary insufficiency. Again, thrombus can be seen in the right pulmonary artery.

**Video 8.3** In this modified apical view, the right ventricle is well seen. There is significant right ventricular systolic dysfunction with apical sparing consistent with McConnell's sign in this patient with a large pulmonary embolism seen on CT scan.

**Video 8.4** A patient with aortic dissection. The abdominal aorta can be seen pulsating with two lumens.

**Video 8.5** Microbubbles can be used to identify the lumens. The true lumen is seen on top of the false lumen. Microbubbles in the true lumen are constantly flowing without a noticeable flow pulsation. In the false lumen, microbubbles can be seen slowly pulsing into the dissection.

**Video 8.6** A patient with large pericardial effusion with cardiac tamponade. The entire heart is swinging within the pericardial cavity. Right atrial diastolic collapse can also be appreciated.

### Chapter 9: Assessment of the Extent of Myocardial Damage

*Vinayak Agrawal*

**Video 9.1** Extensive regional wall-motion abnormalities in the left anterior descending artery territory with significantly reduced left ventricular ejection fraction. The patient also had pericardial effusion.

**Video 9.2** Myocardial contrast echocardiography in apical 4-chamber view in a patient with acute myocardial infarction. There is reduced myocardial perfusion of the lateral wall.

**Video 9.3** Longitudinal strain measurement by 2-dimensional speckle tracking echocardiography.

**Video 9.4** Three-dimensional speckle-tracking echocardiography.

### Chapter 11: Mechanical Complications of Acute Myocardial Infarction

*Sanjay Mittal, Vivek Jain*

**Video 11.1** An example of a ventricular septal rupture. The patient presented 6 days after anterior wall myocardial infarction with shortness of breath. (A) Apical 4-chamber view showing a rent in the apical ventricular septum suggestive of ventricular septal rupture. There is also a large serpentine clot floating in the right atrium. This is likely an embolized clot from deep vein thrombosis in the legs. (B) Color flow through the apical ventricular septal rupture. Note the flow acceleration on the left ventricular side and the turbulent jet on the right ventricular side of the defect. The location is clearly apical. (C) Short-axis view showing left-to-right shunt though the ventricular septal rupture. Note the shunt is located in anterior septum and therefore this was an apicoanterior ventricular septal rupture.

**Video 11.2** Another example of a ventricular septal rupture in a patient with inferior-posterior wall infarct who had presented with cardiogenic shock. (A) Modified apical longitudinal view shows a breach in the mid-ventricular septum. (B) Subcostal long-axis view with color showing left-to-right shunt through mid-posterior septum. This is an example of mid-posterior ventricular septal rupture.

**Video 11.3** Parasternal long-axis view in a patient with posterior wall infarct. Note the wall motion defect in mid-posterior wall along with flail A2 scallop of the anterior mitral leaflet. The fragment of the ruptured papillary muscle head is seen attached to the tip of the anterior mitral leaflet and is freely moving in and out of the left atrium.

**Video 11.4** Transesophageal echocardiography in the same patient as in Video 11.3. (A) Lower esophageal view shows eccentric severe mitral regurgitation directed posteriorly. (B) Flail A1, A2 scallops of the anterior mitral leaflet with ruptured head of papillary muscle seen attached to it. Fragments of ruptured chordae are also seen at the tip of the posterior mitral leaflet. Transesophageal echocardiography is much better in detection and evaluation of papillary muscle rupture.

**Video 11.5** Apical 4-chamber view in a patient with large anterior wall infarct showing apical dyskinetic aneurysm. The aneurysm is seen to expand during systole. There is large layered clot attached to the aneurysm. One can notice the central portion of the clot is echolucent as compared to the periphery. This central echolucency is a marker of dissolving clot as commonly observed in patients on anticoagulants.

**Video 11.6** Zoomed apical 4-chamber view in a patient with anteroapical infarction showing a large apical pseudoaneurysm with a shelf-like structure at its origin. Note the relatively narrow neck of opening and large aneurysmal cavity, which is partially layered with clot. Spontaneous echo contrast is seen in the aneurysm as swirling smoke.

**Video 11.7** Parasternal long-axis view in a patient with posterior wall infarct showing scarred posterior wall with a rupture. There is a pericardial collection posteriorly, which has contained the rupture. The color flow shows to and fro blood movement into the pseudoaneurysm.

### Chapter 13: Stress Echocardiography for Detection of Myocardial Ischemia and Guiding Treatment in Stable Coronary Artery Disease

*Rahul Mehrotra, Ravi R Kasliwal*

**Video 13.1** Dobutamine stress echocardiography showing significant inducible ischemia in left anterior descending artery territory. Compared with the baseline image (upper left), there is impairment of contractility in the septal and apical segments at low-dose itself (upper right) which becomes much more apparent at peak-dose dobutamine (lower left).

**Video 13.2** Apical two-chamber view from the same patient as in Video 13.1. Inducible ischemia is easily apparent in the anterior wall and apex. Basal and mid-inferior wall is akinetic at baseline itself which is suggestive of previous infarct.

**Video 13.3** Significance of recovery images in assessment of myocardial ischemia. In this patient, because of significant left ventricular hypertrophy and reduction in left ventricular cavity size with dobutamine, inducible ischemia is not apparent at peak-dose (lower left) but becomes glaring during recovery phase (lower right).

### Chapter 14: Use of Contrast in Ischemic Heart Disease

*Nitin J Burkule*

**Video 14.1:** An example of normal exercise stress echocardiography. Only systole is shown. The left side images are rest images whereas the right side images are corresponding views obtained immediately after exercise. The upper images show apical 4-chamber view with contrast LVO and the lower images show apical 2-chamber view with contrast LVO.

**Video 14.2:** Abnormal exercise stress echocardiography with stress induced akinesia of posterolateral wall (LCX territory). A-D: Contrast LVO images are shown (A) Apical 4-chamber view at rest (B) Apical 4-chamber view after exercise (C) Apical long-axis view at rest (D) Apical long-axis view after exercise. Note thinning and bulging of posterolateral wall. (E) Coronary angiogram showing complete occlusion of a large obtuse marginal artery.

**Video 14.3:** A patient with chest pain with abnormal stress echocardiogram (A) Non-contrast harmonic 2D 4-chamber and (B) Apical long-axis view do not show RWMA. (C) Contrast LVO 4-chamber and (D) Apical long-axis views show apical septal akinesia.

**Video 14.4:** LV apical clot on contrast LVO

**Video 14.5:** (A) LV apical clot (B) Minimal residual layer of clot after 2 weeks of anticoagulation.

**Video 14.6:** LV pseudoaneurysm identified with the help of contrast LVO (A) Apical long-axis non-contrast 2D harmonic image does not show the pseudoaneurysm. (B) Apical long-axis contrast LVO and (C) Apical short-axis contrast LVO clearly delineate the pseudoaneurysm and the contained rupture.

**Video 14.7:** (A) Contrast LVO (right panel) clearly shows apical displacement of papillary muscle not visualized on non-contrast 2D harmonic imaging (left panel). (B) Apical displacement of papillary muscle confirmed on cardiac MRI.

**Video 14.8:** Stress cardiomyopathy in a patient of road traffic accident admitted in intesnive care unit and on high dose noradrenaline (A) Non-diagnostic bedside 2D echo image on non-contrast 2D harmonic imaging. (B) Bedside contrast LVO clearly shows LV apical ballooning and hypovolemia.

**Video 14.9:** Post CABG patient with hemodynamic instability. (A) Non-diagnostic bedside 2D echo image on harmonic imaging. (B) Bedside contrast LVO clearly shows normally contracting all LV wall segments with hypovolemic LV cavity.

**Video 14.10:** (A) Uniform myocardial opacification of LAD territory on MCE performed 48 hr after primary PCI. (B) Late recovery of systolic function in LAD territory seen on contrast LVO during follow-up. (C) Coronary angiogram prior to PCI. (D) Coronary angiogram immediately after primary PCI.

**Video 14.11:** (A) Takatsubo cardiomyopathy after bereavement. Note typical apical ballooning. (B) MCE shows delayed but uniform myocardial opacification of LAD territory in 12 seconds. (C) and (D) Coronary angiogram confirming absence of significant coronary stenosis.

## Chapter 15: Direct Visualization of Coronary Arteries by Echocardiography

*Ty Whitfield, Ayman A Farag, Navin C Nanda*

**Video 15.1** Live/real time transthoracic echocardiographic assessment of coronary arteries. The moving image shows a plaque in the obtuse marginal artery which is somewhat mobile and "wiggling", indicating its soft consistency and probable propensity to rupture. Please refer to Figure 15.5 for detailed description of the findings.

**Video 15.2** (A) and (B) Live/real time three-dimensional transesophageal echocardiographic assessment of ascending aortic dissection. A mobile dissection flap is seen protruding into the right coronary artery lumen.

## Chapter 16: Chronic Ischemic Mitral Regurgitation

*Raluca Dulgheru, Patrizio Lancellotti*

**Video 16.1** (A) Severe left ventricular systolic dysfunction resulting in symmetrical tenting of mitral valve leaflets leading to non-coaptation. (B) Central jet of severe mitral regurgitation.

**Video 16.2** (A) Asymmetric tethering of mitral valve leaflets causing more marked restriction of the posterior mitral leaflet. (B) Eccentric posteriorly directed jet of mitral regurgitation due to malcoaptation of mitral valve leaflets secondary to asymmetric tethering.

## Chapter 17: Assessment of Myocardial Viability

*Manish Bansal, Ravi R Kasliwal*

**Video 17.1** Apical four-chamber view at different stages during dobutamine echocardiography. Mid and apical lateral segments are hypokinetic at rest (upper left), improve at low-dose (upper right) but worsen at peak-dose (lower left). This is a typical biphasic response and suggests viability with ischemia (hibernation). In comparison, interventricular septum is akinetic (except for a small segment in the mid part) with no response to dobutamine infusion, which is suggestive of nonviable myocardium.

**Video 17.2** Apical two-chamber view at different stages during dobutamine echocardiography in the same patient as in Video 17.1. Typical biphasic response is seen in mid and apical anterior wall.

## Chapter 19: Role of Echocardiography in the Evaluation and Follow-up of Patients Receiving Ventricular Assist Devices

*M Sonia Jain, Sunil Mankad*

**Video 19.1** Perioperative transesophageal echocardiographic images in a patient undergoing LVAD (same as in Figure 19.2). (A) A left to right intra-atrial shunt by color Doppler through a patent foramen ovale pre-LVAD implantation. Closure of the shunt was initially unsuccessful at the time of LVAD implantation. (B) Post-LVAD imaging and now the shunt has reversed and was right to left as shown by color Doppler due to lowering of left atrial pressure with appropriate LVAD function. This led to significant hypoxia postoperatively and the shunt was subsequently closed percutaneously.

**Video 19.2** A zoomed in parasternal long-axis color Doppler image demonstrating moderately-severe aortic regurgitation. This required placement of a "Park's stitch" (suture closure of the aortic valve) at the time of LVAD implantation.

**Video 19.3** (A) The inflow cannula of the LVAD can be seen with no evidence of thrombus. (B) Nice laminar, nonturbulent color Doppler flow.

**Video 19.4** (A) Right parasternal view demonstrating the LVAD outflow cannula entering the aorta. (B) Color Doppler image showing normal flow through the outflow cannula.

**Video 19.5** A transesophageal echocardiographic 4-chamber view demonstrating an LV apical thrombus (same patient as in Figure 19.6). The thrombus was partially obstructing the LVAD inflow cannula which was also at the apex and this led to abnormal LVAD function. This required surgical intervention with restoration of normal LVAD function after removal of the clot.

## Chapter 21: Coronary Anomalies in Pediatric Age Group: Echocardiographic Imaging

*Munesh Tomar*

**Video 21.1** Two-dimensional echocardiography in parasternal short-axis view at the level of great vessels showing origin of left coronary artery from medial aspect of main pulmonary artery. Caution needs to be exercised as the echocardiography seems to give an impression that the left coronary artery is arising from aorta.

**Video 21.2** Two-dimensional echocardiography in apical four-chamber view showing sclerosed dilated left ventricle with severe systolic dysfunction. Mitral valve papillary muscle is also sclerosed.

**Video 21.3** Color flow mapping in parasternal short axis view showing flow reversal in left coronary artery (blue). Please note, the left coronary artery is seen to be originating from the medial aspect of the main pulmonary artery.

**Video 21.4** Parasternal short-axis view with color flow mapping showing flow reversal in left coronary artery (blue color in left anterior descending artery and red in circumflex artery). Left coronary artery is originating from the left lateral aspect of the main pulmonary artery.

**Video 21.5** Apical four-chamber view with color flow mapping showing moderate mitral regurgitation.

## Chapter 22: Coronary Arterial Involvement in Connective Tissue Disorders and Other Diseases

*Divya Malhotra, Raj Kumar*

**Video 22.1** The same patient with systemic lupus erythematosus as in Figure 22.1. There is hypokinesia of mid-anterior septum (A) and left ventricular apex (B and C) with left ventricular ejection fraction around 35%.

**Video 22.2** The same patient as in Video 22.1, but 4 weeks after the initial presentation. All regional wall-motion abnormalities had disappeared and the left ventricular ejection fraction had normalized by this time (A to C).

# Section 1

# Echocardiographic Techniques Used in the Evaluation of Patients with Coronary Artery Disease

# Assessment of Left Ventricular Systolic Function

CHAPTER 1

*Shantanu P Sengupta, Bijoy K Khandheria*

## INTRODUCTION

The most important clinical application of echocardiography has been the evaluation of left ventricular (LV) size, volume, and function. The first signals from the human heart were demonstrated by Edler with the use of A-mode and M-mode.[1] Edler noted that the echo from the posterior wall of the heart moved anteriorly about 1 cm, and that with aortic valve incompetence, the amplitude of motion of this echo increased. These moving signals from the LV posterior wall and from the posterior mitral annulus were correlated with LV function. He also noticed that when the movement of the heart was well, all parts had greater motion than when cardiac function was globally impaired. Subsequently, Harvey Feigenbaum tried to measure LV systolic function by using an index comprising of the anteroposterior dimension of the heart, measured from the chest wall to the posterior LV signal multiplied by the M-mode excursion of the posterolateral mitral annulus measured from the cardiac apex. This index did not work well in all cases, but it was soon appreciated that, in optimal cases, one could see a signal representing the interventricular septum also. Nonetheless, this index was useful in measuring the LV dimensions. The earlier instruments used did not give consistent information. Subsequent improvements in the echocardiography instrumentation helped in better and consistent signals from blood-endocardial interfaces. These echocardiographic instruments delineated anterior right ventricular wall thickness, right ventricular internal dimension, interventricular septum thickness, internal LV dimension, and posterior LV wall thickness.[2] This helped in understanding the cardiac dimensions in real time for the first time noninvasively, which was a reflection of cardiac function.

This was followed by a collaborative study between Feigenbaum and Harold Dodge, which correlated LV volume by angiography with echocardiographic parameters for the first time.[3] Successful attempts were made to use the change in the M-mode LV dimension from diastole to systole as an indication of stroke volume in normally shaped hearts; however, the method was not robust in dilated hearts or in presence of regional wall abnormalities.

Subsequently, M-mode echocardiography was used for estimation of LV volume, stroke volume, and wall thickness with good results in clinical situations.[4,5] At the end of the M-mode era, the Indiana group developed the technique of M-mode scanning that gave a sense of the shape and function of the LV but failed to record the apex and provided no additional quantitative information. The quest for more consistent measurement of cardiac size and function was a major reason for development of two-dimensional (2D) echocardiography.

## TWO-DIMENSIONAL ECHOCARDIOGRAPHY

The first B-mode images from the heart were developed from linear array transducers by Bom et al.[6] The aggregate image on a display screen produced a 2D echocardiogram. Then a group of scientists from Indiana and others worked out systems for rocking a standard M-mode transducer over a 30-degree angular sector of a circular plane to create a narrow real-time 2D echocardiogram.[7] The resulting sector scan was most useful for understanding heart valve disease and pericardial effusion, but the narrow field of view was not optimal for assessing global LV function. Initial studies using this device, however, provided the apical information which was missing in the M-mode scan. Being portable, it helped in assessing significance and complications of acute myocardial infarction.[8] Over a period of time, development of this technology increased the angle of view to approximately 60 degrees. Subsequently, the bioengineering group at Duke University (Durham, NC, USA), and later the Varian Corporation (Palo Alto, CA, USA), developed electronic phased-array 2D echocardiographic imaging systems with a field of view of approximately 90 degrees that encompassed the majority of the heart in most patients when scanned from either the anterior chest wall or the cardiac apex.[9,10] Once the entire LV could be recorded, more accurate quantitation of LV volume was possible using the dimensions and areas contained in these images in a variety of mathematic models. The simple M-mode anteroposterior LV dimension was a reasonably accurate estimate of LV function in patients with symmetric ventricles. However, this simple dimension could

**Table 1.1:** Left ventricular dimensions by 2D echocardiography in males and females

| **Male** | | | | |
|---|---|---|---|---|
| | *Normal* | *Mildly dilated* | *Moderately dilated* | *Severely dilated* |
| LV diastolic diameter/ BSA, cm/m$^2$ | 2.2–3.0 | 3.1–3.3 | 3.4–3.6 | >3.6 |
| LV systolic diameter/ BSA, cm/m$^2$ | 1.2–2.1 | 2.2–2.3 | 2.4–2.5 | >2.5 |
| **Female** | | | | |
| | *Normal* | *Mildly dilated* | *Moderately dilated* | *Severely dilated* |
| LV diastolic diameter/ BSA, cm/m$^2$ | 2.3–3.1 | 3.1–3.3 | 3.4–3.6 | >3.6 |
| LV systolic diameter/ BSA, cm/m$^2$ | 1.3–2.1 | 2.2–2.3 | 2.4–2.6 | >2.6 |

*Abbreviations:* BSA, body surface area; LV, left ventricular.

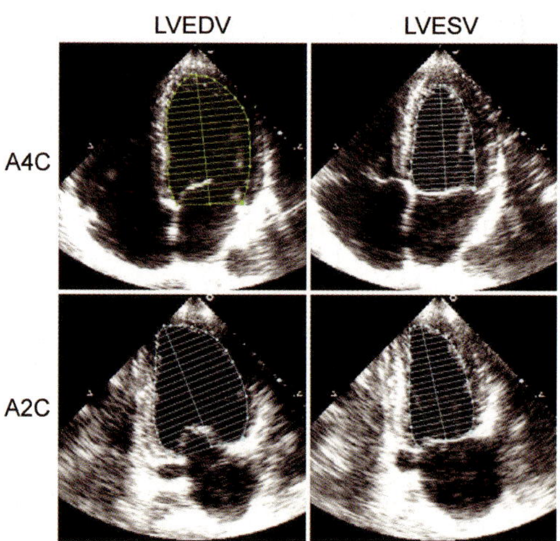


**Figure 1.1:** Two-dimensional measurements for volume calculations using the biplane method of disks (modified Simpson's rule), in the apical 4-chamber (A4C) and apical 2-chamber (A2C) views at end-diastole (LVEDV) and at end-systole (LVESV). Note the papillary muscles should be excluded from the cavity in the tracing.

significantly overestimate or underestimate volume in more irregular ventricles. Hence, the recent chamber guidelines advocate the use of direct 2D linear measurements for quantification of LV internal dimensions, and these values are indexed to body surface area **(Table 1.1)**.[11] Addition of the LV long-axis measurement improved accuracy, while addition of area measurements into the formulas for a variety of geometric figures and the ventricular contours in Simpson's rule calculations incrementally increased measurement accuracy.

The most common method for determining LV volumes currently is the Simpson rule or the "disk summation method". This technique requires recording an apical 4- and 2-chamber view from which the endocardial border is outlined in end-diastole and end-systole. The ventricle is then mathematically divided along its long axis into a series of disks of equal height. Individual disk volume is calculated as height multiplied by disk area where height is assumed to be the total length of the LV long axis divided by the number of segments or disks. The surface area of each disk is determined by the diameter of the ventricle at that point. The ventricular volume is then represented by the sum of the volume of each of the disks which are equally spaced along the long axis of the ventricle **(Figure 1.1)**. If the ventricle is symmetrically contracting, then either the 4- or 2-chamber view will reflect the true ventricular volume. However, in an asymmetrically contracting LV, both the views are needed to obtain accurate volume measurements. In any view, foreshortening of the ventricular apex will result in underestimation of the LV volumes and most often in overestimation of the ejection fraction. The biggest limitation of Simpson's formula is myocardial drop out, which causes difficulty in identifying the endocardial border. Also, many times, the LV apex cannot be easily identified. These can be minimized by the use of contrast to identify the endocardial borders **(Figure 1.2)**.

Numerous studies have validated the accuracy of 2D volumes and ejection fraction measurements by comparison with a variety of reference standards. However, there are various limitations to this: (i) the acquisition and assumed position of short-axis images along the ventricular long axis were based on internal ventricular landmarks and, thus, might not correspond precisely to the placement assumed by the geometric models, (ii) the placement of the transducer was assumed to be over the LV apex, which was often not the case, resulting in foreshortening of the ventricle, (iii) apical views were assumed to be obtained by rotation around the ventricular long axis and separated by known degrees of rotation, which was not always true, and (iv) in any acquisition format, the majority of the ventricular surface was not recorded and, hence, spatial symmetry had to be assumed. The normal values of LV volumes and thresholds for classification into mild, moderate, and severe dilated LV are provided in **Table 1.2**.

## Is Visual Assessment an Alternative?

There is a routine use of visual assessment of LV function in day-to-day practice, for example, by estimating the LV ejection fraction (LVEF) in 5% steps, such as 30–35% or just classifying the LV function as normal, mildly, moderately or severely impaired. This is not recommended in the guidelines

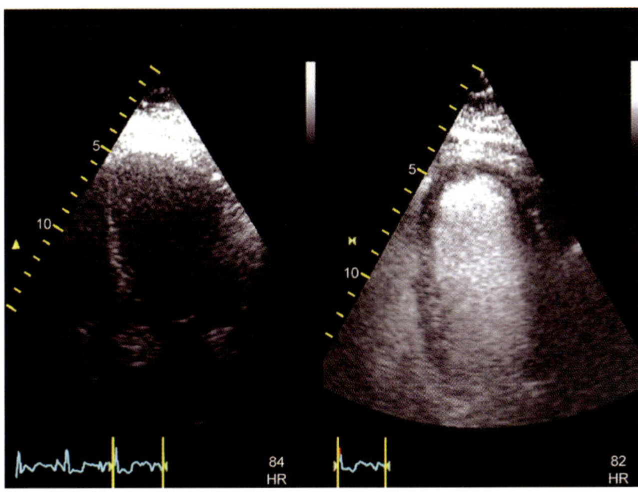


**Figure 1.2:** Contrast echocardiography helps in better delineation of endocardial border.

**Table 1.2:** Left ventricular volumes by 2D echocardiography in males and females[11]

| | | | | |
|---|---|---|---|---|
| **Males** | | | | |
| | *Normal* | *Mildly dilated* | *Moderately dilated* | *Severely dilated* |
| LV diastolic volume/ BSA, mL/m² | 34–74 | 75–89 | 90–100 | >100 |
| LV systolic volume/ BSA, mL/m² | 11–31 | 32–38 | 39–45 | >45 |
| **Female** | | | | |
| | *Normal* | *Mildly dilated* | *Moderately dilated* | *Severely dilated* |
| LV diastolic volume/ BSA, mL/m² | 29–61 | 62–70 | 71–80 | >80 |
| LV systolic volume/ BSA, mL/m² | 8–24 | 25–32 | 33–40 | >40 |

*Abbreviations:* BSA, body surface area; LV, left ventricular.

but is routinely practiced due to time constraints and difficulties in tracing the endocardial borders on still frames. Although visual assessment of global LV systolic function has been reported to be reasonably accurate among experienced readers,[12,13] there is still considerable observer variability.[14] This does not allow the use of visual assessment for follow-up studies of LVEF and volumes. Furthermore, when compared with cardiac MRI, visual assessment has been shown to result in significant underestimation (8.4%) of LVEF.[15] For these reasons, it is recommended to use quantitative analysis for accurate assessment of LV systolic function.

## Strain Imaging

Strain imaging by speckle-tracking echocardiography (STE) has emerged in last decade as a quantitative imaging tool to evaluate regional and global myocardial function by analyzing the motion of speckles identified by 2D or three-dimensional (3D) sonograms. STE uses non-Doppler, angle-independent, objective quantification of myocardial deformation and LV systolic and diastolic dynamics.[16,17] It tracks the displacement of the speckles during the cardiac cycle and generates longitudinal, radial and circumferential strain measurements, and LV twist and torsion.

Strain analysis by STE is principally based on the analysis of speckles during the cardiac cycle. Single speckles are merged in functional units (kernels), which are identifiable given the peculiar disposition of the speckles. Each kernel thus constitutes a sort of ultrasound fingerprint which can be tracked by software during the entire length of the cardiac cycle. The motion is analyzed by the system without using the Doppler signal. This then gives a calculation of displacement, rate of displacement (velocity), deformation (strain) and rate of deformation (strain rate) of the selected myocardial segments, and LV rotation. Assessment is obtained by averaging at least 3 consecutive heart cycles to reduce the noise, setting the frame rate of the routine 2D image acquisition between 60 and 110 frames per second.[18] The STE derived measurements have been validated using sonomicrometry and tagged magnetic resonance imaging (MRI), showing high feasibility and reproducibility.[19] Potential limitations of this technique are its strict dependence on the frame rate and on high-quality 2D images which are necessary for obtaining an optimal definition of the endocardial border.

### *Strain*

Strain is the degree of deformation of the analyzed myocardial segment in relation to its initial dimensions expressed as a percentage. The strain equation (ε) is as follows:

$$\varepsilon = L - L_0/L_0,$$

where L is the length of the object after deformation, and $L_0$ is the basal length.

By convention, lengthening or thickening deformation is given a positive value, whereas a shortening or thinning deformation is given a negative value.

### *Strain Rate*

The strain rate (ε′) represents the rate of myocardial deformation expressed as seconds$^{-1}$. Studies have shown that the strain rate is less dependent on LV load variations than strain. However, because the strain rate signal is noisier and less reproducible, clinical studies still use strain measurements.

### *Longitudinal Strain*

Longitudinal strain represents myocardial deformation directed from the base to the apex in the longitudinal direction. It is a reflection of subendocardial muscle fibers which are predominantly arranged longitudinally. During systole, ventricular myocardial fibers shorten with a translational movement from the base to the apex. Analysis of the longitudinal strain in 4-chamber, 2-chamber, and apical long-axis view helps us in identifying global and regional (17 segments) strain values of the LV **(Figure 1.3)**. Global longitudinal strain has been validated recently as a quantitative parameter of global LV function.

### *Radial Strain*

Radial strain represents myocardial deformation toward the center of the LV cavity and thus indicates the LV thickening and thinning motion during the cardiac cycle. Consequently, during systole, radial strain values are always positive curves. Radial strain values are obtained by STE analysis of both basal, mid and apical LV short-axis views.[20]

### *Circumferential Strain*

Circumferential strain represents LV myocardial deformation along the circular perimeter observed on a short-axis view.[20] Consequently, during systole, circumferential strain measurements are represented by negative curves. As for longitudinal strain, it is possible to obtain a global circumferential strain value.

### *Twist and Torsion*

Earlier, the evaluation of LV twisting had been possible only through MRI. STE has now emerged as a new promising tool for LV twisting analysis.[21] LV twisting is a component of the normal LV systolic contraction that arises from the reciprocal rotation of the LV apex and base during systole.[22,23] STE helps in quantifying LV twist by analyzing the reciprocal rotation of the LV apex and base during systole. The LV twist is the net difference in mean rotation between the apical and basal levels. The LV torsion is defined as LV twisting normalized with the base-to-apex distance.[24]

Of all the components of the STE, longitudinal strain has now been standardized and is in clinical use. The major use of longitudinal strain is in coronary artery disease (CAD), assessing subclinical LV dysfunction in various conditions, cancer chemotherapy, various cardiomyopathies, constrictive pericarditis, and understanding LV function in valvular heart disease.

## THREE-DIMENSIONAL ECHOCARDIOGRAPHY

Earlier acquisition of 3D echocardiography was based on the reconstruction of 2D images.[25] The images were obtained along with the cardiac cycle and were positioned in their proper orientation relative to one another. The quality of the 3D images from the reconstruction methods are a function of the quality and number of images used in the reconstruction. The highest quality images are usually obtained using position-sensing devices because they allow each plane to be aligned independently to achieve optimal target definition. Quantitation of LV volume in 3D was shown to be accurate with a minimum of 8 intersecting, nonparallel 2D images.[26] Although reconstruction methods are time consuming, important studies have used these approaches to demonstrate the improved accuracy of assessment of LV size and function compared with 2D echocardiography.[27,28] In addition, this approach improved our understanding of the shape and spatial relationships of many cardiac structures, such as the mitral valve and its supporting structures.[29]

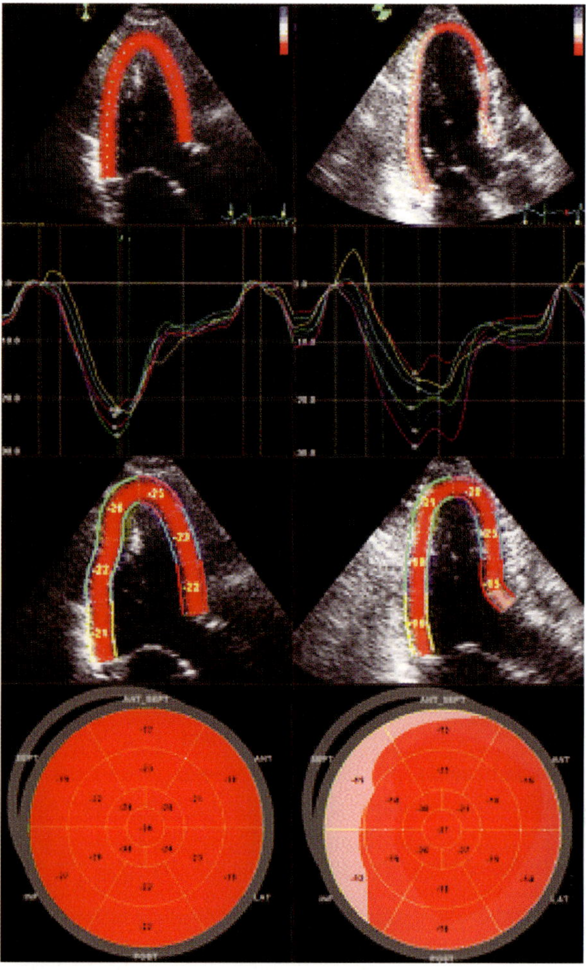

**Figure 1.3:** Speckle-tracking echocardiographic analysis of myocardial deformation by longitudinal strain in 17 segments represented as bull's eye map.

Over the years, there has been an evolution in transducer technology to the development of the matrix-array transducer. This transducer has elements arranged in a grid, and after transmission of a single pulse can acquire data from many lines of sight simultaneously to reconstruct a volume of ultrasound data in real time. The earliest of these transducers was a sparse array with 256 elements which resulted in limitations in spatial and temporal resolution.[28] Currently, these transducers have more than 3,000 elements and enable a 30- to 50-degree volume to be acquired and displayed in real time. Although this is sufficient for visualization of valves, masses, the LV and color Doppler jets, it is typically not a large enough volume. To display and quantify the adult LV, a series of component volumes of the heart are obtained over consecutive cardiac cycles and then combined to obtain a larger volume. Currently, with this approach, 4 or more images are fused resulting in maximal frame rates of 25 Hz.[29] In addition, the matrix-array transducer can record multiple individual planes simultaneously **(Figure 1.4A to D)**.

When this full-volume 3D ultrasound data set is initially displayed, only the outer boundaries of the pyramid can be visualized. This provides minimal or no information. To see the cardiac structures, the volume is then cropped in various planes to define the structures. The LV volume can be calculated from the 3D image in several ways.

For defining the LV volume, the endocardial border is traced either manually from selected planes or auto-matically by a border-tracking algorithm. Alternatively, the machine then automatically defines the LV volume both in systole and diastole from which LVEF is obtained.

Compared with single plane and 2D approaches, 3D echocardiography has been shown to represent and quantify LV volumes and function more accurately.[30] Although the early 3D reconstruction methods provide important data, real-time 3D acquisition has proven more rapid and hence, practical, for clinical application.

The advantage of LV volume calculation with 3D echocardiography over 2D echocardiography is easily explained by the fact that more of the LV endocardial surface is incorporated into the 3D echocardiographic quantification, the position of the transducer over the cardiac apex can be better appreciated, intersecting planes are precisely aligned, and no assumptions of shape are required. As the LV volumes

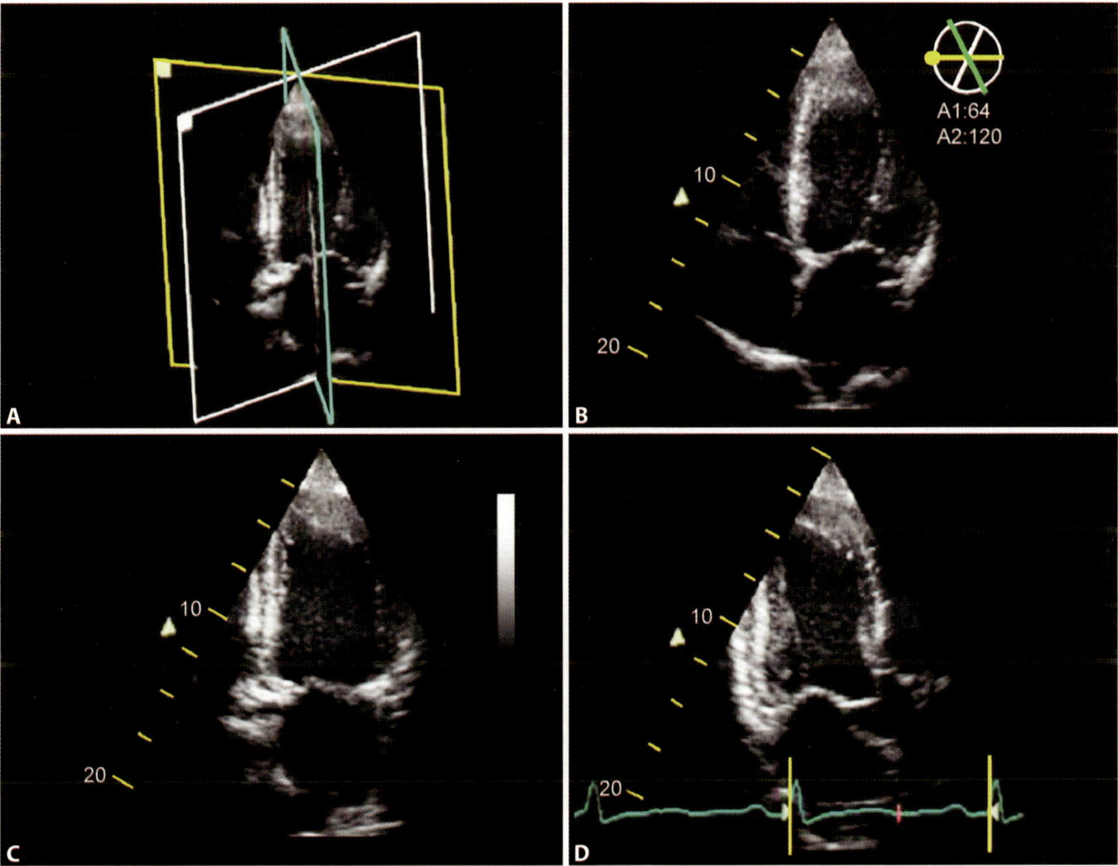


**Figure 1.4A to D:** A triplane view obtained from apical transducer position with matrix–array transducer. Scan planes 0, 60, and 120 degrees (yellow, white, and green planes, respectively) (A) yield familiar apical 4-chamber, 2-chamber, and long-axis images (B to D). The frame shown is end-systolic.

calculated from 3D echocardiograms are more accurate, the LV stroke volume and ejection fraction derived from these volumes are also more accurate **(Figure 1.5)**.[30] This improved accuracy, which is helpful in patients with ventricles that are distorted in shape and in those with regional wall-motion abnormalities caused by CAD. Despite the advantages of 3D echocardiography, there are the following few limitations: (i) image quality is often poor, because despite parallel processing, the line density within the 3D volume is much lower than in a 2D image and more interpolation is necessary, (ii) when the 3D volume is acquired from a fixed point many of the targets within the volume will not be optimally aligned to produce strong echoes and, thus, may be either missing or poorly recorded, (iii) when the entire LV is reconstructed from multiple subvolumes, arrhythmias and respiration can cause movement of the heart between cycles and result in artifacts in the images (stitch artifacts), and (iv) although acquisition time for one volume is much less than for multiple planes, the analysis time to this point has limited general application, and the technique has been primarily used in research studies. It can be anticipated that over the time, 3D image quality will improve, as has been the case with 2D images.

## ASSESSMENT OF REGIONAL MYOCARDIAL CONTRACTION

Since CAD typically affects the myocardium regionally, regional assessment of LV systolic function is of paramount importance in the evaluation of CAD. It not only helps in assessing the extent of myocardial damage, but more importantly, also provides information about the coronary artery involved in the disease process.

Regional LV systolic function is commonly assessed by dividing the LV into 17 segments, a scheme that is agreed to by the echocardiographic, nuclear and magnetic resonance communities. The LV is divided into 6 walls: anterior, anteroseptal, inferoseptal, inferior, inferolateral, and anterolateral. Each wall is divided into basal, mid and apical segments (except for the anteroseptal and the inferolateral walls which are divided only into basal and mid segments), and the apical cap represents the 17th segment **(Figure 1.6)**. In the earlier schemes, apical cap was not recognized as a separate segment, resulting in a 16-segment model. Several echocardiographers continue to use the 16-segement model for LV segmentation, both because of their familiarity with the earlier model and also because of the arguments that the

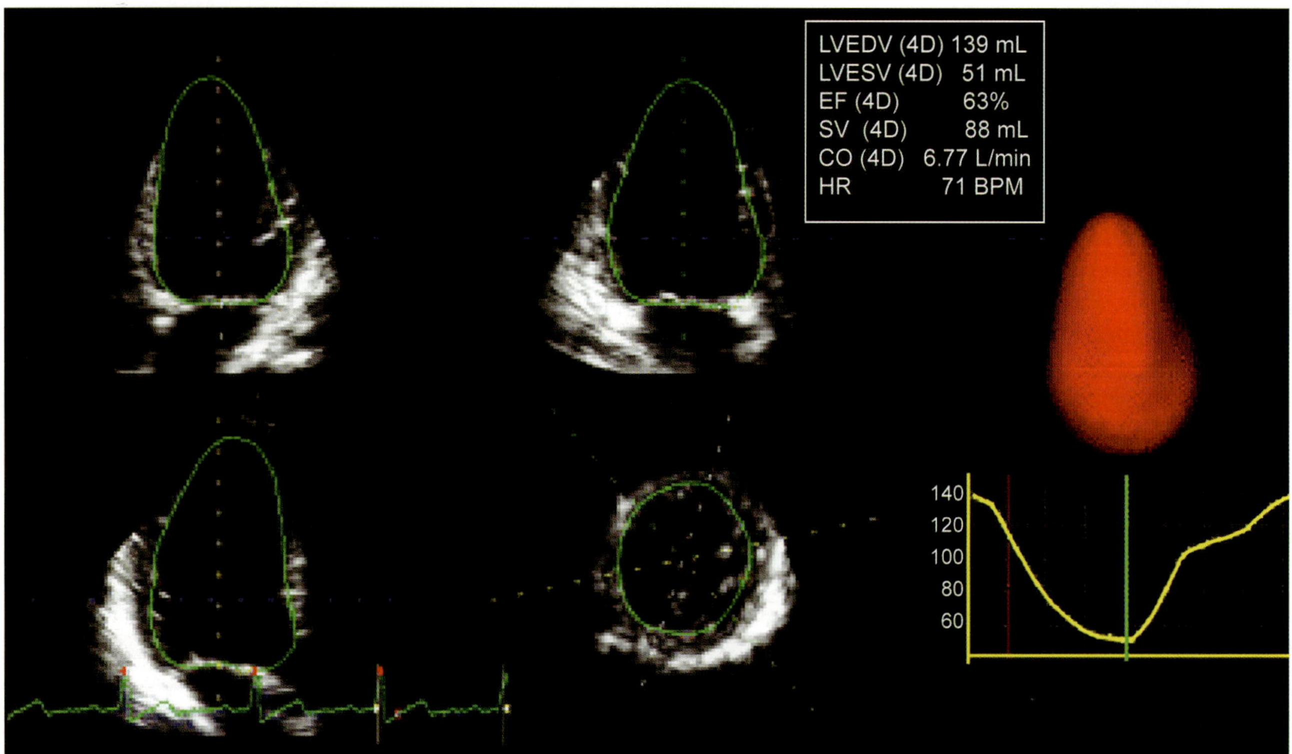


**Figure 1.5:** Example of left ventricular volume assessment by 4D auto-learning vector quantization software. The endocardial border is automatically detected in three dimensions throughout the cardiac cycle.
*Abbreviations:* 4D, four-dimensional (same as three-dimensional); CO, cardiac output; EF, ejection fraction; HR, heart rate; LVEDV, left ventricular end-diastolic volume; LVESV, left ventricular end-systolic volume; SV, stroke volume.

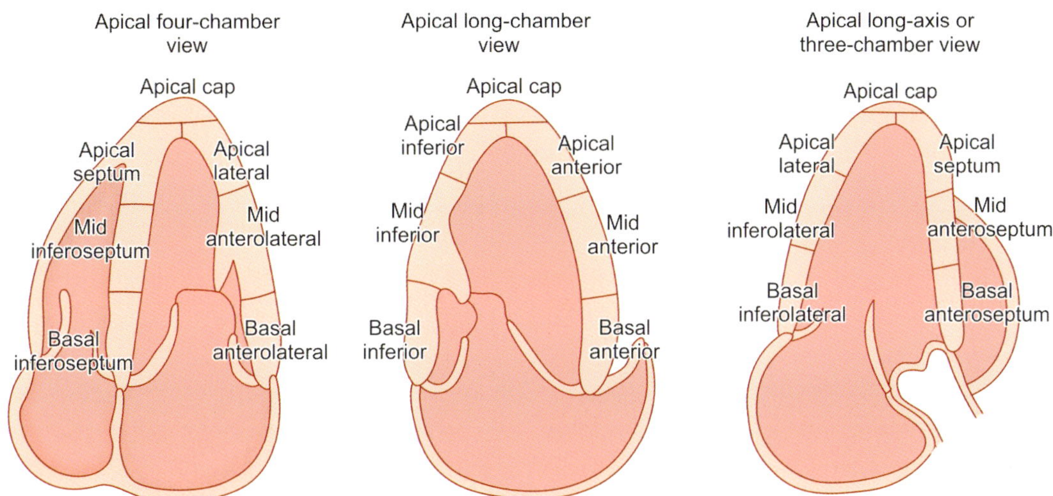


**Figure 1.6:** Approach to left ventricular myocardial segmentation for regional function assessment. The 17-segment model is depicted here. Please note the anteroseptal and the inferolateral walls are divided into two segments (basal and mid) only.

apical cap is beyond the LV cavity and does not really take part in the LV cavity shortening during systole.

Regardless of the model used, each myocardial segment is visually assessed for the extent of endocardial thickening and is classified as normokinetic, hypokinetic (reduced thickening), akinetic (negligible or no thickening at all), or dyskinetic (systolic thinning or stretching). When there is resting outpouching of a myocardial segment during diastole, it is termed as aneurysm. A semiquantitative wall-motion score can also be assigned to each myocardial segment from 1 (normal) to 4 (dyskinetic/aneurysmal), depending on the extent of endocardial thickening.[11] The average of the scores of all analyzed segments provides wall-motion score index (WMSI), which is a semiquantitative measure of overall LV systolic function. Higher is the WMSI, worse is the LV systolic function. This method of regional LV systolic function assessment is obviously observer dependent and has changed little from the initial descriptions of wall-motion abnormalities by echocardiography.[31]

The 17-segment model can also be applied to longitudinal strain analysis by 2D STE which is depicted as bull's-eye imaging (See **Figure 1.3**). However, most STE software use 18-segment model to divide the LV, in which each myocardial wall (including the anteroseptal and the inferolateral walls) is divided into basal, mid and apical segments. Although STE-based regional function assessment still suffers considerable variability, STE would generally show lower longitudinal strain value in areas of ischemia/infarction **(Figure 1.7A and B)**. Further improvements in these newer echocardiographic modalities providing novel insights into myocardial structure may dramatically change the way we assess LV regional systolic function.

Since the regional wall-motion abnormalities in CAD follow distribution of coronary vascular supply, the pattern of regional myocardial dysfunction helps identify the affected coronary artery (**Videos 1.1 and 1.2**). The anteroseptum, anterior wall, apex, and mid-segments of the inferoseptal and the anterolateral walls are generalized supplied by the left anterior descending coronary artery; posterolateral wall and the basal anterolateral segment are usually supplied by the left circumflex artery; and the inferior wall and the basal inferoseptal segment are supplied by the right coronary artery. However, variations are common in this segmental distribution, depending on whether it is a right-dominant system or is left-dominant and also because of the differences in the sizes of the three coronary arteries and their major branches. The atypical distribution of wall-motion abnormalities are also common in patients with previous coronary artery bypass surgery in whom dual sources of blood supply (i.e. native and grafts) alter the myocardial blood-supply pattern.

While regional wall-motion abnormalities are considered to be the sine qua non of CAD, it should be remembered that various noncoronary diseases may also produce regional LV systolic dysfunction. These include intra-ventricular conduction abnormalities (bundle-branch blocks, accessory pathways, paced ventricular rhythms, etc.), post-pericardiotomy state, constrictive pericarditis, right ventricular pressure and volume overload, systemic illnesses, such as sarcoidosis, hemochromatosis, etc., and even nonischemic dilated cardiomyopathy (**Videos 1.3 and 1.4**). However, there are several important clues that can help in differentiating true ischemic wall-motion abnormalities from those seen in the nonischemic conditions. Atypical distribution of the wall-motion abnormalities not conforming to any particular vascular territory, abnormal myocardial motion but preserved myocardial thickening and the wall-motion abnormalities confined only to a brief period of cardiac cycle generally favor nonischemic etiology as the underlying cause.

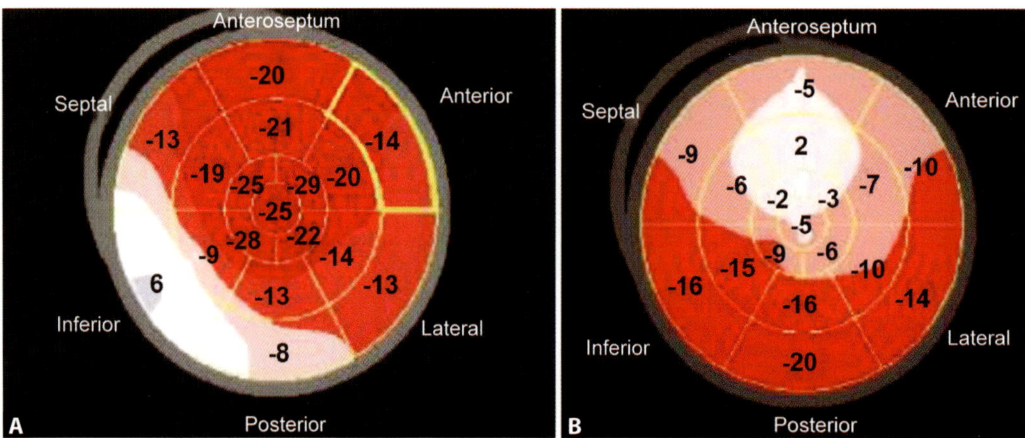


**Figure 1.7A and B:** (A) Strain echocardiography of a patient with inferior wall myocardial infarction because of right coronary obstruction. (B) Strain echocardiography due to left anterior descending artery occlusion causing anterior wall myocardial infarction.

## FUTURE DIRECTIONS

With the advent of time and advances, future machines will see a reduction in the size of many of the components of the echocardiography machine. The future will undoubtedly see a new model of clinical cardiology care that incorporates the equivalent of an ultrasound stethoscope. In addition, as investigators continue to make advances in understanding the molecular and genetic controls over cardiac physiology and disease, they will look to noninvasive imaging with echocardiography to assist in these correlations. Thus, echocardiographic assessment of LV function will be crucial in assessing the results of pharmacologic, molecular, and genetic manipulations of the failing heart to determine whether observations at the bench can be translated to effective therapies in patients.[32,33]

## SUMMARY

Comprehensive and precise assessment of LV systolic and diastolic function is important and one of the most common indications for performing echocardiography in cardiovascular practice. Echocardiography readily assesses LV systolic function; its advantages include that echocardiography is noninvasive, does not require radiation, is portable, rapid, readily available and in competent hands, can provide an accurate and comprehensive assessment of LV systolic and diastolic function. Assessment of LV systolic function is important for diagnosis, prognostication, planning the treatment modality, and for monitoring response to treatment. Echocardiography is widely used to provide vital parameters of LV function, such as ejection fraction, wall-motion score indices, LV volumes, and regional wall-motion assessment. This chapter focuses on the evolution of various echocardiographic methods used in the assessment of LV systolic function.

## VIDEO LEGENDS

**Video 1.1:** Apical 4-chamber view in a patient with previous myocardial infarction. Left ventricular apex and distal parts of mid-inferoseptal and mid-anterolateral segments are akinetic, consistent with involvement of the left anterior descending coronary artery. Left ventricular apical thrombus is also present.

**Video 1.2:** Apical 2-chamber view in a patient with inferior wall myocardial infarction demonstrating akinesia of basal and mid-inferior wall.

**Video 1.3:** Typical septal bounce in a patient with chronic constrictive pericarditis. Marked thickening of the pericardium in the posterior region can also be easily appreciated.

**Video 1.4:** Apical 4-chamber view in a patient with nonischemic dilated cardiomyopathy. Although there is global left ventricular hypokinesia, basal and mid-inferoseptal segments are almost akinetic, giving an impression of regional involvement.

## REFERENCES

1. Edler I. The diagnostic use of ultrasound in heart disease. Acta Med Scand Suppl. 1955;308:32.
2. Popp RL, Wolfe SB, Hirata T, et al. Estimation of right and left ventricular size by ultrasound. A study of the echoes from the interventricular septum. Am J Cardiol. 1969;24:523-30.
3. Feigenbaum H, Popp RL, Wolfe SB, Troy BL, Pombo JF, Haine CL, et al. Ultrasound measurements of the left ventricle. A correlative study with angiocardiography. Arch Intern Med. 1972;129:461-7.
4. Popp RL, Filly K, Brown OR, et al. Effect of transducer placement on echocardiographic measurement of left ventricular dimensions. Am J Cardiol. 1975;35:537-40.
5. Popp RL. Echocardiographic evaluation of left ventricular function. N Engl J Med. 1977;296:856-8.
6. Bom N, Hugenholtz PG, Kloster FE, Roelandt J, Popp RL, Pridie RB, et al. Evaluation of structure recognition with

the multiscan echocardiograph. A cooperative study in 580 patients. Ultrasound Med Biol. 1974;1:243-52.

7. Griffith JM, Henry WL. A sector scanner for real time two-dimensional echocardiography. Circulation. 1974;49:1147-52.
8. Weyman AE, Peskoe SM, Williams ES, et al. Detection of left ventricular aneurysms by cross-sectional echocardiography. Circulation. 1976;54:936-44.
9. Von Ramm OT, Thurstone FL. Thaumascan: Design considerations and performance characteristics. In: White D (Ed): Ultrasound in Medicine. New York, NY: Plenum Press; 1975. pp 373-8.
10. Tajik AJ, Seward JB, Hagler DJ, et al. Two-dimensional real-time ultrasonic imaging of the heart and great vessels. Technique, image orientation, structure identification, and validation. Mayo Clin Proc. 1978;53:271-303.
11. Lang RM, Badano LP, Mor-Avi V, Afilalo J, Armstrong A, Ernande L, et al. Recommendations for cardiac chamber quantification by echocardiography in adults: an update from the American Society of Echocardiography and the European Association of Cardiovascular Imaging. J Am Soc Echocardiogr. 2015; 28:1-39.
12. Gudmundsson P, Rydberg E, Winter R, Willenheimer R. Visually estimated left ventricular ejection fraction by echocardiography is closely correlated with formal quantitative methods. Int J Cardiol. 2005;101:209-212
13. Jensen-Urstad K, Bouvier F, Hojer J, et al. Comparison of different echocardiographic methods with radionuclide imaging for measuring left ventricular ejection fraction during acute myocardial infarction treated by thrombolytic therapy. Am J Cardiol. 1998;81:538-544
14. Blondheim DS, Beeri R, Feinberg MS, Vaturi M, Shimoni S, Fehske W, et al. Reliability of visual assessment of global and segmental left ventricular function: a multicenter study by the Israeli Echocardiography Research Group. J Am Soc Echocardiogr. 2010;23:258-64.
15. Sievers B, Kirchberg S, Franken U, Puthenveettil BJ, Bakan A, Trappe HJ. Visual estimation versus quantitative assessment of left ventricular ejection fraction: A comparison by cardiovascular magnetic resonance imaging. Am Heart J. 2005;150:737-742
16. Perk G, Tunick PA, Kronzon I. Non-Doppler two-dimensional strain imaging by echocardiography—from technical considerations to clinical applications. J Am Soc Echocardiogr. 2007;20:234-43.
17. Geyer H, Caracciolo G, Abe H, Wilansky S, Carerj S, Gentile F, et al. Assessment of myocardial mechanics using speckle tracking echocardiography: fundamentals and clinical applications. J Am Soc Echocardiogr. 2010;23:351-369; Erratum in: J Am Soc Echocardiogr. 2010;23:734.
18. Serri K, Reant P, Lafitte M, Berhouet M, Le Bouffos V, Roudaut R, et al. Global and regional myocardial function quantification by two-dimensional strain: application in hypertrophic cardiomyopathy. J Am Coll Cardiol. 2006;47:1175-81.
19. Amundsen BH, Helle-Valle T, Edvardsen T, Torp H, Crosby J, Lyseggen E, et al. Noninvasive myocardial strain measurement by speckle tracking echocardiography: validation against sonomicrometry and tagged magnetic resonance imaging. J Am Coll Cardiol. 2006;47:789-93.
20. Saito K, Okura H, Watanabe N, Hayashida A, Obase K, Imai K, et al. Comprehensive evaluation of left ventricular strain using speckle tracking echocardiography in normal adults: comparison of three-dimensional and two-dimensional approaches. J Am Soc Echocardiogr. 2009;22:1025-30.
21. Takeuchi M, Nakai H, Kokumai M, Nishikage T, Otani S, Lang RM. Age-related changes in left ventricular twist assessed by two-dimensional speckle-tracking imaging. J Am Soc Echocardiogr. 2006;19:1077-84.
22. Buckberg G, Hoffman JI, Mahajan A, et al. Cardiac mechanics revisited: the relationship of cardiac architecture to ventricular function. Circulation. 2008;118:2571-87.
23. Sengupta PP, Khandheria BK, Korinek J, Jahangir A, Yoshifuku S, Milosevic I, et al. Left ventricular isovolumic flow sequence during sinus and paced rhythms: new insights from use of high-resolution Doppler and ultrasonic digital particle imaging velocimetry. J Am Coll Cardiol. 2007;49:899-908.
24. Rüssel IK, Götte MJ, Bronzwaer JG, Knaapen P, Paulus WJ, van Rossum AC. Left ventricular torsion: an expanding role in the analysis of myocardial dysfunction. JACC Cardiovasc Imaging. 2009;2:648-55.
25. Dekker DL, Piziali RL, Dong E Jr. A system for ultrasonically imaging the human heart in three dimensions. Comput Biomed Res. 1974;7:544-53.
26. King DL, Harrison MR, King DL Jr, Gopal AS, Martin RP, DeMaria AN. Improved reproducibility of left atrial and left ventricular measurements by guided three-dimensional echocardiography. J Am Coll Cardiol. 1992;20:1238-45.
27. Levine RA, Handschumacher MD, Sanfilippo AJ, Hagege AA, Harrigan P, Marshall JE, et al. Three-dimensional echocardiographic reconstruction of the mitral valve, with implications for the diagnosis of mitral valve prolapse. Circulation. 1989;80:589-98.
28. Snyder JE, Kisslo J, von Ramm O. Real-time orthogonal mode scanning of the heart. I. System design. J Am Coll Cardiol. 1986;7:1279-85.
29. Corsi C, Lang RM, Veronesi F, Weinert L, Caiani EG, MacEneaney P, et al. Volumetric quantification of global and regional left ventricular function from real-time three-dimensional echocardiographic images. Circulation. 2005;112:1161-70.
30. Fleming SM, Cumberledge B, Kiesewetter C, et al. Usefulness of real-time three-dimensional echocardiography for reliable measurement of cardiac output in patients with ischemic or idiopathic dilated cardiomyopathy. Am J Cardiol. 2005;95:308-10.
31. Heger JJ, Weyman AE, Wann LS, et al. Cross-sectional echocardiography in acute myocardial infarction: detection and localization of regional left ventricular asynergy. Circulation. 1979;60:531-8.
32. Hataishi R, Rodrigues AC, Neilan TG, Morgan JG, Buys E, Shiva S, et al. Inhaled nitric oxide decreases infarction size and improves left ventricular function in a murine model of myocardial ischemia-reperfusion injury. Am J Physiol Heart Circ Physiol. 2006;291:H379-84.
33. Neilan TG, Blake SL, Ichinose F, Raher MJ, Buys ES, Jassal DS, et al. Disruption of nitric oxide synthase 3 protects against the cardiac injury, dysfunction, and mortality induced by doxorubicin. Circulation. 2007;116:506-14.

# Assessment of Left Ventricular Diastolic Function in Coronary Artery Disease

2
CHAPTER

*SK Parashar*

## INTRODUCTION

Diastolic dysfunction of the left ventricle has assumed considerable importance in the last several years, because of the recognition that isolated left ventricular (LV) diastolic dysfunction can itself result in heart failure (HF). It is now well known that almost 40–50% of all patients in the Western population with clinically diagnosed HF have normal LV ejection fraction (LVEF).[1,2] This form of HF, which occurs in the absence of significant valvular lesion or pericardial disease, is now referred to as HF with preserved ejection fraction (HFpEF). Clinical conditions usually responsible for HFpEF include hypertension, cardiomyopathy, coronary artery disease (CAD), diabetes mellitus, obesity, sleep apnea, etc. Patients with HFpEF may have a better short-term prognosis as compared to those with systolic HF, but the long-term mortality and incidence of recurrent hospitalizations are almost the same in both the groups.[1-5]

CAD with its varying presentations is one of the leading causes of morbidity and mortality universally. Traditionally, CAD has been considered to result mainly in LV systolic dysfunction by causing ischemic myocardial damage. However, LV diastolic dysfunction is an equally integral part of the pathophysiology of CAD. Some degree of LV diastolic dysfunction is invariably present in all patients with LV systolic dysfunction. In addition, LV diastolic dysfunction can occur as an independent entity also, in absence of LV systolic dysfunction.[1,3] The presence of LV diastolic dysfunction in patients with CAD not only contributes to their symptomatology and clinical presentation, but also has great prognostic implications. Accordingly, assessment of LV diastolic function is an important part of echocardiographic evaluation of every patient with CAD.

## HEMODYNAMIC CHANGES DURING LEFT VENTRICULAR DIASTOLE AND THE MECHANISMS OF DIASTOLIC DYSFUNCTION

LV diastole starts with the closure of the aortic valve and ends with the closure of the mitral valve. It encompasses the following main phases:

- Isovolumic relaxation phase
- Rapid ventricular filling phase
- Diastasis
- Late diastolic filling due to atrial contraction.

The isovolumic relaxation phase starts with the aortic valve closure and ends with the mitral valve opening. During this phase, the LV pressure falls rapidly to the lowest level, whereas the left atrial (LA) pressure rises because of the incoming pulmonary venous return. Due to these changes, and also due to ventricular suction effect, an atrioventricular gradient develops which leads to the opening of the mitral valve and the subsequent rapid ventricular filling. Approximately 80% of the LV filling occur during this phase. With rapid ventricular filling, the LV pressure increases resulting in deceleration of mitral inflow and eventual equalization of LA and LV pressures. Once the LA and LV pressures equalize, active LV filling ceases, and there is only minimal forward flow occurring passively with left atrium acting only as a conduit. This is known as diastasis. The diastasis phase ends with the onset of atrial contraction during late diastole that results in increase in LA pressure once again. A second phase of rapid ventricular filling ensues contributing to almost 20% of the LV filling in normal subjects. However, the relative contribution of early and late phases of diastole to LV filling varies from person-to-person and depends on several factors, including elastic recoil (suction) of the LV, the rate of myocardial relaxation, chamber compliance, and the LA pressure.

### What is Diastolic Dysfunction?

Normal physiology is such that the left ventricle fills without much increase in LV end-diastolic pressure (LVEDP). Therefore, diastolic dysfunction refers to a state wherein an abnormal increase in LVEDP occurs for a given LV end-diastolic volume. Since left atrium and left ventricle are in continuity during diastole, any increase in LVEDP is translated into a concomitant increase in mean LA pressure which in turn results in increase in pulmonary capillary wedge pressure (PCWP). In absence of any pulmonary venous or mitral inflow obstruction, LVEDP, mean LA pressure and PCWP are nearly identical and interchangeably referred to as LV filling pressure (LVFP). LVFP is considered to be elevated when mean PCWP is greater than 12 mm Hg.

LV diastolic dysfunction may result from the abnormalities of active relaxation or of passive stretch (i.e. LV compliance or stiffness) or both. Since myocardial relaxation is an active, energy-dependent process, impairment of myocardial relaxation occurs immediately with the onset of myocardial ischemia. In fact, diastolic dysfunction is one of the earliest abnormalities seen in the ischemic cascade (**Flow chart 2.1**). However, the mechanisms underlying post-myocardial infarction (MI) LV diastolic dysfunction are more complex and remain incompletely understood. Presumably, cell necrosis and microvascular dysfunction affect active relaxation, whereas interstitial edema, fibrocellular infiltration, and scar formation impair LV compliance. This combination of relaxation abnormality of the myocardium along with increased LV chamber stiffness leads to increase in LVEDP.

## ECHOCARDIOGRAPHIC ASSESSMENT OF LEFT VENTRICULAR DIASTOLIC FUNCTION

Although invasive hemodynamic assessment is considered to be the gold-standard for evaluation of LV diastolic function, it requires cardiac catheterization and is technically challenging requiring creation of pressure-volume curves using high fidelity micromanometer catheters. In comparison, echocardiography is noninvasive, safe and provides reasonably accurate estimation of LVFP. Moreover, echocardiography offers the ability to perform serial assessments, which is a great advantage, particularly in hemodynamically labile patients. For these reasons, echocardiography has now become the modality of choice for assessment of LV diastolic function and for estimation of LVFP in clinical practice.

**Flow chart 2.1:** Ischemic cascade

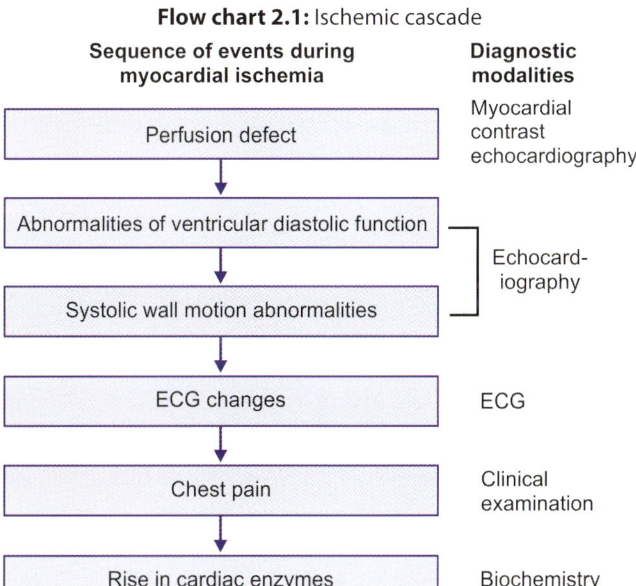


A baseline assessment of LV diastolic function must be performed in all patients with CAD undergoing echocardiography for any indication. This is particularly relevant for patients presenting with acute MI in whom several key therapeutic decisions are based on the state of LVFP and overall intracardiac hemodynamics.

There are a number of echocardiographic parameters used for assessment of LV diastolic function which include[6]:

- Mitral inflow velocities and timing
- Effect of Valsalva maneuver on mitral inflow pattern
- Mitral annular velocities
- Pulmonary vein flow pattern
- Isovolumic relaxation time (IVRT)
- LA volume and function
- Mitral inflow color propagation velocity
- Early diastolic strain rate, peak untwist rate, time to LV untwist, etc.
- Pulmonary arterial systolic, diastolic, and mean pressures.

Of these, the commonly used methods are discussed below.

### Transmitral Inflow Velocity Pattern

For assessment of mitral inflow, pulsed-wave Doppler is used with sample volume placed at the tips of the mitral leaflets in one of the apical views. Recording is made at end-expiration at a sweep speed of 50-100 mm/sec and is averaged over three cardiac cycles. The mitral inflow pattern typically shows an early diastolic wave (E) and a late diastolic wave (A) (**Figure 2.1**). As explained earlier, the 'E' velocity depends upon the early diastolic transmitral pressure gradient between LA and LV.

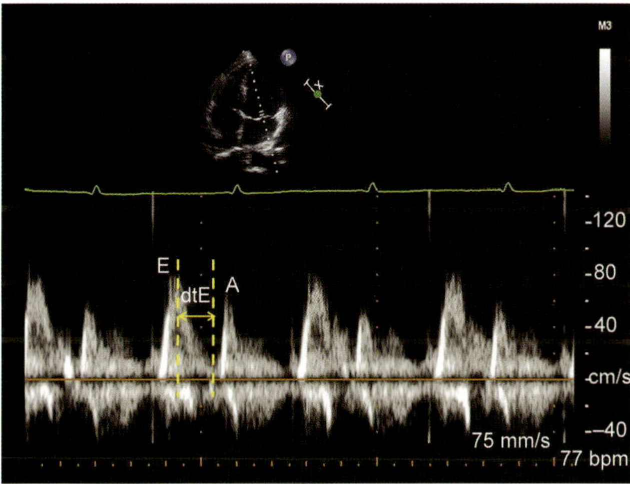


**Figure 2.1:** Mitral inflow pulse-wave Doppler.
*Abbreviations:* A, late diastolic mitral inflow velocity; dtE, deceleration time of early diastolic mitral inflow velocity; E, early diastolic mitral inflow velocity.

**Table 2.1:** Summary of echocardiographic findings in various stages of left ventricular diastolic dysfunction

| | *Normal* | *Grade 1* | *Grade 2* | *Grade 3a* | *Grade 3b* |
|---|---|---|---|---|---|
| LV relaxation<br>LV compliance<br>LA pressure | Normal<br>Normal<br>Normal | Impaired<br>N/↓<br>Normal | Impaired<br>↓↓<br>↑↑ | Impaired<br>↓↓↓<br>↑↑↑ | Impaired<br>↓↓↓↓<br>↑↑↑↑ |
| Mitral E/A ratio | 1.0–1.5 | <0.75–1.0 | 1.0–2.0 | >2.0 | >2.0 |
| IVRT (msec) | 70–100 | >100 | <100 | <70 | <70 |
| dtE (msec) | 160–220 | >220 | >140 | <140 | <140 |
| PV S/D ratio | >1.0 | N/<1 | <1 | <<1 | <<1 |
| PV Ar velocity (cm/sec) | <35 | <35* | >35 | >35 | >35 |
| PV Ar – mitral A duration (msec) | <30 | <30* | >30 | >30 | >30 |
| Mitral E/e' | <10 | <10* | >10 | >15 | >15 |
| Effect of Valsalva maneuver | Overall ↓ inflow velocities | Overall ↓ inflow velocities | Changes to grade 1 | Changes to grade 1–2 | No change |

* These values may be increased in presence of elevated left ventricular end-diastolic pressure.

*Abbreviations:* A, late diastolic mitral inflow velocity; Ar, pulmonary venous atrial reversal wave; D, pulmonary venous diastolic wave; dtE, deceleration time of early diastolic mitral inflow velocity; E, early diastolic mitral inflow velocity; e', early diastolic mitral annular velocity; IVRT, isovolumic relaxation time; LA, left atrial; LV, left ventricular; PV, pulmonary venous; S, pulmonary venous systolic wave.

With higher atrioventricular pressure gradient, the 'E' wave becomes progressively taller. The slope of the 'E' wave depicts the rapidity with which LA and LV pressures equalize after the initial rapid filling. With impairment of active LV relaxation, equalization of the pressures is delayed resulting in longer deceleration time of the E wave (dtE, measured from the peak of the E wave to the end of the E wave). However, with increase in the LA pressure, dtE is progressively shortened. During late diastole, when left atrium contracts, LA pressure rises once again and exceeds LV pressure resulting in a late-diastolic gradient between left atrium and left ventricle. This is responsible for the 'A' wave seen on Doppler tracing. Since most of the LV filling has already occurred and LA has already emptied before the onset of the 'A' wave, the 'A' wave usually has a low velocity. Consequently, the E/A ratio is usually between 1.0 and 1.5.

It can thus be summarized that mitral 'E' wave reflects LA–LV pressure gradient in early diastole and is affected by LV relaxation and pre-load. In contrast, the 'A' wave reflects LA–LV pressure gradient in late diastole and is affected by LA compliance and contractility.

**Table 2.1** summarizes mitral inflow Doppler findings in different stages of LV diastolic dysfunction.

## Mitral Annular Velocities

Pulsed-wave tissue Doppler imaging (TDI) is used for recording tissue velocities from medial or lateral mitral annulus in apical 4-chamber view (**Figure 2.2**). Since the LV apex is relatively fixed throughout the cardiac cycle, it is the LV base which moves longitudinally during the cardiac cycle. Thus, the early diastolic annular velocity (e') reflects LV relaxation and is inversely correlated with invasively determined parameters of LV relaxation. The e' velocity decreases with age, but generally it is ≥10 cm/s at medial annulus and ≥15 cm/s at lateral annulus. The lateral annular velocity is higher than medial annular velocity because of greater excursion of LV free wall during systole, which is due to greater density of longitudinal fibers in the lateral wall as compared to the ventricular septum and also because lateral wall is relatively free to move. Since e' is a reflection of myocardial relaxation, it gets reduced in all stages of LV diastolic dysfunction. Abnormalities in e' wave precede mitral inflow abnormalities by almost 10 years.

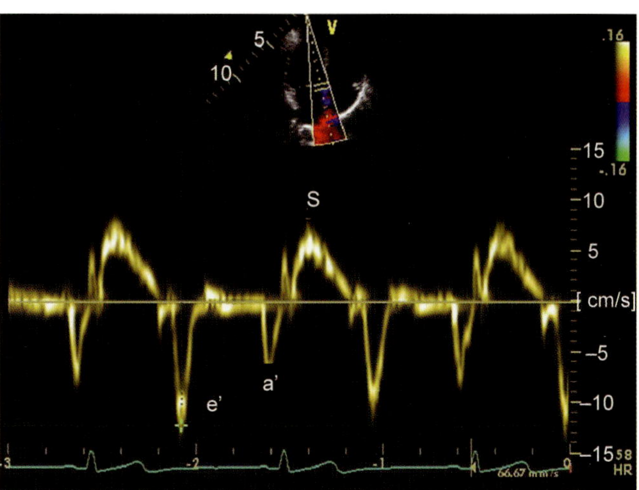


**Figure 2.2:** Tissue-Doppler imaging from medial mitral annulus. *Abbreviations:* a', late diastolic mitral annular velocity; e', early diastolic mitral annular velocity; S, systolic mitral annular velocity.

The late diastolic mitral annular a' wave is generated because of LA contraction and is, therefore, influenced by LA systolic function and LVEDP. Increased LA contractility enhances a' velocity and increased LVEDP reduces it.

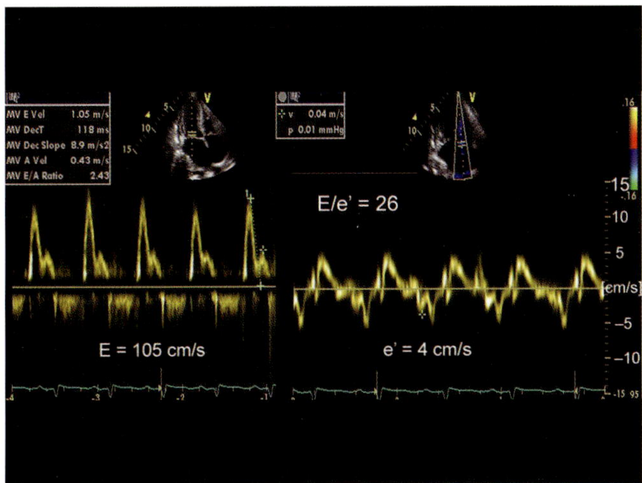


**Figure 2.3:** A patient with advanced left ventricular diastolic dysfunction. The ratio of mitral inflow early diastolic velocity (E) to early diastolic medial mitral annular velocity (e') is 26, suggestive of very high left ventricular filing pressure. Also note shortened deceleration time of mitral E wave.

Instead of using absolute e' velocities, more commonly mitral E/e' ratio is used for assessing LV diastolic function and for estimating LVFP (**Figure 2.3**). The ratio minimizes the effects of aging, LV relaxation and LV pre-load on mitral E and e' individually and thus provides more accurate estimation of LVFP.[6-9] The normal value of mitral E/e' is <8, whereas a value of ≥15 indicates elevated LVFP when medial e' is used, ≥12 when lateral e' is used and ≥13 when the average of the two is used.[6] However, in the 2016 American Society of Echocardio-graphy (ASE) guidelines for assessment of LV diastolic function, these cut-off values have been revised as >15, >13, and >14 for medial, lateral and average e' respectively.[10]

In the setting of MI, the E/e' ratio has several advantages over mitral inflow pattern for assessment of LV diastolic function. First, in patients presenting with MI, loading conditions keep changing very rapidly. In these circumstances, mitral E/e', being relatively pre-load independent, provides more accurate assessment of LVFP as compared to mitral E/A ratio.[6] Second, in many patients with acute MI, LVEF is well preserved. Mitral E/e' has been shown to correlate better with LVFP than mitral E/A ratio in presence of preserved LVEF.[6] And finally, E/e' ratio can be applied even in situations like sinus tachycardia and atrial fibrillation (AF) which are commonly encountered in acute MI patients.[11,12]

However, there are certain situations in which mitral E/'e may not be a reliable indicator of LVFP:

- Severe primary mitral regurgitation, as it leads to increased 'E' velocity due to increased flow volume across mitral valve
- Lateral/septal wall motion abnormality
- Mitral valve disease, including annular calcification
- Abnormal interventricular septal motion like postcardiac surgery, left bundle-branch block (LBBB), cardiac pacing, right ventricular volume overload, etc. In these conditions, measurement of mitral 'e' is often inaccurate because of cardiac translational motion, asynchronous LV contraction and/or increased insonation angle.

Mitral E/e' is also less accurate in normal, healthy young individuals as they often have excellent ventricular relaxation, vigorous elastic recoil (suction) and good ventricular compliance. This results in tall physiological 'E' wave velocity and small 'A' wave.

### *Mitral 'L' Wave*

Although the phase of diastasis is usually quiescent on Doppler examination, a forward wave can sometimes be seen during this period. This is known as 'L' wave and can be recorded on both mitral inflow Doppler and TDI of mitral annular motion (**Figure 2.4A and B**).[13,14] 'L' wave is in fact a relatively common finding but is usually unnoticed. It can be an important clue to raised filling pressure and is a precursor for HF.[12,13] Sometimes, small 'L' waves can also be seen in normal individuals, particularly in presence of bradycardia. But a pathological 'L' wave is characterized by (a) velocity more than 20 cm/sec, (b) reduction or disappearance with Valsalva maneuver (**Figure 2.5**), and (c) concomitant elevated E/e' ratio.[13] 'L' wave occurs mainly due to prolonged active relaxation in presence of increased LV stiffness and raised LA pressure. The prolonged relaxation lowers LV pressure in mid-diastole, which in the presence of increased LA pressure, leads to mid-diastolic filling.

## Pulmonary Vein Flow Pattern

Pulmonary veins are interrogated from apical 4-chamber view utilizing color-flow mapping. The sample volume is placed within one of the pulmonary veins, about 1 cm from its orifice, and velocities are recorded. The Doppler tracing thus obtained comprises of the following waves: systolic wave (S), diastolic wave (D), and a small end-diastolic atrial reversal wave (Ar) (**Figure 2.6**). Sometimes, especially in patients with bradycardia, two systolic waves can be recorded. The first antegrade systolic wave is due to decline in LA pressure during atrial relaxation, which results in a pressure gradient between pulmonary vein and left atrium. The second antegrade systolic wave is due to increased pulmonary venous return during late systole. With early diastolic LA emptying, the LA pressure declines leading to an early diastolic D wave which changes in parallel with mitral 'E' velocity. During late-diastolic LA contraction, LA pressure increases more than the pulmonary vein leading to atrial reversal (Ar). The velocity of

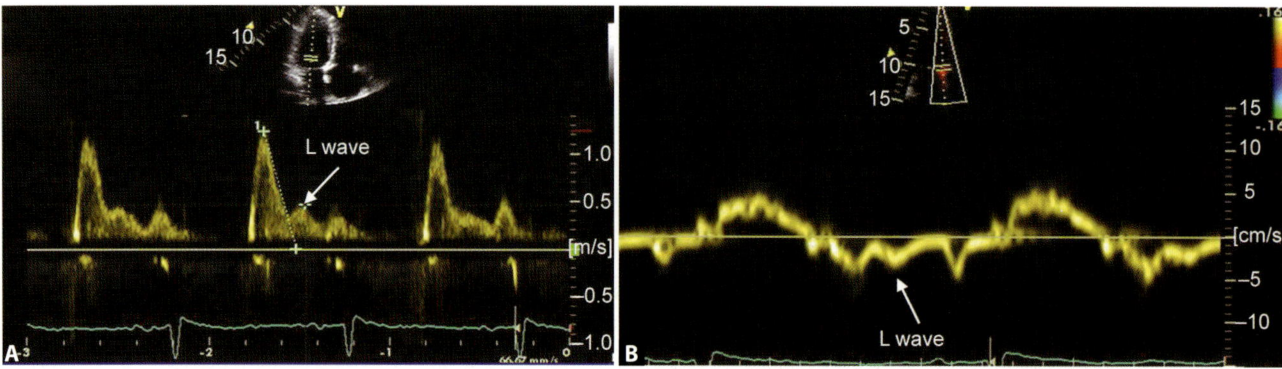


**Figure 2.4A and B:** Mid-diastolic 'L' wave recorded on (A) mitral inflow spectral Doppler and (B) mitral annular tissue Doppler imaging.

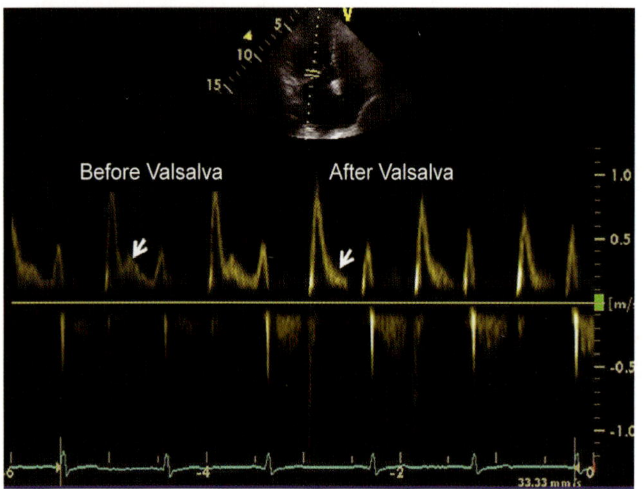


**Figure 2.5:** Blunting of mid-diastolic mitral inflow 'L' wave with Valsalva maneuver.

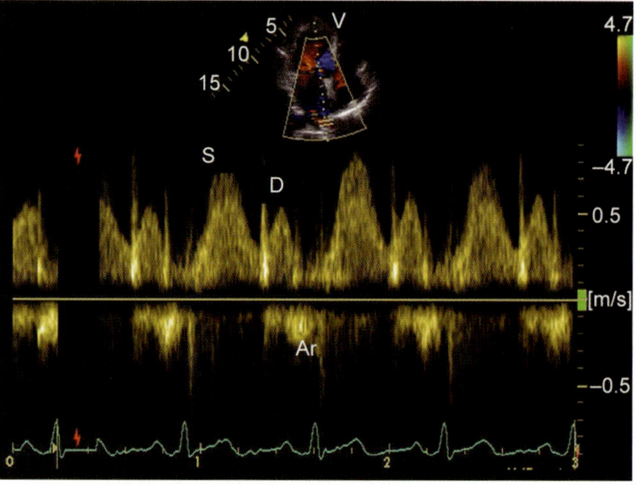


**Figure 2.6:** Pulmonary vein flow pattern.
*Abbreviations:* Ar, pulmonary venous atrial reversal wave; D, pulmonary venous diastolic wave; S, pulmonary venous systolic wave.

'Ar' wave is normally less than 35 cm/sec, and its duration is within 30 msec of mitral 'A' wave duration.

In normal left ventricle, the pulmonary venous S/D ratio is more than 1.0. With progressive LV diastolic dysfunction, there is increased LA pressure leading to decreased pulmonary vein-left atrium gradient. Consequently, systolic wave velocity decreases and most of the filling occurs in diastole resulting in reversal of S/D ratio. While the pulmonary venous S/D ratio reflects mean LA pressure, the Ar wave more closely reflects LVEDP. When left atrium contracts against elevated LV diastolic pressure, blood will preferentially flow backwards into the pulmonary veins, as opposed to transmitrally into the left ventricle. As a result, Ar velocity increases (>35 cm/sec) and becomes prolonged (longer than mitral 'A' velocity by >30 msec). Accordingly, Ar-A duration is a measure of LVEDP (**Figure 2.7A and B**).

It should however be noted that good quality pulmonary vein flow tracing may not be obtainable in about 20% cases, especially during transthoracic echocardiography. It may also be difficult to discern Ar wave in presence of atrial contraction artifacts. Finally, Ar is also not a reliable measure of LVFP in presence of impaired LA contractility.

## Isovolumic Relaxation Time

IVRT is the time interval between the closure of the aortic valve and the opening of the mitral valve. It is usually recorded from apical long-axis view or apical 5-chamber view, preferably using continuous wave Doppler. The Doppler beam is aligned between LV outflow and mitral inflow, thus permitting recording of both the signals simultaneously. From the spectral Doppler signal thus obtained, IVRT is measured as the time interval from the termination of aortic outflow signal

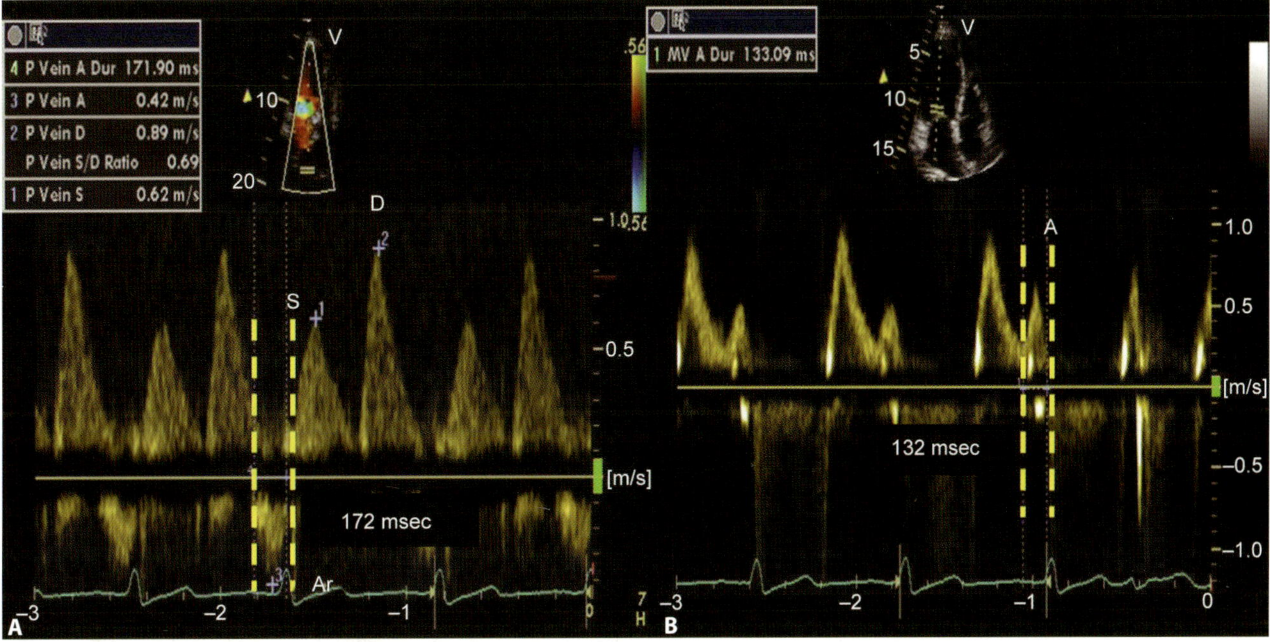


**Figure 2.7A and B:** Pulmonary vein flow pattern (A) and mitral inflow pattern (B) in a patient with grade 2 left ventricular diastolic dysfunction. Pulmonary venous systolic (S) and diastolic (D) ratio is reversed and the atrial reversal wave (Ar) is accentuated and prolonged. The difference between pulmonary venous Ar duration and mitral inflow late diastolic 'A' wave is increased (40 msec).

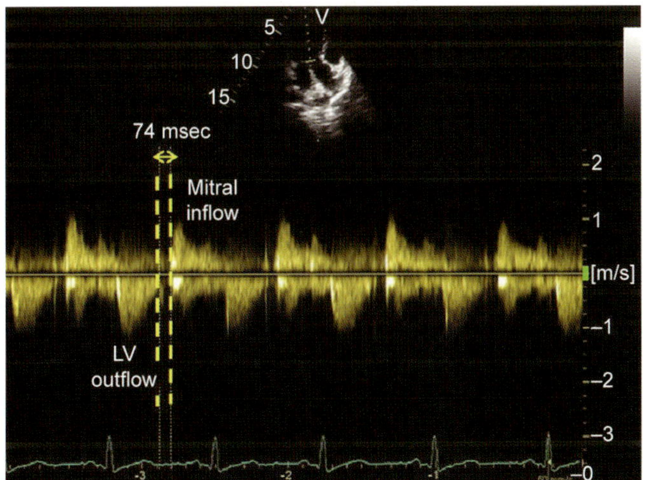


**Figure 2.8:** Measurement of isovolumic relaxation time from apical long-axis view. The time interval from the end of aortic outflow signal to the beginning of mitral inflow signal is measured.
*Abbreviation:* LV, left ventricular.

to onset of mitral inflow (**Figure 2.8**). Normal value of IVRT is 70–100 msec. When there is impaired LV relaxation, mitral valve opens later, resulting in prolongation of IVRT. However, when LA pressure is elevated, it leads to earlier opening of the mitral valve and thus, shortening of IVRT. If IVRT is <60 msec, then in the presence of an underlying heart disease, it can be concluded that LA pressure is increased.

### *IVRT/$T_{E-e'}$*

Since IVRT is a load-dependent parameter, it is integrated into another parameter IVRT/$T_{E-e'}$ to provide more accurate, load-independent estimate of LVFP. To obtain $T_{E-e'}$, the time intervals from the beginning of the QRS complex to the onset of mitral E wave and the onset of e' are measured separately. The former value is then subtracted from the latter (**Figure 2.9A and B**). This value depends on LV relaxation and LA pressure. The longer the interval, more severe is the LV diastolic dysfunction. In contrast, IVRT decreases with increasing filling pressure. Thus, IVRT/$T_{E-e'}$ is inversely related to mean LA pressure. The normal value of IVRT/$T_{E-e'}$ is >2 and a value <2 is indicative of raised mean LA pressure.[6] It is noteworthy that IVRT/$T_{E-e'}$ remains accurate in many of the conditions in which other parameters become fallacious.[6]

## Left Atrial Volume

In the last few years, there has been growing evidence that LA size has robust diagnostic and prognostic implications in a variety of clinical conditions.[15-21] Its value as an indicator of LV diastolic dysfunction is immense because during diastole, the thin wall left atrium is directly exposed to increased LV pressure through the mitral valve. When persistently exposed to elevated LVFP, LA gets stretched and enlarged. Thus, increased LA size reflects cumulative effect of elevated LVFP

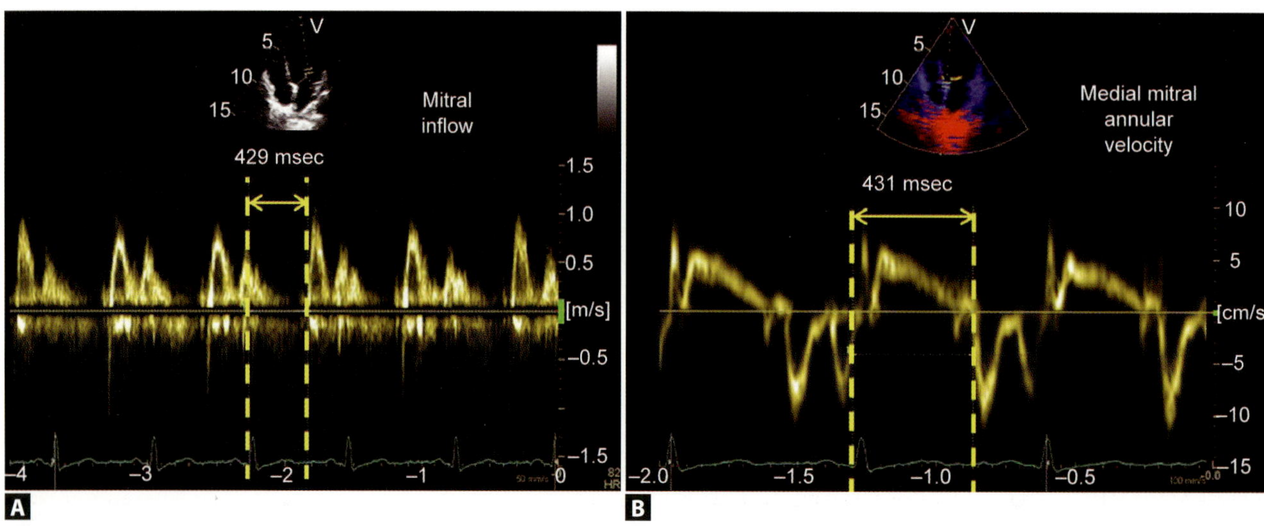


**Figure 2.9A and B:** Measurement of $T_{E-e'}$. mitral inflow Doppler (A) and mitral annular tissue Doppler (B) are recorded separately. Time intervals from the onset of the QRS complex on ECG to the beginning of mitral inflow early diastolic velocity (E) and the beginning of early diastolic annular velocity (e') are measured, and the former is subtracted from the latter to obtain $T_{E-e'}$.

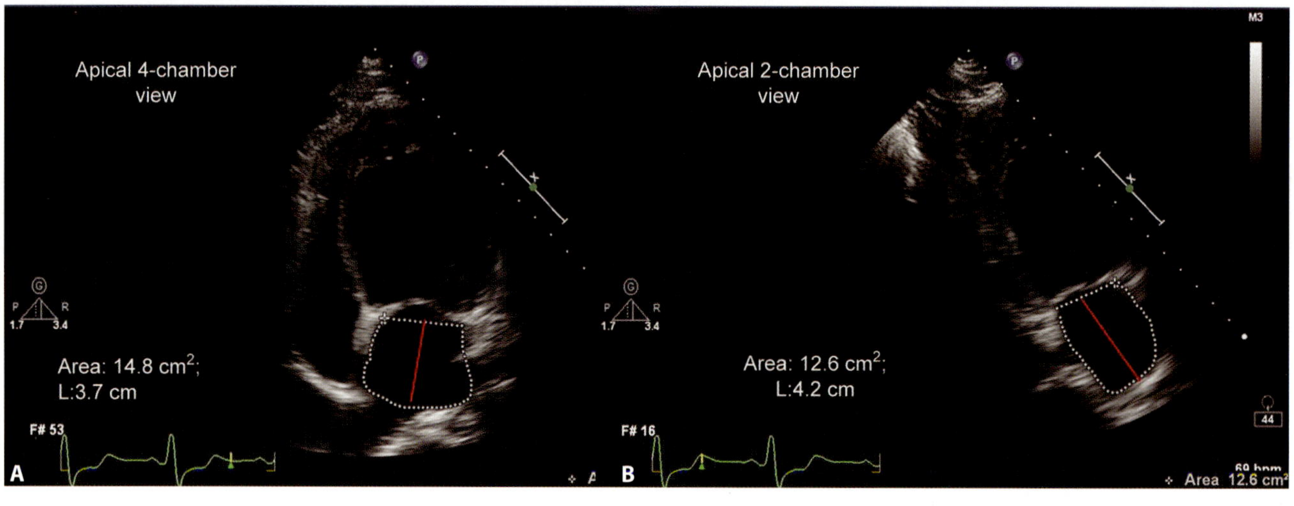


$$\begin{aligned}\text{LA volume} &= 0.85 \times A1 \times A2/L \\ &= 0.85 \times 14.8 \times 12.6/3.7 \\ &= 42.8 \text{ mL}\end{aligned}$$

**Figure 2.10A and B:** Measurement of left atrial (LA) volume by area–length method. $A_1$ and $A_2$ are LA areas in apical 4- and 2-chamber views. L is the length of the left atrium which is recorded in both the views, but shorter of the two is used for the calculation. The calculated LA volume needs to be indexed to body-surface area.

over time and is a measure of chronic LV diastolic dysfunction, unlike mitral inflow and annular velocities which reflect instantaneous LVFP.

LA volume is a more accurate measure of LA size than anteroposterior dimension because (a) Left atrium is not a symmetrical-shaped structure, and (b) LA enlargement may occur eccentrically and not necessarily in anteroposterior dimension. It has been shown that patients with normal LA dimension can have LA volumes varying between 27.5 mL and 106 mL.[22]

Area-length method is the recommended echocardiographic method for estimation of LA volume.[23] Apical 4- and 2-chamber views are obtained at the end of ventricular systole, just prior to mitral valve opening, to obtain maximum LA dimension. If apical 2-chamber view is not satisfactorily visualized, then apical long-axis view can be utilized. LA area is planimetered in both these views by tracing the inner border of the left atrium while excluding the inlets of pulmonary veins, LA appendage and area under the mitral annulus (**Figure 2.10A and B**). LA length is also recorded in both the views as the distance between the mitral annular plane and the posterior wall of the left atrium and the shorter of the two is used. LA volume is then calculated using the formula $0.85 \times A_1 \times A_2 / L$, where $A_1$ and $A_2$ are the two LA areas and L is the shortest LA length. All LA measurements need to be indexed to body surface area. The upper normal limit for two-dimensional echocardiographic LA volume is 34 mL/m$^2$ for both men and women.[23]

It should be noted that though LA volume is an important index of LV diastolic dysfunction, there are several situations in which it may be less reliable. These include chronic AF, mitral valve disease, anemia, elite athletes, bradycardia, etc. In chronic AF, LA enlargement can occur even in the absence of significant elevation of LA pressure.[15] It has therefore been suggested that LA volume has a better negative— as opposed to positive- predictive value for significant LV diastolic dysfunction and HF, i.e. a normal or small left atrium usually excludes significant raised LVFP, while a large LA volume may occur even in the absence of significant LV diastolic dysfunction.

## Integrating Echocardiographic Variables for Accurate Assessment of Left Ventricular Diastolic Function and Left Ventricular Filling Pressure

Unfortunately, none of the parameters described above is accurate enough to be used in isolation for assessment of LV diastolic dysfunction. Moreover, not infrequently, these various parameters appear to conflict with each other. Therefore, as a rule, multiple echocardiographic parameters of LV diastolic function should be assessed in every patient and integrated to reach a more accurate estimation of LVFP. The associated cardiac abnormalities, such as mitral valve disease, pericardial disease, etc. should also be taken into account. The ASE has published guidelines outlining step-wise approach to assessment of LV diastolic function in patients with and without LV systolic dysfunction (**Flow chart 2.2**).[6,10] Using this algorithmic approach, LV diastolic dysfunction can be categorized as normal or abnormal and when abnormal, can be graded as grade 1 (impaired relaxation), 2 (pseudonormal pattern) or 3 (restrictive pattern).

## Assessment of Diastolic Dysfunction in Certain Special Situations

### *Atrial Fibrillation*

Assessment of LV diastolic function in AF is challenging because in AF, there is (a) loss of atrial mechanical function, (b) mitral inflow 'A' wave is not seen, (c) cardiac cycle length is highly variable, (d) Doppler waves are chaotic, and (e) applicability of LA volume is doubtful, as AF can itself lead to LA enlargement independent of LA pressure.

**Flow chart 2.2:** Estimation of left ventricular filling pressure in patients with and without left ventricular systolic dysfunction

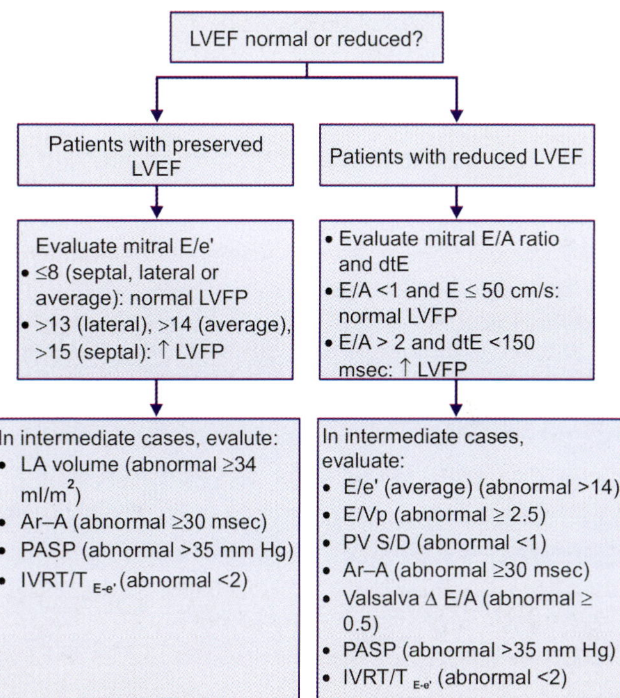


*Abbreviations:* A, late diastolic mitral inflow velocity; Ar, pulmonary venous atrial reversal wave; D, pulmonary venous diastolic wave; dtE, deceleration time of early diastolic mitral inflow velocity; E, early diastolic mitral inflow velocity; e', early diastolic mitral annular velocity; IVRT, isovolumic relaxation time; LA, left atrial; LV, left ventricular; LVEF, left ventricular ejection fraction; LVFP, left ventricular filling pressure; PASP, pulmonary arterial systolic pressure; PV, pulmonary venous; S, pulmonary venous systolic wave; $V_p$, propagation velocity of mitral inflow.

The parameters that have been shown to be useful for assessment of LV diastolic function in presence of AF include[6,12]:

- Mitral dtE <150 msec (especially in presence of LV systolic dysfunction)
- Mitral E/e' ≥11
- IVRT (≤65 msec)
- Deceleration time of pulmonary venous 'D' wave ≤220 msec (a value <150 msec suggests PCWP >18 mm Hg with 100% sensitivity and 96% specificity), and
- The ratio of mitral 'E' velocity to mitral inflow propagation velocity ≥1.4.

Due to significant beat-to-beat variability in intracardiac flow during AF, all parameters should be recorded over at least 5–10 cardiac cycles. Cardiac cycles may not be consecutive but should be of good quality signal and the cycle length should preferably be equivalent to a heart rate of 60–80 beats/

min. If there is a lack of significant beat-to-beat variability in various Doppler parameters during AF, it does itself provide an indirect clue towards elevated LVFP.

### *Sinus Tachycardia*

During sinus tachycardia, the evaluation of LV diastolic function becomes difficult due to fusion of early and late diastolic Doppler waves. However, a ratio of mitral inflow peak E-wave velocity to lateral mitral e' >10 indicates a mean PCWP >12 mm Hg with 78% sensitivity and 95% specificity in this situation.[11] If only a single wave is identifiable on mitral inflow Doppler and mitral annular TDI due to complete merging of the early and late diastolic waves, the peak velocity of these single waves can be used for estimating LVFP with fair degree of accuracy.[24]

## CLINICAL RELEVANCE OF ASSESSMENT OF LEFT VENTRICULAR DIASTOLIC FUNCTION IN CORONARY ARTERY DISEASE

### Diagnostic Significance and Role in Guiding Management

In CAD patients who have preserved LV systolic function, the presence of significant LV diastolic dysfunction with raised LVFP may be an indirect clue to the underlying CAD, apart from also offering a mechanistic explanation for their symptoms. In many of these patients, LVFP is normal at rest but rises rapidly as the patient exercises. Appropriate management of CAD is required in these patients to correct these abnormalities as the conventional pharmacological management of HF has not been shown to be of much benefit in these patients.[1,3,4]

In those who present with acute MI with LV systolic dysfunction, the assessment of LV diastolic function provides important information about intracardiac hemodynamics which is crucial for their optimum management. The need for diuretics, intravenous fluids, inotropes, vasodilators, etc., timing of introduction of beta-blockers, timing of coronary intervention, ambulation and mobilization of the patients after acute MI, etc. are important clinical decisions that are all guided by the status of LVFP. Furthermore, being an important prognostic marker, LVFP is also helpful in determining the aggressiveness of the treatment in these patients.

### Prognostic Significance of Left Ventricular Filling Pressure

During the early phase of MI, about 38% of patients have impaired myocardial relaxation and about 24% patients have an advanced diastolic dysfunction in the form of restrictive LV filling pattern.[25] The prognostic significance of advanced diastolic dysfunction, i.e. raised LVFP or restrictive physiology, has been reported by several investigators. It was initially reported by Oh et al. as early as in 1992.[26] In a study of 62 patients, restrictive filling pattern was found to be associated with a high incidence of in-hospital HF. Several other workers have confirmed this initial observation. Nijland et al. studied 95 patients with first acute MI and found that raised LVFP was associated with 22% survival rate at 3 years compared with 100% in the nonrestrictive group.[27] Other large studies have also shown that a dtE <140 msec is an independent predictor of all-cause mortality in patients with ST-elevation MI (STEMI).[28-30] It is the elevation of LVFP that is the important link between diastolic dysfunction and prognosis, as milder forms of diastolic dysfunction do not seem to portend an adverse prognosis in MI.[30]

Although the prevalence and severity of filling abnormalities correlate with the severity of LV systolic dysfunction, a considerable proportion of patients present with Doppler signs of elevated filling pressures despite only mildly reduced LVEF. Even in these patients, LVFP is a predictor of morbidity and mortality as the prognostic value of LVFP in acute MI is independent of LVEF. In a study involving 395 patients with MI, only restrictive transmitral filling pattern, LA volume and Killip class were found to be independent predictors of death on multivariate analysis.[31] LVEF or wall motion score index did not provide any additional prognostic information.

Increased LA size and volume have also been reported to be associated with higher all-cause mortality rate in MI patients.[30,31] Beinart et al. studied 395 consecutive patients of acute MI within 48 hours of hospital admission.[31] It was found that the 5 years mortality rate was 34.4% in those with LA volume >32 mL/m$^2$ as compared to only 14.2% in those with LA volume <32 mL/m$^2$. Additionally, those with a higher LA volume had higher incidence of cardiac failure, mitral regurgitation and LV systolic dysfunction. Similarly, Moller et al. studied 314 patients of acute MI and followed them for a mean duration of 15 months.[30] Overall, 15% of the patients died during this follow-up. There were 27 patients who had LVEF <40% and LA volume <32 mL/m$^2$. Out of these, only one died. In contrast, 22 of the 55 patients who had similar LVEF but enlarged left atrium (i.e. LA volume >32 mL/m$^2$) died. All these studies confirm the prognostic significance of LA volume in acute MI.

Increased LA size also predisposes to the development of AF which in turn increases the risk of various embolic complications. As per Framingham study, a 5 mm increase in LA diameter is associated with a 39% increase in the risk of developing AF.[32]

Apart from LA size, LA function also has prognostic value in acute MI. Dogan et al. studied 90 consecutive patients of STEMI who underwent primary percutaneous coronary intervention (PCI).[33] LA contractile function was assessed using speckle-tracking echocardiography. It was observed that LA systolic strain was consistently impaired in STEMI patients as compared to healthy controls. In addition, LA systolic strain had significant positive correlation with LVEF and negative correlation with mitral E/e', LA volumes and the circulating levels of brain natriuretic peptide levels. It is thus evident that regardless of the parameter used for assessment of LVFP, any direct or indirect evidence of raised LVFP is associated with adverse prognosis in patients presenting with acute MI.

Importantly, LV diastolic function seems to be favorably affected by timely institution of reperfusion therapy in acute MI. Wang et al. studied 340 consecutive STEMI patients who underwent primary PCI.[34] Door-to-balloon time was <90 minutes in 232 patients and ≥90 minutes in the remaining 108 patients. All subjects underwent a detailed echocardiographic examination within 48 hours of hospitalization. Mean LVEF was almost similar in both the groups and the comorbidities were also similar. However, the proportion of the patients having mitral E/e' >15 was much greater among those who had longer door-to-balloon times (i.e. >90 minutes) as compared to those with shorter door-to-balloon times (44.4% vs. 30.6%). The effect was more pronounced in elderly patients with age >65 years. This study emphasizes the importance of shortening door-to-balloon time to preserve LV diastolic function in STEMI patients undergoing primary PCI.

## CONCLUSION

Assessment of LV diastolic function has important diagnostic, prognostic, and therapeutic implications in patients with CAD. It is particularly more important in the setting of STEMI as it helps in risk stratification of these patients and identifies those who are likely to be benefited by aggressive treatment, such as early revascularization. Detailed echocardiographic examination including two-dimensional imaging, spectral Doppler, TDI, and speckle-tracking echocardiography permits a comprehensive assessment of LV diastolic function in most patients. Information derived using all these modalities needs to be integrated to obtain the most accurate assessment of LV diastolic function and LVFP.

## REFERENCES


1. Yancy CW, Jessup M, Bozkurt B, et al. 2013 ACCF/AHA guideline for the management of heart failure: A report of the American College of Cardiology Foundation/American Heart Association task force on practice guidelines. J Am Coll Cardiol. 2013;62:e147-239.
2. Owan TE, Hodge DO, Herges RM, Jacobsen SJ, Roger VL, Redfield MM. Trends in prevalence and outcome of heart failure with preserved ejection fraction. N Engl J Med. 2006;355:251-9.
3. Komajda M, Lam CS. Heart failure with preserved ejection fraction: A clinical dilemma. Eur Heart J. 2014;35:1022-32.
4. Gupta DK, Solomon SD. Imaging in heart failure with preserved ejection fraction. Heart Fail Clin. 2014;10:419-34.
5. Butler J, Fonarow GC, Zile MR, et al. Developing therapies for heart failure with preserved ejection fraction: Current state and future directions. JACC Heart failure. 2014;2:97-112.
6. Nagueh SF, Appleton CP, Gillebert TC, et al. Recommendations for the evaluation of left ventricular diastolic function by echocardiography. J Am Soc Echocardiogr. 2009;22:107-33.
7. Sohn DW, Chai IH, Lee DJ, et al. Assessment of mitral annulus velocity by Doppler tissue imaging in the evaluation of left ventricular diastolic function. J Am Coll Cardiol. 1997;30:474-80.
8. Nagueh SF, Middleton KJ, Kopelen HA, et al. Doppler tissue imaging: A noninvasive technique for evaluation of left ventricular relaxation and estimation of filling pressures. J Am Coll Cardiol. 1997;30:1527-33.
9. Ommen SR, Nishimura RA, Appleton CP, et al. Clinical utility of Doppler echocardiography and tissue Doppler imaging in the estimation of left ventricular filling pressures: a comparative simultaneous Doppler-catheterization study. Circulation. 2000;102:1788-94.
10. Nagueh SF, Smiseth OA, Appleton CP, et al. Recommendations for the evaluation of left ventricular diastolic function by echocardiography: An update from the American Society of Echocardiography and the European Association of Cardiovascular Imaging. J Am Soc Echocardiogr. 2016;29:277-314
11. Nagueh SF, Mikati I, Kopelen HA, Middleton KJ, Quinones MA, Zoghbi WA. Doppler estimation of left ventricular filling pressure in sinus tachycardia: a new application of tissue Doppler imaging. Circulation. 1998;98:1644-50.
12. Nagueh SF, Kopelen HA, Quinones MA. Assessment of left ventricular filling pressures by Doppler in the presence of atrial fibrillation. Circulation. 1996;94:2138-45.
13. Ha JW, Ahn JA, Moon JY, et al. Triphasic mitral inflow velocity with mid-diastolic flow: The presence of mid-diastolic mitral annular velocity indicates advanced diastolic dysfunction. Eur J Echocardiogr. 2006;7:16-21.
14. Ha JW, Oh JK, Redfield MM, Ujino K, Seward JB, Tajik AJ. Triphasic mitral inflow velocity with middiastolic filling: Clinical implications and associated echocardiographic findings. J Am Soc Echocardiogr. 2004;17:428-31.
15. Abhayaratna WP, Seward JB, Appleton CP, et al. Left atrial size: Physiologic determinants and clinical applications. J Am Coll Cardiol. 2006;47:2357-63.
16. Zile MR, Gottdiener JS, Hetzel SJ, et al. Prevalence and significance of alterations in cardiac structure and function in patients with heart failure and a preserved ejection fraction. Circulation. 2011;124:2491-501.
17. Shah AM, Shah SJ, Anand IS, et al. Cardiac structure and function in heart failure with preserved ejection fraction: Baseline findings from the echocardiographic study of the treatment of preserved cardiac function heart failure with an aldosterone antagonist trial. Circ Heart Fail. 2014;7:104-15.
18. Tsang TS, Abhayaratna WP, Barnes ME, et al. Prediction of cardiovascular outcomes with left atrial size: is volume superior to area or diameter? J Am Coll Cardiol. 2006;47:1018-23.

19. Benjamin EJ, D'Agostino RB, Belanger AJ, et al. Left atrial size and the risk of stroke and death: the Framingham heart study. Circulation. 1995;92:835-41.
20. Moller JE, Hillis GS, Oh JK, et al. Left atrial volume: a powerful predictor of survival after acute myocardial infarction. Circulation. 2003;107:2207-12.
21. Meris A, Amigoni M, Uno H, et al. Left atrial remodelling in patients with myocardial infarction complicated by heart failure, left ventricular dysfunction, or both: the VALIANT echo study. Eur Heart J. 2009;30:56-65.
22. Parashar SK. LV diastolic function evaluation: What is practical? In: Chopra HK (ed). Cardiology Society of India Cardiology Update 2014. New Delhi: Jaypee Brothers Medical Publishers; 2014. pp 271-82.
23. Lang RM, Badano LP, Mor-Avi V, et al. Recommendations for cardiac chamber quantification by echocardiography in adults: An update from the American Society of Echocardiography and the European Association of Cardiovascular Imaging. J Am Soc Echocardiogr. 2015;28:1-39.e14.
24. Sohn DW, Kim YJ, Kim HC, Chun HG, Park YB, Choi YS. Evaluation of left ventricular diastolic function when mitral e and a waves are completely fused: Role of assessing mitral annulus velocity. J Am Soc Echocardiogr. 1999;12:203-8.
25. Poulsen SH, Jensen SE, Egstrup K. Longitudinal changes and prognostic implications of left ventricular diastolic function in first acute myocardial infarction. Am Heart J. 1999;137:910-8.
26. Oh JK, Ding ZP, Gersh BJ, et al. Restrictive left ventricular diastolic filling identifies patients with heart failure after acute myocardial infarction. J Am Soc Echocardiogr. 1992;5:497-503.
27. Nijland F, Kamp O, Karreman AJ, et al. Prognostic implications of restrictive left ventricular filling in acute myocardial infarction: A serial Doppler echocardiographic study. J Am Coll Cardiol. 1997;30:1618-24.
28. Schwammenthal E, Adler Y, Amichai K, et al. Prognostic value of global myocardial performance indices in acute myocardial infarction: Comparison to measures of systolic and diastolic left ventricular function. Chest. 2003;124:1645-51.
29. Temporelli PL, Giannuzzi P, Nicolosi GL, et al. Doppler-derived mitral deceleration time as a strong prognostic marker of left ventricular remodeling and survival after acute myocardial infarction: Results of the GISSI-3 echo substudy. J Am Coll Cardiol. 2004;43:1646-53.
30. Moller JE, Egstrup K, Kober L, Poulsen SH, Nyvad O, Torp-Pedersen C. Prognostic importance of systolic and diastolic function after acute myocardial infarction. Am Heart J. 2003;145:147-53.
31. Beinart R, Boyko V, Schwammenthal E, et al. Long-term prognostic significance of left atrial volume in acute myocardial infarction. J Am Coll Cardiol. 2004;44:327-34.
32. Vaziri SM, Larson MG, Benjamin EJ, et al. Echocardiographic predictors of nonrheumatic atrial fibrillation. The Framingham heart study. Circulation. 1994;89:724-30.
33. Dogan C, Ozdemir N, Hatipoglu S, et al. Relation of left atrial peak systolic strain with left ventricular diastolic dysfunction and brain natriuretic peptide level in patients presenting with ST-elevation myocardial infarction. Cardiovasc Ultrasound. 2013;11:24.
34. Wang YC, Wu HP, Lo PH, et al. Impact of prolonged door-to-balloon times on the diastolic function in acute ST-elevation myocardial infarction patients undergoing primary percutaneous coronary intervention. Acta Cardiol Sin. 2015;31:281-91.

# Echocardiographic Evaluation of the Right Atrium and Right Ventricle

*Anuj Mediratta, Francesco Maffessanti, Karima Addetia, Roberto M Lang*

## INTRODUCTION TO THE RIGHT HEART

Understanding the echocardiographic evaluation of the right atrium and right ventricle is essential in patients with coronary artery disease. Previously thought of as a passive conduit or a "bystander" to the left heart, right-sided abnormalities are now known to have significant impact on the morbidity and mortality of patients with cardiovascular disease. Generally, principles of echocardiography applied to the left heart are similar in the right side; however, there are several unique aspects which need to be considered when performing an echocardiogram on the right heart. This chapter highlights the unique characteristics of the right heart and describes how to appropriately use echocardiography to evaluate right ventricle and right atrium in patients with cardiovascular diseases.

Due to its complex shape and location, the right heart imaging planes are less standardized and more difficult to reproduce. Though the importance of right heart function has historically been minimized, interest in the right heart and related structures has increased over the last decade and continues to be a focus of cardiovascular research. Relative to the left heart, clinical data and reference values for the right atrium and right ventricle are significantly lacking; however, quantitative evaluation of the right heart should be part of every transthoracic echocardiographic (TTE) examination.

## ANATOMY AND PHYSIOLOGY OF THE RIGHT HEART

The right ventricle is situated just posterior to the sternum inferior to the great vessels. From an echocardiographic perspective, the right heart is visualized in sections starting with the right ventricular (RV) inflow, main RV body and RV outflow tract (RVOT) regions with focused views of specific structures. The right ventricle specifically is further separated either into three sections—basal, mid and apical, or by specific walls into septal, anterior, inferior or lateral. The shape of the right ventricle is different than the ellipsoid shape of the left ventricle taking on more of a triangular shape in the long-axis and a crescent shape in the short-axis. Main anatomic features defining the right ventricle include the coarse trabeculations, a large moderator band, greater number of papillary muscles and the more apically situated tricuspid annulus.[1]

Functionally, the right heart collects systemic deoxygenated blood and delivers to the pulmonary circulation for oxygenation by the lungs. This is done typically under a relatively low resistance system. Because of the low-pressure system, external forces, such as normal respiration cause important alterations of RV filling and contraction.[1]

The right ventricle is a relatively thin-walled chamber including the respective portion of the interventricular septum. Although the mass of the right ventricle is significantly less than that of the left ventricle, RV volumes are typically similar to or greater than those of the left ventricle. Systolic contraction of the right ventricle occurs in a "segmental" manner with forces occurring in multiple directions: lateral forces from RV free wall contraction, longitudinal contraction and medial forces as a result from contraction of the interventricular septum. Resulting in segmental contraction, RV myocyte depolarization occurs from both the right and left bundle branches with the right bundle branch depolarizing the free wall and the left bundle branch depolarizing the interventricular septum. Notably different, the right ventricle relies predominantly on longitudinal contraction as opposed to the more balanced radial, longitudinal and circumferential deformation of the left ventricle.[1,2]

## BLOOD SUPPLY TO THE RIGHT HEART

The right ventricle primarily receives blood flow via the right coronary artery (RCA) in both right dominant and codominant anatomic variants. Less often (7% of the time), the left circumflex artery supplies to the RV free wall. The left anterior descending (LAD) coronary artery typically supplies to the moderator band via the first septal perforator and part of the RV apex **(Figure 3.1)**. The dual blood supply to the right ventricle is an important distinction from the single blood supply to the left ventricle for patients with coronary artery disease.[3,4]

Furthermore, the right ventricle has distinctive physiology allowing it to be relatively resistant to ischemia. During baseline conditions, the RV demand for oxygen is lower due to the thin myocardium (and lower oxygen extraction)

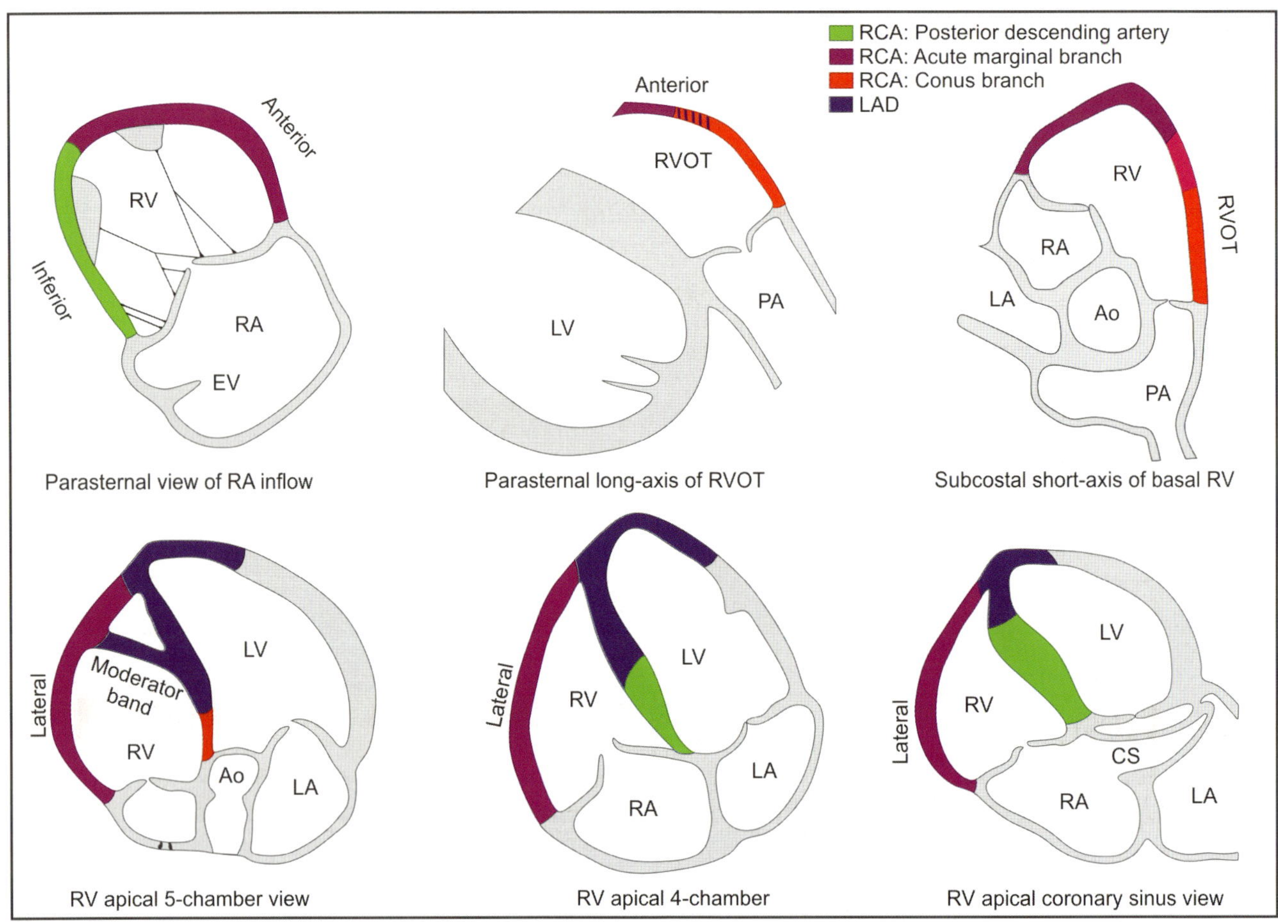


**Figure 3.1:** Right ventricular walls and corresponding coronary artery territory.

*Abbreviations:* Ao, aorta; CS, coronary sinus; EV, Eustachian valve; LA, left atrium; LAD, left anterior descending artery; LV, left ventricle; PA, pulmonary artery; RA, right atrium; RCA, right coronary artery; RV, right ventricle; RVOT, right ventricular outflow tract.

*Courtesy:* Rudski LG, Lai WW, Afilalo J, et al. Guidelines for the echocardiographic assessment of the right heart in adults. J Am Soc Echocard. 2010, *with permission.*

and low resistance system. Because of the large pressure differences, coronary blood flow in the RCA is present in both systole and diastole, whereas flow in the left coronary artery is only present in diastole; thus, heart rate typically has less of an effect on RV ischemia than on left ventricular (LV) ischemia. Furthermore, the dual blood supply of the RV from both left and right coronary arteries allows for compensatory flow from the less diseased vessel either via vasodilation or collateral formation. In the assessment of a possible RV acute coronary syndrome, several echocardiographic clues may suggest the presence of an RV myocardial infarction, including acute changes in RV diameter, RV:LV ratio, as well as worsening in the surrogates of RV function.[3,4]

## Blood Supply to RV Walls (Figure 3.1)

1. RVOT/infundibulum—dual supply from the conus branch of RCA and LAD, least susceptible to ischemia.
2. Anterior free wall—dual supply from the acute marginal and branches of LAD, least susceptible to ischemia.
3. Lateral wall—supply predominantly from the acute marginal branches from RCA only. Most susceptible to ischemia.
4. Inferior wall—supplied mostly from RCA if right dominant [though acute marginal and posterior descending artery]. Most susceptible to ischemia.
   - Moderator band largely supplied by septal perforator of LAD.

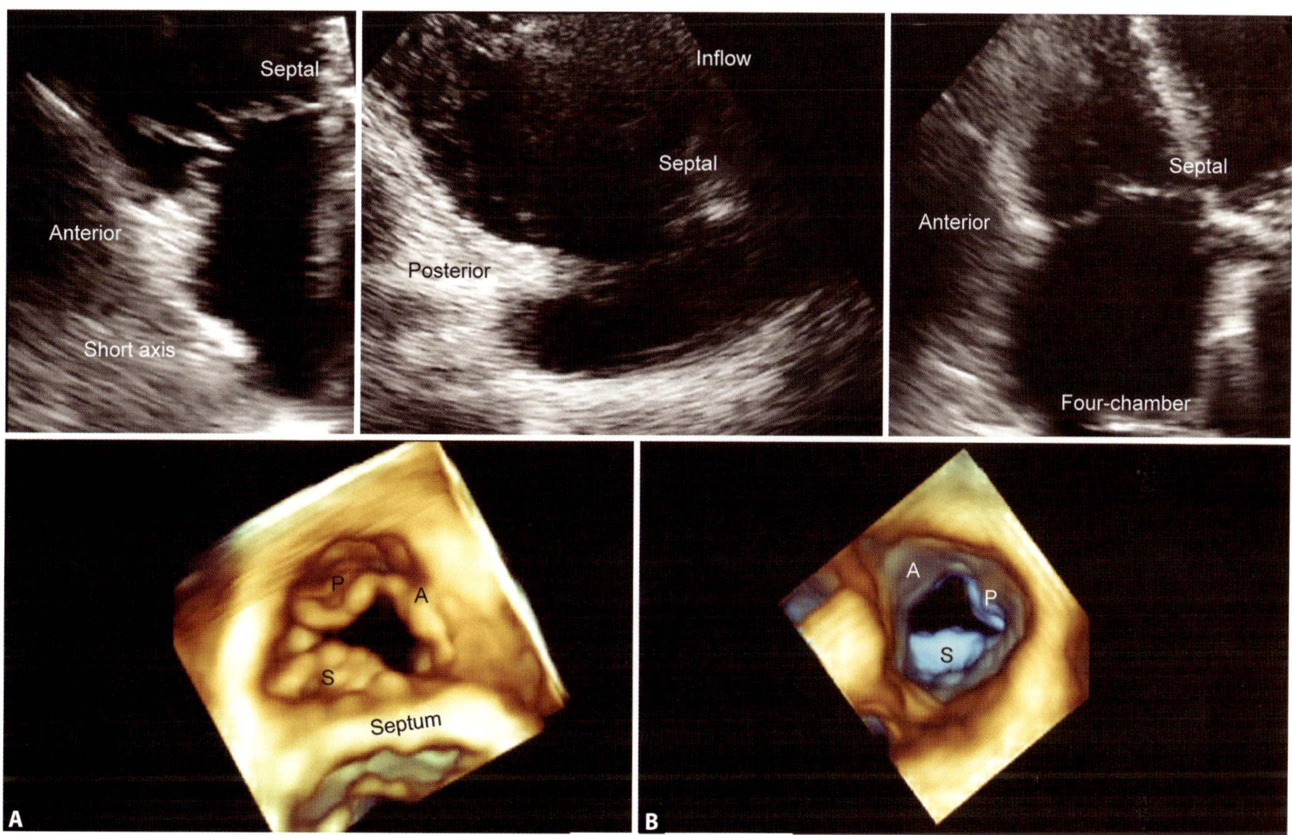


**Figure 3.2A and B:** The tricuspid valve from transthoracic echocardiography with two-dimensional imaging (upper panel) and 3-dimensional (3D) imaging (lower panel). (A) 3D zoom from ventricular perspective. (B) 3D zoom from ventricular perspective. *Abbreviations:* A, anterior; P, posterior; S, septal.

## VALVES IN THE RIGHT HEART

Within the right heart, assessment of tricuspid and pulmonic valve function is a crucial part of the echocardiographic evaluation. Appropriately named, the tricuspid valve (TV) is a trileaflet atrioventricular valve comprised of anterior, posterior and septal leaflets. As an anterior structure, the TV is best imaged using TTE, because of its position closer to the transthoracic probe. Two-dimensional (2D) imaging of the TV requires that the valve be imaged in at least three different probe positions to allow imaging of all three leaflets. With three-dimensional (3D) echocardiography, simultaneous visualization of all three leaflets is possible with a single 4–6 beat full-volume or zoom dataset obtained in held respiration **(Figure 3.2A and B, Video 3.1)**. The TV is the most proximal valve in the direction of blood-flow; thus, TV function is affected by the downstream valves often causing tricuspid regurgitation (TR). While trace TR is normal or physiologic, more significant TR is often a marker of left heart disease or primary right heart disease, i.e. pathology within the valve itself. In cardiovascular patients, new or worsening TR can be a sign of acute myocardial infarction of the right ventricle or left ventricle or any process that causes changes in RV afterload, such as pulmonary embolism or ischemic mitral regurgitation.[5]

The pulmonic valve (PV) is a semilunar valve located between the RVOT and the main pulmonary artery. Of the cardiac valves, the pulmonic valve is the least likely to have pathology requiring intervention in the adult patient; however, in congenital heart disease, pathologic changes may often require echocardiographic evaluation. Because of its position posterior to the sternum, the PV is the valve that is more difficult to image using either TTE or transesophageal echocardiography (TEE). For this reason, the PV leaflets are not typically visualized. Similar to the presence of minimal TR, trace PV regurgitation is a normal finding.[5]

### Imaging and Views

The standard right heart evaluation should include focused views with both quantitative and qualitative assessment of size, function, wall motion and estimations of RV systolic pressure (RVSP) and RA pressure, including inferior vena cava (IVC) evaluation.

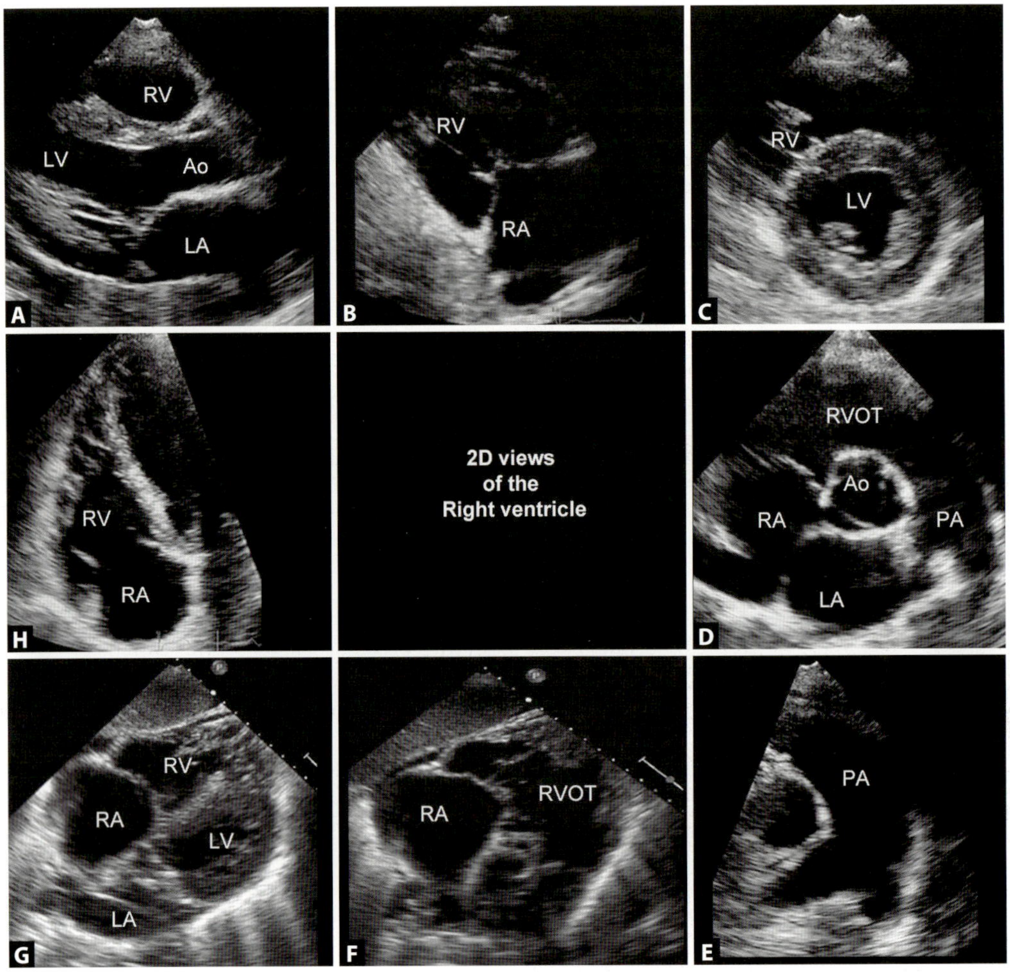

**Figure 3.3A to H:** Standard transthoracic views of the right heart from the parasternal (A to E), subcostal (F and G) and apical (H) positions. Due to shape and location, multiple views are required to fully image the right heart.
*Abbreviations:* Ao, aorta; CS, coronary sinus; EV, Eustachian valve; LA, left atrium; LAD, left anterior descending artery; LV, left ventricle; PA, pulmonary artery; RA, right atrium; RCA, right coronary artery; RV, right ventricle; RVOT, right ventricular outflow tract.

Standard imaging of the right ventricle should include views acquired from the left parasternal, apical and subcostal transducer positions. The RV inflow and outflow **(Videos 3.2 to 3.4)**, right ventricle focused apical **(Video 3.5)** and subcostal views provide general qualitative assessment, whereas Doppler imaging provides details of valvular function. Quantitative evaluation of RV function requires specific indices discussed in detail later in this chapter. The RA size is best assessed from the apical 4-chamber view or the subcostal views **(Figure 3.3A to H)**.[4]

## MEASUREMENTS, DIMENSIONS AND QUANTIFICATION OF RIGHT HEART

Guidelines recommend the quantification of RV and RA with linear dimensions, assessment of RV function using a variety of indices, and estimation of RVSP using an estimation of RA pressure derived from IVC size.

### Right Atrium

Qualitative assessment of the right atrium often is performed by comparison to the indexed LA volume. Quantitative assessment includes measurement of the area and both major and minor dimensions. The minor dimension extends from the RA lateral wall to the interatrial septum, perpendicular to the major dimension, which extends from the TV annulus to the posterior wall of the right atrium **(Figure 3.4A and B)**. *New guidelines recommend volume acquisition of the RA using area-length or method of disks with normal range of 25 +/- 7 mL/m² for males and 21 +/- 6 mL/m² for females.*[6]

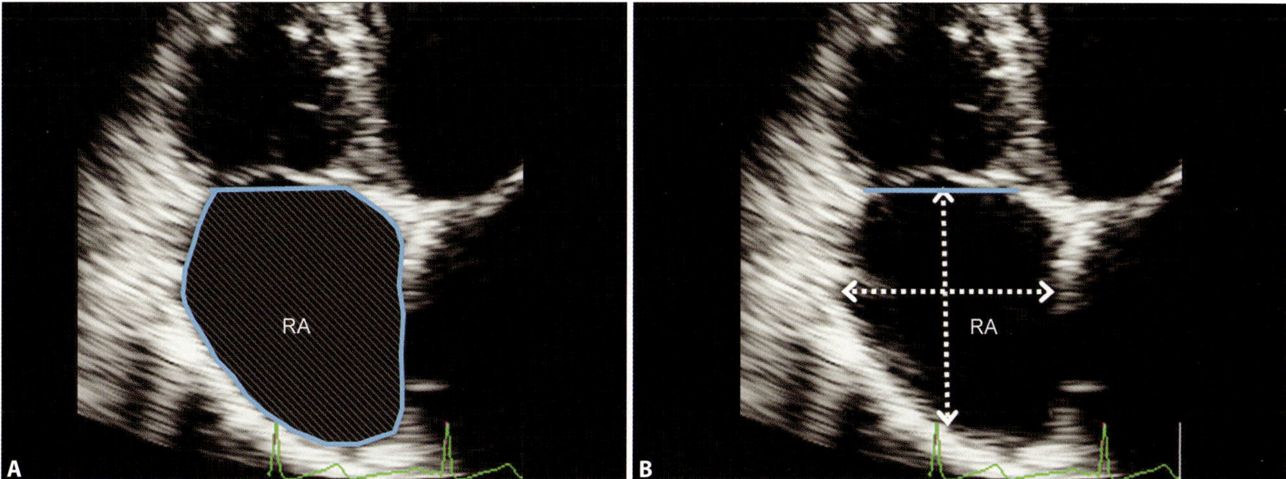


**Figure 3.4A and B:** Quantitative assessment of the right atrium (RA), measured at end-systole. (A) Manual tracing of right atrial borders for volumetric evaluation using method of disks. (B) Right atrial linear dimensions showing minor (horizontal arrow) and major (vertical arrow) dimensions.

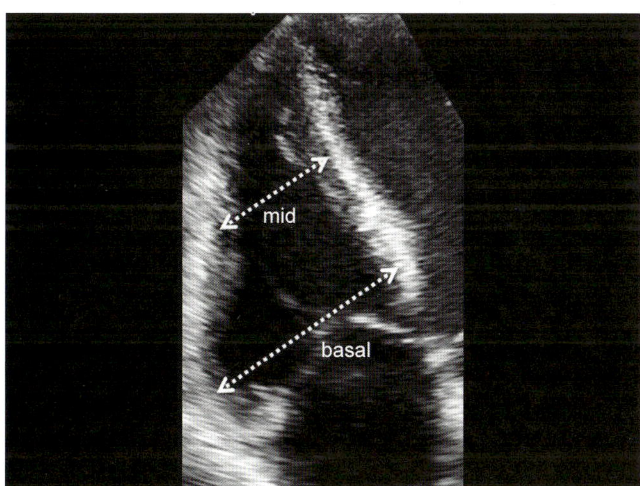


**Figure 3.5:** Apical 4-chamber focused right ventricular view with mid-chamber and basal ventricle measurements at end-diastole.

## Right Ventricle

The right ventricle size should be assessed quantitatively with an RV-focused view from the apical 4-chamber view. The basal diameter should be measured at an end-diastole where the entire RV free wall can be seen. The alignment should be such that the LV apex is in the center of the vector to avoid foreshortening. *The diameter at the base and at the mid-portion should be less than 41 mm and 35 mm, respectively* **(Figure 3.5)**.[6]

The evaluation of RV wall thickness from echocardiography is challenging, both due to lack of normal values and often difficult imaging. When possible, RV free wall thickness should be measured from the subcostal view or parasternal views either with M-mode or standard 2-dimensional imaging, at end-diastole. *An RV thickness greater than 0.5 cm is considered abnormal and should be reported when present.*[4]

## Inferior Vena Cava

Visualization of the IVC during an echocardiogram is a part of the assessment of the right heart function as a surrogate for RA pressures. From the subcostal views in the supine position, the diameter of the IVC is assessed in standard and M-mode views to determine the diameter of the IVC and the percent of collapsibility with a "sniff" maneuver. Notably, IVC assessment can overestimate RA pressures in young healthy athletes and does not follow normal respiratory changes in patients with positive pressure ventilation. *Using a cutoff diameter of 2.1 cm and a collapsibility of 50%, the RA pressures are estimated. The current guidelines suggest estimation of RA pressure as follows: 0–5 mm Hg (IVC <2.1 cm, >50% collapse), 10–20 mm Hg (IVC >2.1, <50% collapse) and 5–10 mm Hg if either diameter is <2.1 cm or if the collapse is >50%, but not both* **(Figure 3.6A and B)**.[4,6]

## Right Ventricular Systolic Pressure

Doppler assessment of the TV allows for the estimation of RVSP. Using the peak velocity TR jet, the modified Bernoulli equation can be used to estimate the RVSP that is as follows:

RVSP in mm Hg = 4 ($V^2$) + RA pressure, where V is peak velocity from TR in centimeters (or meters) per second.

*RVSP greater than 25 mm Hg is abnormal and RVSP greater than 40 mm Hg or 2/3 systemic blood pressures signifies*

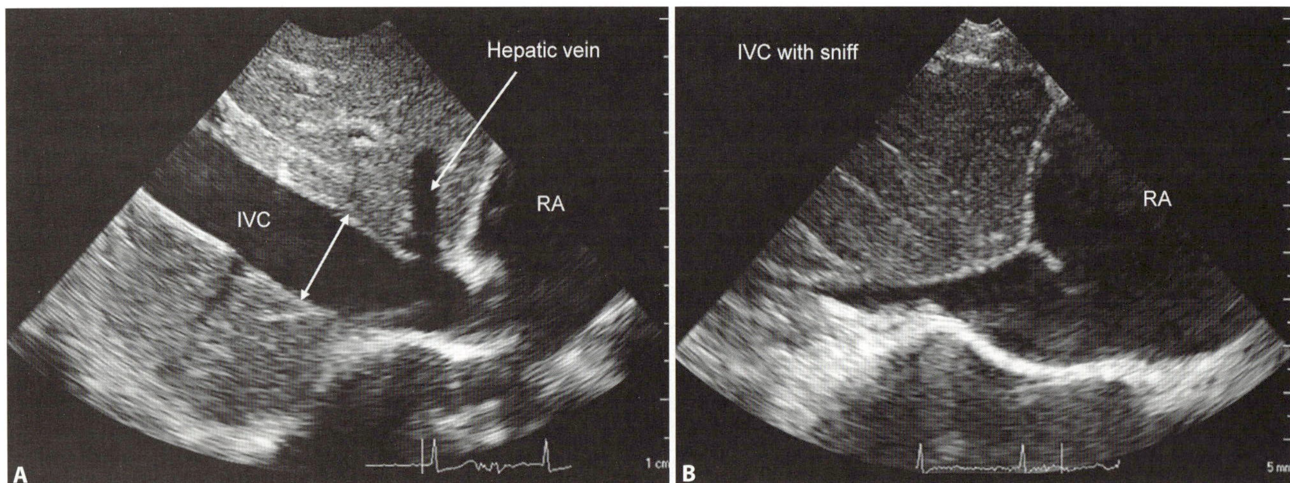


**Figure 3.6A and B:** Junction of right atrium (RA) and inferior vena cava (IVC) inflow from subcostal view. (A) The IVC should be measured 1.5 cm proximal to the RA-IVC junction (double arrow). (B) "Sniff" maneuver to assess compressibility of IVC.

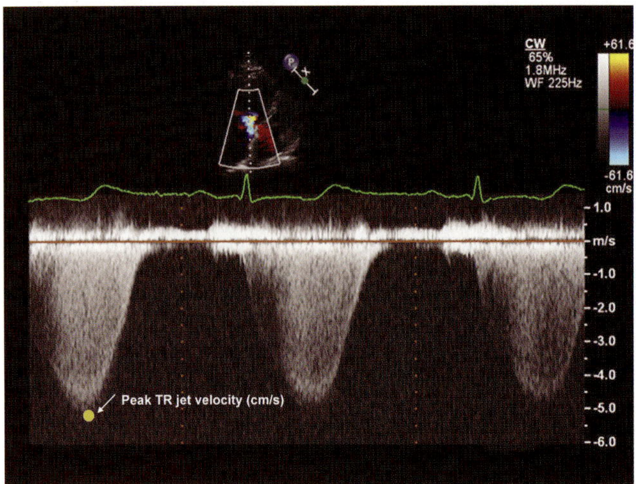


**Figure 3.7:** Peak velocity (yellow dot) from tricuspid regurgitation (TR). Using modified Bernoulli equation right ventricular systolic pressure can be estimated using peak velocity and right atrial pressure (from inferior vena cava).

*severely abnormal pulmonary resistance and should be further evaluated* **(Figure 3.7)**.[7]

## Right Ventricular Systolic Function

All patients undergoing a complete echocardiogram should have a quantitative assessment of RV systolic function. Each of the parameters has strengths and limitations. Thus, a single quantitative method should not be in isolation; rather, an approach with multiple quantitative parameters should be used in concert with the qualitative assessment.

1. *Tricuspid annular peak systolic excursion (TAPSE):* It is widely used as index of RV global systolic function. This measurement is taken from a standard apical 4-chamber window by placing the M-mode cursor optimally aligned with the direction of movement of the lateral tricuspid annulus. The TAPSE mostly reflects RV longitudinal function at basal level, and an incorrect alignment of the sampling line with the longitudinal motion of the annulus may result with an underestimation of the motion. Also, TAPSE is, by definition, a regional index, and it describes the longitudinal function of lateral basal wall of the right ventricle, and it may not be representative of the global RV systolic function. *A cutoff of 17 mm is usually considered the lower reference value for TAPSE.* Because of the angle (and load) dependence, TAPSE may under- or overestimate the motion of the lateral tricuspid annulus, as the motion relative to the transducer position may be influenced by overall cardiac translation.[4]
2. *Tissue Doppler imaging (TDI):* It is routinely used to measure the velocity of the basal portion of the RV free wall from an apical 4-chamber window. This can be accomplished using pulsed tissue Doppler or color-coded tissue Doppler. The sampling cursor or region should be placed in the basal lateral segment or in correspondence of the lateral tricuspid annulus, looking for the optimal alignment with the direction of motion to avoid underestimation of the peak systolic velocity or S'. *Generally a cutoff of TDI S' <10 cm/s is considered abnormal.* Like TAPSE, this measurement is angle dependent and uses the basal segment to extrapolate entire RV function, making this less useful with regional wall motion, such as in MI or in pulmonary embolism.[4]

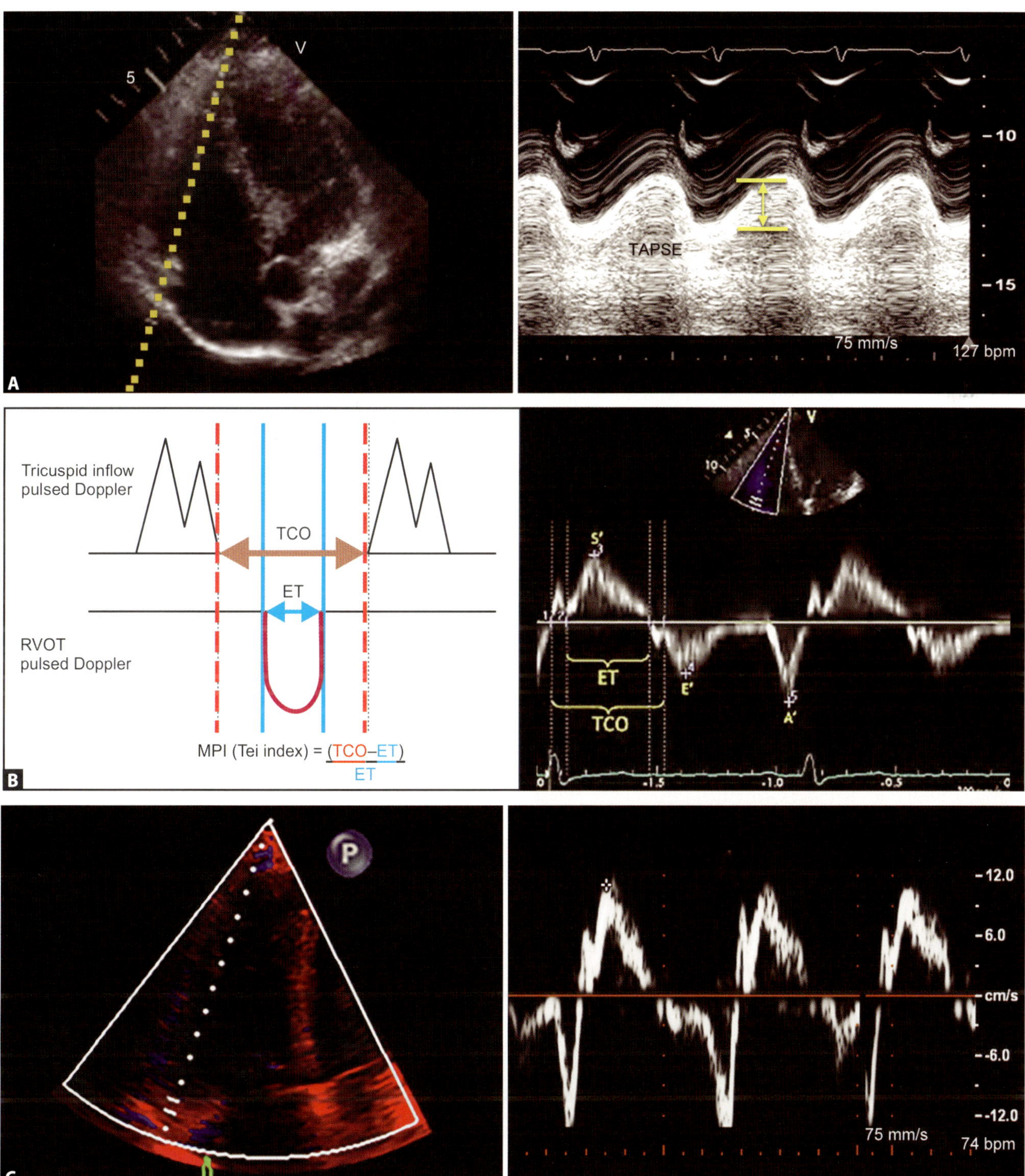


**Figure 3.8A to C:** Quantitative assessment of right ventricular systolic function using the following: (A) Tricuspid annular peak systolic excursion (TAPSE). (B) Myocardial performance index (MPI). (C) Tissue Doppler imaging of peak systolic velocity (TDI S′).

*Abbreviations:* ET, ejection time; TCO, tricuspid closure opening time; RVOT, right ventricular outflow tract.

*Source:* Rudski LG, Lai WW, Afilalo J, et al. Guidelines for the echocardiographic assessment of the right heart in adults. J Am Soc Echocard. 2010, *with permission.*

3. *Myocardial performance index (MPI):* Also known as Tei index or RV index of myocardial performance (RIMP), the MPI is an index of global RV performance that reflects both systolic and diastolic RV function. The index is defined as the ratio between the isovolumetric (contraction and relaxation) times and the ejection time **(Figure 3.8A to C)**. An MPI can be obtained either using pulsed-wave (PW) Doppler or TDI methods. When using the PW Doppler, the ejection time should be measured by sampling the outflow tract, while the isovolumetric times can be obtained as the interval between TV closure and opening measured sampling the tricuspid inflow. Alternatively, in presence of TR, the isovolumetric times can be estimated as the difference between the time from the onset and cessation of TR as from the continuous Doppler and the ejection time. Care should be taken when assessing MPI using PW, as measurements are taken in different heart beats, and especially in presence of atrial fibrillation, this may affect the accuracy of the MPI value. As using TDI allows to overcome this limitation, isovolumetric and ejection times are estimated from the velocity of the tricuspid annulus. *The correlation between MPI values obtained using tissue and pulse wave Doppler has been shown to be suboptimal and led to the definition of different normal ranges: the upper values for MPI is 0.40 and 0.55 for PW and TDI, respectively.*

   An MPI should not be used in presence of abnormally high RA pressure, as in this condition, it is associated with shortening of the isovolumetric relaxation time, and thus lower values.

   In conclusion, MPI is a simple method for the assessment of RV performance, especially when performed using TDI and should be combined with other quantitative measurements of RV function. It should be avoided when the patient presents rhythm disturbance or increased RA pressure. [4]

4. *RV dP/dt:* The dP/dt is one of the simple parameters used to describe RV systolic function. The physiological idea behind this index is that the slope of the pressure curve is a measurement of RV contractility. In clinical routine, dP/dt is measured by sampling the TR jet using continuous wave Doppler, i.e. under the assumptions of the simplified Bernoulli equation, the increase in velocity from 1 to 2 m/s is associated with an increase in pressure of 12 mm Hg. Therefore, dP/dt is calculated as the ratio between 12 mm Hg and the time required to TR jet to accelerate from 1 to 2 m/s. *A value of dP/dt equal to 400 mm Hg/s is considered to be the lower range for normal RV systolic function.*

   Despite its high feasibility and easiness of use, this index is highly load dependent and may not be reliable in presence of significant TR, where the hypotheses behind the simplified Bernoulli equation are not met and RA pressure is increased.[4]

5. *Fractional area change (FAC):* It is an index of global RV systolic function and reflects the fraction of blood present in the RV cavity at end-diastole that is ejected during systole. Using 2D images, the end-diastolic area (EDA) and end-systolic area (ESA) are assumed to reflect the end-diastolic and end-systolic volumes, and FAC is defined as EDA–ESA/EDA × 100. An EDA and ESA should be measured in a standard apical 4-chamber window including the entire right ventricle, and care should be taken to include the trabeculae when tracing the RV endocardial borders.[4] *RV FAC <35% indicates RV systolic dysfunction* **(Figure 3.9A and B)**.[4,6]

6. *Right ventricular train:* Strain assessment in the right ventricle allows for assessment of function both in the free wall (regional) and globally as in global longitudinal strain (GLS). Using speckle-tracking echocardiography, a percentage of myocardial shortening of segments and the entire free wall are assessed during systole. Likewise, the strain rate is the rate of shortening which can be followed by segment or globally. The longitudinal strain in the right ventricle is often vendor specific with variable cutoffs for abnormal, depending on the software. *Currently, limited data suggest a global longitudinal strain of the RV free wall of greater than –20 is abnormal; however, this should be taken into context of the strain software used.* Like with any strain assessment, an effort should be made to assure adequate tissue tracking using strain curves.[6]

   Though RV strain is a relatively new tool, it has been shown to be associated with clinical outcomes in multiple patient populations. In those with known or suspected pulmonary hypertension, RV free wall strain was both feasible in 88% of patients and was predictive of both cardiac events and mortality.[8] In patients with heart failure with LV systolic dysfunction, abnormal RV GLS was predictive of adverse events after adjusting for LV ejection fraction (LVEF) and diastolic dysfunction.[9] Furthermore, in patients with LV systolic dysfunction, RV strain was predictive of RV failure in patients undergoing LV assist device implantation **(Figure 3.10)**.[10]

7. *Right ventricular volumetric measurements, ejection fraction with 3D echocardiography:* Quantitation of RV volumes can be challenging with conventional 2D echocardiography; however, using 3D echocardiography the RV volume can be measured such that an RV ejection fraction (RVEF) can be calculated. RV systolic performance can be assessed using volumetric tracings from full-volume 3D echocardiographic acquisition. 3D acquisitions of the right ventricle over multiple beats are obtained from the right ventricle focused apical 4-chamber view. Care should be taken to approximate true endocardial border including trabeculations, papillary muscles and moderator band. The assessment can be used in all patients where 3D echocardiography

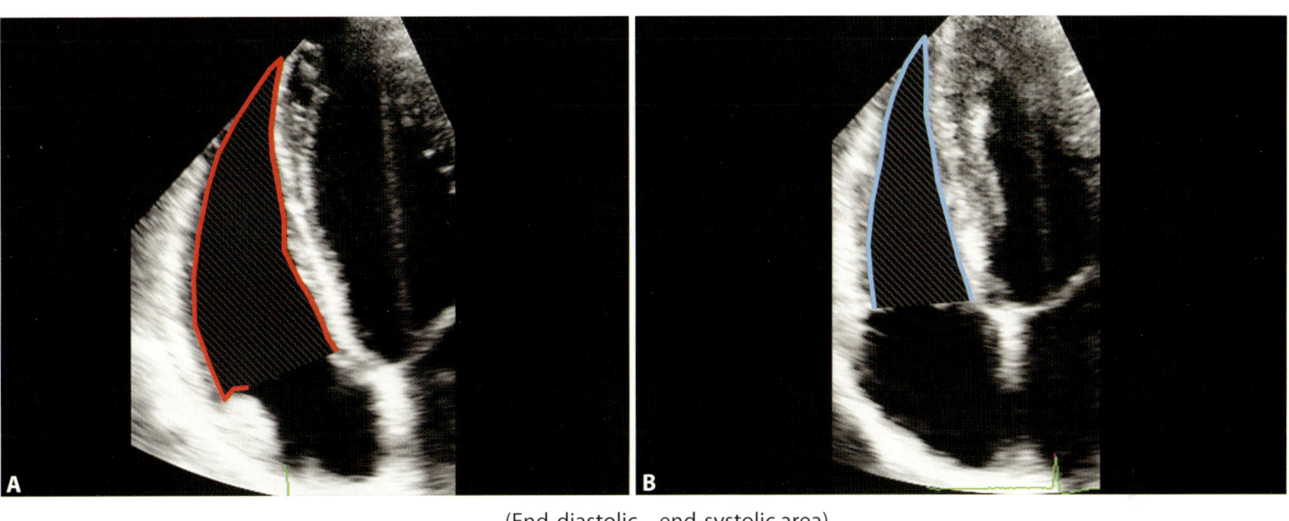


$$\text{FAC} = \frac{\text{(End-diastolic} - \text{end-systolic area)}}{\text{End-diastolic area}}$$

**Figure 3.9A and B:** Right ventricular systolic function evaluation by fractional area change (FAC). (A) Right ventricle area measurement at end-diastole. (B) Right ventricle area measurement at end-systole.

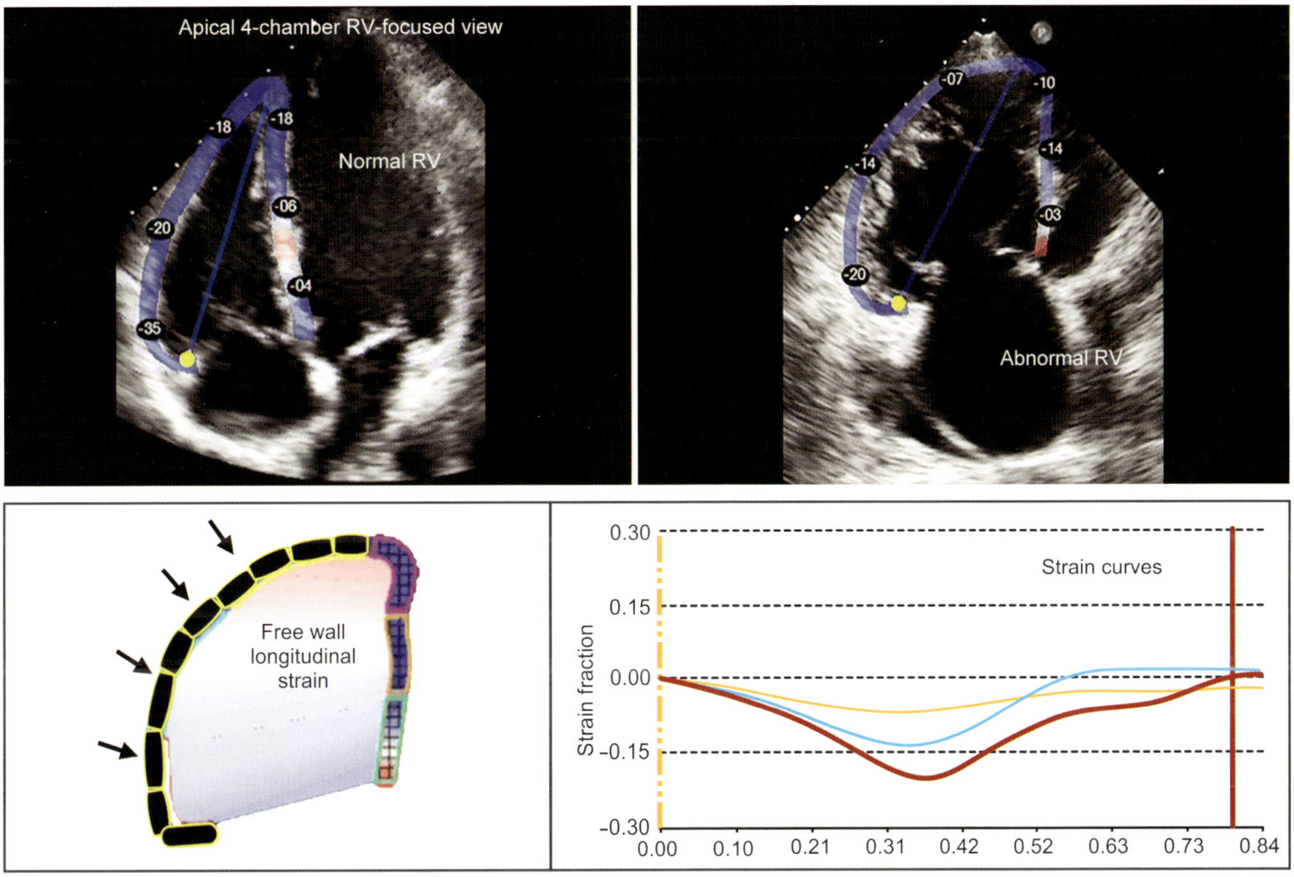

**Figure 3.10:** Right ventricular (RV) systolic function evaluation using right ventricular free wall longitudinal strain.

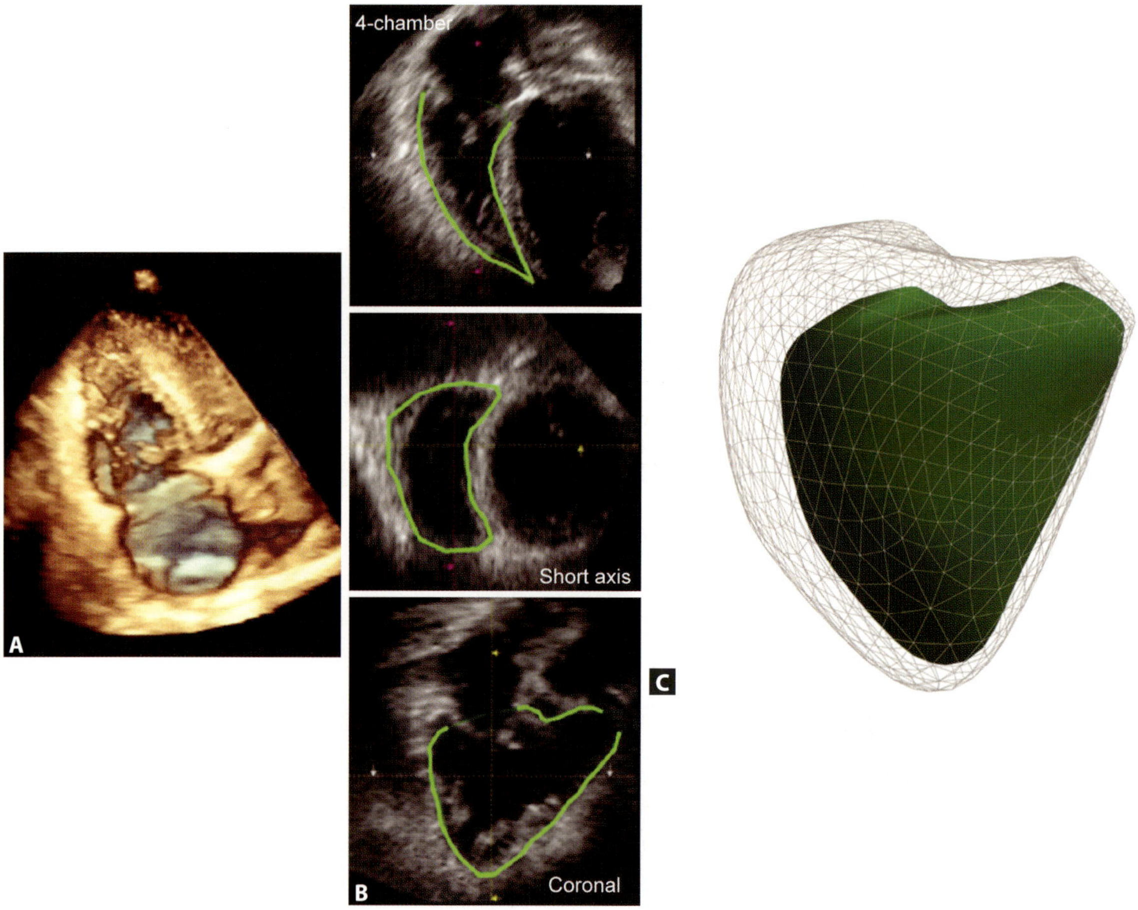

**Figure 3.11A to C:** Right ventricular (RV) systolic function performance using RV ejection fraction with the following: (A) Three-dimensional (3D) full volume RV acquisition from apical 4-chamber focused RV view; (B) Cut planes with endocardial tracings (green lines) acquired from RV 3D full volume acquisition; (C) 3D volumetric reconstructions at end-systole (green) and end-diastole (black).

is available and RV views are adequate; it is particularly helpful in those where conventional RV systolic function indices fail as such with post-cardiac surgery. Using end-systolic and end-diastolic values, RVEF can be calculated as with LVEF, using the formula:

$$[(EDV - ESV)/EDV] \times 100$$

Compared to cardiac magnetic resonance (CMR) imaging, 3D echocardiographic assessment of the right ventricle tends to underestimate volumes. In a meta-analysis of 807 subjects, the differences in volumes between 3D echocardiography and CMR were statistically significant, whereas the differences in RVEF were not. The greatest underestimation of volumes was in patients with larger RV volumes.[11] *Generally speaking, an RVEF <45% is considered abnormal* **(Figure 3.11A to C)**.[6]

## CONCLUSION

It is slowly being appreciated that quantitative 2D echocardiographic analysis as outlined in this chapter is insufficient to fully describe the impact of disease on the right ventricle. 3D echocardiography, a relatively recent advancement, allows the determination of RV volumes and ejection fraction and will likely, together with 2D speckle tracking longitudinal strain, help improve the assessment and follow-up of RV dysfunction in the future.

Previous work suggests that LV shape analysis provides insight into extent of LV dysfunction that is independent of size and function data.[12] Recent data have shown that it is possible with 3D echocardiography to study RV shape using indices of curvature where a curvature value of zero defines a flat surface; a negative value signifies concavity and a positive

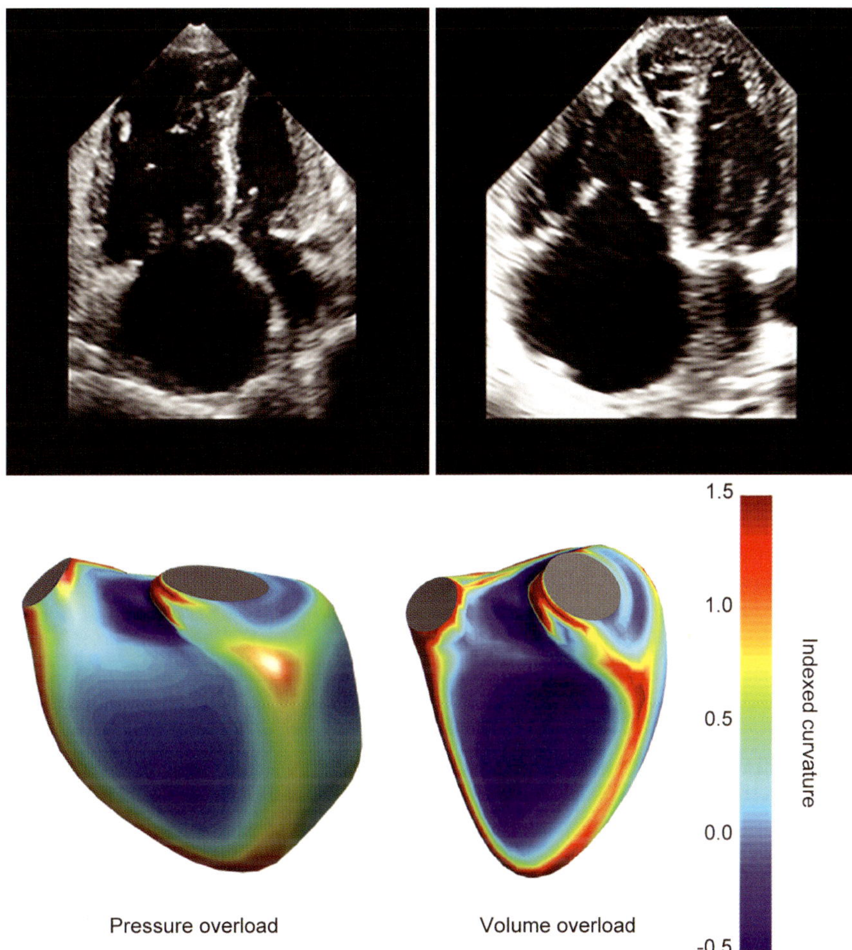


**Figure 3.12:** Two-dimensional echocardiographic images of a patient with pulmonary arterial hypertension (pressure overload, top left) and a patient with chronic severe tricuspid regurgitation (volume overload, top right). Corresponding curvature maps superimposed on three-dimensional endocardial surfaces as seen from the septal perspective are shown in the bottom panel. Dark blue illustrates that the septum has a negative curvature, a concave surface (see legend, right)

value, convexity. Using this index, a pressure overloaded right ventricle, for example, can be distinguished from a volume loaded right ventricle **(Figure 3.12).** Work in this area is in its infancy, but the concept opens up a whole new way of visualizing the right heart.

## VIDEO LEGENDS

**Video 3.1:** Three-dimensional echocardiographic imaging of tricuspid valve. All the three valve leaflets are visualized simultaneously.

**Video 3.2:** Parasternal right ventricular inflow view.

**Video 3.3:** Parasternal right ventricular outflow view.

**Video 3.4:** Parasternal short axis view showing both right ventricular inflow and outflow.

**Video 3.5:** Right ventricular focused apical four-chamber view.

## REFERENCES

1. Haddad F, Hunt SA, Rosenthal DN, Murphy DJ. Right Ventricular Function in Cardiovascular Disease, Part I: Anatomy, Physiology, Aging, and Functional Assessment of the Right Ventricle. Circulation. 2008;117:1436-48.
2. Petitjean C, Rougon N, Cluzel P. Assessment of Myocardial Function: a Review of Quantification Methods and Results using tagged MRI. J Cardiovasc Magn Reson. 2005;7(2):501-16.
3. Rallidis LS, Makavos G, Nihoyannopoulos P. Right Ventricular Involvement in Coronary Artery Disease: Role of Echocardiography for Diagnosis and Prognosis. J Am Soc Echocardiogr. 2014;27:223-9.
4. Rudski LG, Lai WW, Afilalo J, Hua L, Handschumacher MD, Chandrasekaran K, et al. Guidelines for the Echocardiographic Assessment of the Right Heart in Adults: a report from the American Society of Echocardiography endorsed by the

European Association of Echocardiography, a registered branch of the European Society of Cardiology, and the Canadian Society of Echocardiography. J Am Soc Echocardiogr. 2010;23:685-713.

5. Zoghbi WA, Enriquez-Sarano M, Foster E, Grayburn PA, Kraft CD, Levine RA, et al. Recommendations for Evaluation of the Severity of Native Valvular Regurgitation with Two-dimensional and Doppler Echocardiography. J Am Soc Echocardiogr. 2003;16:777-802.
6. Lang RM, Badano LP, Afilalo J, Armstrong A, Ernande L, Flachskampf FA, et al. Recommendations for the Cardiac Chamber Quantification by Echocardiography: An Update from the American Society of Echocardiography and the European Association of Cardiovascular Imaging. J Am Soc Echocardiogr; 2014. *In Press.*
7. McLaughlin VV, Archer SL, Badesch DB, Barst RJ, Farber HW, Lindner JR, et al. ACCF/AHA 2009 expert consensus document on pulmonary hypertension: a report of the American College of Cardiology Foundation Task Force on Expert Consensus Documents and the American Heart Association developed in collaboration with the American College of Chest Physicians; American Thoracic Society, Inc.; and the Pulmonary Hypertension Association. J Am Coll Cardiol. 2009;53:1573-619.
8. Fine NM, Chen L, Bastiansen PM, Frantz RP, Pellikka P, Oh JK, et al. Outcome Prediction by Quantitative Right Ventricular Function Assessment in 575 Subjects Evaluated for Pulmonary Hypertension. Circ Cardiovasc Imaging. 2013;6:711-21.
9. Motoki H, Borowski AG, Shrestha K, et al. Right Ventricular Global Longitudinal Strain Provides Prognostic Value Incremental to Left Ventricular Ejection Fraction in Patients with Heart Failure. J Am Soc Echocardiogr. 2014;27:726-32.
10. Grant ADM, Smedira NG, Starling RC, Marwick TH. Independent and Incremental Role of Quantitative Right Ventricular Evaluation for the Prediction of Right Ventricular Failure After Left Ventricular Assist Device Implantation. J Am Coll Cardiol. 2012;60:521-8.
11. Shimada YJ, Shiota M, Siegel JF, et al. Accuracy of Right Ventricular Volumes and Function Determined by Three-Dimensional Echocardiography in Comparison with Magnetic Resonance Imaging: A Meta-Analysis Study. J Am Soc Echocardiogr. 2010;23:943-53.
12. Maffessanti F, Caiani EG, Tamborini G, et al. Serial changes in left ventricular shape following early mitral valve repair. Am J Cardiol. 2010;106(6):836-42.

# Pharmacologic Stress Echocardiography

*Srikanth Sola*

## INTRODUCTION

Stress echocardiography is a well-validated, versatile noninvasive imaging modality that has proven utility in the detection of myocardial ischemia, viability, determining prognosis, and evaluating therapy.[1] Compared to other imaging modalities, stress echocardiography is less costly, avoids the use of ionizing radiation or iodinated contrast agents, is widely available and is easy to perform. We discuss common clinical indications for pharmacologic stress testing, review protocols for the different pharmacologic stress agents available, and discuss pitfalls in image acquisition which can impact the test's accuracy.

## CLINICAL INDICATIONS AND CHOICE OF MODALITIES

The most common clinical indications for pharmacologic stress testing include evaluation for ischemia, typically in a patient with baseline ECG abnormalities who is unable to exercise, a previous nondiagnostic exercise treadmill test, or cardiac chest pain in patients with prior surgical or percutaneous revascularization. Other important but less frequent indications for pharmacologic stress testing include assessment of myocardial viability, and finally, low gradient low flow aortic stenosis. In most patients, exercise testing is the preferred test for ischemia over pharmacologic stress testing, as exercise capacity measured in metabolic equivalents (METs) provides important prognostic information. In addition, exercise results in a higher rate-pressure product (>25,000) vs. dobutamine (average 20,000) or pacing (<20,000).[2,3] However, pharmacologic stress testing is preferred when the patient is unable to exercise, most commonly due to neurologic, orthopedic, or other impairments that limit the ability to exercise. Many echocardiography laboratories also prefer pharmacologic stress testing, particularly, dobutamine stress echocardiography (DSE) in patients with baseline left ventricular (LV) systolic dysfunction. In such patients, the typical biphasic response to dobutamine in ischemic segments or lack of improved contractile response in nonviable segments is more easily assessed with DSE than with exercise or vasodilator stress echocardiography.

In some patients, pharmacologic stress testing is preferred as the hyperventilation and excessive chest wall movement after exercise can limit the echocardiographic examination of the heart. This degrades image quality, increases inter-reader variability, and reduces the diagnostic accuracy of exercise stress echocardiography. Some indications for stress testing, however, are better evaluated by symptom-limited exercise stress echocardiography. These include aortic regurgitation, aortic stenosis (asymptomatic, with normal systolic function), mitral regurgitation, mitral stenosis, hypertrophic cardiomyopathy to assess for provocable LV outflow tract (LVOT) gradients, pulmonary hypertension and the diastolic stress test. Important contraindications to pharmacologic stress echocardiography are listed in **Table 4.1**.

The decision regarding which stress echocardiography protocol (exercise, dobutamine, or vasodilator) to use depends on both the clinical indication and the experience of the echo lab. However, it is advisable that labs develop expertise with all 3 protocols, as no single protocol is suitable

**Table 4.1:** Contraindications to pharmacologic stress echocardiography

- Ongoing chest pain in patients with acute coronary syndromes
- Acute decompensated heart failure
- Unstable brady- or tachyarrhythmia
- Severe hypertension
- Hypotension
- Acute myocarditis
- Acute aortic syndromes (aortic dissection, intramural hematoma, or penetrating ulcer)
- Acute pulmonary embolism
- Mobile intracardiac thrombus
- High degree atrioventricular block
- Additional contraindications for vasodilator stress:
  - Active bronchospasm or significant asthma (usually requiring home $O_2$, oral steroids, prior history of intubation, or ongoing exacerbation)

for all patients. For example, a DSE test that is stopped early due to a hypertensive response to dobutamine will yield a nondiagnostic result, whereas in a lab with proficiency in vasodilator stress, the patient can then be rescheduled to complete a vasodilator stress test comfortably.

## DOBUTAMINE STRESS ECHOCARDIOGRAPHY PROTOCOL

### Pharmacology of Dobutamine

Dobutamine is a synthetic catecholamine agent which has a very short plasma half-life (<2 minutes), requiring that it should be given as a continuous intravenous infusion. The effects of dobutamine vary depending on the dose at which it is given. At *lose dose dobutamine* (<10 μg/kg/min), it has a predominant inotropic effect (without tachycardia) via its effect on $\beta_1$-adrenergic receptors in the heart. In addition, it has a relatively lesser effect on the $\beta_2$-adrenergic receptors and $\alpha_1$-adrenergic receptors in the peripheral vasculature, which at low doses, balance any changes in systemic vascular resistance and lead to a neutral effect on blood pressure.[4]

At higher doses, however, the inotropic and chronotropic effects of dobutamine increase, leading to progressive increases in heart rate (average increase 40–50 beats/min) and contractility of the heart, thus increasing cardiac output, blood pressure, and myocardial oxygen demand. However, there is also a greater effect on the $\beta_2$-adrenergic receptors at higher dobutamine doses, which can lead to peripheral vasodilation and, in some patients, a decrease in blood pressure and even hypotension. Bradycardia with high dose dobutamine is less common and is due to a reflex response to increased blood pressure, activation of mechanoreceptors due to increased myocardial contractility, or both.[5]

### Dobutamine Protocols

The 2007 guidelines from the American Society of Echocardiography and the 2008 guidelines of the European Association of Echocardiography recommend dobutamine as the first-line agent for the performance of pharmacologic stress echocardiography.[6,7] The specific dobutamine protocol used depends on the clinical indication and whether the patient has a pacemaker. *For ischemia testing,* dobutamine infusion is started at 5 μg/kg/min for three minutes, followed sequentially by 10 μg/kg/min, 20 μg/kg/min, 30 μg/kg/min, and 40 μg/kg/min for 3 minute stages each or until 85% of the age predicted maximum heart rate is achieved. Some echo labs forgo the 5 μg/kg/min stage and start dobutamine at 10 μg/kg/min, particularly, in patients with a normal resting ejection fraction. For patients who fail to achieve 85% age predicted maximum heart rate at the dose of 40 μg/kg/min stage; adjunctive agents, such as atropine and hand grip exercise can be used (see section on Hand-grip Exercise further).

*For viability testing,* protocols vary widely but dobutamine infusion is typically started at 2.5–5 μg/kg/min, followed by 10 μg/kg/min and ending at 20 μg/kg/min. These low doses of dobutamine provide a predominant inotropic effect with minimal chronotropy. Therefore, no target heart rate is required for viability testing when this protocol is used. In patients with LV systolic dysfunction and suspected ischemia, the complete DSE protocol, starting with the 2.5–5 μg/kg/min stage and extending until indication for termination of the test is reached, allows for the assessment of both viability and ischemia (i.e. the classic biphasic response). The latter protocol is more frequently used, as this also has a higher positive predictive value for the assessment of myocardial viability than a low dose protocol.[8] In patients with low gradient low-flow aortic stenosis, only the low-dose dobutamine protocol is used (up to 20 μg/kg/min), along with measurements of aortic valve gradients and cardiac output at each stage.

*For patients with permanent pacemakers,* the dobutamine protocol is combined with changes in the patient's paced rate to achieve an adequate stress. Typically, dobutamine is started at 5 μg/kg/min for 3 minutes, then 10 μg/kg/min for 3 minutes, and 20 μg/kg/min. At the end of the 20 μg/kg/min stage, the pacemaker is adjusted as follows: If the patient's heart is already paced, then pacing is adjusted to 70% of age predicted maximal heart rate while dobutamine is continued at 20 μg/kg/min for 3 minutes. If the patient's heart is not paced, the heart is paced at just above resting heart rate for 3 minutes, then increased to 70% of age predicted maximal heart rate while dobutamine is continued at 20 μg/kg/min for 3 minutes. Finally, the pacing rate is increased to 85% of the age-predicted maximum heart rate for 3 minutes (in all patients) while dobutamine is continued at 20 μg/kg/min for 3 minutes. For recovery, dobutamine is discontinued and the pacemaker returned to its normal baseline settings.

Atrial pacing is preferred to ventricular pacing as the latter results in asynchronous ventricular pacing that can cause difficulties in interpretation, particularly, in the interventricular septum. An alternate protocol to dobutamine plus pacing is to use pacing alone, usually to a target rate of 160 beats/min. Unlike dobutamine, the resulting tachycardia with pacing alone is accompanied by unchanged loading conditions and stable blood pressure, resulting in better hemodynamic control than with dobutamine.[9] The disadvantage of pacing alone protocols is that the absence of an increased blood pressure response leads to at best only a modest increment in the rate-pressure product.

For all dobutamine protocols, the test is terminated when the patient (i) reaches target heart rate (and completes imaging at that stage), (ii) develops new regional wall motion abnormalities in at least 2 contiguous segments, (iii) completes the study protocol (40 μg/kg/min for ischemia or 20 μg/kg/min for viability alone), or (iv) experiences an adverse event that necessitates discontinuation of the infusion and supportive or emergent care. Adverse events that would necessitate stopping the study include hypotension (systolic blood pressure <90 mm Hg or decrease in systolic blood pressure >20 mm Hg from baseline), severe hypertension (>220 mm Hg systolic or >120 mm Hg diastolic), anginal chest pain, ST depression >2 mm on ECG, or sustained ventricular tachycardia. Isolated nonsustained ventricular tachycardia can be a side effect of dobutamine administration and does not necessarily require termination of the test if the patient is hemodynamically stable and asymptomatic.

After completion of the dobutamine infusion and when recovery images are obtained, patients are typically monitored in either the stress echo room or recovery area until the heart rate returns to within 20 minutes of baseline, all new wall motion abnormalities have returned to baseline, and the patient is asymptomatic.

## OTHER ADJUNCTIVE AGENTS

### Atropine

Atropine is an anticholinergic drug that, among other effects, increases the heart rate. Atropine can be used in doses of 0.25–0.3 mg (depending on how it is supplied) every minute up to a maximum of 2 mg. Many echo laboratories have moved toward early administration of atropine to improve time to target heart rate. A common atropine protocol would be to give one dose of atropine under the following conditions: (i) if heart rate is less than 90 beats/min at the end of the 20 µg/kg/min stage, or (ii) if the heart rate is less than 70% of the age predicted maximum heart rate at the end of the 30 µg/kg/min stage. Additional doses of atropine (up to 2 mg maximum) can be given if the heart rate is less than 85% of the age predicted maximum heart rate at the end of the 40 µg/kg/min stage.

Atropine has additional benefits in DSE beyond reaching target heart rate. Patients taking β blockers can experience blunting of the effects of dobutamine, reducing the double-product to 14,000. This can be prevented by the administration of atropine.[10] In addition, the combined use of dobutamine and atropine can prevent vagal activation, and the depression of heart rate occurs due to a hypertensive reaction or stimulation of the cardiac mechanoreceptors.

Atropine has a half-life of 3.5 hours, which means that the tachycardia effect of this agent can continue even after the cessation of dobutamine administration. Intravenous β blockers are commonly used to return heart rate to within 20 beats/min of baseline in patients with adequate blood pressure. Patients should be warned that atropine dilates the pupil which can lead to visual disturbance and intolerance to light. Sensations of thirst and dry mouth are frequent. Some patients may experience giddiness and staggering, and therefore, they should avoid driving a vehicle or operating machinery for 6 hours after receiving atropine. Atropine is contraindicated in patients with acute-angle glaucoma, paralytic ileus, and severe benign prostatic hypertrophy with urinary retention, although these patients are infrequently seen in the stress echo laboratory.

### Hand-grip Exercise

Hand grip increases afterload, causing a small incremental increase in heart rate and blood pressure, leading to a modest increase in myocardial $O_2$ demand.[11] Hand grip is usually performed at the end of the 40 µg/kg/min stage of a DSE test or the last stage of exercise stress echo test, typically when the patient fails to reach target heart rate. At some centers, a tennis or soft cricket ball is used as an aid to the hand grip, and the patient is asked to squeeze the ball with 30% of his or her maximum strength for 30 seconds. Specially designed devices for isometric hand grip exercises are popular in some European echo labs, as they require a calibrated amount of hand pressure leading to a more reliable increase in afterload. In patients with extensive coronary artery disease (CAD), hand-grip exercise alone can cause regional wall motion abnormalities, although it is rarely used for diagnostic purposes in this manner.

### Nitroglycerin-Dobutamine Stress-Echocardiography for Viability

A small body of literature exists to support the use of nitroglycerin enhanced DSE testing for viability. Ling et al. have shown that nitroglycerin can be used in addition to dobutamine and can enhance the accuracy of detecting hibernating myocardium.[12] Nitroglycerin was given as a 0.4 mg sublingual spray, followed 5 minutes later by rest images, and the standard DSE protocol. Nitroglycerin alone increases regional thickening in approximately 20% of akinetic but viable segments, whereas the combination of nitroglycerin plus dobutamine had the best specificity for viability compared with intracoronary myocardial contrast echo and rest-redistribution thallium-201 single photon emission computed tomography (SPECT). Although infrequently used for DSE viability testing, nitroglycerin has been used to increase contractility of akinetic but viable segments on ventriculography,[13] enhance radionuclide uptake in 18F-fluoro-2-deoxy-D-glucose positron emission tomography (FDG-PET) and SPECT,[14] and augment wall thickening in dobutamine stress magnetic resonance imaging.[15] The mechanism of nitroglycerin in viability assessment by DSE is not clear, but it may be related to effects of vasodilation leading to recruitment of collateral circulation or improvement of loading conditions.[16,17]

## VASODILATOR STRESS ECHOCARDIOGRAPHY PROTOCOL

Vasodilator stress echocardiography is an alternative to DSE and is more commonly used at some European centers. Three vasodilators are approved for use in vasodilator stress protocols: dipyridamole, adenosine, and regadenoson. Dipyridamole acts by increasing endogenous adenosine levels, whereas both adenosine and regadenoson (an $A_{2A}$ adenosine receptor agonist) act directly on adenosine receptors in the vasculature to cause vasodilation. All of these agents produce a modest tachycardia, a small decrease in blood pressure, and a minor increase in ventricular systolic function. Of these three agents, only adenosine is available commercially in South Asia.

Adenosine is most commonly given as a continuous infusion at a dose of 140 µg/kg/min for 6 minutes. For patients who fail to respond to adenosine, as determined by an increase in heart rate by at least 10 beats/min above baseline, the dose of adenosine is increased to 180, then finally 210 µg/kg/min over 3 minute stages until the expected increase in heart rate is achieved. Atropine may be given during vasodilator administration to increase heart rate and myocardial oxygen demand, resulting in improved diagnostic sensitivity.[18] Patients must be counseled to avoid caffeinated beverages, including tea, coffee, colas, and energy drinks, as well as chocolate and xanthine derivative medications, such as deriphylline for 24–48 hours prior to the study, as these interfere with the effects of adenosine and lead to a false-negative test.

## IMAGING ACQUISITION PROTOCOLS

The diagnostic accuracy of stress echocardiography is dependent on the quality of image acquisition and optimal image display. Guidelines from the American Society of Echocardiography provide details on image acquisition and display in stress echocardiography.[6] The physio setting on the echo machine should be adjusted so that ECG triggering is used for imagine acquisition. Tissue harmonic imaging should be employed routinely, as this enhances the definition of the endocardial to LV cavity interface and reduces near field noise. Gain and time gain compensation settings, focus, transducer frequency, and sector width should be optimized for imaging the left ventricle. Active collaboration between the patient and sonographer, including brief breath holds at mid inspiration or mid expiration, can help maintain the echocardiographic window and avoid respiratory motion artifacts. Common mistakes made by less experienced operators include using too high a depth, too narrow a sector, foreshortening of the LV apex on apical windows, and opening up the LVOT or aortic valve on the apical 4-chamber view **(Figure 4.1A to E)**.

For patients who have not undergone a recent echo study, baseline images should screen for pathology beyond the left ventricle which may be related to the patient's symptoms. These include assessment for valvular stenosis and regurgitation, diastolic function, pulmonary hypertension, the ascending aorta (for dissection or dilation), and pericardial effusion. If asymmetric hypertrophy or systolic anterior motion of the mitral valve is present, then assessment of LVOT gradients using continuous wave Doppler at rest and with amyl nitrate should be performed to exclude unrecognized hypertrophic cardiomyopathy. Findings on pre-stress screening which may lead to cancelation of the test include hypertrophic cardiomyopathy with a resting or provocable gradient of more than 50 mm Hg, aortic stenosis which is moderate or greater in severity, thoracic aortic aneurysm or dissection, severe LV systolic dysfunction (except when DSE is being done for viability), large pericardial effusion, and LV or left atrial thrombus.

Transthoracic echocardiography images are acquired at rest, at each stage of dobutamine infusion, and during recovery. At each stage, images should include the parasternal long-axis, parasternal short-axis at mid-papillary level, apical 4-chamber, apical 2-chamber, and apical long-axis views. To ensure accurate comparison between the rest images and subsequent dobutamine and recovery stages, care should be taken to ensure that all images are in the same imaging planes and depth as the baseline images. Anatomic landmarks, such as the papillary muscle heads in the parasternal mid short-axis levels or thickened valve chordae on the parasternal long-axis view, can facilitate this. For the parasternal long-axis view, moving the probe laterally 3–4 cm away from the sternum will allow the mid segments of the left ventricle to be seen. The apical windows allow imaging of the LV apex, but care must be taken to avoid foreshadowing on the apical 4-chamber and 2-chamber views. The anterior and anteroseptal walls can be difficult to visualize on the apical windows. Breath holding by the patient, steep lateral decubitus positioning (facilitated by an examination bed with a cut out for apical windows), and steep angulation of the transducer can facilitate this. When two or more contiguous segments cannot be visualized, then contrast can be used (see section on Echo Contrast further).

In some echocardiography laboratories, additional views include the basal and apical parasternal short-axis views. Since display software for multistage acquisition typically allows for only one parasternal short-axis view (usually the mid-papillary level is chosen since all three coronary territories are seen), the additional short-axis views are archived for later review if more detailed analysis is required. The subcostal short-axis views can be substituted for the parasternal window when views are limited, but this requires patient repositioning when moving from apical to subcostal windows, and obtaining the subcostal short-axis view at

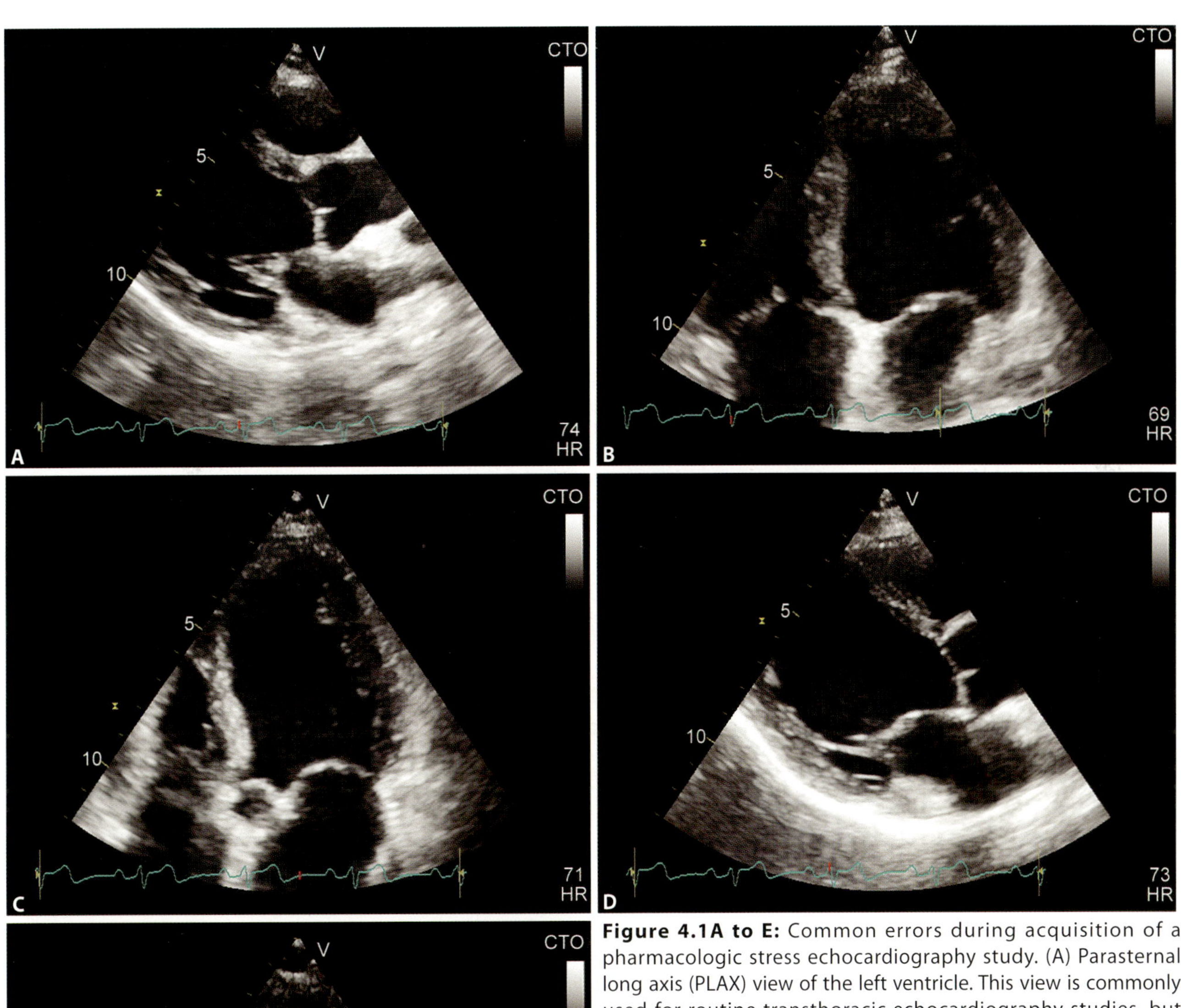


**Figure 4.1A to E:** Common errors during acquisition of a pharmacologic stress echocardiography study. (A) Parasternal long axis (PLAX) view of the left ventricle. This view is commonly used for routine transthoracic echocardiography studies, but is not good for stress echocardiography studies as it excludes the mid portions of the left ventricle. (B) Apical 4-chamber view showing too much of the left atrium (depth has not been optimized). In addition, a portion of the apical anterolateral wall is not seen in the sector. This can cause errors during analysis for regional wall motion abnormalities and strain measurements. (C) Apical 4-chamber view with the left ventricular outflow tract seen. The probe is tilted too far cranially in this example. (D) Good PLAX view for stress echocardiography studies. The probe shifted is laterally (away from the sternum) allowing the mid segments of the left ventricle to be better seen. Apical segments are usually not visible from the PLAX view. (E) Good apical 4-chamber view for stress echocardiography studies. Depth and sector are optimized to show mainly the left ventricle, without excess emphasis on the right ventricle or left atrium.

the same level for each stage of the study can sometimes be challenging.

Additional information, which may be required depending on the clinical scenario, include transmitral inflow and TDI of the mitral annulus (for diastolic stress testing), estimated right ventricular systolic pressure (in suspected pulmonary hypertension, mitral stenosis), vena contracta and effective regurgitant orifice area for patients with mitral or tricuspid regurgitation, and pulse waved Doppler/continuous wave Doppler of the LVOT and aortic valve, respectively, plus cardiac output for patients with paradoxical low-flow low-gradient aortic stenosis. Except for the latter indication, however, most of these additional views are more common with exercise-stress echocardiography.

## DISPLAY PROTOCOLS

Upon completion of the study, the sonographer should select the best images for each view, ensuring that all images are labeled with the correct window name and include the ECG tracing. Images acquired during ventricular ectopic beats should be excluded, as these can cause difficulty in interpretation.

Images are displayed in either a standard quad-screen format (DSE) or split screen (vasodilator stress) on the echocardiography machine or the workstation. For DSE studies, rest, low-dose, pre-peak, and peak images are displayed simultaneously. Recovery images are viewed separately and are used to assess for post-stress (late) ischemia. Newer echocardiography machines provide additional display options. However, the image size in these other display formats must be adequate for image interpretation.

## ADJUNCTIVE MODALITIES

### Strain DSE

Longitudinal, circumferential, and radial strain as assessed by either two-dimensional (2D) or three-dimensional (3D) speckle tracking echocardiography quantitatively analyzes global and regional myocardial function. It presents an objective, semiautomatic, and angle-independent analysis of myocardial deformation based on speckle tracking and provides a single bull's-eye summary of the LV segmental wall strain.

Recent studies have shown that strain analysis, when added to standard diagnostic criteria for ischemia (e.g. new or worsening wall motion abnormalities), improves the diagnostic accuracy of DSE testing compared with standard diagnostic criteria alone. Arnold et al. conducted a multi-centered study of 102 patients who underwent concurrent DSE and invasive coronary angiography.[19] While global longitudinal strain (GLS) alone was as accurate as wall motion score index (WMSI) for the diagnosis of ischemia, the result from the combination of GLS and WMSI highest sensitivity, specificity, and accuracy was 100%, 87.5%, and 96.3%, respectively.

In our laboratory, analysis of global longitudinal strain and peak segmental strain is routinely done for DSE studies with adequate image quality. Training of the sonographer and/or physician performing the study and analyzing the image data is needed to ensure high quality images and avoid artifacts that would affect interpretation. In addition, care is needed to avoid loss of image data in the anterior and anteroseptal walls on the apical windows. We do not use strain analysis in exercise stress echocardiography studies (due to respiratory motion artifact) or when contrast is used. However, measurement of longitudinal segmental strain 5 minutes after cessation of exercise (i.e. during the recovery phase) can be a useful adjunct for detection of ischemia during exercise stress echocardiography.

## 3D ECHOCARDIOGRAPHY

Advances in hardware and postprocessing for 3D echocardiography have led to impressive improvements in temporal and spatial resolution in the past 2–3 years. Two approaches are currently in use for 3D echocardiography based DSE. The first and simpler technique is to utilize the multiplanar capability of the 3D transthoracic probe to acquire the required apical and parasternal views using a single acquisition from each of these windows (e.g. the probe is positioned once on the apex and the apical 4-chamber, apical 2-chamber, and apical long-axis views are acquired simultaneously using a 3D triplane acquisition). This has the theoretical advantage of improving acquisition time and workflow, although there is a steep but short learning curve for sonographers or physicians new to 3D echocardiography particularly as very high quality images are typically required for DSE.

The second, a more comprehensive approach, utilizes the full volume capability of 3D echocardiography to acquire the entire left ventricle from the apical window. The resulting volume can then be sliced into multiple short axis, 4-chamber, 2-chamber, and apical long-axis views, allowing a more detailed analysis of wall motion compared with the limited views available from current 2D DSE imaging planes. Foreshortening of the LV apex is avoided using the volumetric approach, imaging planes can be easily standardized across stages, and imaging time is reduced since only a single apical acquisition is required at each stage. Commercially available 3D DSE viewing systems are now available which simplify workflow and interpretation.

Limitations of full volume 3D DSE include lower temporal resolution compared to 2D echocardiography, which can potentially reduce the ability to detect subtle wall motion abnormalities, including tardokinesis. In addition, multibeat acquisitions, if used to improve temporal resolutions, can lead to stitch artifacts due to patient respiration. This is an obvious limitation of 3D echocardiography during exercise stress echocardiography, but is not so problematic for DSE where breath holds of 3–7 heartbeats are feasible for most patients. As 3D echocardiography continues to advance, it is likely that the majority of DSE studies in the future will be performed using this modality.

## ECHO CONTRAST AND MYOCARDIAL CONTRAST ECHOCARDIOGRAPHY

Ultrasound contrast agents for LV opacification are indicated when two contiguous segments cannot be adequately visualized. At some centers, however, contrast is used when only one segment cannot be adequately visualized at rest, since high-quality stress images are typically more difficult to obtain than are rest images (particularly with exercise).

Myocardial contrast echocardiography (MCE) can be used to assess coronary perfusion and microvascular integrity, making it a potential adjunct in the assessment of ischemia and viability.[20] An MCE can be performed with either dobutamine or vasodilators, and adds incremental predictive value to traditional wall motion assessment.[21] However, MCE has still not received widespread adoption at most echocardiography laboratories, despite more than two decades of research.

## SAFETY CONCERNS

Pharmacologic stress echocardiography using dobutamine or vasodilator stress is widely regarded as a safe, noninvasive imaging modality for the heart. The American Society of Echocardiography guidelines note that DSE has been demonstrated to be safe in patients with severe LV dysfunction,[22] abdominal aortic aneurysms,[23] cerebral aneurysms,[24] and implantable cardioverter defibrillators.[25]

For dobutamine, significant side effects, which cause termination of the study, occur in a minority of patients (5%) and most commonly include severe hypertension (2%), symptomatic hypotension (0.5%), severe chest pain (1%), nausea (0.5%), and cardiac arrhythmias (1%).[26] In most cases these side effects are self-limiting and cease after termination of drug infusion. Even clinically important side effects, such as cardiac arrhythmias and systolic hypotension, are usually well-tolerated and are not associated with myocardial ischemia or LV dysfunction.[27] However, due to the potential adverse effects of dobutamine, the patient's heart rate and ECG must be continuously monitored, and blood pressure measured at rest, at each stage of dobutamine, and during recovery.

Hypotension during dobutamine infusion is easily managed by discontinuing the infusion and, in some cases, administering intravenous fluids. Hypertension and tachyarrhythmias are most frequently treated by intravenous esmolol or metoprolol. Esmolol is a short-acting β blocker that can be given in doses of 0.5 mg/kg. Metoprolol has a longer half-life and slower onset of action and is typically given in doses of 5 mg as a slow IV push. Up to 3 doses of IV metoprolol can be given, each dose 5 minutes apart (15 mg IV metoprolol is equivalent to 50 mg oral metoprolol). Chest pain can be treated by a sublingual nitroglycerin spray or tablet, plus IV β blocker as needed. Vomiting can often be prevented by giving metoclopramide 5 mg injection as soon as nausea occurs. Metoclopramide should not be used in patients with Parkinson's disease. A kidney basin or emesis tray must be kept near the patient's head during the study, or can be quickly provided as soon as nausea or vomiting occurs.

Adenosine is a short-acting agent that can occasionally cause chest pain, headache, nausea, and hypotension. Patients should be counseled prior to starting the test that these symptoms can occur as a result of medication administration and that they should avoid excessive movement if possible during that time, as this would interfere with the quality of the echo images. These adverse effects typically resolve within 15–30 seconds of discontinuing the infusion. Unlike adenosine, regandenason has a longer half-life (2–3 minutes) but a very favorable side effect profile. When side effects do occur, they can be treated by a slow injection of IV aminophylline (required in approximately 3% of patients).

Regardless of which pharmacologic agent is used, the cardiac rhythm must be monitored continuously during the study. A 12-lead electrocardiogram and noninvasive blood pressure measurements are obtained at baseline, at each stage of stress, and during the recovery phase. An emergency resuscitation cart, defibrillator, intubation equipment, including suction catheters, portable oxygen, patient trolley, and other emergency equipment are mandatory for any stress echo lab and must be maintained in good working order. At our lab, we routinely conduct emergency drills in the stress echo lab to ensure that all of our medical and administrative staff are proficient with code blue (cardiac arrest) procedures.

### Quality Assurance

Pharmacologic stress echocardiography requires a higher level of expertise, both in terms of acquisition as well as interpretation, than routine transthoracic echocardiography. For each sonographer or physician who routinely performs stress echocardiography, peer review of 5–10 studies should be performed annually to assess image quality and adherence to protocols for image acquisition.[28]

## SUMMARY

Pharmacologic stress echocardiography is a valuable non-invasive modality to assess patients with suspected myocardial ischemia, determine viability, and evaluate patients with low-flow low-gradient aortic stenosis. Knowledge of the pharmacologic stressors and adjunctive agents used, as well as imaging protocols and pitfalls in acquisition can improve image quality and enhance diagnostic accuracy.

## REFERENCES

1. Douglas PS, Garcia MJ, Haines DE, et al. ACCF/ASE/AHA/ASNC/HFSA/HRS/SCAI/SCCM/SCCT/SCMR 2011 appropriate use criteria for echocardiography. J Am Coll Cardiol. 2011;57;1126-66.
2. Beleslin BD, Ostojic M, Stepanovic J, et al. Stress echocardiography in the detection of myocardial ischemia: Head-to-head comparison of exercise, dobutamine, and dipyridamole tests. Circulation. 1994;90;1168-76.
3. Marwick TH, D'Hondt AM, Mairesse GH, et al. Comparative ability of dobutamine and exercise stress in inducing myocardial ischaemia in active patients. Br Heart J. 1994;72:31-8.
4. Sawada SG, Segar DS, Ryan T, et al. Echocardiographic detection of coronary artery disease during dobutamine infusion. Circulation. 1991;83:1605-14.
5. Marwick T, D'Hondt AM, Baudhuin T, et al. Optimal use of dobutamine stress for the detection and evaluation of coronary artery disease: Combination with echocardiography or scintigraphy, or both? J Am Coll Cardiol. 1993;22: 159-67.
6. Pellikka P, Naueh SF, Elhendy AA, et al. American Society of Echocardiography recommendations for performance, interpretation, and application of stress echocardiography. J Am Soc Echocardiogr. 2007;20:1021-41.
7. Sicari R, Nihoyannopolous P, Evangelista A, et al. EAE guidelines: Stress echocardiography consensus statement. Eur J Echocardiog. 2008;9:415-37.
8. Afridi I, Kleiman NS, Raizner AE, et al. Dobutamine echocardiography in myocardial hibernation. Optimal dose and accuracy in predicting recovery of ventricular function after coronary angioplasty. Circulation. 1995;91:663-70.
9. McKay RG, Aroesty JM, Heller GV, et al. The pacing stress test re-examined: correlation of pacing-induced hemodynamic changes with the amount of myocardium at risk. J Am Coll Cardiol. 1984;3:1469-81.
10. Chen L, Ma L, de Prada VA, et al. Effects of beta-blockade and atropine on ischemic responses to left ventricular regions subtending coronary stenosis during dobutamine stress echocardiography. J Am Coll Cardiol. 1996;28:1866-76.
11. Khan IA, et al. Adjunctive hand-grip during dobutamine stress echocardiography: invasive assessment of myocardial oxygen consumption in humans. Clin Cardiol. 2005;28(7): 349-52.
12. Ling LH, Christian TF, Mulvagh SL, et al. Determining myocardial viability in chronic ischemic left ventricular dysfunction: a prospective comparison of rest-redistribution thallium 201 single-photon emission computed tomography, nitroglycerin-dobutamine echocardiography, and intracoronary myocardial contrast echocardiography. Am Heart J. 2006;151:882-9.
13. Helfant RH, Pine R, Meister SG, et al. Nitroglycerin to unmask reversible asynergy. Correlation with post-coronary bypass ventriculography. Circulation. 1974;50:108-13.
14. Perrone-Filardi P, Bacharach SL, Dilsizian V, et al. Regional left ventricular wall thickening. Relation to regional uptake of 18 fluorodeoxyglucose and $^{201}$Tl in patients with chronic coronary artery disease and left ventricular dysfunction. Circulation. 1992;86:1125-37.
15. Martinez RR, Bennett J, Eikman EA, et al. Comparison of nitroglycerin magnetic resonance imaging with dobutamine echocardgraphy for predicting recovery of function after revascularization. Am J Cardiol. 2000;85:1250-2.
16. Fujita M, Yamanishi K, Hirai T, et al. Significance of collateral circulation in reversible left ventricular asynergy by nitroglycerin in patients with relatively recent myocardial infarction. Am Heart J. 1990;120:521-8.
17. Greco C, Tanzilli G, Ciavolella M, et al. Nitroglycerin-induced changes in myocardial sestamibi uptake to detect tissue viability: radionuclide comparsion before and after revascularization. Coron Artery Dis. 1996;7:877-84.
18. Picano E, Pinitore A, Conti U, et al. Enhanced sensitivity for detection of coronary artery disease by addition of atropine to dipyridamole echocardiography. Eur Heart J. 1993;14:1216-22.
19. Ng ACT, Sitges M, Pham PN, et al. Incremental value of 2-dimensional speckle tracking strain imaging to wall motion analysis for detection of coronary artery disease in patients undergoing dobutamine stress echocardiography. Am Heart J. 2009;158:836-44.
20. Porter TR, Xie F. Myocardial perfusion imaging with contrast ultrasound. J Am Coll Cardiol Imag. 2010;2:176-87.
21. Tsutsui JM, Elhendy A, Anderson JR, et al. Prognostic value of dobutamine stress myocardial contrast perfusion echocardiography. Circulation. 2005;112:1444-50.
22. Cornel J, Balk A, Boersma E, et al. Safety and feasibility of dobutamine-atropine stress echocardiography in patients with ischemic left ventricular dysfunction. J Am Soc Echocardiogr. 1996;9:27-32.
23. Pellikka P, Roger V, Oh J, et al. Safety of performing dobutamine stress echocardiography in patients with abdominal aortic aneurysm 4 cm in diameter. Am J Cardiol. 1996;77:413-6.
24. Takhtehchian D, Novaro G, Barnett G, et al. Safety of dobutamine stress echocardiography in patients with unruptured intracranial aneurysms. J Am Soc Echocardiogr. 2002;15:1401-4.
25. Elhendy A, Windle J, Porter T. Safety and feasibility of dobutamine stress echocardiography in patients with implantable cardioverter defibrillators. Am J Cardiol. 2003;92:475-7.
26. Mertes H, Sawada SG, Ryan T, et al. Symptoms, adverse effects, and complications associated with dobutamine stress echocardiography. Experience in 1118 patients. Circulation. 1993;88:15-9. doi: 10.1161/01.CIR.88.1.15
27. Lattanzi F, Picano E, Adamo E, et al. Dobutamine stress echocardiography: safety in diagnosing coronary artery disease. Drug Saf. 2000;22(4):251-62.
28. Picard HR, Adam D, Bierig M, et al. American Society of Echocardiography recommendations for quality echocardiography laboratory operations. J Am Soc Echocardiog. 2011;24:1:1-10.

# Nonpharmacologic Stress Echocardiography

*Asrar Ahmed, Roxy Senior*

## CASE SCENARIO

A 57-year-old female with a background of hypertension, raised cholesterol, and elevated body mass index (29.6 kg/$m^2$) presents to the rapid access chest pain clinic with chest discomfort for last six months. The chest pain is not necessarily related to exertion and is sometimes present at rest also. She is able to perform most of her activities of daily living without any support and has no disabling comorbidity. She is a smoker and has strong family history of ischemic heart disease. Her recent echocardiogram showed normal left ventricular (LV) ejection fraction (EF) and mild LV hypertrophy, which was evident on electrocardiogram as well. She underwent an exercise stress echocardiogram as part of initial assessment based on her intermediate pretest probability of coronary artery disease (CAD) by age, gender, and symptoms.

## INTRODUCTION

Evaluation of CAD is currently the most common indication of stress echocardiography and is based on the fundamental relationship of LV wall motion abnormality (WMA) mirroring stress-induced myocardial ischemia. The use of exercise stress and simultaneous M-mode ultrasound imaging of the left ventricular wall was first reported almost 40 years ago by a group led by Feigenbaum.[1] Around the same time, Wann et al. applied two-dimensional echocardiography to show ischemic WMA during exercise.[2] Over the past two decades, stress echocardiography has evolved into a reliable and readily accessible tool for clinical decision making in patients with known or suspected CAD. This has been made possible mainly because of rapid advances in imaging technology and digital acquisition techniques: continuous quad loop format for side-by-side display of rest and stress images, harmonic imaging as well as development of intravenous contrast agents for better endocardial border definition. All these factors have contributed to greater accuracy, increased sensitivity and improved prognostic value of stress echocardiography in day-to-day clinical practice.[3-5]

Among different stress echocardiographic modalities, exercise remains the preferred technique as it is safer and more physiological. It also provides valuable information regarding functional status which adds to the overall prognostic value of the test. Therefore, according to all current guidelines, exercise stress echocardiogram/echocardiography (ESE) must be the first choice for patients who are able to exercise.[6,7]

## EXERCISE STRESS ECHOCARDIOGRAPHY

Exercise is the prototype of demand-driven ischemic stress. Traditionally, exercise test using 12-lead ECG monitoring has been used in the evaluation of suspected CAD at low to intermediate pretest probability. This is due to its simplicity and widespread availability. However, published data suggest limited sensitivity (45–50%) of exercise ECG when used as a stand-alone screening test for ischemia detection.[6] Furthermore, exercise ECG has limited accuracy, especially in women and in patients with baseline ECG abnormalities.[8] For these reasons, current guidelines suggest stress echocardiography to be more appropriate and yield greatest diagnostic and prognostic value when used in patients with nondiagnostic, ambiguous or inconclusive exercise ECG.[9] Published data[10] suggest that stress echocardiography when used as an initial diagnostic test reduces downstream costs because of overall improved risk stratification.

ESE simply involves the addition of echocardiography to conventional exercise stress ECG. It provides additional physiological data, such as exercise time and workload, as well as information about changes in heart rate, blood pressure, and ECG (ST segment); useful clinical information that has both diagnostic and prognostic value. Exercise ECG remains inferior to ESE even when risk assessment scores like Duke Treadmill score are incorporated into decision making.[11] Moreover, a recent study found that 1 in 6 patients with suspected or known CAD who had a completely normal exercise ECG test, ischemia could be detected at peak exercise by echocardiography.[12] These patients were at higher risk of overall mortality and major cardiac events as compared with those without ischemia (5-year mortality rate of 12.1%

vs 6.4%; 5-year major cardiac event rate of 10.1% vs 4.2%). Therefore, ESE allows more accurate risk stratification and prognostic value in patients with a normal exercise ECG.

## Methodology

### General Test Protocol

During ESE, ECG and blood pressure are monitored as for conventional exercise ECG test. Echocardiographic imaging is typically performed from the three apical views (4-chamber, 2-chamber, long-axis) and two parasternal views (long- and short-axis). In some cases, subcostal images are used. Images are recorded in resting condition and peak- or post-exercise from all views and captured digitally. Intravenous contrast should be used for improved endocardial border definition when two or more segments are not well visualized. Analysis and scoring of the study is usually performed using a 16- or 17-segment model of the left ventricle.[13] Echocardiographic signs of ischemia, particularly the four-grade scale of regional wall motion analysis as described later in this chapter, are evaluated when comparing the rest and stress images.

Patients are candidates for exercise testing, if they are capable of performing at least moderate physical functioning (i.e. moderate household, yard, or recreational work and most of the activities of daily living) and have no disabling comorbidity. As for exercise ECG test, it is important to know diagnostic end points of ESE:[9]

- Maximum workload or achievement of target heart rate [220-age (years)]
- Obvious echocardiographic positivity (with akinesia of ≥2 LV segments)
- Severe chest pain
- Obvious ECG positivity (>2 mV ST segment shift).

Submaximal nondiagnostic end points of ESE include:

- Nontolerable symptoms
- Limiting asymptomatic side effects like systolic blood pressure >220 mm Hg or diastolic blood pressure >120 mm Hg, symptomatic hypotension with >40 mm Hg drop in blood pressure, supraventricular arrhythmias (e.g. atrial fibrillation) and complex ventricular arrhythmias (e.g. ventricular tachycardia or frequent, polymorphic premature ventricular beats).

For ESE, following technical requirements are mandatory to optimize image acquisition and interpretation:[14]

- A direct ECG wire connection between the echocardiography machine and the ergometer to obtain well-registered cardiac cycles.
- A continuous image acquisition system, which allows the acquisition of multiple cardiac cycles during several minutes. After the test, the highest quality loops of corresponding views are chosen for image interpretation.
- A quad screen format to compare rest and peak stress images. The current echocardiography machines are equipped with these requirements.
- An off-line station to read, store, and retrieve the studies.

### Specific Exercise Protocols

Exercise echocardiography is most often performed using either treadmill or bicycle (upright or semi-supine) protocol. Patients should be able to achieve 85% of age-predicted maximum heart rate. However, symptom limited exercise according to a standardized protocol in which the workload is gradually increased in stages is recommended.[3] Whatever the method used, it is imperative that images are acquired at peak stress as peak imaging is more sensitive for the diagnosis of CAD.[15] In addition, the prognostic value of peak imaging is higher than that of postexercise imaging.[16]

### Treadmill

Treadmill exercise is the most common form of stress testing **(Figure 5.1)**. The Bruce protocol is most commonly used (change in speed and slope every 3 minutes; modified occasionally to suit a particular patient) and the expected exercise level for a given age and sex can be expressed as functional aerobic capacity or in metabolic equivalents. Imaging is performed at rest and immediately after completion of exercise (scanning during exercise is not feasible). It is important that postexercise imaging is accomplished as soon as possible (within 60 seconds from cessation of exercise). This is done by moving the patient immediately from the treadmill to the imaging bed and placed in the left lateral

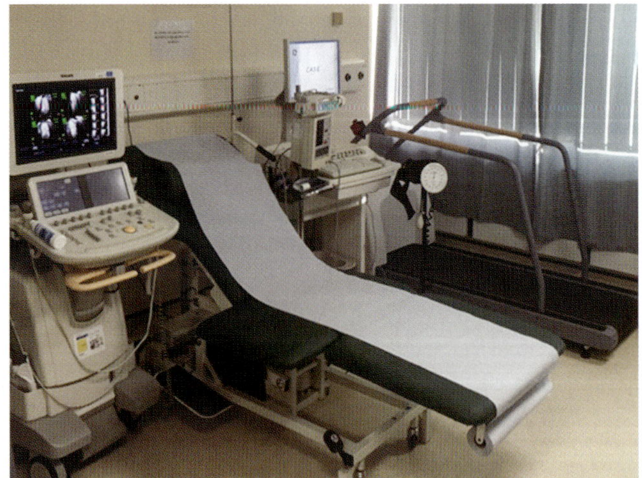

**Figure 5.1:** The set-up for treadmill exercise stress echocardiography. Images are obtained with the patient in the left lateral decubitus position on the specifically designed examination couch. Close proximity of the treadmill and the examination bed facilitated rapid acquisition of postexercise images.

position so that imaging is completed as soon as possible (within 60 seconds), to reduce false-negative results (as WMAs can recover quickly). Treadmill offers the advantage of widespread availability, operator familiarity, and greater feasibility than bicycle. Simultaneous information on exercise capacity, heart rate response, blood pressure changes and ECG are obtained and together with wall motion analysis, becomes the part of overall interpretation.

### *Bicycle*

Bicycle stress echocardiography is performed with either supine or upright ergometry. With the commonly used supine bicycle protocol, imaging is performed at baseline, at an initial workload of 25 watts, at peak stress, and in recovery. The workload is increased at increments of 25 W every 2–3 minutes. It is important that with increasing workload, the patient pedals at a constant cadence (usually 60 rpm). Successful bicycle stress testing requires cooperation of the patient (to maintain the correct cadence) and coordination (to perform the pedalling action). The most important advantage of bicycle exercise is the chance to obtain images at peak exercise (rather than relying on post-exercise imaging). With the patient in the supine posture, it is relatively easy to record images from multiple views during graded exercise. With the development of ergometers that permit leftward tilting of the patient, the ease of acquiring images has been further improved. In the upright posture, imaging is generally limited to apical and subcostal views which can be improved by asking the patient to lean forward or backward, respectively.

The treadmill has several advantages over the bicycle, including achievement of higher $O_2$ consumption, and the fact that all patients able to exercise can effectively walk on the treadmill. Ineffective pedaling is common in patients not familiar with cycling, while muscular pain or discomfort before achievement of submaximal age-predicted heart rate is a common reason for stopping exercise on a bicycle. This is more commonly seen with supine ergometry.[14] This limitation is overcome in part by occurrence of ischemia at a lower workload with supine position, resulting from higher end-diastolic volume and higher mean arterial blood pressure for a given level of stress.[17] This fundamental difference contributes to a higher wall stress and associated increase in myocardial $O_2$ demand compared with an upright bicycle.

## Echocardiographic Signs of Ischemia

The normal LV wall motion shows uniform inward endocardial movement along with preserved systolic thickening (normokinesis) and is normally completed within initial one-third of systole. Ischemic myocardium characteristically has segmental distribution corresponding to the coronary tree, and the cardinal sign observed is the transient regional WMA.

The stress echocardiographic sign of ischemia is the stress-induced worsening of functions or wall motion in a region contracting normally at baseline **(Figure 5.2 and 5.3, Videos 5.1A and B)**. This can range from hypokinesis (reduced wall motion and systolic thickening) to akinesis (absence of wall motion and systolic thickening) and, more severely, dyskinesis (paradoxical outward motion associated with systolic thinning). Although this description is arbitrary and prone to interobserver variability, the latter two markers of wall motion correlate to the severity and transmural extent of flow deficit. A fixed WMA (at rest and during stress) represents a scar, while a resting WMA that worsens with stress indicates mixed scar and ischemia which may develop in the same or a different territory (ischemia at a distance).

A semiquantitative scale is used to calculate wall motion score by dividing the left ventricle into 16 or 17 segments[12] and assigning a score of 1-normal, 2-hypokinesia, 3-akinesia and 4-dyskinesia. The sum of all the scores divided by the number of visualized segments is the wall motion score index (WMSI). LVEF at rest and peak stress is also calculated.

Sometimes, less sensitive but highly specific signs of ischemia can be observed that would point towards extensive CAD and confer poor prognostic outcome.[9] These include as follows:

- Transient dilatation of the LV cavity (>20% from baseline of end-systolic diameter, or >17% increase in end-systolic volume (ESV) from rest)
- Development of acute mitral insufficiency
- Reduced stroke volume with stress
- An increase in ultrasound lung comets, a sign of extravascular lung water accumulation (detectable by chest ultrasonography by placing probe on the third right intercostal space, and
- Reduced amplitude of S-wave by strain rate tissue Doppler imaging.

For the detection of angiographically significant CAD (>50% luminal stenosis), ESE has an overall sensitivity and specificity of 83% and 85%,[8] respectively. The specificity is similar to dobutamine echocardiogram but lower than dipyridamole echocardiography, and higher for all forms of stress echocardiography compared to single-photon emission computed tomography.[18]

## Prognostic Value

A normal exercise echocardiogram result is associated with an annual event rate of cardiac death and nonfatal myocardial infarction (MI) of less than 1%, equivalent to that of an age- and sex-matched population. These patients do not require further diagnostic evaluation unless there is a change in clinical status.[3] On the other hand, an abnormal stress echocardiogram, defined as new or worsening WMA, substantially increases the likelihood of a coronary event

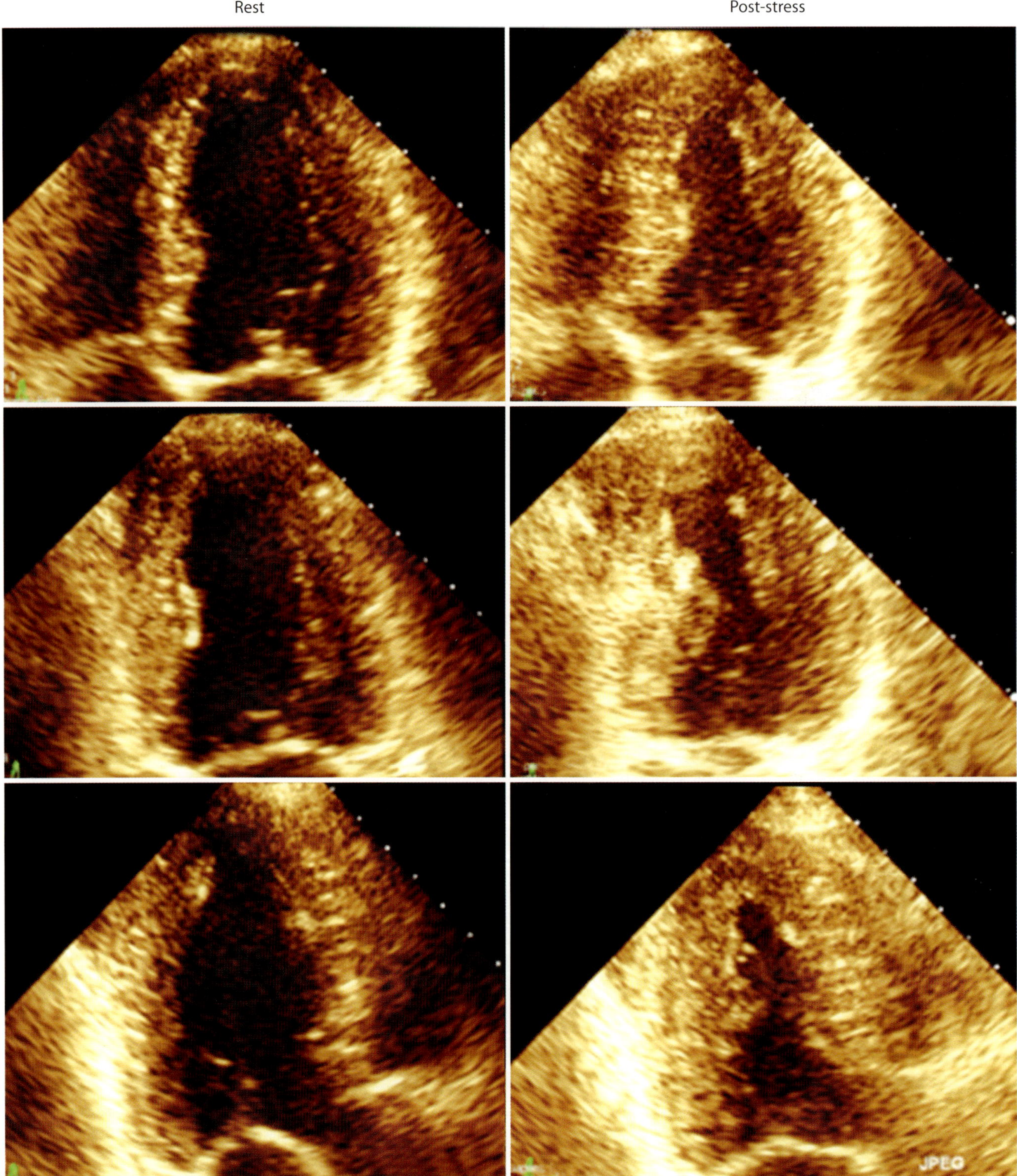


**Figure 5.2:** Resting (left) and post-exercise (right) images in a patient with normal exercise stress echocardiogram.

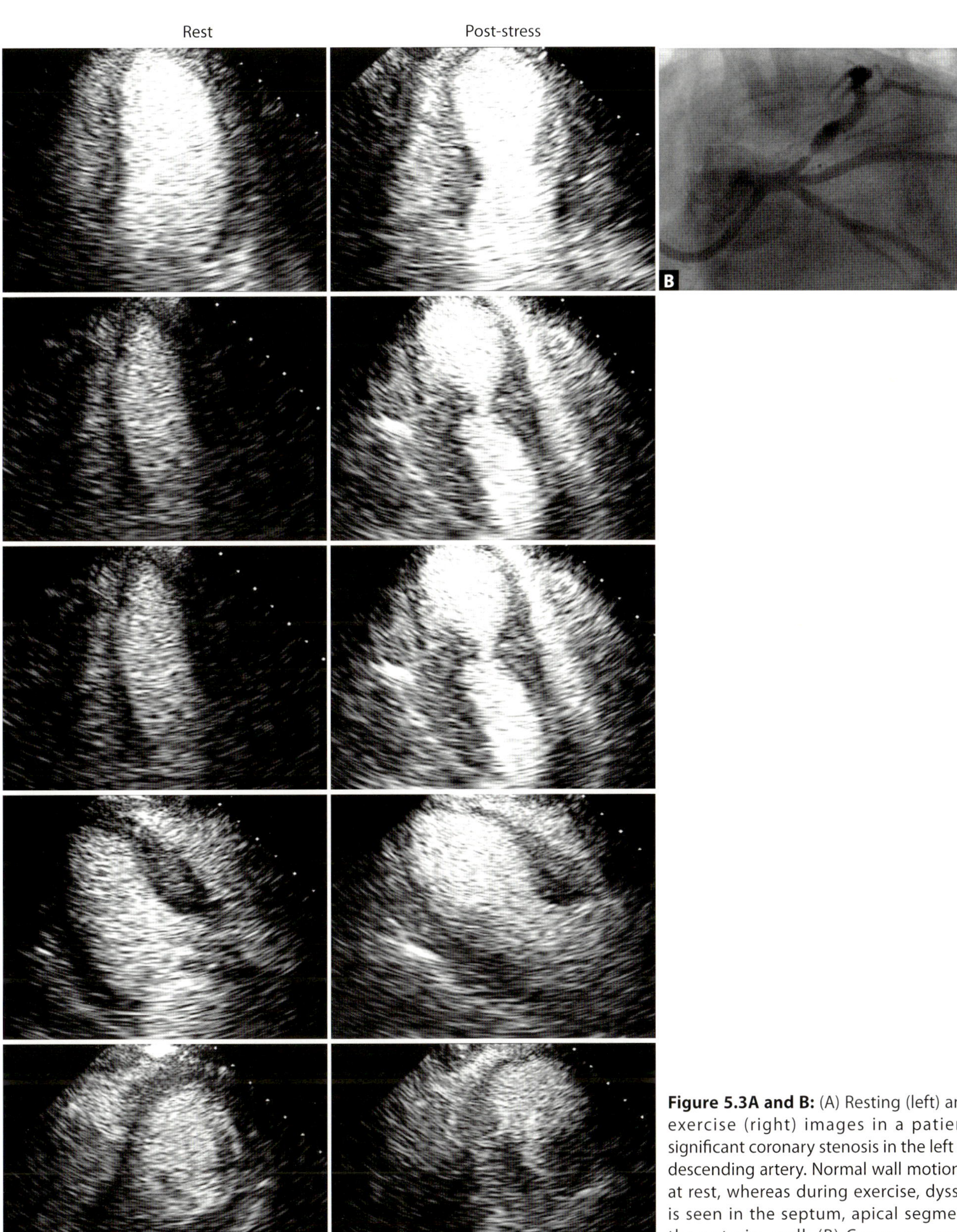


**Figure 5.3A and B:** (A) Resting (left) and post-exercise (right) images in a patient with significant coronary stenosis in the left anterior descending artery. Normal wall motion is seen at rest, whereas during exercise, dyssynergia is seen in the septum, apical segments and the anterior wall. (B) Coronary angiogram confirmed critical proximal left anterior descending artery disease.

**Table 5.1:** Studies evaluating the value of exercise stress echocardiography in predicting outcome

| *Author* | *Number of patients* | *Patient characteristics* | *Mean or median follow-up (years)* | *End point* | *Echocardiographic parameters* |
|---|---|---|---|---|---|
| Arruda-Oslon et al. 2002[19] | 5798 | Known or suspected CAD | 3.2 | Cardiac death/MI | Exercise WMSI |
| Marwick et al. 2001[20] | 5375 | Known or suspected CAD | 5.5 | All deaths | Extent of resting WMA; extent of ischemia |
| Bergeron et al. 2004[21] | 3260 | Chest pain or dyspnea | 3.1 | Mortality and morbidity | Change in WMSI |
| Elhendy et al. 2001[22] | 563 | Diabetes | 3 | Cardiac death/MI | EF, extent of ischemia |
| Arruda et al. 2001[23] | 2632 | Elderly (>65 years) | 2.9 | Cardiac death/MI | Change of EF and ESV |
| Elhendy et al. 2003[24] | 483 | LVH by echocardiographic criteria | 3 | Cardiac death/MI | Resting WMSI, EF response |
| Arruda et al. 2001[25] | 718 | Previous coronary artery bypass grafting | 2.9 | Cardiac death/MI | Change of EF and ESV |
| Bouzas-Mosquera et al. 2010[26] | 2159 | Elderly (>70 years) with known or suspected CAD | 3.5 | Cardiac death/MI | WMSI |
| Peteiro J et al. 2010[27] | 1107 | LV systolic dysfunction (EF <50%) | 4.1 | All-cause mortality/ major cardiac events | WMSI |
| Peteiro J et al. 2010[28] | 1058 | LVH by echocardiographic criteria (LV mass) | 4.6 | All-cause mortality/ major cardiac events | WMSI |
| Bouzas-Mosquera et al. 2009[29] | 609 | Left bundle branch block | 4.6 | All-cause mortality/ major cardiac events | WMSI |

*Abbreviations:* CAD, coronary artery disease; EF, ejection fraction; ESV, end-systolic volume; LV, left ventricular; LVH, left ventricular hypertrophy; MI, myocardial infarction; WMA, wall motion abnormality; WMSI, wall motion score index.

during the follow-up period. Variables associated with adverse outcome include extensive ischemia in a multivessel distribution, patients with peak WMSI >1.5, exercise EF <50% or failure to reduce ESV with exercise, a low ischemic threshold, and ischemia in presence of concomitant anti-ischemic therapy. Furthermore, development of new mitral regurgitation or worsening of pre-existing mitral regurgitation during exercise is associated with a poor outcome as well as predictive of mortality independent of the ESE results.

**Table 5.1** summarizes major studies that reported the prognostic use of ESE in patients with known or suspected CAD. Overall, the presence, site, extent and severity of exercise-induced WMAs has a clearly proven prognostic impact—ranging from patients with normal or reduced baseline function to those with underlying left bundle branch block, women, elderly or hypertensive subjects. The prognostic value of ESE is comparable to other forms of pharmacological (dobutamine or vasodilator) stress echocardiography and stress nuclear imaging.[9]

## Safety and Cost Effectiveness

The safety of ESE has a strong evidence base resulting from multicenter trials, meta-analyses and registries data.[8] Death occurs on an average in 1 in 10,000 tests,[30] while major life-threatening events (including MI, arrhythmias, and stroke) were reported in 1 in 6,000 patients,[31] five-fold less than vasodilator SE and ten-fold less than with dobutamine SE, although with the caveat that 'sicker' patients who are unable to exercise are usually referred for pharmacologic stress.

Marwick et al.[32,33] demonstrated that ESE was more cost effective than exercise ECG. This was due to better risk stratification with the former which resulted in lower downstream costs with ESE. Patients deemed to be low risk by exercise ECG had higher rate of cardiac catheterization and revascularization on follow-up. Also, ESE was superior to exercise ECG in risk stratification of patients evaluated in chest pain units, resulting in less diagnostic uncertainty, fewer referrals for further unnecessary investigations, and hence, a significant cost benefit over exercise ECG testing.[34]

Despite wide availability, not all patients can be referred for an ESE and a proper selection is mandatory. As discussed earlier, patients with resting ECG abnormalities, known CAD or intermediate pretest probability of CAD are preferentially referred for ESE.

## Limitations

The contraindications to exercise echocardiography are similar to exercise stress test and include unstable hemodynamic conditions, uncontrolled hypertension and of course, inability to exercise adequately due to any reason. Even when appropriate, presence of poor acoustic window in some patients is a major limitation of ESE and results in inadequate assessment of segmental wall motion. With the use of harmonic imaging and, specifically, the ultrasonic contrast agents, improved image quality through improved endocardial border definition has resulted in better visualization of regional WMAs and increased reader confidence as well as accuracy of diagnosis.[4] Current guidelines recommends use of contrast agent when at least 2 myocardial segments are nonvisualized.[4]

Compared to pharmacologic stress, acquisition of postexercise images is challenging, because of lung and motion artefacts as well as limited time window after exercise. Therefore, appropriate training is required to acquire the necessary expertise to perform peak exercise studies on a treadmill with confidence.[9] With the current imaging equipment and occasionally the use of contrast agents, the feasibility is, however, excellent, although use on a routine basis may not be cost effective. At the same time, up to one-third of patients who exercise may not achieve the age-predicted maximal heart rate response and thus considered to have inconclusive test. This percentage can be reduced by using atropine during exercise, therefore, reducing the need for pharmacological stress.[35] Atropine is particularly useful for patients with reduced resting heart rate as a result of β-blocker therapy, peripheral artery disease, or arthropathies.

## NEWER IMAGING MODALITIES

ESE can be complemented by the addition of newer imaging modalities. With the use of contrast agents for improving endocardial border delineation, it is now possible to assess myocardial perfusion at the same time using myocardial contrast echocardiography.[4] Stress-induced perfusion defect precedes WMA, thereby, improving the sensitivity of the stress test for detection of ischemia, albeit at the expense of specificity. It should be noted that assessment of myocardial perfusion during ESE is not without certain technical limitations.

Tissue Doppler imaging and speckle imaging can assess myocardial velocities and strain during stress, improving the accuracy of wall motion assessment by less experienced operators. Speckle imaging can be effectively used to assess torsional movement of the myocardium, which is altered during ischemic conditions.[36] However, the clinical application of the assessment of LV torsion remains to be refined. Speckle imaging may also be used to assess tardokinesis (delayed contraction), which is difficult to observe visually. In a recent ESE study, delayed strain was found to be more sensitive than WMA for detection of CAD. While WMA usually recovered in less than 2 minutes, strain delay recovery lasted as long as 10 minutes.[37]

Finally, real-time three-dimensional (3D) echocardiography can be used during stress testing and provides not only a potential for more accurate assessment of wall motion, but also allows for rapid acquisition of images over a few cardiac cycles. With real-time 3D echocardiography, time required to obtain all the essential views is decreased, thus allowing acquisition closer to peak heart rate.[38] This makes it ideal for ESE. However, the application of real-time 3D echocardiography to stress testing is still limited with lower feasibility in clinical practice. Relatively, long time is required to crop the images offline, while use of contrast is technically limited, because of increased bubble destruction by 3D transducer. Moreover, suboptimal image quality and stitch artifacts can make image interpretation difficult.

## CONCLUSION

Stress echocardiography using exercise protocol plays a valuable role in the evaluation of angina or anginal equivalents. Its advantages include low cost, good safety, excellent diagnostic accuracy, and lack of radiation exposure. It is the first indication for patients with resting ECG abnormalities or for those with inconclusive exercise ECG test results. With studies showing better risk stratification and improved prognostic value over exercise ECG, it is highly likely that ESE will become the recommended first-line procedure in all patients with suspected or confirmed CAD, and who are able to exercise. Furthermore, the combined evaluation of functional capacity as well as Doppler data during and after exercise makes it useful in a wide spectrum of patients.

### What Do the Guidelines Suggest?

#### *European Society of Cardiology 2013 Guidelines for Stable Coronary Artery Disease*[6]

- Stress imaging is recommended as the initial test option for establishing a diagnosis of stable CAD in patients with symptoms of angina and intermediate (15-65%) pre-test probability of CAD, if local expertise and availability permits *(Class I, Level C)*.
- Exercise stress testing is recommended rather than pharmacologic testing whenever possible. *(Class I, Level C)*.
- An imaging stress is recommended as the initial test for diagnosing stable CAD if the pre-test probability is between 66 and 85% or if LVEF is <50% in patients without angina *(Class 1, Level B)*.
- An imaging stress test is recommended in patients with resting ECG abnormalities which prevent accurate interpretation of ECG changes during stress *(Class 1, Level B)*.

### *American College of Cardiology/ American Heart Association 2012 Guidelines*[7]

- Exercise stress with echocardiography [or nuclear myocardial perfusion imaging (MPI)] is recommended for patients with an intermediate to high pre-test probability of ischemic heart disease who have an *uninterpretable* ECG and at-least moderate physical functioning or no disabling comorbidity (*Class I, Level B).*
- Exercise stress with echocardiography (or nuclear MPI) is recommended for patients with an intermediate to high pre-test probability of ischemic heart disease who have an *interpretable* ECG and at least moderate physical functioning or no disabling comorbidity (*Class IIa, Level B).*
- Exercise with echocardiography (or nuclear MPI) is recommended in patients with known stable CAD who have new or worsening symptoms not consistent with unstable angina and who have (a) at least moderate physical functioning or no disabling comorbidity but (b) an uninterpretable ECG (*Class I, Level B).*
- Exercise with echocardiography (or nuclear MPI) is reasonable in patients with known stable CAD who have new or worsening symptoms not consistent with unstable angina and who have (a) at least moderate physical functioning and no disabling comorbidity, (b) previously required imaging with exercise stress, or (c) known multivessel disease or high risk for multivessel disease (*Class IIa, Level B).*

## VIDEO LEGEND

**Video 5.1:** (A) Contrast-enhanced images showing parasternal long-axis (upper left), parasternal short-axis (upper right), apical four-chamber (lower left) and apical two-chamber (lower right) views at rest. There is no regional wall motion abnormality at rest. (B) Same views obtained immediately after exercise stress demonstrating akinesia of mid anteroseptum, apex and mid anterior wall indicative of a significant stenosis in the left anterior descending coronary artery.

## REFERENCES

1. Wann LS, Weiss JL, Weisfeldt ML, et al. Exercise echocardiography in detection of wall motion abnormalities during ischemia heart disease. Circulation. 1979;59:50-4.
2. Wann LS, Faris JV, Childress RH, et al. Exercise cross sectional echocardiography in detection of ischemic heart disease. Circulation. 1979;60:1300-8.
3. Pellika PA, Nagueh SF, Elhendy AA, et al. American Society of Echocardiography Recommendations for Performance, Interpretation, and Application of stress Echocardiography. J Am Soc Echocardiogr. 2007;20(9):1021-41.
4. Senior R, Becher H, Monaghan M, et al. Contrast echocardiography: evidence based recommendations by European Association of Echocardiography. Eur J Echocardiogr. 2009;2:194-212.
5. Chelliah R, Anantharam B, Burden L, et al. Independent and incremental value of stress echocardiography over clinical and stress echocardiographic parameters for the prediction of hard cardiac events in new-onset suspected angina with no history of coronary artery disease. Eur J Echocardiogr. 2010;11:875-82.
6. Montalescot G, Sechtem U, Achenbach S, et al. 2013 ESC guidelines on the management of stable coronary artery disease. The Task Force on the management of stable coronary artery disease of the European Society of Cardiology. Eur Heart J. 2013;34:2949-3003.
7. Fihn SD, Gardiin JM, Abrams J, et al. 2012 ACCF/AHA/ACP/AATS/PCNA/SCAI/STS Guidelines for the Diagnosis and Management of Patients With Stable Ischemic Heart Disease: Executive Summary. A Report of the American College of Cardiology Foundation/American Heart Association Task Force on Practice Guidelines, and the American College of Physicians, American Association for Thoracic Surgery, Preventive Cardiovascular Nurses Association, Society for Cardiovascular Angiography and Interventions, and Society of Thoracic Surgeons. J Am Coll Cardiol. 2012;60(24):2564-603.
8. Morise AP, Diamond GA. Comparison of the sensitivity and specificity of exercise electrocardiography in biased and unbiased populations of men and women. Am Heart J. 1995; 130:741-7.
9. Sicari R, Nihoyannopoulos P, Evangelista A, et al. Stress echocardiography expert consensus statement. European Association of Echocardiography (EAE) (a registered branch of ESC). Eur J Echocardiogr. 2008;9:415-37.
10. Marwick TH, Shaw L, Case C, et al. Clinical and economic impact of exercise electrocardiography and exercise echocardiography in clinical practice. Eur Heart J. 2003; 24:1153-63.
11. Peteiro J, Monserrate L, Pineiro M, et al. Comparison of exercise echocardiography and the Duke treadmill score for risk stratification in patients with known or suspected coronary artery disease and normal resting electrocardiogram. Am Heart J. 2006;151:1324e1-10.
12. Bouzas-Mosquera A, Peteiro J, Alcarez-Gracia N, et al. Prediction of mortality and major cardiac events by exercise echocardiography in patients with normal exercise electrocardiographic testing. J Am Coll Cardiol. 2009;53: 1981-90.
13. Cerqueira MD, Weissman NJ, Dilsizian V, et al. AHA Writing group on myocardial segmentation and registration for cardiac imaging. Standardized myocardial segmentation and nomenclature for tomographic imaging of the heart: a statement for healthcare professionals from the Cardiac Imaging Committee of the Council on Clinical Cardiology of the American Heart Association. Circulation. 2002;105:539-42.
14. Peteiro J, Bouzas-Mosquera A. Exercise echocardiography. World J Cardiol. 2010;2(8):223-32.
15. Peteiro J, Fabregas R, Montserrat L, et al. Comparison of treadmill exercise echocardiography before and after exercise in the evaluation of patients with known or suspected coronary artery disease. J Am Soc Echocardiogr. 1999;12:1073-19.

16. Peteiro J, Bouzas-Mosquera A, Broullon FJ, et al. Prognostic value of peak and post-exercise treadmill exercise echocardiography in patients with known or suspected coronary artery disease. Eur Heart J. 2010;31:187-95.
17. Currie PJ, Kelly MJ, Pitt A. Comparison of supine and erect bicycle exercise electrocardiography in coronary artery disease: accentuation of exercise-induced ischemic ST segment depression by supine posture. Am J Cardiol. 1983;52: 1167-73.
18. Heijenbrok-Kal MH, Fleischmann KE, Hunink MG. Stress echocardiography, stress SPECT and electron beam computed tomography for the assessment of coronary artery disease: a meta-analysis of diagnostic performance. Am Heart J. 2007;154:415-23.
19. Arruda-Olson A, Juracan E, Mahoney D, et al. Prognostic value of exercise echocardiography in 5,798 patients: Is there a gender difference? J Am Coll Cardiol. 2002;39:625-31.
20. Marwick T, Case C, Vasey C, et al. Prediction of mortality by exercise echocardiography: a strategy for combination with the Duke treadmill score. Circulation. 2001;103:2566-71.
21. Bergeron S, Ommen S, Bailey K, et al. Exercise echocardiography findings and outcome of patients referred for evaluation of dyspnea. J Am Coll Cardiol. 2004;43:2242-6.
22. Elhendy A, Arruda A, Mahoney D, et al. Prognostic stratification of diabetic patients by exercise echocardiography. J Am Coll Cardiol. 2001;37:1551-7.
23. Arruda A, Das F, Roger R, et al. Prognostic value of exercise echocardiography in 2632 patients ≥65 years of age. J Am Coll Cardiol. 2001;37:1036-41.
24. Elhendy A, Modesto K, Mahoney D, et al. Prediction of mortality in patients with left ventricular hypertrophy by clinical, exercise stress, and echocardiographic data. J Am Coll Cardiol. 2003;41:129-35.
25. Arruda A, McCully R, Oh J, et al. Prognostic value of exercise echocardiography in patients after coronary artery bypass surgery. Am J Cardiol. 2001;87:1069-73.
26. Bouzas-Mosquera A, Peteiro J, Broullon FJ, et al. Value of exercise echocardiography for predicting mortality in elderly patients. Eur J Clin Invest. 2010;40(12):1122-30.
27. Peteiro J, Bouzas-Mosquera A, Pazos P, et al. Prognostic value of exercise echocardiography in patients with left ventricular systolic dysfunction and known or suspected coronary artery disease. Am Heart J. 2010;160(2):301-7.
28. Peteiro J, Bouzas-Mosquera A, Pazos P, et al. Treadmill exercise echocardiography as a predictor of events in patients with left ventricular hypertrophy. Am J Hypertens. 2010; 23(7):794-801.
29. Bouzas-Mosquera A, Peteiro J, Alvarez-Gracia N, et al. Prognostic value of exercise echocardiography in patients with left bundle branch block. JACC Cardiovasc Imaging. 2009; 2(3):251-9.
30. Fletcher GF, Balady GJ, Masuda T, et al. Exercise standards for testing and training: a statement for healthcare professionals from the American Heart Association. Circulation. 2001;104: 1694-740.
31. Varga A, Gracia MA, Picano: International stress echo complication registry. Safety of stress echocardiography. Am J Cardiol. 2006;98:541-3.
32. Marwick TH, Shaw L, Case C, et al. Clinical and economic impact of exercise electrocadiography and exercise echocardiography in clinical practice. Eur Heart J. 2003; 24:1153-63.
33. Marwick TH, Anderson T, Williams MJ, et al. Exercise echocardiography is an accurate and cost effective technique for detection of coronary artery disease in women. J Am Coll Cardiol. 1995;26:335-41.
34. Jeetley P, Burden L, Stoykova B, et al. Clinical and economic impact of stress echocardiography compared with exercise electrocardiography in patients with suspected acute coronary syndrome but negative troponin: a prospective randomized controlled study. Eur Heart J. 2007;28:204-11.
35. Peteiro J, Garrido I, Monserrat L, et al. Exercise echocardiography with addition of atropine. Am J Cardiol. 2004;94:346-8.
36. Helle-Valle T, Crosby J, Edvarsden T, et al. New non-invasive method for assessment of left ventricular rotation: speckle tracking echocardiography. Circulation. 2005;112: 3149-356.
37. Ishii K, Imai M, Suyama T, et al. Exercise induced post-ischemic left ventricular delayed relaxation or diastolic stunning: is it a reliable marker in detecting coronary artery disease? J Am Coll Cardiol. 2009;53:698-705.
38. Sugeng L, Kirkpatrick J, Lang RM, et al. Biplane stress echocardiography using a prototype matrix-array transducer. J Am Soc Echocardiogr. 2003;16:937-41.

# Contrast Echocardiography

6

CHAPTER

*Adrian Chong, Sudhir Wahi*

## INTRODUCTION AND BASIC PRINCIPLES

Echocardiography is the most widely utilized noninvasive imaging modality for the assessment of cardiac structure and function. In clinical practice today, the use of microbubble ultrasound contrast should be viewed as a routine extension of the standard clinical echocardiography laboratory. Left ventricular opacification (LVO; for delineation of structural abnormalities) and improvement of endocardial border delineation (EBD; when ≥2 contiguous myocardial segments are not adequately visualized on noncontrast images) are standard approved indications when presented with technically challenging studies or suboptimal images as recommended by the American Society and European Association of Echocardiography.[1-3]

The first generation contrast echocardiography agents included Echovist (Schering AG), Albunex (Molecular Biosystems Inc.), and Levovist (Schering AG) produced microbubbles, which were either too large and unable traverse the pulmonary vasculature to opacify the left ventricle or were not sufficiently durable to provide a sustainable echogenic contrast effect to allow adequate imaging over time, largely due to the escape of their highly diffusible air content following a peripheral venous injection.[4-6] Commercially available second generation echocardiographic contrast agents currently in use include Sonovue® (Bracco Imaging), Optison® (GE Healthcare) and Definity® or Luminity® (Lantheus Medical Imaging). Sonovue® is a sulfur hexafluoride-based agent with the latter two utilizing perfluoropropane gas with outer shells of serum albumin (Optison®, perflutren protein-type A microspheres) or phospholipid (Definity®). Definity® requires mechanical agitation using the Vialmix® (Lantheus Medical Imaging) in order to "emulsify" the microbubbles prior to intravenous administration. These microbubbles are <10 μm in size allowing transpulmonary passage into the left-sided cardiac chambers and real-time evaluation of intracardiac blood flow. The common essential elements of these microbubbles are the use of high-molecular weight low-solubility gases to minimize diffusion and thereby dissolution, and high elasticity shells to reduce acoustic bubble destruction. These characteristics maximize microbubble stability and persistence in the circulation, while optimizing the intrinsic nonlinear contrast backscatter properties, thus overcoming the limitations of the first generation agents.[7,8]

Contrast-specific ultrasound imaging techniques are required to obtain optimal contrast-enhanced echocardiographic images. Most commercially available machines have vendor-specific presets for this particular purpose. Injected microbubbles within the insonating ultrasound beam undergo asymmetric oscillation (alternating compression and expansion with inverse changes in radius and stiffness) as a consequence of the compression and rarefaction bands. The multiple gas-liquid interfaces formed by the microbubbles increases the amount of nonlinear ultrasound backscatter.[1,6,9] The reflected ultrasound waves returning to the transducer will be comprised of a combination of higher multiples of the transmitted fundamental frequency, more widely known as harmonics.[7] The strength of these harmonic frequencies is dependent on the acoustic power output or mechanical index (MI). Soft tissue structures, such as myocardium are predominantly linear reflectors that produce a lesser degree of tissue harmonic frequencies from sound wave propagation. High-MI settings (with high peak negative pressures) used for standard non-contrast diagnostic studies result in significant microbubble disruption. Real-time contrast echocardiography utilizes low-MI (<0.2–0.3) harmonic imaging to minimize microbubble destruction, improve intracavitary contrast intensity for LVO and EBD, while maintaining a relatively high signal-to-noise ratio with the filtering of linear tissue backscatter and harmonics.[10]

The effect of high-MI imaging causing microbubble destruction has been exploited for the non-FDA approved indication of assessing myocardial perfusion or myocardial contrast echocardiography (MCE). Intermittent harmonic imaging at progressively increasing pulsing intervals, using dual triggered high-MI pulsed ultrasound, induces microbubble destruction on the background of a continuous intravenous infusion of contrast agent which then allows measurement of the replenishment rate and peak intensity in order to extrapolate the myocardial microbubble velocity as a surrogate of myocardial blood flow (MBF).[11] Low-MI MCE techniques, including power pulse inversion, power modulation and coherent contrast imaging were developed with the added advantages of improved signal-to-noise ratio, image resolution, and the potential for simultaneous assessment of myocardial thickening and wall motion which was previously not possible with triggered imaging (although frame rates may still be suboptimal).[1,12,13] This latter technique still requires high-MI pulses to deplete the microbubbles, but continuous low-MI imaging is used to monitor contrast replenishment as a marker of microcirculatory or capillary flow.

## RATIONALE FOR USE

Despite the advances in echocardiography technology since its inception, there remains a subset of patients who are technically challenging to image. This may result in diagnostic errors and unnecessary downstream testing with potential negative impacts on patient outcome and economic costs.[14] Current established indications for the use of echocardiography contrast in resting transthoracic echocardiography (TTE) are LVO and enhancement of left ventricular (LV) EBD for wall motion assessments, improvement in the accuracy and precision of quantitative ventricular chamber volumes and ejection fractions, diagnosis of LV structural abnormalities (e.g. apical thrombus, hypertrophic cardiomyopathy (HCM), and non-compaction), and detection of postmyocardial infarction pseudoaneurysms.[1,2,15,16] Microbubble contrast is recommended in the performance of stress echocardiography when ≥2 contiguous segments are not adequately visualized to improve the identification and interpretation of the extent of segmental wall motion abnormalities, accuracy and confidence of the readers, and thereby minimizing the proportion of nondiagnostic examinations.[17] Off-label indications also include MCE in perfusion imaging and Doppler signal enhancement.

In the current health economic climate, where appropriate and cost-effective use of diagnostic imaging resources are critical for sustainable healthcare budgets, the need to improve diagnostic accuracy remains crucial, and any avenues for potential cost-containment need to be explored and embraced. Microbubble contrast enhancement has undergone cost-effective analysis in multiple clinical setting with recognized benefits both from financial savings and reduction in the need for further more expensive or invasive downstream investigations as a result of nondiagnostic studies. A secondary analysis of an Optison phase III clinical trial performed by Shaw et al. demonstrated a 2.7-fold increase in echocardiographic diagnostic accuracy with the use of intravenous contrast, decreased need for follow-up confirmatory invasive or nuclear testing due to inadequate noncontrast studies, and translating to an estimated $269 savings per patient.[18]

Technically challenging TTE studies are common in the critical care setting, because of both patient and environmental factors. Yong et al. concluded that contrast enhancement for EBD improved the accuracy, reproducibility and cost-effectiveness of LV ejection fraction (LVEF) assessment in the intensive care unit (ICU), resulting in a $423 savings for every 1% increase in diagnostic accuracy per 100 patients, and avoiding the need for transesophageal echocardiography (TEE) that is not without its own inherent risks and limitations.[19] Assessment for ischemia by stress echocardiography is conventionally based upon the visual interpretation of endocardial excursion and wall thickening at rest and during stress. Appropriate use of microbubble contrast reduced further need for nuclear stress testing as a result of suboptimal noncontrast stress imaging and offered an incremental saving of $238 per patient even after accounting for the additional cost of the contrast agent.[20]

## SAFETY AND CONTRAINDICATIONS

Microbubble ultrasound contrast echocardiography is safe when its use is appropriately indicated. Reports of serious cardiopulmonary reactions and deaths during or within 30 minutes of the administration of Definity® contrast, resulted in a labeling revision and the Food and Drug Administration (FDA) issuing a black box warning for perflutren-based agents, contraindicating their use in the setting of unstable cardiopulmonary status (acute coronary syndromes, acute myocardial infarction, worsening or unstable heart failure) and pulmonary hypertension in October 2007.[21] Accordingly, the FDA required all patients receiving microbubble contrast to undergo physiologic monitoring (vitals, including cutaneous oxygen saturations, and electrocardiography) during and for 30 minutes after the contrast injection.

Despite the apparent temporal relationship with contrast administration, there was no definite evidence of causality established and these adverse events were attributed to likely pseudocomplications related to the underlying disease states. Subsequently, multiple retrospective studies, a meta-analysis and a large multicenter registry have repeatedly published the absence of any statistically significant difference in mortality between patients who underwent contrast-enhanced and noncontrast echocardiographic examinations (a 24% reduction in "crude mortality" was even noted).[22-26] In July 2008, the black box warning for Definity® and Optison® was revised where the 30-minute monitoring requirement remained mandatory but limited to patients with pulmonary hypertension (no clear degree of severity specified) or unstable cardiopulmonary conditions.

The safety of contrast agents in stress echocardiography, even with coexistent pulmonary hypertension, has also since been well validated.[27-29] Given the ongoing concern of microbubble contrast causing pulmonary capillary obstruction or secondary vasoconstriction resulting in exacerbation of pulmonary hypertension and potential circulatory compromise, Wei et al. undertook a small prospective invasive hemodynamic study to further resolve this issue.[30] The study demonstrated no clinically or statistically significant changes in pulmonary or systemic hemodynamic parameters following bolus administration of Definity® contrast in those with normal pulmonary artery systolic pressures (PASP ≤35 mm Hg; mean PASP 30.4 ± 3.4 mm Hg) and more importantly in patients with baseline pulmonary hypertension (PASP >35 mm Hg; mean PASP 50.9 ± 10.3 mm Hg). Of note, however, patients with severely elevated pulmonary pressures (PASP >75 mm Hg) were excluded from this study. Nonetheless, further reassurance was derived from the results of a large multicenter retrospective analysis of over 1500 inhospital patients across a range of pulmonary hypertension [mild (PASP 35–49 mm Hg), moderate (PASP 50–69 mm Hg), and severe (PASP ≥70 mm Hg)] undergoing contrast-enhanced resting or stress echocardiograms where the documented adverse event rate was only 0.002%.[31] The FDA recommendation for postadministration monitoring was removed from the Definity® product label in October 2011.

Postmarketing surveillance of ultrasound contrast agents has estimated the risk of a serious life-threatening adverse reaction to be approximately <1 in 100,000.[32] The majority of these are anaphylactoid reactions or complement-mediated pseudoallergies and, depending on the severity, may require antihistamines, intravenous fluids, and/or adrenaline. Other infrequent side effects noted in clinical trials have included headaches, nausea/vomiting, flushing or warm sensation, dizziness, back pain, chest pain, taste perversion, hyperglycemia, paresthesia, and injection site reactions.[2,33] These are often mild and self-limiting and may be managed symptomatically.

Contraindications to the use of microbubble contrast are a known hypersensitivity to the contrast agent or any of its components (blood products in the case of Optison®) and intracardiac shunts (right-to-left, bidirectional or transient right-to-left shunts). There is a move towards removing the contraindication against "known or suspected cardiac shunts", but this proposal by the International Contrast Ultrasound Society has not received formal approval or endorsement by the FDA at this point in time.[15,34] Intra-arterial administration of contrast is not FDA-approved, but intracoronary injections (to correctly locate septal perforators) during echocardiographic guidance of transcatheter alcohol septal ablation for the treatment of LV outflow tract obstruction in hypertrophic obstructive cardiomyopathy are recommended by current international societal guidelines.[34-36]

## INTRODUCING A CONTRAST PROGRAM

A team approach is crucial for the successful implementation of a contrast program into an echocardiography laboratory.[1,37] The key team players are the cardiac sonographer, echocardiographer (fellow or physician), and a registered nurse who is able to obtain intravenous access and administer the intravenous contrast agent. As there is no specific legislation or formal accreditation required, sonographers must be appropriately trained and credentialed. The supervising physicians should be, as a minimum, competent American Society of Echocardiography level 2 (or equivalent) echocardiographers with skills in basic and advanced life support to ensure the appropriate, safe and efficient introduction of microbubble contrast use.

It is recommended that independent interpreting physicians should have adequate instruction in instrumentation and have participated in supervised reporting of at least ≥20 LVO contrast studies for EBD (MCE will require additional advanced training).[38] This basic experience is necessary to develop a sound understanding of contrast physics, indications for use, and contrast-specific image optimization techniques to obtain high quality and diagnostic images. A preceptorship training model in a reference laboratory performing high-volume contrast studies, with adequate exposure to a wide range of pathologies, would be an acceptable means of acquiring the necessary skill and expertise. Members of the team must also be prepared and equipped to manage any patient adverse reactions that may potentially arise from the use of intravenous ultrasound contrast agents **(Table 6.1)**.

### Basic Set-up and Equipment

The same readily available equipment required for an agitated saline contrast study will suffice for the basic preparation and administration of ultrasound contrast agents. These include syringes, normal saline (sterile for injections), large gauge needles for "venting" and drawing up the contents of the contrast vial, alcohol pads or swabs, gloves, intravenous cannulae, three-way taps, gauze pads and medical tape.[39,40] Contrast agents require storage in an appropriate medication refrigerator. Standard institutional needle collection and disposal systems must also be available for discarding the contaminated sharps. Despite the rarity of serious adverse reactions, a regularly updated resuscitation trolley with airway equipment, emergency drugs for advanced life support, and an external defibrillator must be available in the event of any cardiorespiratory compromise.

**Table 6.1: Example of echocardiography laboratory protocol for contrast administration for resting LVO[48]**

**Basic equipment**
- Sterile syringes
- Sterile normal saline solutions
- Sterile large gauge needles for venting and drawing up (≥21 G)
- Standard equipment required for intravenous cannulae insertion (preferably ≥20 G) and maintenance of universal precautions
- Three-way stopcock
- Fully-equipped resuscitation trolley (basic and advanced life support)
- Appropriate facilities for postadministration monitoring where indicated
- Refrigerator for storage of contrast vials
- Agitator (VialMix®) for Definity® contrast "activation"

**Patient identification**
- Ideally sonographer-driven based on both clinical indication(s) and technical difficulty of the study
- Early recognition of challenging studies based upon patient characteristics, previous echocardiograms, or by screening with apical views at start of the routine examination
- Notify attending physician of need for contrast, exclude contraindications, obtain consent (process based on local institutional guidelines) and secure intravenous access

**Contrast protocol**
- *Prepare or "activate" contrast agent as per product information:*
  - Contrast from a single vial of Definity® (~1.3–1.5 mL) can be diluted to 10 mL in total with normal saline
- *Instrument settings (use vendor contrast-specific presets where available):*
  - Harmonic imaging
  - Reduce MI (Start with 0.2–0.4 to minimize microbubble destruction)
  - Increase receiver gains
  - Adjust compression and dynamic range
  - Optimize image to visualize the left ventricle
  - Move focus to level of the mitral annulus
- *Contrast administration and image acquisition:*
  - Bolus approach is easy to use and time-efficient (as per the ASE contrast recommendation 2014):
    - Definity® 0.5 mL bolus of diluted solution OR Optison® 0.3 mL of undiluted solution 0.3–0.5 mL initial bolus followed by 3 mL normal saline flush over 10 seconds
    - Repeated titrated boluses of 0.5–1.0 mL administered as required
  - Image from apical windows first
    - Orientate image using landmarks (e.g. ventricular or atrial cavities or aortic root) or alternate between standard harmonic and contrast-specific imaging presets
- *Practical tips for common pitfalls:*
  - Far-field attenuation
    - Wait for contrast to spontaneously dilute and clear
    - Induce microbubble destruction by transiently increasing MI
    - Smaller subsequent boluses of contrast
  - Swirling
    - Increase dose or rate of bolus injections
    - Decrease MI further
  - Lateral rib artifact
    - Move probe footprint

*Abbreviations:* ASE, American Society of Echocardiography, MI, mechanical index.

## Early Recognition

The cardiac sonographer is key to the early recognition of the need for contrast enhancement.[37] Timely identification of a technically difficult study, where microbubble contrast is clinically indicated, will allow a more efficient process to be followed whereby inherent delays associated with the setting up and administration of the intravenous contrast agent can be minimized. During the initial introductory period of contrast use in an echocardiography laboratory, the decision to administer microbubble contrast should be determined directly by the attending physician on an individual basis following recommendation by the sonographer.

As experience and expertise develop or, as in the case of accredited laboratories, a sonographer-directed protocol may even be implemented whereby qualified sonographers with "contrast skills", certification to obtain intravenous access and inject the contrast agent, may be able to independently facilitate the entire process in accordance with strictly pre-defined clinical criteria established by the laboratory director and medical staff.[39,40] Such expansion of scopes of practice will be institutional-dependent but offers the potential benefits of limiting disruption to patient scheduling and the laboratory workflow.[41] Another sonographer-directed initiative involves screening with imaging from the apical window to determine if contrast enhancement would be required and thereby allowing early modification of the study protocol to incorporate contrast administration.[42] Where post-injection monitoring is indicated, the recommended 30-minute interval can be undertaken following the initial administration of the microbubble contrast, during which the remainder of the routine study is being completed.

## Administering Ultrasound Contrast Agents

Following the decision to proceed with contrast administration and explanation of the procedure, benefits and risks by trained personnel, informed consent must then be obtained from the patient (either verbal or written depending on the institutional requirements). Contrast preparation is agent-dependent: Sonovue® and Optison® are "activated" by hand agitation, whereas Definity® must be agitated using the manufacturer supplied VialMix® for 45 seconds. Once activated, care must be taken to minimize microbubble destruction even from the earliest stages. "Venting" the vials with a large gauge sterile needle (18–21 G) or vent spike prior to slow aspiration of the contents with a second needle and syringe is necessary to avoid unwanted disruption of the microspheres. A large forearm or antecubital vein should ideally be cannulated with a ≥20 G cannulae and, using a 3-way tap, boluses of contrast can then be injected directly through the unobstructed in-line port (with the vein) while normal saline flushes are delivered via the 90° side-port.[43]

There are two methods for the intravenous administration of the microbubble ultrasound contrast agent. The bolus approach is the most commonly used technique due to its relative ease and practicality of delivery for resting LVO studies.[40,43] The contents of a vial of Definity® is diluted to 10 mL with sterile normal saline (~1.3–1.5 mL of undiluted contrast solution with ~8.5 mL of saline) with an initial 0.5 mL bolus or a 0.3 mL bolus of undiluted Optison® followed by a slow 3–5 mL flush of normal saline over 5–10 seconds to clear the line of any contrast agent.[15] Depending on the quality and persistence of the contrast enhancement, further boluses of 0.5–1.0 mL must then be titrated to the individual to achieve and maintain the desired uniform bright LV cavity for real-time imaging.

Significant variations in contrast intensity and artifacts can be avoided by ensuring good communication between the sonographer and contrast injector with regards to timing and optimizing the volume of the delivered boluses and flushes. The importance of this is further highlighted in stress echocardiography, where contrast boluses must be administered in an anticipatory fashion in order to achieve timely and optimal LVO during image acquisition at the different stages. The main advantage of continuous infusions is the ability to produce a more consistent and uniform contrast effect with minimal artifacts once the "correct" infusion rate is achieved.[44,45] Although this technique may potentially be more beneficial during stress echocardiography and MCE studies, it is time and labor intensive with the need for infusion pumps, rate titration, and continual manual agitation of the contrast syringe.[46]

## Instrumentation for Contrast-specific Imaging and Overcoming Common Pitfalls

The basic principles behind acquiring the optimal contrast-enhanced image have not changed significantly in the past decade. Standard low-MI (<0.3) harmonic imaging system presets for LVO are readily available from commercial vendors. In addition there are now also various vendor-specific real-time very low-MI (<0.2) imaging software designed to maximize the contrast enhancement while suppressing tissue signals.[15]

The goal of contrast-specific imaging is to minimize microbubble destruction and artifacts while optimizing microbubble persistence and image resolution. Similar to noncontrast echocardiographic examinations, continuous fine instrument adjustments for each individual patient are also necessary for contrast-enhanced imaging. Starting with the default LVO settings is useful, but minor modifications to the transducer frequency, transmit power or MI, receiver gains, and the compression or dynamic range will be required for image optimization.[47,48]

The initial precontrast image should ideally include a dark LV cavity with faintly visible myocardium in the background and the focal zone (where available) is placed at the level of the mitral annulus. Alternate landmarks including the aortic root, atria, and ventricular cavities will then need to be used for image orientation as the mitral and tricuspid valves are no longer well visualized in the contrast setting. Images during LVO for enhanced EBD are primarily acquired from the apical views (standard 4-chamber, 2-chamber and long-axis views). The parasternal window is usually regarded as secondary as the LV cavity may be shadowed as a result of far-field attenuation from the persisting circulating contrast within the anteriorly positioned right ventricle. Following delivery of an intravenous bolus or commencement of the infusion of contrast agent image acquisition should occur at peak LV cavity opacification where there is maximum "contrast" between the bright blood pool and dark myocardium. Homogeneous opacification of the left ventricle with excellent EBD may also occur with the initial appearance of contrast within the cavity, the so-called "first-pass effect", and often produces diagnostic images that are well worth acquiring before any far-field attenuation occurs.

Cardiac sonographers are not strangers to ultrasound artifacts, and contrast imaging is no exception. Attenuation, swirling, and rib artifacts during LVO are common and sonographers need to be equipped to deal with them.[43,47-49] Attenuation results from accumulation of microbubbles in high concentration in the cardiac apex (or any other near-field cavity) causing acoustic shadowing of far-field structures (e.g. basal segments of the left ventricle). This is more often an issue with bolus injection techniques. Options for the sonographer to overcome this include simply waiting for the contrast agent to dilute and dissipate or induce microbubble destruction by manually increasing the MI or if available, using a high-MI flash impulse. For the team member administering the contrast reducing subsequent bolus amounts or slowing the infusion rate will prevent this from recurring. Swirling arises from inadequate opacification of the LV cavity, which may be due to either insufficient amount of contrast being administered or an excessive amount of microbubble destruction. The sonographer in this situation may attempt to reduce the MI or, alternatively, increasing the bolus dose or infusion rate of the contrast agent. Finally, the lateral artifact encountered on the apical 4-chamber view as a consequence of "obstruction" to the transmission of ultrasound in the lateral scan plane by the ribs requires repositioning of the transducer footprint.

## CLINICAL INDICATIONS

### Left Ventricular Structure and Function

#### *Quantification of Left Ventricular Ejection Fraction*

Quantitative assessment of LVEF is fundamental to the diagnosis and prognosis of cardiac disease and is well established as a guide for device-based therapies.[50,51] Re-evaluation with echocardiography is appropriate when there has been a clinical change in the absence of a clear precipitant and also to guide antifailure management.[3] Cardiotoxicity of chemotherapeutic agents is an increasing area of interest globally. While chemotherapy offers a potential prognostic advantage in patients with various malignancies, this can easily be offset by the cardiotoxic risk and worsening LV function. Longitudinal surveillance of LVEF is mandatory in many of these patients.[52] By virtue of its accessibility, cost-effectiveness and safety profile, echocardiography is pivotal in the follow-up of these patients. There is a large body of evidence supporting the use of contrast-enhanced echocardiography for LVO to improve LVEF correlation with cine or radionuclide ventriculography and cardiac magnetic resonance imaging (cMRI), and the overall intra- and interobserver reliability and reproducibility.[14,33,53-57] Contrast LVO has also been demonstrated to reduce the underestimation of LV volumes by noncontrast two-dimensional (2D) echocardiography in comparison to cMRI.[58]

#### *Enhancement of EBD and Wall Motion Assessment (Resting and Stress Echocardiography)*

The incidence of nondiagnostic TTE studies due to poor EBD may be as high as 20% in routine clinical practice.[14,59,60] Technically, difficult examinations can be due to both patient and environmental factors. Obesity, lung disease (e.g. chronic obstructive airways disease), chest wall deformities, and the clinical need for studies to be performed in the emergency department or critical care settings are all commonly encountered scenarios that place limitations on the quality of the acoustic windows available for imaging. The use of microbubble contrast for LVO to enhance EBD in these situations has been shown to improve diagnostic accuracy, interpreter confidence, and interobserver variability for assessment of global LV function and regional wall motion abnormalities.[61-64] Microbubble contrast has been reportedly able to "salvage" up to 48% of previously nondiagnostic studies (defined as ≥4 nonevaluable segments in either the apical 4- or 2-chamber views) and resulted in an average of 4 additional evaluable segments in comparison to the technically difficult noncontrast baseline images.[65] This conversion rate of nondiagnostic to diagnostic studies is even more relevant in mechanically ventilated patients in the intensive care unit (ICU) environment.[66-68] As previously mentioned, contrast LVO with harmonic imaging on TTE is also a cost-effective and safer alternative to the invasive transesophageal approach for assessment of wall motion and LVEF in ICU patients.[19]

Stress echocardiography is a routine noninvasive test for the diagnosis and risk stratification of myocardial ischemia due to obstructive coronary artery disease.[17,69] Reliable interpretation of regional wall motion abnormalities based on endocardial excursion and segmental myocardial thickening requires clear endocardial definition. Up to 30% of exercise stress echocardiograms (ESE) may be suboptimal, and the interobserver agreement for dobutamine stress echocardiograms (DSE), even among experienced stress echocardiographers, can be significantly influenced by image quality.[70,71] Microbubble contrast use during DSE has been demonstrated on numerous occasions to improve the assessment of poorly visualized segments and, therefore, increase the diagnostic accuracy and interpreter's confidence.[72-76] Extent of ischemia detected with contrast during DSE is also predictive of adverse cardiac events.[77]

Using coronary angiography as the reference standard, a small randomized cross-over study investigating the improvement in diagnostic yield of contrast-enhanced DSE over noncontrast studies confirmed the improved accuracy with contrast use.[78] Jung et al. assessed the additional diagnostic value of contrast-enhanced DSE for the detection of the hemodynamic significance of intermediate coronary stenosis.[79] This subset of patients poses a greater challenge in determining the need for revascularization. Contrast-enhanced DSE, in comparison to standard imaging, improved the sensitivity and accuracy for detection of ischemia from those coronary lesions, which were determined to be hemodynamically relevant by pressure-derived myocardial fractional flow reserve.

## *Diagnosis of Left Ventricular Structural Abnormalities*

It is often difficult to image abnormalities in the LV apex due to foreshortening of the images or near-field artifacts. In early 2-dimensional echocardiographic studies, LV apical thrombi were reported in 27% of patients who suffered an anterior myocardial infarction in the thrombolysis era and 36% of chronic dilated cardiomyopathy patients.[80,81] The most feared complication of this is systemic embolization with a resultant stroke (0.7–11% in those studies). The corollary to this is long-term anticoagulation with its associated risk of bleeding. Consequently, the accurate identification of apical thrombi is critical. However, up to 46% of studies reviewed in one series by Thanigaraj et al. were regarded as inconclusive for this purpose.[82] The diagnosis may further be confounded by the presence of apical trabeculae, apically displaced papillary muscles, false tendons, or near-field artifacts including clutter or reverberations. Administration of Optison® contrast resulted in 90% of those suboptimal studies became diagnostic thereby allowing appropriate clinical decision making and anticoagulation **(Figure 6.1 to 6.3 and Videos 6.1 to 6.3)**.

In a study using cMRI as a reference standard for the detection of LV thrombus in a high-risk population of patients, contrast-enhanced echocardiography had almost double the sensitivity (61% vs 33%, $p < 0.05$) and not unexpectedly higher diagnostic accuracy (92% vs 82%, $p < 0.01$) in comparison to noncontrast studies and was comparable to cine-MRI.[83] However, it should be noted that 39% of thrombi identified on delayed-enhancement MRI were not noted with contrast echocardiography but were more likely mural (concave in shape similar to the endocardial contour [compare intracavitary thrombi that appear as irregular intraluminal filling defects]) and smaller in size when in the apical position. Echocardiographic contrast perfusion imaging has also been demonstrated to assist with the differentiation of intracardiac masses.[84] Malignant and vascular tumors exhibit hyperenhancement and relatively more perfusion when compared with the adjacent myocardium, stromal tumors partially enhance and show less perfusion, while thrombi being avascular show no contrast enhancement.

Multiple variations of the distribution of hypertrophy in apical HCM have been described, including abrupt "shelf-like" or gradual transitions from the normal basal septal thickness, to true apical involvement with hypertrophy confined to below the level of the papillary muscles, and other variants with circumferential or asymmetrical apical hypertrophy (apical septum or apical lateral).[85] The myocardial definition in the apex may be difficult to visualize even with standard harmonic imaging because of its position in the near-field limiting the degree of soundwave propagation needed for generation of tissue harmonics. The diagnostic criteria for apical HCM includes asymmetric LV hypertrophy, predominantly confined to the LV apex, with

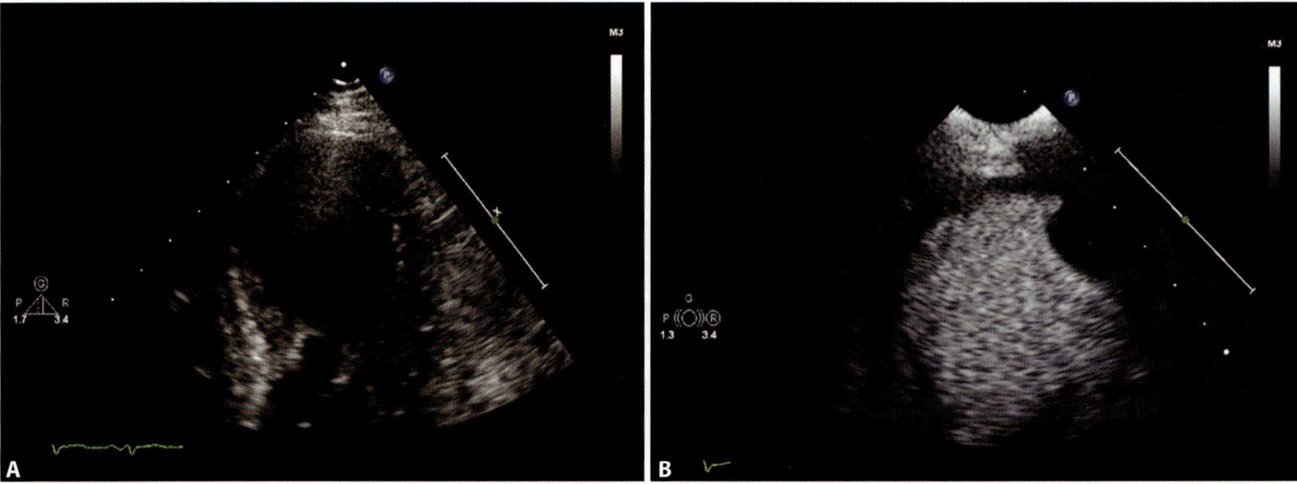


**Figure 6.1A and B:** Apical aneurysm and thrombus. (A) Standard two-dimensional apical 4-chamber view demonstrating an aneurysmal left ventricular apex with near-field clutter and a possible apical thrombus. (B) Contrast enhancement confirming the presence of an intraluminal filling defect in the apical lateral region consistent with an intracavitary thrombus.

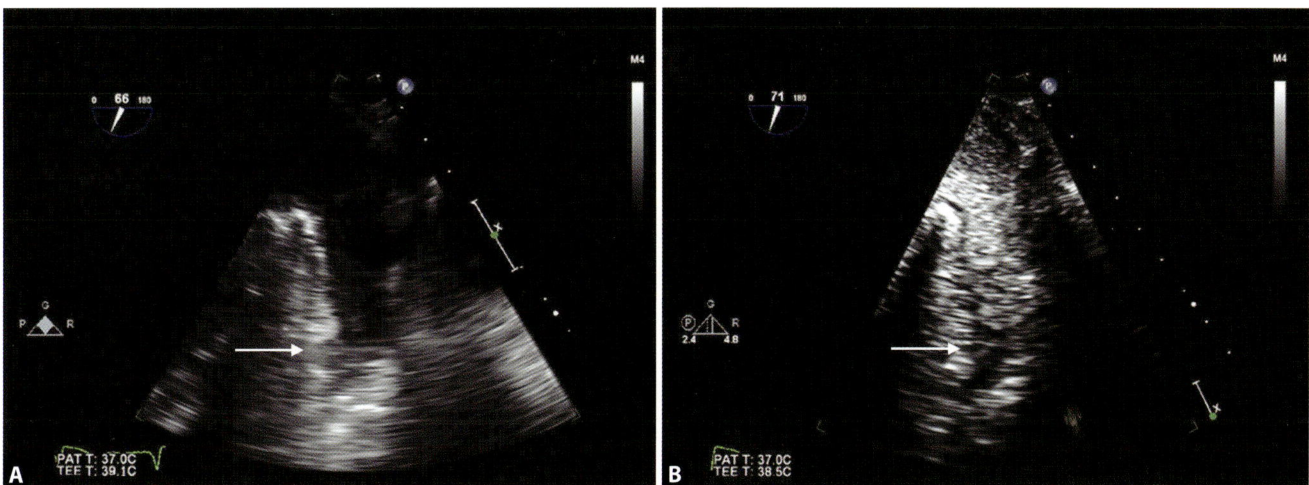

**Figure 6.2A and B:** Left atrial appendage thrombus. (A) two-dimensional transesophageal echocardiographic assessment of the left atrial appendage demonstrating an echodensity suspicious for a thrombus (arrow). (B) Off-label use of Definity contrast confirms the presence of an intraluminal filling defect at the base of the left atrial appendage consistent with a thrombus (arrow) with a layered extension to the opening of the appendage.

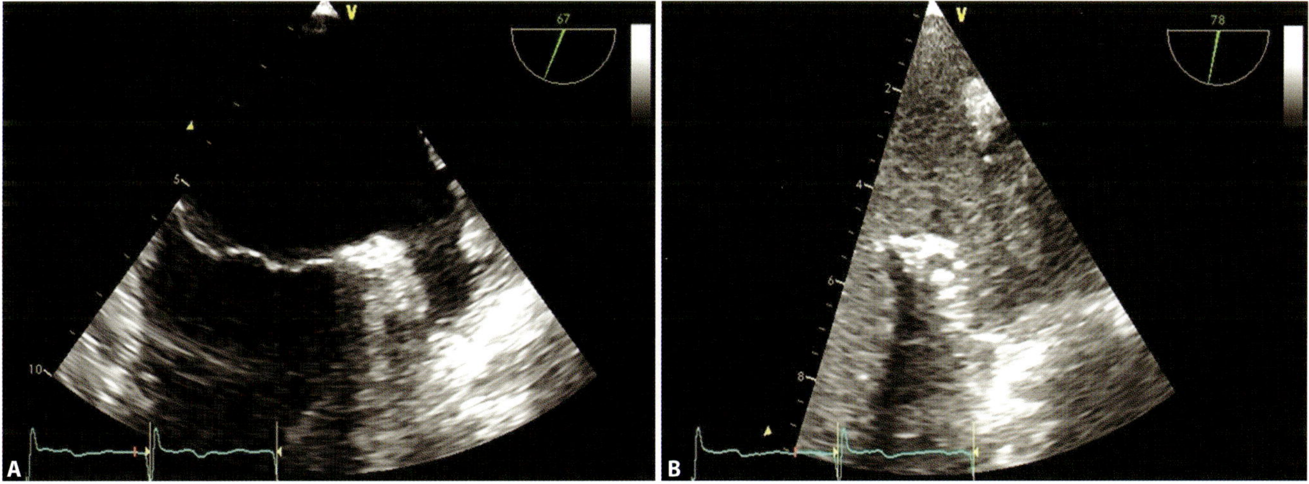

**Figure 6.3A and B:** Left atrial appendage artefact prior to direct current cardioversion for atrial fibrillation. (A) two-dimensional transesophageal echocardiographic assessment demonstrating an echodensity in the left atrial appendage suspicious for a potential thrombus in the setting of suboptimal anticoagulation. (B) Definity contrast was administered resulting in full opacification of the left atrial appendage with no evidence of a filling defect to suggest thrombus. The patient was successfully cardioverted with no adverse outcome.

an apical wall thickness of >15 mm and a ratio of maximal apical to posterior wall thickness of ≥1.5 as measured by cMRI or echocardiography.[86] Contrast-enhancement is able to establish the diagnosis of apical HCM **(Figure 6.4A and B, Videos 6.4A and B)** and should be routinely used if the condition is suspected clinically or unable to be excluded with standard 2D harmonic imaging techniques.[87,88] The classic end-diastolic "spade-like" appearance of the LV apex can be clearly outlined without the need for alternative diagnostic imaging including left ventriculography or cMRI.

LV noncompaction (LVNC) is a form of congenital cardiomyopathy characterized by a "spongy" LV myocardium which results from an arrest of normal embryonic endomyocardial morphogenesis.[89] The earliest case report of isolated persistent myocardial sinusoids was published by Engberding et al. in 1984 and may present clinically with the triad of heart failure, ventricular arrhythmias, and systemic emboli.[90,91] Jenni et al. proposed four echocardiographic criteria for isolated LVNC that include as follows: (i) the absence of coexisting cardiac structural abnormalities,

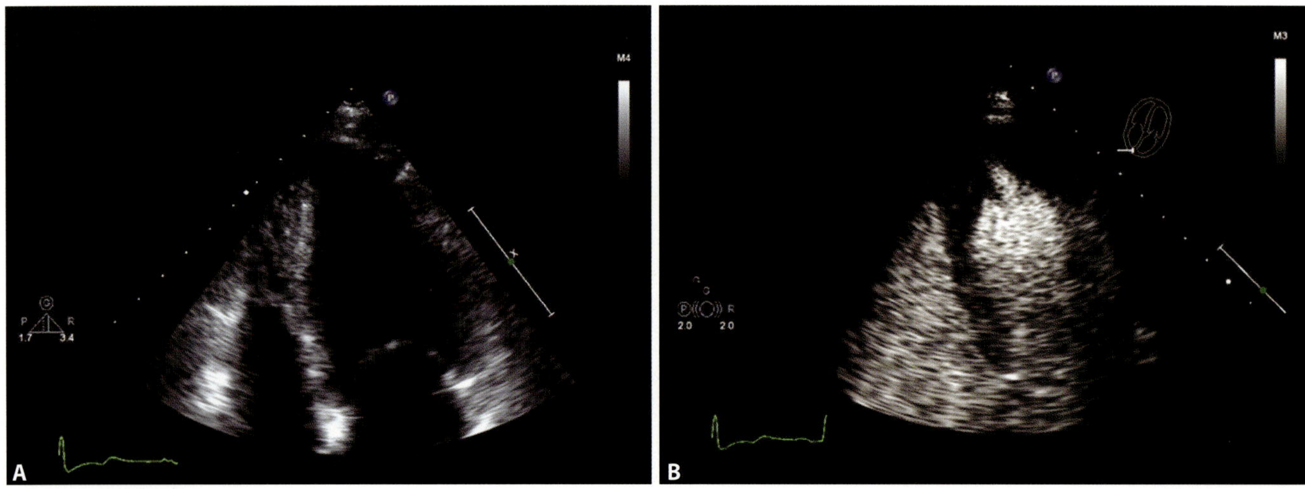

**Figure 6.4A and B:** Apical hypertrophic cardiomyopathy. (A) Standard two-dimensional apical 4-chamber view with suboptimal endocardial definition and poor delineation of the left ventricular apex. (B) Contrast enhancement demonstrating hypertrophy of the apical myocardium with the classic end-diastolic spade-shaped appearance of apical hypertrophic cardiomyopathy.

(ii) a double-layer appearance of the myocardium with a thinner compacted epicardium and thick noncompacted endocardium composed of prominent trabeculae with characteristic deep inter-trabecular recesses (end-systolic ratio of noncompacted to compacted layers of >2:1), (iii) evidence of blood flow by color Doppler into these recesses in communication with the ventricular cavity, and (iv) a predilection for the apex, mid-lateral, and mid-inferior LV segments.[92] Alternatively, cMRI criteria uses the ratio of noncompacted to compacted myocardium of >2.3 in end-diastole (sensitivity 86%, specificity 99%, negative-predictive value 75%, and positive-predictive value 99%).[93] The use of contrast during routine echocardiography improves detection and definition of these diagnostic features, especially in the apical region, which is often obscured during standard imaging techniques, thereby avoiding the potential underdiagnosis of this rare but significant form of cardiomyopathy **(Figure 6.5A and B, Videos 6.5A and B)**.[94,95]

Differentiating postmyocardial infarction pseudoaneurysm (free wall rupture) from an aneurysm with thinned, fibrotic, and scarred myocardium is prognostically significant. Pseudoaneurysms are pathologically defined by containment of the rupture by epicardium or overlying adherent pericardium and are typically associated on imaging studies with an inferior or posterior location, a relatively narrow connection or neck between the LV cavity and pseudoaneurysm **(Figure 6.6A and B, Videos 6.6A and B)**, and the presence of turbulent or bidirectional flow between the ventricle and extracardiac space.[96] Recognizing the echo-free space of the pseudoaneurysm sac is not difficult, but when echocardiographic images are suboptimal, localizing the narrow neck or myocardial discontinuity or estimating the true size in the presence of thrombus can be very challenging. Pseudoaneurysms may spontaneously rupture, and prompt bedside diagnosis is time critical. Microbubble ultrasound agents used for standard LVO imaging will allow immediate and direct visualization of contrast extravasation through the myocardial defect into the pericardial space.[97-99] The operative mortality has been previously estimated at ~7%, and thus presurgical confirmation is mandatory.[100] Apical aneurysms that are missed due to foreshortening can also be clearly outlined and definitively diagnosed with contrast enhancement.

## Off-label Uses

### *Doppler Signal Enhancement*

Estimation of the right ventricular systolic pressure (RVSP), regarded as an equivalent of PASP in the absence of right ventricular outflow tract obstruction, is calculated by the simplified Bernoulli equation (RVSP = $4v^2$ + right atrial pressure) using the peak tricuspid regurgitation (TR) jet velocity measured on continuous wave Doppler. The severity of pulmonary hypertension has a poor correlation with the severity of TR. Trivial amounts of regurgitation can coexist with severely elevated pulmonary pressures. Incomplete TR Doppler spectral signals can result in underestimation of the right ventricular-to-right atrial pressure gradient and therefore the PASP. Intravenous contrast can be used to optimize the TR envelope (defined as a smooth parabolic well-defined signal) and to ensure that the true peak TR velocity is obtained **(Figure 6.7A and B)** and measured.[101]

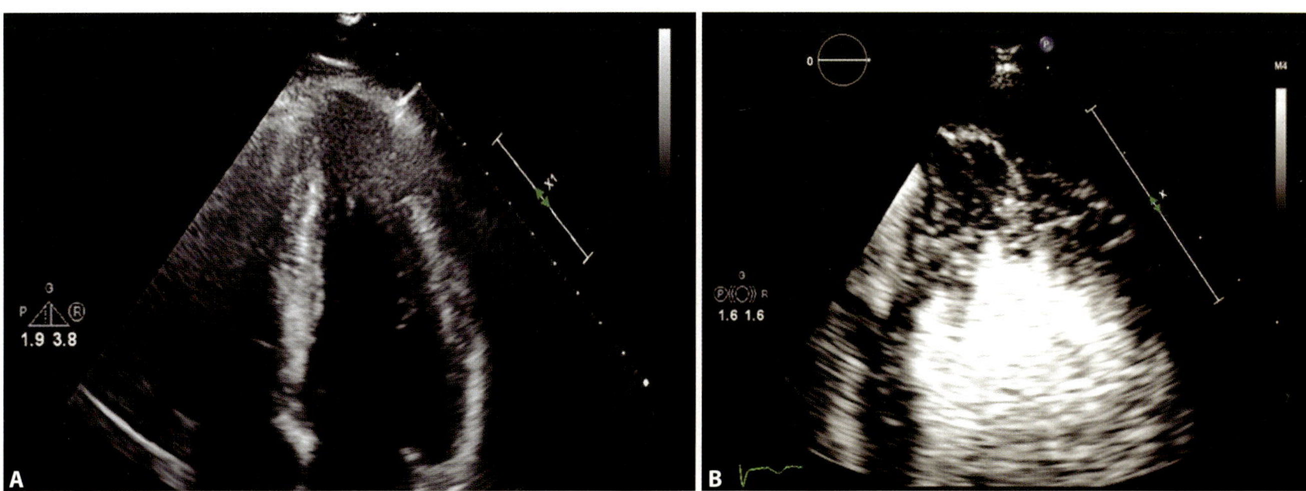


**Figure 6.5A and B:** Noncompaction. (A) Standard two-dimensional apical 4-chamber view demonstrating an ill-defined echodensity in the left ventricular apex. (B) Contrast enhanced focused apical view revealing the prominent trabeculae and deep intertrabecular recesses typical of noncompaction cardiomyopathy.

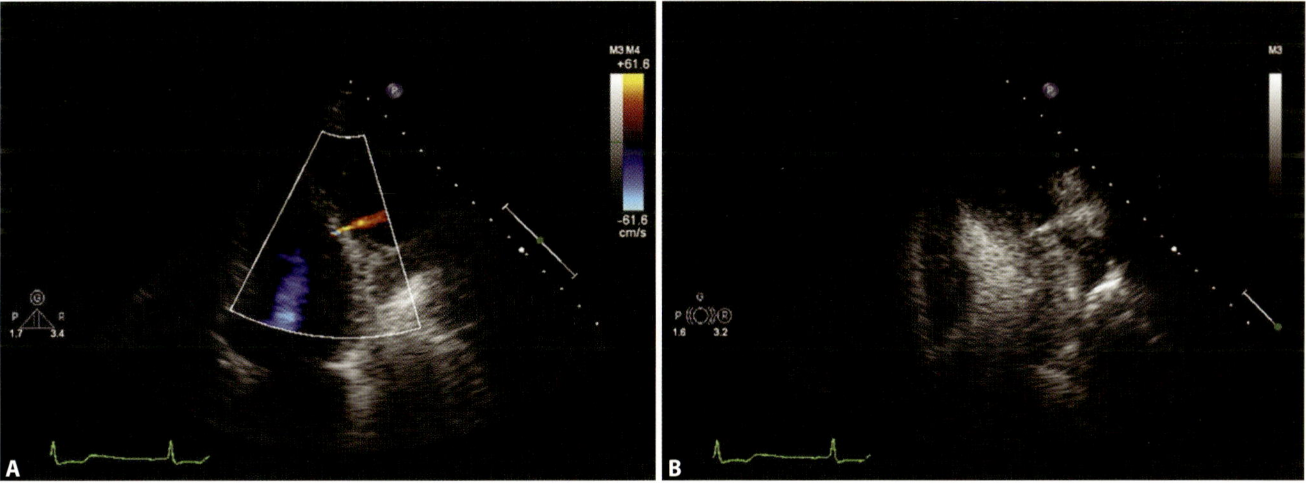


**Figure 6.6A and B:** Pseudoaneurysm. (A) Standard two-dimensional apical 4-chamber view with color Doppler demonstrating a communication between the left ventricular cavity and an echo-free extracardiac collection through the anterolateral wall. (B) Contrast extravasation through a narrow neck consistent with a left ventricular free wall rupture or pseudoaneurysm.

On the left side of the heart, degenerative aortic stenosis (AS) is currently the most common native valvular disease in developed countries. The peak aortic jet velocity on echocardiography remains one of the key diagnostic criteria in the assessment of AS severity.[102] Higher peak aortic jet velocities (≥5.5 m/sec) have previously been shown to predict poorer outcomes, higher event rates and accelerated functional decline within the subset of patients with otherwise clearly defined severe AS.[103] Intravenous contrast agents may also enhance the continuous wave spectral Doppler signals from the aortic valve permitting more accurate quantification of the transvalvular gradients and improved correlation with invasive hemodynamics.[104,105] When used for spectral Doppler signal enhancement (this remains an off-label use), a "blooming" artifact often occurs because of the strong acoustic backscatter from the microbubbles. Using very small boluses of contrast (or waiting for its progressive dilution over circulating time) and decreasing the overall Doppler gain are effective approaches to optimize the signal.

## Myocardial Contrast Echocardiography

Myocardial perfusion is physiologically the MBF at the capillary level within the myocardium and is the product

**Figure 6.7A and B:** Tricuspid regurgitation continuous-wave Doppler signal. (A) Standard noncontrast continuous wave Doppler spectral tracing in pulmonary arterial hypertension. (B) Contrast enhanced tricuspid regurgitation spectral Doppler signal.

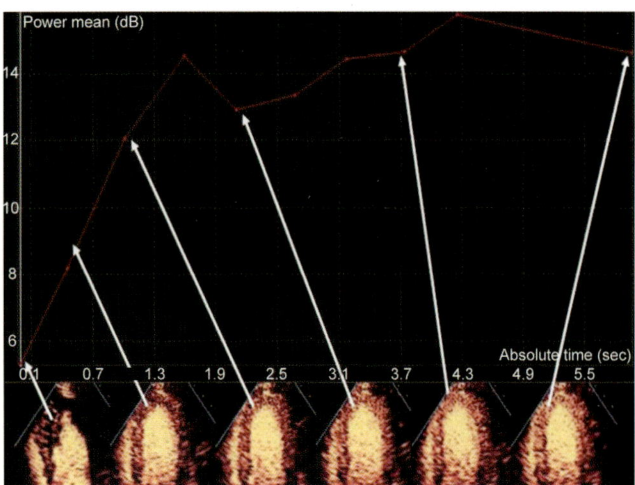


**Figure 6.8:** Myocardial perfusion. The raw signal intensity data from the apical septal segment is plotted against time after destruction.

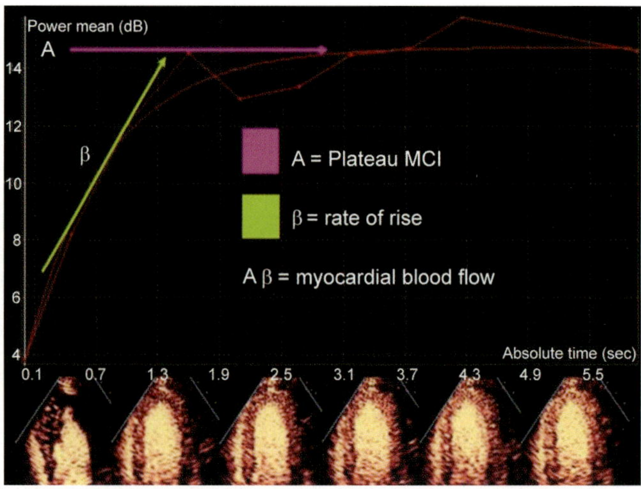


**Figure 6.9:** An exponential function curve is applied to allow calculation of A, β, and Aβ.
*Abbreviation:* MCI, myocardial contrast intensity.

of the volume of blood within the capillaries and the blood flow velocity.[46] Ninety percent of myocardial blood volume is contained at the capillary level.[106] Contrast microbubbles are ideal flow tracers as they are contained within the intravascular space and are able to circulate through the microvasculature. A method for quantification of MBF was first published by Wei et al.[11] The investigators administered a continuous intravenous infusion of microbubble contrast at a constant rate to obtain a steady state, delivered high-intensity ultrasound pulses to cause microbubble destruction, and then measured the reappearance rate using a time-intensity curve.[11] The rate of contrast replenishment represents mean MBF velocity (β) and can be extrapolated from the slope of the time-intensity curve while the peak plateau video intensity (A) reflects the microvasculature cross-sectional area. Therefore, for a constant ultrasound beam thickness or elevation, the product of A ($cm^2$) × β (cm/sec) equates to MBF (mL/sec) **(Figure 6.8 and 6.9)**.[107,108] Imaging during the reappearance phase can be performed with intermittent (high-MI) or continuous (low-MI) imaging techniques as previously discussed. Normal contrast replenishment by qualitative visual assessment is defined as homogenous enhancement within 5 seconds following microbubble destruction at rest or within 2 seconds at stress.[107] The rate and intensity of contrast reappearance would be reduced in the context of a hemodynamically significant coronary artery stenosis where the flow limitation exceeds the coronary flow reserve.

The main roles of MCE for evaluation of MBF have been in the diagnosis of underlying stable coronary artery disease, risk stratification in acute coronary syndromes, and assessment for myocardial viability. The MCE has been repeatedly demonstrated to offer comparable concordance with or noninferiority to $^{99m}$Tc-sestamibi single-photon emission computed tomography (SPECT) on resting, exercise and pharmacologic stress for the detection of coronary artery disease.[46,106,109] The MCE for myocardial perfusion was found to be more accurate than wall motion analysis in detecting significant coronary artery disease, and Shimoni et al. suggested that the combination of MCE and wall motion analysis offered the optimal balance of sensitivity (86%), specificity (88%), and accuracy (86%).[110,111] Tsuitsui et al. further went on to show the incremental prognostic benefit of myocardial perfusion by MCE over standard clinical risk assessment and wall motion analysis for coronary artery disease during DSE. The 3-year event free survival was 95% when both wall motion and perfusion were normal, 82% when wall motion was normal but perfusion was abnormal, and 68% when both were abnormal.[112]

In the acute setting, the consensus definition of myocardial infarction requires fulfilment of evidence of myonecrosis (rise and/or fall in biomarkers) and at least one of consistent clinical symptoms, electrocardiographic changes, imaging evidence of myocardial damage, or the presence of intracoronary thrombus at time of cardiac catheterization.[113] Contrast LVO and MCE has been studied in a prospective cohort of patients presenting to the emergency department with potential acute coronary syndromes and was found to provide 17% incremental information by composite scores for prediction of cardiac events beyond standard clinical and electrocardiographic assessment.[114] The same group of investigators and others have also applied the thrombolysis in myocardial infarction risk score to this group of patients and confirmed the additional value of LVO and MCE.[115,116] The proposed benefit was earlier triaging of these patients with chest pain, and no diagnostic electrocardiographic changes before the availability of cardiac biomarker results that are inherently delayed. Contrast enhanced wall motion analysis and myocardial perfusion also has excellent concordance with SPECT imaging in assessment of acute coronary syndrome patients in the emergency room.[117] Finally, in the postmyocardial infarction phase, MCE had equivalent sensitivity to Thallium 201 scintigraphy scintigraphy (90% and 92%, respectively) but higher specificity (63% and 45%, respectively) for the identification of hibernating myocardium and therefore predict functional recovery following revascularization.[118] The extent of infarction or residual myocardial viability assessed by MCE following a presentation with an acute myocardial infarction has also been an independent predictor of cardiac death and/or nonfatal reinfarction and LV remodeling.[119,120] The highlighted benefit of MCE for viability assessment over other imaging modalities (radionuclide perfusion imaging and cMRI) is the relative portability of echocardiography and also the ability of MCE to assess viability at rest, without the need for DSE, and with a higher level of sensitivity.

### Cardiac Structural Interventions

Hypertrophic obstructive cardiomyopathy is associated with asymmetrical septal hypertrophy and systolic anterior motion (SAM) of the mitral valve apparatus. This combination of pathological features results in a dynamic intraventricular or LV outflow tract obstruction or gradient. Alcohol septal ablation or chemical myectomy was introduced as a method of treatment for patients with HCM almost 15 or 20 years ago.[121] The intracoronary injection of 100% ethanol into the septal perforator branch of the left anterior descending artery, produces a controlled myocardial injury and infarction in the septum, resulting in a reduction of the septal thickness and the obstruction. However, the feasibility and success of this procedure depend on correctly identifying the septal perforator branch supplying the SAM–septal contact point on echocardiography and defining the region of myocardium supplied to quantify the extent of injury likely to be produced.

MCE has been used to guide the procedure and quantify the myocardial perfusion from the targeted septal perforator branch before the injection of intracoronary alcohol. However, despite its recognized role and safety,[122] the intra-arterial injection of ultrasound contrast agents remains an off-label use of the agent. An alternate approach adopted by many interventionalists is the use of agitated radiocontrast to opacify the myocardium supplied by the septal branch to guide the procedure.

## AGITATED SALINE CONTRAST

Despite all the advances in the newer generation microbubble ultrasound contrast agents, agitated saline contrast remains a key tool for the screening and diagnosis of intracardiac right-to-left shunts, intrapulmonary shunts (e.g. pulmonary arteriovenous malformations) and persistent left-sided superior vena cava (where bilateral upper limb intravenous injections should be performed). This method of bolus air microbubble contrast uses the "limitation" of the large injected bubbles being unable to transit across the pulmonary circulation into the left heart in the absence of an anatomical shunt.

A recommended method of preparation of the saline contrast is the use of 8 mL of sterile saline with 1 mL of air and 1 mL of the patient's blood drawn into a 10 mL syringe, connected via a 3-way stopcock to another 10 mL syringe, and then "agitating" the mixture by maximally pushing the contents from one to the another back and forth.[15,123-125] This cocktail produces better contrast enhancement in comparison to a simple air-saline combination alone. Alternatively, an admixture of air and intravenous colloid sterile solutions can also be used following the same agitation process. Following a forceful injection of the admixture into a peripheral vein, the appearance of bubbles within the left heart within 3 (up to 5) cardiac cycles following complete right atrial opacification is suggestive of an interatrial shunt [patent foramen ovale (PFO) or atrial septal defect]. Confirming the simultaneous leftward septal bowing and dense contrast filling the area adjacent to the right atrial aspect of interatrial septum is necessary to assess the diagnostic adequacy of the bubble study.[125] Late appearance of bubbles in the setting of a PFO may still occur in hypodynamic circulations, atrial fibrillation with atrial dilatation, or as a result of delayed spontaneous respirophasic (inspiratory) increase in right atrial pressure necessary for gradient reversal beyond the designated 3–5 cardiac cycles.[124] Conversely, large intrapulmonary shunts can also result in the early appearance of bubbles in the left heart. Interatrial shunting, especially in the case of PFOs, are dynamic and dependent on the relative difference between left and right atrial pressures, right and left ventricular diastolic pressures, respiration and the patient's intravascular status.[126,127]

Following a negative resting study, a proper Valsalva maneuver (forced expiration against a closed glottis) should be performed, ideally with a demonstrable leftward bulging of the interatrial septum on the release phase, to detect the presence of transient right-to-left shunting through a PFO that may have been otherwise interpreted as a false- negative finding.[128-130] Other common causes for false-negative studies include an inadequate Valsalva, elevated left heart filling pressures, reduced right atrial pressure due to intravascular depletion from preprocedural fasting, or the presence of a persistent eustachian valve "preventing" the inflow of contrast from an upper limb injection contacting the interatrial septum.[131] Where the Valsalva is suboptimal, coughing as a provocative measure can be considered as it has been demonstrated to induce the same hemodynamic reversal of the interatrial pressure gradient.[132] Femoral vein injection of contrast has been shown to improve the detection of PFOs due to a "streaming" effect where inferior vena caval flow is directed towards the fossa ovalis.[133] The trade-off for this increased sensitivity is the relatively invasive nature of femoral vein cannulation and thus limiting its use to select situations. All of the above are equally applicable to either TTE or TEE, although TEE with color Doppler and contrast enhancement is regarded as the gold standard for assessment of interatrial shunts, especially in the era of percutaneous device closures, meticulous preparation, and performance of the saline contrast study as well as repeated injections (recommended up to 5 and with the Valsalva maneuver) are still prerequisites to ensure the highest diagnostic sensitivity.[134-136] Residual shunts following device closure can also be assessed with the same approach. The mixture of 10% air–10% blood–80% saline agitated admixture can also be used to enhance suboptimal continuous wave Doppler TR signals for the estimation of PASP resulting in excellent correlation (r = 0.92) with invasive hemodynamic measurements.[137] Lastly, agitated saline contrast can also be used during echocardiographic-guided pericardiocentesis procedures to safely confirm the correct position of the sheath within the pericardial space.[138,139]

## CONCLUSION

Microbubble contrast enhancement where indicated for LVO (LVEF quantification or assessment of LV structural abnormalities) and improvement of EBD (during resting and stress echocardiography) should be the standard care in all echocardiography laboratories. Contrast enhancement improves the accuracy, reproducibility, and confidence of reading physicians with proven cost-effectiveness and cost-savings by reducing the need for downstream investigations as a result of nondiagnostic studies. Microbubble contrast agents can be safely and efficiently used by credentialed sonographers and accredited echocardiographers with the implementation of simple contrast-specific imaging protocols.

## VIDEO LEGENDS

**Video 6.1:** (A) Standard 2D apical 4-chamber view demonstrating an aneurysmal left ventricular apex with near-field clutter and a possible apical thrombus. (B) Contrast enhancement confirming the presence of an intraluminal filling defect in the apical lateral region consistent with an intracavitary thrombus.

**Video 6.2:** (A) 2D transesophageal echocardiographic assessment of the left atrial appendage demonstrating an echodensity suspicious for a thrombus. (B) Off-label use of Definity contrast confirms the presence of an intraluminal filling defect at the base of the left atrial appendage consistent with a thrombus with a layered extension to the opening of the appendage.

**Video 6.3:** (A) 2D transesophageal echocardiographic assessment demonstrating an echodensity in the left atrial appendage suspicious for a potential thrombus in the setting of suboptimal anticoagulation. (B) Definity contrast was administered resulting in full opacification of the left atrial appendage with no evidence of a filling defect to suggest thrombus. The patient was successfully cardioverted with no adverse outcome.

**Video 6.4:** (A) Standard 2D apical 4-chamber view with suboptimal endocardial definition and poor delineation of the left ventricular apex. (B) Contrast enhancement demonstrating hypertrophy of the apical myocardium with the classic end-diastolic spade-shaped appearance of apical hypertrophic cardiomyopathy.

**Video 6.5:** (A) Standard 2D apical 4-chamber view demonstrating an ill-defined echodensity at the left ventricular apex. (B) Contrast enhanced focused apical view revealing the prominent trabeculae and deep intertrabecular recesses typical of noncompaction cardiomyopathy.

**Video 6.6:** (A) Standard 2D apical 4-chamber view with color Doppler demonstrating a communication between the left ventricular cavity and an echo-free extracardiac collection through the anterolateral wall. (B) Contrast extravasation through a narrow neck consistent with a left ventricular free wall rupture or pseudoaneurysm.

## REFERENCES


1. Mulvagh SL, Rakowski H, Vannan MA, Abdelmoneim SS, Becher H, Bierig SM, et al. American Society of Echocardiography Consensus Statement on the Clinical Applications of Ultrasonic Contrast Agents in Echocardiography. J Am Soc Echocardiogr. 2008;21(11):1179-201.
2. Senior R, Becher H, Monaghan M, Agati L, Zamorano J, Vanoverschelde JL, et al. Contrast echocardiography: evidence-based recommendations by European Association of Echocardiography. Eur J Echocardiogr. 2009;10(2):194-212.
3. Douglas PS, Garcia MJ, Haines DE, Lai WW, Manning WJ, Patel AR, et al. ACCF/ASE/AHA/ASNC/HFSA/HRS/SCAI/SCCM/SCCT/SCMR 2011 Appropriate Use Criteria for Echocardiography. A Report of the American College of Cardiology Foundation Appropriate Use Criteria Task Force, American Society of Echocardiography, American Heart Association, American Society of Nuclear Cardiology, Heart Failure Society of America, Heart Rhythm Society, Society for Cardiovascular Angiography and Interventions, Society of Critical Care Medicine, Society of Cardiovascular Computed Tomography, and Society for Cardiovascular Magnetic Resonance Endorsed by the American College of Chest Physicians. J Am Coll Cardiol. 2011;57(9):1126-66. doi: 10.1016/j.jacc.2010.11.002
4. Feinstein SB, Cheirif J, Cate Ten FJ, et al. Safety and efficacy of a new transpulmonary ultrasound contrast agent: initial multicenter clinical results. J Am Coll Cardiol. 1990; 16(2):316-24.
5. Nanda NC. History of echocardiographic contrast agents. Clin Cardiol. 1997;10 (Suppl 1):I7-11.
6. Kaul S. Myocardial contrast echocardiography: 15 years of research and development. Circulation. 1997;96(10):3745-60.
7. McCulloch M, Gresser C, Moos S, Odabashian J, Jasper S, Bednarz J, et al. Ultrasound contrast physics: A series on contrast echocardiography, article 3. J Am Soc Echocardiogr. 2000;13(10):959-67.
8. Raisinghani A, DeMaria AN. Physical principles of microbubble ultrasound contrast agents. Am J Cardiol. 2002;90(10A): 3J-7J.
9. Mulvagh SL, DeMaria AN, Feinstein SB, Burns PN, Kaul S, Miller JG, et al. Contrast echocardiography: current and future applications. J Am Soc Echocardiogr. 2000;13(4):331-42.
10. Allen MR, Pellikka PA, Villarraga HR, Klarich KW, Foley DA, Mulvagh SL, et al. Harmonic imaging: echocardiographic enhanced contrast intensity and duration. Int J Card Imaging. 1999;15(3):215-20.
11. Wei K, Jayaweera AR, Firoozan S, Linka A, Skyba DM, Kaul S. Quantification of myocardial blood flow with ultrasound-induced destruction of microbubbles administered as a constant venous infusion. Circulation. 1998;97(5):473-83.
12. Tiemann K, Lohmeier S, Kuntz S, Köster J, Pohl C, Burns P, et al. Real-Time Contrast Echo Assessment of Myocardial Perfusion at Low Emission Power: First Experimental and Clinical Results Using Power Pulse Inversion Imaging. Echocardiography. 1999;16(8):799-809.
13. Sieswerda GT, Yang L, Boo MB-D, Kamp O. Real-time perfusion imaging: a new echocardiographic technique for simultaneous evaluation of myocardial perfusion and contraction. Echocardiography. 2003;20(6):545-55.
14. Yu EH, Sloggett CE, Iwanochko RM, Rakowski H, Siu SC. Feasibility and accuracy of left ventricular volumes and ejection fraction determination by fundamental, tissue harmonic, and intravenous contrast imaging in difficult-to-image patients. J Am Soc Echocardiogr. 2000;13(3):216-24.
15. Porter TR, Abdelmoneim S, Belcik JT, McCulloch ML, Mulvagh SL, Olson JJ, et al. Guidelines for the cardiac sonographer in the performance of contrast echocardiography: a focused update from the American Society of Echocardiography. J Am Soc Echocardiogr. 2014;27(8):797-810.
16. Lang RM, Badano LP, Mor-Avi V, Afilalo J, Armstrong A, Ernande L, et al. Recommendations for cardiac chamber quantification by echocardiography in adults: an update from the American Society of Echocardiography and the European Association of Cardiovascular Imaging. J Am Soc Echocardiogr. 2015;28(1): 1-39.e14.
17. Pellikka PA, Nagueh SF, Elhendy AA, Kuehl CA, Sawada SG. American Society of Echocardiography. American Society of Echocardiography recommendations for performance, interpretation, and application of stress echocardiography. J Am Soc Echocardiogr. 2007;20(9):1021-41.
18. Shaw LJ, Gillam L, Feinstein S, et al. Use of an intravenous contrast agent (Optison) to enhance echocardiography: efficacy and cost implications. Optison Multicenter Study Group. Am J Manag Care. 1998;4 Spec No:SP169-76.
19. Yong Y, Wu D, Fernandes V, Kopelen HA, Shimoni S, Nagueh SF, et al. Diagnostic accuracy and cost-effectiveness of contrast echocardiography on evaluation of cardiac function in technically very difficult patients in the intensive care unit. Am J Cardiol. 2002;89(6):711-8.
20. Thanigaraj S, Nease RF, Schechtman KB, Wade RL, Loslo S, Pérez JE. Use of contrast for image enhancement during stress echocardiography is cost-effective and reduces additional diagnostic testing. Am J Cardiol. 2001;87(12):1430-2.
21. Main ML, Goldman JH, Grayburn PA. Thinking outside the "box-"the ultrasound contrast controversy. J Am Coll Cardiol. 2007;50(25):2434-7.
22. Kusnetzky LL, Khalid A, Khumri TM, Moe TG, Jones PG, et al. Acute mortality in hospitalized patients undergoing echocardiography with and without an ultrasound contrast agent: results in 18,671 consecutive studies. J Am Coll Cardiol. 2008;51(17):1704-6.
23. Wei K, Mulvagh SL, Carson L, Davidoff R, Gabriel R, Grimm RA, et al. The safety of deFinity and Optison for ultrasound image

enhancement: a retrospective analysis of 78,383 administered contrast doses. J Am Soc Echocardiogr. 2008;21(11):1202-6.

24. Main ML, Ryan AC, Davis TE, Albano MP, Kusnetzky LL, Hibberd M. Acute mortality in hospitalized patients undergoing echocardiography with and without an ultrasound contrast agent (multicenter registry results in 4,300,966 consecutive patients). Am J Cardiol. 2008;102(12):1742-6.
25. Dolan MS, Gala SS, Dodla S, Abdelmoneim SS, Xie F, Cloutier D, et al. Safety and efficacy of commercially available ultrasound contrast agents for rest and stress echocardiography a multicenter experience. J Am Coll Cardiol. 2009;53(1):32-8.
26. Khawaja OA, Shaikh KA, Al-Mallah MH. Meta-analysis of adverse cardiovascular events associated with echocardiographic contrast agents. Am J Cardiol. 2010;106(5):742-7.
27. Timperley J, Mitchell ARJ, Thibault H, Mirza IH, Becher H. Safety of contrast dobutamine stress echocardiography: a single center experience. J Am Soc Echocardiogr. 2005;18(2):163-7.
28. Shaikh K, Chang SM, Peterson L, Rosendahl-Garcia K, Quinones MA, Nagueh SF, et al. Safety of contrast administration for endocardial enhancement during stress echocardiography compared with noncontrast stress. Am J Cardiol. 2008;102(11):1444-50.
29. Abdelmoneim SS, Bernier M, Scott CG, Dhoble A, Ness SAC, Hagen ME, et al. Safety of contrast agent use during stress echocardiography in patients with elevated right ventricular systolic pressure: a cohort study. Circulation: Cardiovascular Imaging. 2010;3(3):240-8.
30. Wei K, Main ML, Lang RM, Klein A, Angeli S, Panetta C, et al. The effect of Definity on systemic and pulmonary hemodynamics in patients. J Am Soc Echocardiogr. 2012;25(5):584-8.
31. Wever-Pinzon O, Suma V, Ahuja A, Romero J, Sareen N, Henry SA, et al. Safety of echocardiographic contrast in hospitalized patients with pulmonary hypertension: a multi-center study. European Heart J Cardiovasc Imag. 2012;13(10):857-62.
32. Lindner JL, Wei K. Action or over-reaction. J Am Coll Cardiol. 2008.
33. Bhatia VK, Senior R. Contrast echocardiography: evidence for clinical use. J Am Soc Echocardiogr. 2008.
34. Parker JM, Weller MW, Feinstein LM, Adams RJ, Main ML, Grayburn PA, et al. Safety of ultrasound contrast agents in patients with known or suspected cardiac shunts. Am J Cardiol. 2013;112(7):1039-45.
35. Gersh BJ, Maron BJ, Bonow RO, et al. 2011 ACCF/AHA Guideline for the Diagnosis and Treatment of Hypertrophic Cardiomyopathy: a report of the American College of Cardiology Foundation/American Heart Association Task Force on Practice Guidelines. Developed in collaboration with the American Association for Thoracic Surgery, American Society of Echocardiography, American Society of Nuclear Cardiology, Heart Failure Society of America, Heart Rhythm Society, Society for Cardiovascular Angiography and Interventions, and Society of Thoracic Surgeons. J Am Coll Cardiol. 2011;58(25):e212-60. doi: 10.1016/j.jacc.2011.06.011. Epub 2011 Nov 8.
36. Authors/Task Force members, Elliott PM, Anastasakis A, Borger MA, Borggrefe M, Cecchi F, et al. 2014 ESC Guidelines on diagnosis and management of hypertrophic cardiomyopathy: the Task Force for the Diagnosis and Management of Hypertrophic Cardiomyopathy of the European Society of Cardiology (ESC). Euro Heart J. 2014; pp. 2733-79.
37. Waggoner AD, Ehler D, Adams D, Moos S, Rosenbloom J, Gresser C, et al. Guidelines for the cardiac sonographer in the performance of contrast echocardiography: recommendations of the American Society of Echocardiography Council on Cardiac Sonography. Journal of the American Society of Echocardiography : official publication of the American Society of Echocardiography. 2001; pp. 417-20.
38. Ryan T, Armstrong WF, Khandheria BK. American Society of Echocardiography. Task force 4: training in echocardiography endorsed by the American Society of Echocardiography. J Am Coll Cardiol. 2008. pp. 361-7.
39. Moos S, Odabashian J, Jasper S, Bednarz J, Burgess P, Carney D, et al. Incorporating ultrasound contrast in the laboratory: a series on contrast echocardiography, article 1. J Am Soc Echocardiogr. 2000; 13(3):240-7.
40. Burgess P, Moore V, Bednarz J, Carney D, Floer S, Gresser C, et al. Performing an echocardiographic examination with a contrast agent: a series on contrast echocardiography, article 2. J Am Soc Echocardiogr. 2000;13(6):629-34.
41. Castello R, Bella JN, Rovner A, Swan J, Smith J, Shaw L. Efficacy and time-efficiency of a "sonographer-driven" contrast echocardiography protocol in a high-volume echocardiography laboratory. Am Heart J. 2003;145(3):535-41.
42. Lester SJ, Miller FA, Khandheria BK. Contrast echocardiography: beyond a black box warning? J Am Soc Echocardiogr. 2008;21(5):417-8.
43. Witt S. Implementing microbubble contrast in the echocardiography laboratory: a sonographer's perspective. Am J Cardiol. 2002.
44. Weissman NJ, Cohen MC, Hack TC, Gillam LD, Cohen JL, Kitzman DW. Infusion versus bolus contrast echocardiography: a multicenter, open-label, crossover trial. Am Heart J. 2000; 139(3):399-404.
45. Kuersten B, Nahar T, Vannan MA. Methods of contrast administration for myocardial perfusion imaging: continuous infusion versus bolus injection. Am J Cardiol. 2002;90(10A): 35J-37J.
46. Senior R, Monaghan M, Main ML, Zamorano JL, Tiemann K, Agati L, et al. Detection of coronary artery disease with perfusion stress echocardiography using a novel ultrasound imaging agent: two Phase 3 international trials in comparison with radionuclide perfusion imaging. Eur J Echocardiogr. 2009;10(1):26-35.
47. Witt SA, McCulloch M, Sisk E, Gresser C, Moos S, Odabashian J, et al. Achieving a diagnostic contrast-enhanced echocardiogram: a series on contrast echocardiography, article 4. J Am Soc Echocardiogr. 2001;14(4):327-34.
48. Chong A, Haluska B, Wahi S. Clinical application and laboratory protocols for performing contrast echocardiography. Ind Heart J. 2013;65(3):337-46.
49. Stewart MJ. Contrast echocardiography. Heart. 2003;89(3): 342-8.
50. Jessup M, Abraham WT, Casey DE, Feldman AM, Francis GS, Ganiats TG, et al. 2009 focused update: ACCF/AHA Guidelines for the Diagnosis and Management of Heart Failure in Adults: areport of the American College of Cardiology Foundation/

American Heart Association Task Force on Practice Guidelines: developed in collaboration with the International Society for Heart and Lung Transplantation. Circulation. 2009;119(14):1977-2016.

51. Epstein AE, DiMarco JP, Ellenbogen KA, Estes NA 3rd, Freedman RA, Gettes LS, et al. 2012 ACCF/AHA/HRS focused update incorporated into the ACCF/AHA/HRS 2008 guidelines for device-based therapy of cardiac rhythm abnormalities: a report of the American College of Cardiology Foundation/American Heart Association Task Force on Practice Guidelines and the Heart Rhythm Society. J Am Coll Cardiol. 2013; 61(3):e6-75.
52. Bovelli D, Plataniotis G, Roila F, ESMO Guidelines Working Group. Cardiotoxicity of chemotherapeutic agents and radiotherapy-related heart disease: ESMO Clinical Practice Guidelines. Annals of oncology: official Journal of the European Society for Medical Oncology/ESMO. 2010; pp. v277-82.
53. Hundley WG, Kizilbash AM, Afridi I, Franco F, Peshock RM, Grayburn PA. Administration of an intravenous perfluorocarbon contrast agent improves echocardiographic determination of left ventricular volumes and ejection fraction: comparison with cine magnetic resonance imaging. J Am Coll Cardiol. 1998;32(5):1426-32.
54. Nahar T, Croft L, Shapiro R, Fruchtman S, Diamond J, Henzlova M, et al. Comparison of four echocardiographic techniques for measuring left ventricular ejection fraction. Am J Cardiol. 2000;86(12):1358-62.
55. Dias BF, Eric HC, Sloggett CE, Iwanochko RM, Rakowski H, Siu SC. Contrast-enhanced quantitation of left ventricular ejection fraction: what is the best method? J Am Soc Echocardiogr. 2001;14(12):1183-90.
56. Hoffmann R, Bardeleben von S, Cate ten F, Adrian C Borges, Jaroslaw Kasprzak, Christian Firschke, et al. Assessment of systolic left ventricular function: a multi-centre comparison of cineventriculography, cardiac magnetic resonance imaging, unenhanced and contrast-enhanced echocardiography. Eur Heart J. 2005;26(Issue 6):607-16.
57. Lim TK, Burden L, Janardhanan R, Ping C. Improved accuracy of low-power contrast echocardiography for the assessment of left ventricular remodeling compared with unenhanced harmonic echocardiography. J Am Coll Echocarrdiogr. 2005.
58. Malm S, Frigstad S, Sagberg E, Larsson H, Skjaerpe T. Accurate and reproducible measurement of left ventricular volume and ejection fraction by contrast echocardiography: a comparison with magnetic resonance imaging. J Am Coll Cardiol. 2004;44(5):1030-5.
59. Freeman AP, Giles RW, Walsh WF, Fisher R, Murray IP, Wilcken DE. Regional left ventricular wall motion assessment: comparison of two-dimensional echocardiography and radionuclide angiography with contrast angiography in healed myocardial infarction. Am J Cardiol. 1985.56(1):8-12.
60. Grayburn PA, Mulvagh S, Crouse L. Left ventricular opacification at rest and during stress. Am J Cardiol. 2002; 90(10A): 21J-27J.
61. Crouse LJ, Cheirif J, Hanly DE, Kisslo JA, Labovitz AJ, Raichlen JS, et al. Opacification and border delineation improvement in patients with suboptimal endocardial border definition in routine echocardiography: results of the Phase III Albunex Multicenter Trial. J Am Coll Cardiol. 1993;22(5):1494-500.
62. Lindner JR, Dent JM, Moos SP, Jayaweera AR, Kaul S. Enhancement of left ventricular cavity opacification by harmonic imaging after venous injection of Albunex. Am J Cardiol. 1997;79(12):1657-62.
63. Daniel GK, Chawla MK, Sawada SG, Gradus-Pizlo I, Feigenbaum H, Segar DS. Echocardiographic imaging of technically difficult patients in the intensive care unit: use of optison in combination with fundamental and harmonic imaging. J Am Soc Echocardiogr. 2001;14(9):917-20.
64. Sorrell VL, Ross WD, Kumar S, Kalra N. Left ventricular endocardial and epicardial border length delineation with perflutren contrast during transthoracic echocardiography. Echocardiography. 2011; 28(7):761-6.
65. Kitzman DW, Goldman ME, Gillam LD, Cohen JL, Aurigemma GP, Gottdiener JS. Efficacy and safety of the novel ultrasound contrast agent perflutren (definity) in patients with suboptimal baseline left ventricular echocardiographic images. Am J Cardiol. 2000;86(6):669-74.
66. Reilly JP, Tunick PA, Timmermans RJ, Stein B, Rosenzweig BP, Kronzon I. Contrast echocardiography clarifies uninterpretable wall motion in intensive care unit patients. J Am Coll Cardiol. 2000;35(2):485-90.
67. Nguyen TT, Dhond MR, Sabapathy R, Bommer WJ. Contrast microbubbles improve diagnostic yield in ICU patients with poor echocardiographic windows. Chest. 2001;120(4): 1287-92.
68. Costa JM, Tsutsui JM, Nozawa E, Morhy SS, Andrade JL, Ramires JF, et al. Contrast echocardiography can save nondiagnostic exams in mechanically ventilated patients. Echocardiography. 2005;22(5):389-94.
69. Fleisher LA, Beckman JA, Brown KA. 2009 ACCF/AHA focused update on perioperative beta blockade incorporated into the ACC/AHA 2007 guidelines on perioperative cardiovascular evaluation and care for noncardiac surgery. J Am Coll Cardiol. 2009;54(22):e13-e118.
70. Marwick TH, Nemec JJ, Pashkow FJ, Stewart WJ, et al. Accuracy and limitations of exercise echocardiography in a routine clinical setting. Journal of the American College of Cardiology. 1992;19(1):74-81.
71. Hoffmann R, Lethen H, Marwick T, Arnese M, Fioretti P, Pingitore A, et al. Analysis of interinstitutional observer agreement in interpretation of dobutamine stress echocardiograms. J Am Coll Cardiol. 1996;27(2):330-6.
72. Porter TR, Xie F, Kricsfeld A, et al. Improved endocardial border resolution during dobutamine stress echocardiography with intravenous sonicated dextrose albumin. J Am Coll Cardiol. 1994;23(6):1440-3.
73. Falcone RA, Marcovitz PA, Pérez JE, Dittrich HC, Hopkins WE, Armstrong WF. Intravenous albunex during dobutamine stress echocardiography: enhanced localization of left ventricular endocardial borders. Am Heart J. 1995;130(2):254-8.
74. Rainbird AJ, Mulvagh SL, Oh JK, McCully RB, Klarich KW, Shub C, et al. Contrast dobutamine stress echocardiography: clinical practice assessment in 300 consecutive patients. J Am Soc Echocardiogr. 2001;14(5):378-85.

75. Dolan MS, Riad K, El-Shafei A, Puri S, Tamirisa K, Bierig M, et al. Effect of intravenous contrast for left ventricular opacification and border definition on sensitivity and specificity of dobutamine stress echocardiography compared with coronary angiography in technically difficult patients. Am Heart J. 2001;142(5):908-15.
76. Senior R, Dwivedi G, Hayat S. Clinical benefits of contrast-enhanced echocardiography during rest and stress examinations. Eur J Echocardiogr. 2005;Suppl 2:S6-13.
77. Wake R, Takeuchi M, Yoshitani H, Miyazaki C, Otani S, Yoshiyama M, et al. Role of contrast-enhanced dobutamine stress echocardiography in predicting outcome in patients with known or suspected coronary artery disease. Echocardiography. 2006;23(8):642-9.
78. Plana JC, Mikati IA, Dokainish H, Lakkis N, Abukhalil J, Davis R, et al. A randomized cross-over study for evaluation of the effect of image optimization with contrast on the diagnostic accuracy of dobutamine echocardiography in coronary artery disease The OPTIMIZE Trial. JACC Cardiovasc Imaging. 2008;1(2):145-52.
79. Jung PH, Rieber J, Störk S, Hoyer C, Erhardt I, Nowotny A, et al. Effect of contrast application on interpretability and diagnostic value of dobutamine stress echocardiography in patients with intermediate coronary lesions: comparison with myocardial fractional flow reserve. Eur Heart J. 2008;29(20):2536-43.
80. Gottdiener JS, Gay JA, VanVoorhees L, DiBianco R, Fletcher RD. Frequency and embolic potential of left ventricular thrombus in dilated cardiomyopathy: assessment by 2-dimensional echocardiography. Am J Cardiol. 1983;52(10):1281-5.
81. Kontny F, Dale J, Hegrenaes L, Lem P, Søberg T, Morstøl T. Left ventricular thrombosis and arterial embolism after thrombolysis in acute anterior myocardial infarction: predictors and effects of adjunctive antithrombotic therapy. Eur Heart J. 1993;14(11):1489-92.
82. Thanigaraj S, Schechtman KB, Pérez JE. Improved echocardiographic delineation of left ventricular thrombus with the use of intravenous second-generation contrast image enhancement. J Am Soc Echocardiogr. 1999;12(12):1022-6.
83. Weinsaft JW, Kim RJ, Ross M. Contrast-enhanced anatomic imaging as compared to contrast-enhanced tissue characterization for detection of left ventricular thrombus. JACC. 2009.
84. Kirkpatrick JN, Wong T, Bednarz JE, Spencer KT, Sugeng L, Ward RP, et al. Differential diagnosis of cardiac masses using contrast echocardiographic perfusion imaging. J Am Coll Cardiol. 2004;43(8):1412-9.
85. Louie EK, Maron BJ. Apical hypertrophic cardiomyopathy: clinical and two-dimensional echocardiographic assessment. Ann Intern Med. 1987;106(5):663-70.
86. Eriksson MJ, Sonnenberg B, Woo A, Rakowski P, Parker TG, Wigle ED, et al. Long-term outcome in patients with apical hypertrophic cardiomyopathy. J Am Coll Cardiol. 2002;39(4):638-45.
87. Soman P, Swinburn J, Callister M, Stephens NG, Senior R. Apical hypertrophic cardiomyopathy: bedside diagnosis by intravenous contrast echocardiography. J Am Soc Echocardiogr. 2001;14(4):311-3.
88. Thanigaraj S, Pérez JE. Apical hypertrophic cardiomyopathy: echocardiographic diagnosis with the use of intravenous contrast image enhancement. J Am Soc Echocardiogr. 2000;13(2):146-9.
89. Maron BJ, Towbin JA, Thiene G, Antzelevitch C, Corrado D, Arnett D, et al. Contemporary definitions and classification of the cardiomyopathies: an American Heart Association Scientific Statement from the Council on Clinical Cardiology, Heart Failure and Transplantation Committee; Quality of Care and Outcomes Research and Functional Genomics and Translational Biology Interdisciplinary Working Groups; and Council on Epidemiology and Prevention. Circulation. 2006;113(14):1807-16.
90. Engberding R, Bender F. Identification of a rare congenital anomaly of the myocardium by two-dimensional echocardiography: persistence of isolated myocardial sinusoids. Am J Cardiol. 1984;53(11):1733-4.
91. Elliott P, Andersson B, Arbustini E, Bilinska Z, Cecchi F, Charron P, et al. Classification of the cardiomyopathies: a position statement from the European Society of Cardiology Working Group on Myocardial and Pericardial Diseases. Eur Heart J. 2008;29(2):270-6.
92. Jenni R, Oechslin E, Schneider J, et al. Echocardiographic and pathoanatomical characteristics of isolated left ventricular non-compaction: a step towards classification as a distinct cardiomyopathy. Heart. 2001;86(6):666-71.
93. Petersen SE, Selvanayagam JB, Wiesmann F, Robson MD, Francis JM, Anderson RH, et al. Left ventricular non-compaction: insights from cardiovascular magnetic resonance imaging. J Am Coll Cardiol. 2005;46(1):101-5.
94. Koo BK, Choi D, Ha J-W, Kang S-M, Chung N, Cho S-Y. Isolated noncompaction of the ventricular myocardium: contrast echocardiographic findings and review of the literature. Echocardiography. 2002;19(2):153-6.
95. Chow C-M, Lim K-D, Wu L, et al. Images in cardiovascular medicine. Isolated left ventricular noncompaction enhanced by echocontrast agent. Circulation. 2007;116(4):e90-1.
96. Brown SL, Gropler RJ, Harris KM. Distinguishing left ventricular aneurysm from pseudoaneurysm. A review of the literature. Chest. 1997;111(5):1403-9.
97. Thanigaraj S, Pérez JE. Diagnosis of cardiac rupture with the use of contrast-enhanced echocardiography. J Am Soc Echocardiogr. 2000;13(9):862-5.
98. Moreno R, Zamorano JL, Almería C, Rodrigo JL, Villate A, Serra V, et al. Usefulness of contrast agents in the diagnosis of left ventricular pseudoaneurysm after acute myocardial infarction. Eur J Echocardiogr. 2002;3(2):111-6.
99. Mittle S, Makaryus AN, Mangion J. Role of contrast echocardiography in the assessment of myocardial rupture. Echocardiography. 2003;20(1):77-81.
100. Yeo TC, Dujardin KS, Tei C, et al. Value of a Doppler-derived index combining systolic and diastolic time intervals in predicting outcome in primary pulmonary hypertension. Am J Cardiol. 1998;81(9):1157-61.
101. Byrd BF, O'Kelly BF, Schiller NB. Contrast echocardiography enhances tricuspid but not mitral regurgitation. Clin Cardiol. 1991;14(11 Suppl 5):V10-4.
102. Baumgartner H, Otto CM. Aortic Stenosis Severity. J Am Coll Cardiol. 2009;54(11):1012-3.

103. Rosenhek R, Zilberszac R, Schemper M, Czerny M, Mundigler G, Graf S, et al. Natural history of very severe aortic stenosis. Circulation. 2010;121(1):151-6.
104. Nakatani S, Imanishi T, Terasawa A, Beppu S, Nagata S, Miyatake K. Clinical application of transpulmonary contrast-enhanced Doppler technique in the assessment of severity of aortic stenosis. J Am Coll Cardiol. 1992;20(4):973-8.
105. Dwivedi G, Hickman M, Senior R. Accurate assessment of aortic stenosis with intravenous contrast. Eur J Echocardiogr. 2006;7(2):165-7.
106. Kaul S, Jayaweera AR. Coronary and myocardial blood volumes: noninvasive tools to assess the coronary microcirculation? Circulation. 1997;96(3):719-24.
107. Dijkmans PA, Senior R, Becher H, Porter TR, Wei K, Visser CA, et al. Myocardial contrast echocardiography evolving as a clinically feasible technique for accurate, rapid, and safe assessment of myocardial perfusion: the evidence so far. J Am Coll Cardiol. 2006;48(11):2168-77.
108. Moir S, Marwick TH. Combination of contrast with stress echocardiography: A practical guide to methods and interpretation. Cardiovasc Ultrasound. 2004;2:15.
109. Jeetley P, Hickman M, Kamp O, Lang RM, Thomas JD, Vannan MA, et al. Myocardial contrast echocardiography for the detection of coronary artery stenosis: a prospective multicenter study in comparison with single-photon emission computed tomography. J Am Coll Cardiol. 2006;47(1):141-5.
110. Tsutsui JM, Elhendy A, Xie F, O'Leary EL, McGrain AC, Porter TR. Safety of dobutamine stress real-time myocardial contrast echocardiography. J Am Coll Cardiol. 2005;45(8): 1235-42.
111. Shimoni S, Zoghbi WA, Xie F, Kricsfeld D, Iskander S, Gobar L, et al. Real-time assessment of myocardial perfusion and wall motion during bicycle and treadmill exercise echocardiography: comparison with single photon emission computed tomography. J Am Coll Cardiol. 2001; 37(3):741-7.
112. Tsutsui JM, Elhendy A, Anderson JR, Xie F, McGrain AC, Porter TR. Prognostic value of dobutamine stress myocardial contrast perfusion echocardiography. Circulation. 2005;112(10): 1444-50.
113. Thygesen K, Alpert JS, Jaffe AS, Simoons ML, Chaitman BR, White HD, et al. Third universal definition of myocardial infarction. 2012; 2020-35.
114. Kaul S, Senior R, Firschke C, Wang X-Q, Lindner J, Villanueva FS, et al. Incremental value of cardiac imaging in patients presenting to the emergency department with chest pain and without ST-segment elevation: a multicenter study. Am Heart J. 2004;148(1):129-36.
115. Tong KL, Kaul S, Wang X-Q, Rinkevich D, Kalvaitis S, Belcik T, et al. Myocardial contrast echocardiography versus Thrombolysis In Myocardial Infarction score in patients presenting to the emergency department with chest pain and a nondiagnostic electrocardiogram. J Am Coll Cardiol. 2005;46(5):920-7.
116. Jeetley P, Burden L, Greaves K, et al. Prognostic value of myocardial contrast echocardiography in patients presenting to hospital with acute chest pain and negative troponin. Am J Cardiol. 2007;99(10):1369-73.
117. Kontos MC, Hinchman D, Cunningham M, Miller JJ, Cherif J, Nixon JV. Comparison of contrast echocardiography with single-photon emission computed tomographic myocardial perfusion imaging in the evaluation of patients with possible acute coronary syndromes in the emergency department. Am J Cardiol. 2003;91(9):1099-102.
118. Shimoni S, Frangogiannis NG, Aggeli CJ, Shan K, Verani MS, Quinones MA, et al. Identification of hibernating myocardium with quantitative intravenous myocardial contrast echocardiography: comparison with dobutamine echocardiography and thallium-201 scintigraphy. Circulation. 2003;107(4):538-44.
119. Dwivedi G, Janardhanan R, Hayat SA, et al. Prognostic value of myocardial viability detected by myocardial contrast echocardiography early after acute myocardial infarction. J Am Coll Cardiol. 2007;50(4):327-34.
120. Galiuto L, Garramone B, Scarà A, Rebuzzi AG, Crea F, La Torre G, et al. The extent of microvascular damage during myocardial contrast echocardiography is superior to other known indexes of post-infarct reperfusion in predicting left ventricular remodeling: results of the multicenter AMICI study. J Am Coll Cardiol. 2008; 51(5):552-9.
121. Faber L, Seggewiss H, Gleichmann U. Percutaneous transluminal septal myocardial ablation in hypertrophic obstructive cardiomyopathy: results with respect to intra-procedural myocardial contrast echocardiography. Circulation. 1998;98(22):2415-21.
122. Nagueh SF, Lakkis NM, He ZX, Middleton KJ, Killip D, Zoghbi WA, et al. Role of myocardial contrast echocardiography during nonsurgical septal reduction therapy for hypertrophic obstructive cardiomyopathy. J Am Coll Cardiol. 1998;32(1): 225-9.
123. Fan S, Nagai T, Luo H, Atar S, Naqvi T, Birnbaum Y, et al. Superiority of the combination of blood and agitated saline for routine contrast enhancement. J Am Soc Echocardiogr. 1999; 12(2):94-8.
124. Attaran RR, Ata I, Kudithipudi V, et al. Protocol for optimal detection and exclusion of a patent foramen ovale using transthoracic echocardiography with agitated saline microbubbles. Echocardiography. 2006;23(7):616-22.
125. Soliman OII, Geleijnse ML, Meijboom FJ, Nemes A, Kamp O, Nihoyannopoulos P, et al. The use of contrast echocardiography for the detection of cardiac shunts. Eur J Echocardiogr. 2007;8(3):S2-12.
126. Johansson MC, Eriksson P, Guron CW, et al. Pitfalls in diagnosing PFO: characteristics of false-negative contrast injections during transesophageal echocardiography in patients with patent foramen ovales. J Am Soc Echocardiogr. 2010; 23(11):1136-42.
127. Thanigaraj S, Valika A, Zajarias A, et al. Comparison of transthoracic versus transesophageal echocardiography for detection of right-to-left atrial shunting using agitated saline contrast. Am J Cardiol. 2005;96(7):1007-10.
128. Lynch JJ, Schuchard GH, Gross CM, et al. Prevalence of right-to-left atrial shunting in a healthy population: detection by

Valsalva maneuver contrast echocardiography. Am J Cardiol. 1984;53(10):1478-80.

129. Lam Y-Y, Yu C-M, Zhang Q, et al. Enhanced detection of patent foramen ovale by systematic transthoracic saline contrast echocardiography. Intern J Cardiol. 2011;152(1):24-7.
130. Marriott K, Manins V, Forshaw A, et al. Detection of right-to-left atrial communication using agitated saline contrast imaging: experience with 1162 patients and recommendations for echocardiography. J Am Soc Echocardiogr. 2013; 26(1):96-102.
131. Woods TD, Patel A. A critical review of patent foramen ovale detection using saline contrast echocardiography: when bubbles lie. J Am Soc Echocardiogr. 2006;19(2):215-22.
132. Dubourg O, Bourdarias JP, Farcot JC, Gueret P, Terdjman M, Ferrier A, et al. Contrast echocardiographic visualization of cough-induced right to left shunt through a patent foramen ovale. J Am Coll Cardiol. 1984; 4(3):587-94.
133. Gin KG, Huckell VF, Pollick C. Femoral vein delivery of contrast medium enhances transthoracic echocardiographic detection of patent foramen ovale. J Am Coll Cardiol. 1993; 22(7):1994-2000.
134. Schneider B, Zienkiewicz T, Jansen V, Hofmann T, Noltenius H, Meinertz T. Diagnosis of patent foramen ovale by transesophageal echocardiography and correlation with autopsy findings. Am J Cardiol. 1996;77(14):1202-9.
135. Seiler C. How should we assess patent foramen ovale? Heart. 2004;90(11):1245-7.
136. Johansson MC, Helgason H, Dellborg M, et al. Sensitivity for detection of patent foramen ovale increased with increasing number of contrast injections: a descriptive study with contrast transesophageal echocardiography. J Am Soc Echocardiogr. 2008; 21(5):419-24.
137. Jeon D-S, Luo H, Iwami T, Miyamoto T, Brasch AV, Mirocha J, et al. The usefulness of a 10% air-10% blood-80% saline mixture for contrast echocardiography: Doppler measurement of pulmonary artery systolic pressure. J Am Coll Cardiol. 2002; 39(1):124-9.
138. Tsang TS, Freeman WK, Sinak LJ, et al. Echocardiographically guided pericardiocentesis: evolution and state-of-the-art technique. Mayo Clin Proc. 1998;73(7):647-52.
139. Tsang TSM, Enriquez-Sarano M, Freeman WK, Barnes ME, Sinak LJ, Gersh BJ, et al. Consecutive 1127 therapeutic echocardiographically guided pericardiocenteses: clinical profile, practice patterns, and outcomes spanning 21 years. Mayo Clin Proc. 2002;77(5):429-36.

# Tissue Doppler Imaging and Acoustic Speckle Tracking: Technical Considerations

7
CHAPTER

*Jagdish C Mohan, Vishwas Mohan*

## INTRODUCTION

The heart as an organ continues to surprise us as we explore its function in health and disease and carry that knowledge from bench to bedside. The intricate layout of muscle fibers from inside to outside, from right to left, and from base to apex is designed for mechanical efficiency of extreme proportions at low energy consumption. Many techniques like diffusion tensor magnet resonance imaging (MRI), sonomicrometry, tagged MRI, tissue velocity imaging (TVI), acoustic speckle tracking, Doppler echocardiography, high fidelity intracardiac pressure recording, etc. have helped us in understanding this complexity. The heart is an intricate mechanical organ that undergoes cyclic changes in multiple dimensions that ultimately bring a change in chamber volume that results in ejection of blood. In simple terms, it is called multi-dimensional motion or movement. Primary motion of heart muscle secondary to electromechanical coupling provides passive motion to blood. Movement of blood or flow has been studied for long by use of the Doppler principle. Myocardial function assessment is essential for determining the health of the myocardium. Global assessment of myocardial function is widely performed, but many common cardiac diseases initially affect the myocardium on a regional, rather than global basis. Regardless of imaging technique, the holy grail of heart motion or action called "ejection fraction (EF)," which is a sum total of the heart motion, is unable to provide information on the underlying myocardial mechanical activity. Also, ejection fraction reflects the sum contribution of several regions only during systole and does not provide information on regional function. Regional function assessed visually is subjective and prone to error. The most difficult part of regional function by conventional imaging method has been the study of diastolic function and isovolumic phase function with temporal and spatial evaluation. Focal estimation of the regional function has been subject of much research. Tissue Doppler imaging (TDI) and acoustic speckle tracking are the two methods which precisely and accurately depict degree, type, and rate of regional and global myocardial motion at specific points in the heartbeat. These two methods have almost found prime-time utility in assessment of global and regional myocardial function with certain caveats.

## BIOPHYSICS OF THE HEART MUSCLE

The heart muscle is arranged as a syncytium with viscoelastic character and changes its size and shape with every phase of cardiac cycle. It is incompressible and has a definite architecture.[1] It is an almost synchronous generator of bidirectional force for suction and ejection. Cohesive and sequential integration of motion and deformation optimises filling and ejection, the two of its fundamental functions.[2] To some extent, it follows the laws governing motion, material deformation, tension and force.[3] The motion and deformation parameters can be assessed by echocardiography and can be applied to clinical conditions to get information which is otherwise not available from images and intracardiac flow. Myocardial motion and deformation are the complex resultants of intrinsic contractile forces and extrinsic loading forces applied to tissue with varying elastic properties.[2] Motion and deformation parameters provide incremental and unique information of the heart muscle. There are three fundamental intrinsic properties of myocardium:

1. *Self-bracing:* Some distinct areas move more relative to other parts. Motion is differential and region-defined. This is akin to physiological mechanical asynchrony.
2. *Self-restraining:* Autoregulation of the onset, velocity, amount and termination of systolic wall thickening and diastolic wall thinning.
3. *Self-shaping:* This helps in determining intraventricular resistance to flow in various phases of cardiac cycle.

Further description largely applies to the left ventricular (LV) myocardium unless stated otherwise.

### Myocardium: Architecture and Function

Ventricular myocardium possesses the freedom of motion, and the ability for shaping and conformational self-controlling that is unique to this organ. The pumping action of the ventricular myocardium is determined by the

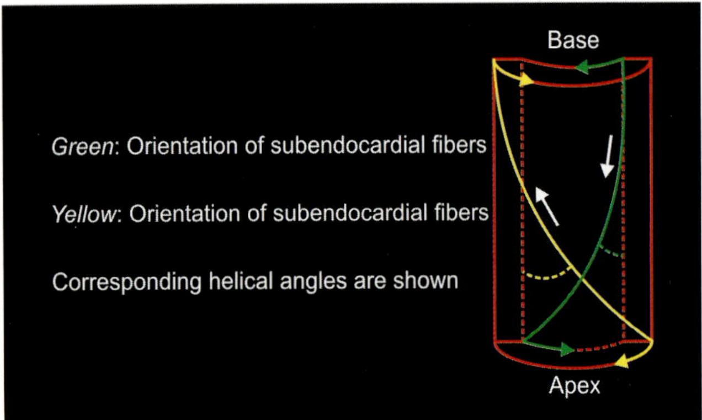


**Figure 7.1:** Orientation of myofiber aggregates

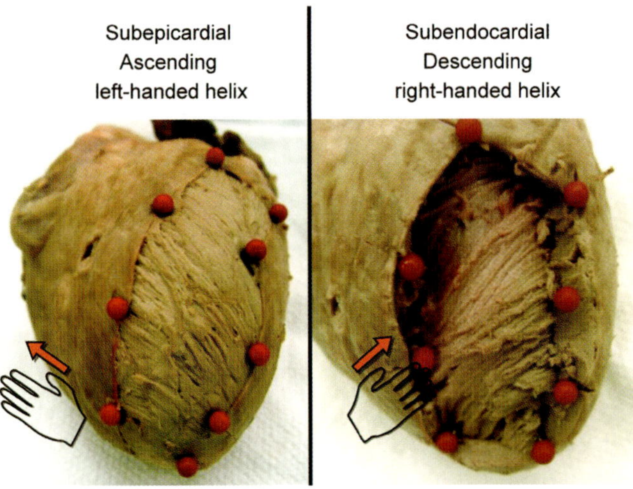


**Figure 7.2:** Gross anatomical arrangement of myofibers in the heart in the form of two helices

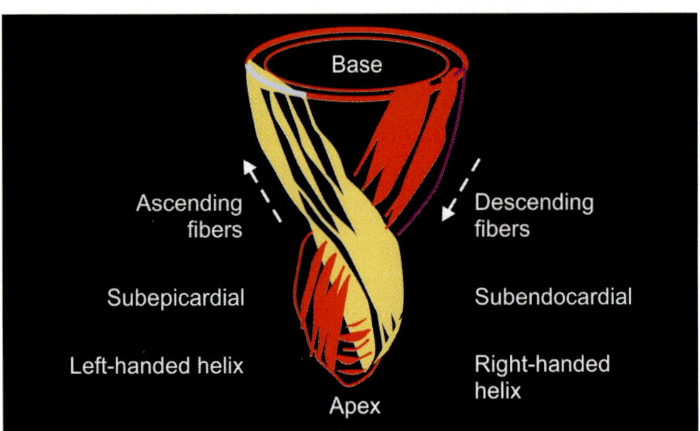


**Figure 7.3:** The unique 3-demensional organization of myocardial fibers of the mammalian ventricle composed of circumferential and longitudinal fibers and also of obliquely running fibers that form a helical spiral from base to apex. When viewed from the apex of the left ventricle, the orientation of fibers changes smoothly from left-handed helical fiber in the subepicardium to circumferential fibers in the mid wall to right-handed helical fiber in the subendocardium. This structure is a key determinant of ventricular mechanical properties, including torsion, strain and stress, and structure adaptation.

three-dimensional (3D) arrangement of the individual myocytes aggregated together within their supporting fibrous matrix. Contractile units of the myocytes are called sarcomere. There is no well-defined beginning and ending of the contractile chains within the myocardium, unlike the situation seen in skeletal muscle. Axial coupling of myocytes on the one hand, and spatial netting on the other hand, produce the histological picture of a meshwork.[4] The prevailing orientation is parallel to the epicardial and endocardial surfaces, with the angle of inclination changing from about 55° upward to about 55° downward **(Figure 7.1)**.

It is the 3D netting of the myocardium which serves as a substrate for disparately distributed afterloads, which cause some degrees of disparity in the amount and timing of regional shortening. Myocytes are aggregated together in reciprocal helices in the subendocardial and subepicardial parts of the walls,[5] whereas they are aggregated predominantly in circular fashion within the middle parts of the walls and the septum **(Figure 7.2 and 7.3)**.

The orientation of these aggregated myocytes can be described in terms of their helical and intruding angles, the latter also being called transverse angle.[6]

Several studies have translated these 3D angulations of the aggregated myocytes to mechanical aspects of cardiac function. The helical angle is the one made between the aggregated myocytes and the ventricular equator, while the so-called intruding or transverse angle measures the extent to which the aggregates angulate from the epicardium toward the endocardium as they penetrate the ventricular wall. The importance of the helical angles in producing centripetal forces and constricting actions during ventricular systole is well recognized. Increasing attention is being paid to the influence of the intruding angles.

At various depths of the ventricular wall, it is possible to note an ordered gradation in the overall long axis of the myocardial aggregates relative to the equator of the ventricular mass. It is also possible to distinguish an obvious circular array of myocardial aggregates arranged parallel to the LV equator **(Figure 7.4)**.

It is the basic 3D arrangement of interweaving longitudinal arrays of myocytes, most aligned tangentially, but some intruding into the ventricular wall which underscores the concept of dualistic ventricular function.[7] Structure of the cardiac muscle influences the electrical propagation and force development throughout the myocardium. This is due

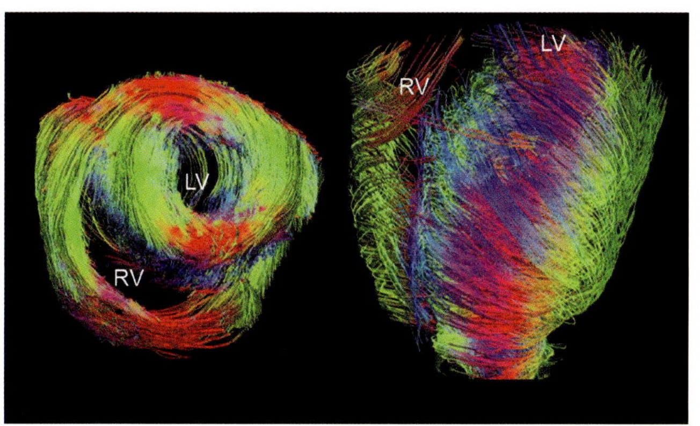


**Figure 7.4:** Diffusion tensor magnetic resonance imaging showing normal myoarchitecture with helical arrangement longitudinally and circular arrangement parallel to the equator.
*Abbreviations:* LV, left ventricle; RV, right ventricle.

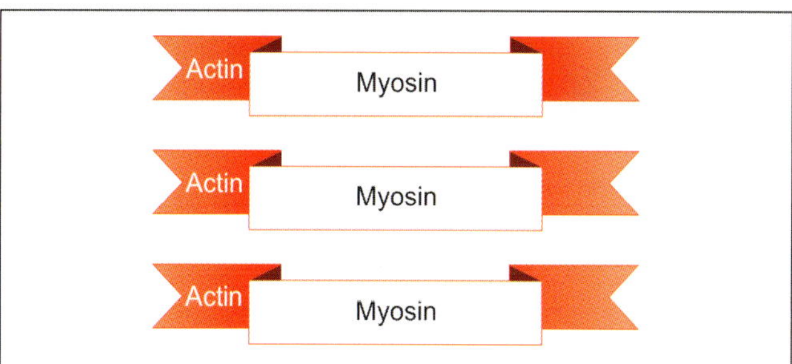


**Figure 7.5:** A sarcomere which is a unit of contraction

to the anisotropy of the electrical and mechanical properties. The conductivity and contractility of ventricular tissue is determined by the direction of the fibers and is highest in the direction of their longitudinal axis.

## Myocardial Form and Function

Sarcomere is the fundamental unit of contraction in the heart muscle. Each sarcomere is attached to at least 15 other sarcomeres. Following electro-mechanical activation, the myocardium deforms during systole due to sarcomere shortening.[2] Sarcomeric unidirectional shortening results in multidirectional change in size and shape of the tissue and this is called myocardial deformation **(Figure 7.5)**.

1. With the onset of systole , there is sarcomere shortening resulting in reduction of intracavitary size and myocardium deformation **(Figure 7.6)**.[2]
2. Since the myocardial tissue is almost incompressible, the volume of ventricular wall and the myocardial mass remain constant in every phase of cardiac cycle .
3. The deformation occurs in three dimensions which are expressed along three ventricular coordinates: a longitudinal and circumferential shortening and a radial thickening **(Figure 7.7 to 7.10, Box 7.1)**. The ventricular myocardium simultaneously shortens in the longitudinal and circumferential planes and thickens in the radial plane, with reciprocal changes in diastole.
4. The fourth form of deformation is rotation which is the angular motion at two ends of the ventricle, and the difference between the two is twist or torsion. Rotation or torsion are indicators of shear strain **(Figure 7.11 to 7.14)**.
5. The deformation is calculated based on the relative change of the length of myocardial fibers during cardiac cycle[3,4] and is expressed in a uni-dimensional parameter termed strain (ε).

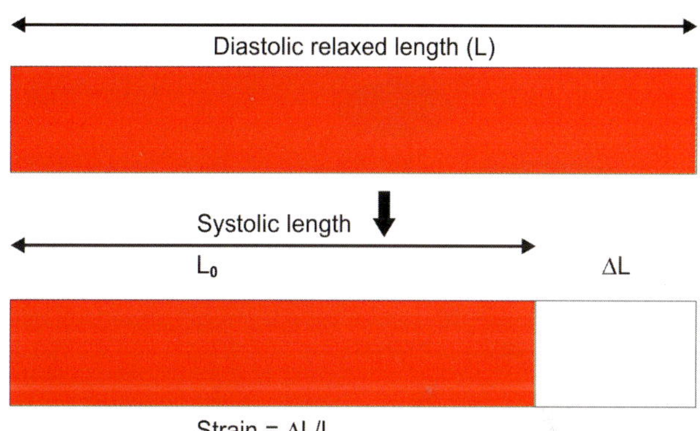


**Figure 7.6:** Graphic description of deformation (strain). Strain is spatial derivation of displacement.

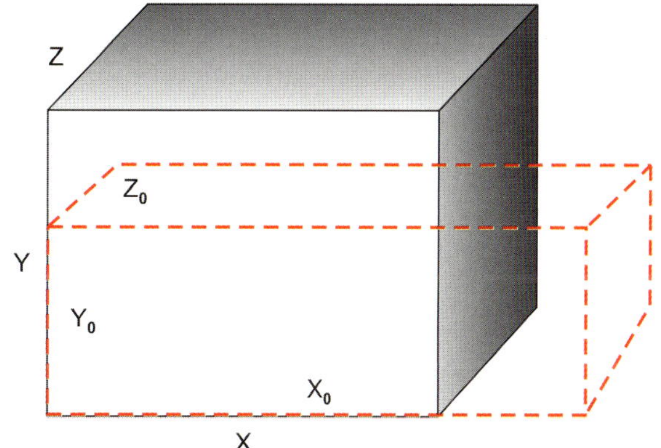


**Figure 7.7:** Depiction of three coordinates of deformation. Deformation in three different planes occurring simultaneously are $X–X_0/X$ , $Y–Y_0/Y$ and $Z–Z_0/Z$.

6. The local end-systolic strain value reflects the regional EF and the global LV end-systolic strain reflects the overall systolic function.[3]

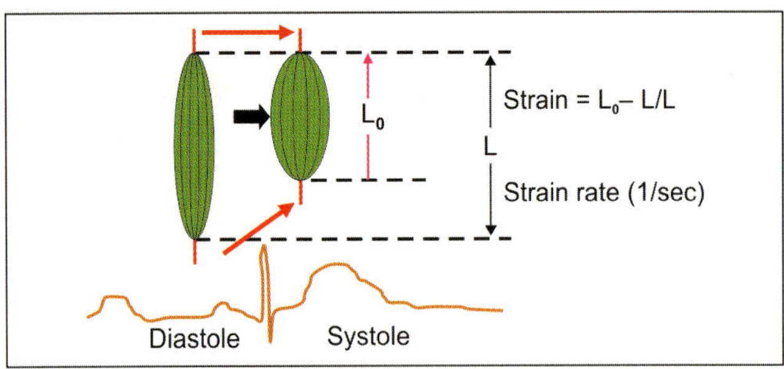


**Figure 7.8:** Graphic diagram showing a single myofiber and its length during diastole (L) and at end-systole ($L_0$). Percentage longitudinal shortening is strain and rate of shortening is strain rate.

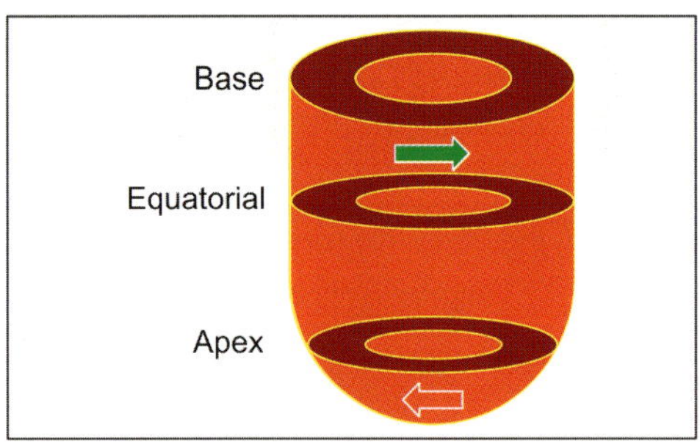


**Figure 7.11:** Myocardial twist. During systole, base rotates clockwise while the apex rotates anticlockwise when viewed from the apex.

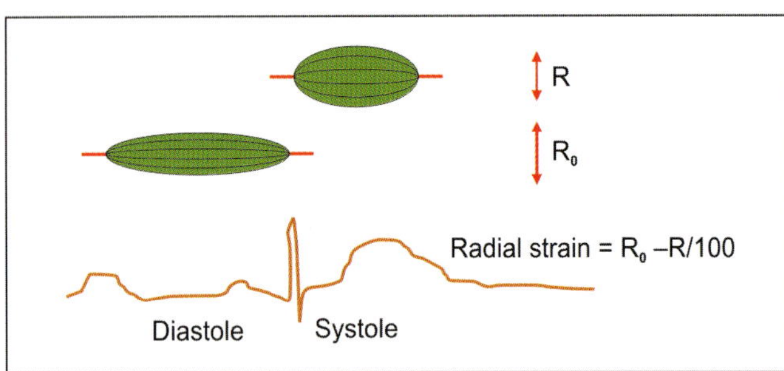


**Figure 7.9:** Graphic description of myofiber width (short-axis diameter) during diastole (R) and during end-systole ($R_0$). Radial strain is the percentage increase in width.

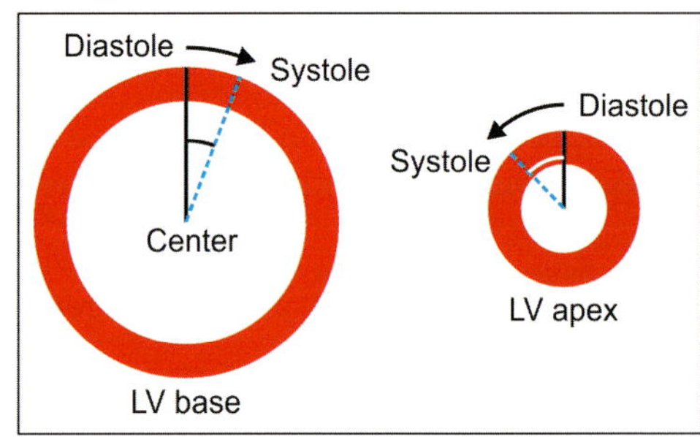


**Figure 7.12:** Diagram to depict clockwise rotation of the base and anticlockwise rotation of the apex.
*Abbreviation:* LV, left ventricular.

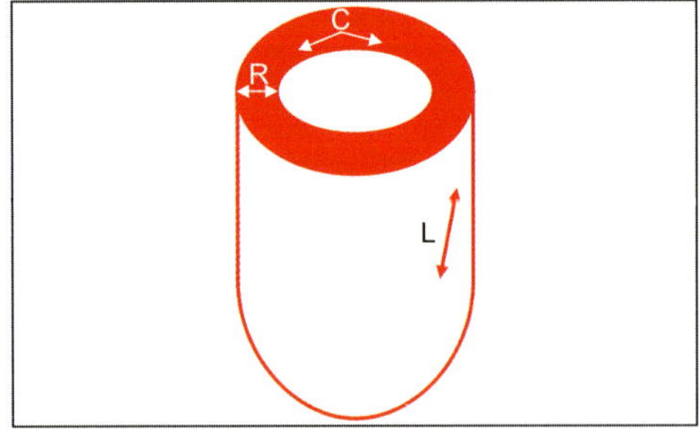


**Figure 7.10:** Simultaneous graphic depiction of three vectors of the heart muscle motion.
*Abbreviations:* C, circumferential; L, longitudinal; R, radial.

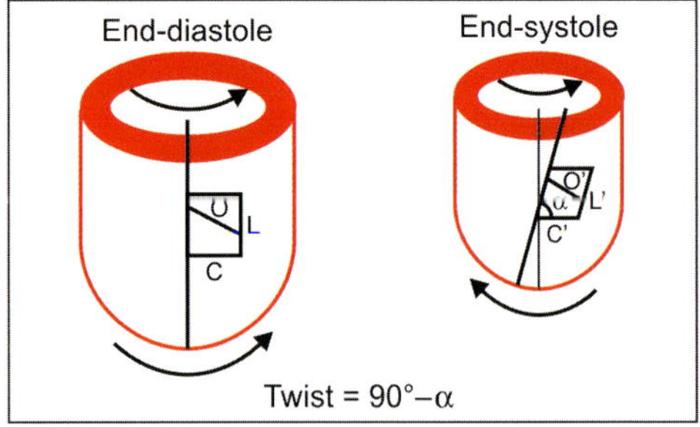


**Figure 7.13:** Measuring angle of the myocardial twist.

**Box 7.1: Vectors of cardiac movement**

- Longitudinal shortening (compression strain) and lengthening (tensile strain)
- Transverse or radial thickening and thinning
- Circumferential shortening and lengthening
- Rotation (twist and untwist)

## DESCRIPTIVE TERMS

*Velocity:* Speed of motion with direction (positive or negative velocity). Color velocity imaging shows red hue while shortening and blue while lengthening. Velocity is a vectoral physical quantity; both magnitude and direction are required to define it.

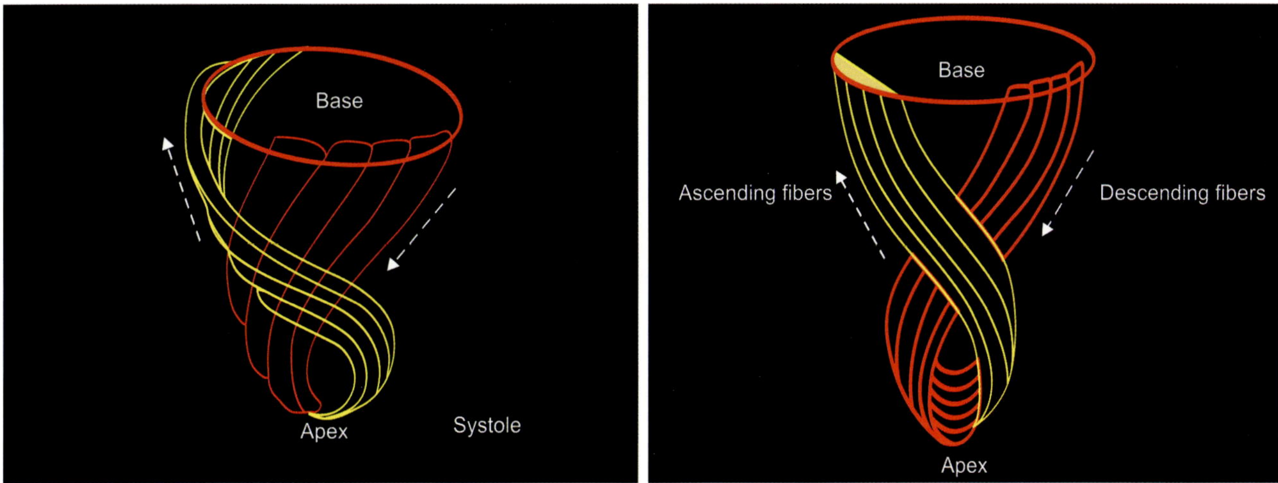


**Figure 7.14:** Composite movement vectors of the left ventricle.

*Displacement:* A displacement is the shortest distance from the initial to the final position of a point. In ultrasound terms, it is time integral of velocity (velocity X time). Displacement imaging also called tissue tracking uses different hues for degree of displacement.

*Elasticity:* It describes materials that return to their resting shape after the force is removed.

*A viscoelastic material* can be simply modeled as an elastic component coupled with a viscous component which acts as a damper that delays the stress–strain response (time-dependent stress–strain relationship). The healthy myocardium has viscoelasticity (hysteresis on contraction and relaxation).

*Deformation:* Change in shape and size of an elastic or viscoelastic object when a force is applied. Deformation is the change in the metric properties of a continuous body. If after a displacement of the continuum, there is a relative displacement between particles, a deformation has occurred.

Strain and strain rate are examples of deformation imaging.

*Strain:* It is a normalized measure of deformation representing the displacement between particles in the body relative to a reference length. Strain is dimensionless and is usually expressed as a decimal fraction, a percentage or in parts per notation. Strain measures how much a given deformation differs locally from a rigid body deformation. Thus, strain is a tensor quantity.

*Meaning of strain:* Tissue strain is a surrogate for tissue stiffness. Low tissue strain corresponds to high tissue stiffness and vice versa. Tissue stiffness corresponds to ischemia, fibrosis, muscle fiber disarray, infiltration, etc.

**Table 7.1:** Types of strain

| *Normal strain* | *Shear strain* |
|---|---|
| a. Longitudinal | a. Longitudinal-circumferential |
| b. Radial | b. Longitudinal-radial |
| c. Circumferential | c. Circumferential-radial |
| | d. Radial-circumferential |
| | e. Radial-longitudinal |
| | f. Circumferential-longitudinal |

*Components of strain:* The amount of stretch or compression along line elements or fibers is the *normal strain*, and the amount of distortion associated with the sliding of plane layers over each other is the *shear strain*, within a deforming body **(Table 7.1)**. Area strain is the combined, longitudinal-circumferential normal strain in a given area and measured by 3D imaging.

*Strain rate:* Regional myocardial velocity gradient is the strain rate. in TDI, strain rate imaging has several hues, e.g. green color denotes no strain rate while orange-red hue indicates negative strain rate; blue color indicates positive strain rate (color hues are reverse of TVI).

*Acceleration:* Rate of velocity over a region (velocity/time). "Deceleration" is called a "negative acceleration".

*Momentum:* Integral of mass and velocity; rarely used in TDI although more common in flow Doppler studies.

*TDI or TVI:* An imaging technique which provides qualitative and quantitative information about regional velocities using pulsed wave Doppler with good temporal resolution.

*Spectral pulsed TDI:* It is online velocity determination from a single point by placing a small sample volume. It has the

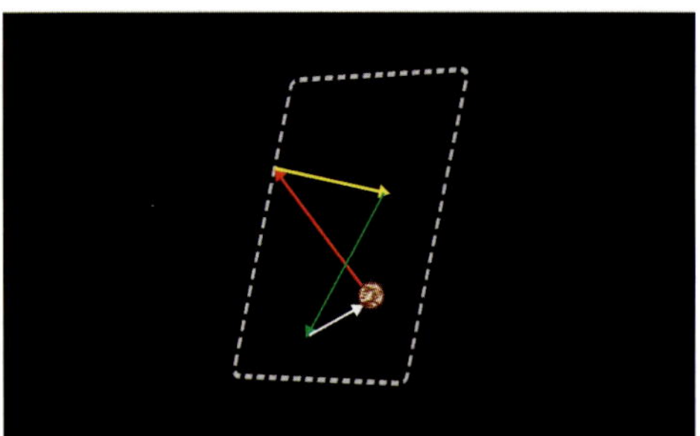

**Figure 7.15A:** Complex motion of a natural acoustic reflector in different planes during a single cardiac cycle. Length and direction of the arrow denote the quantum of displacement. It is tracked by sum-of-absolute differences algorithm.

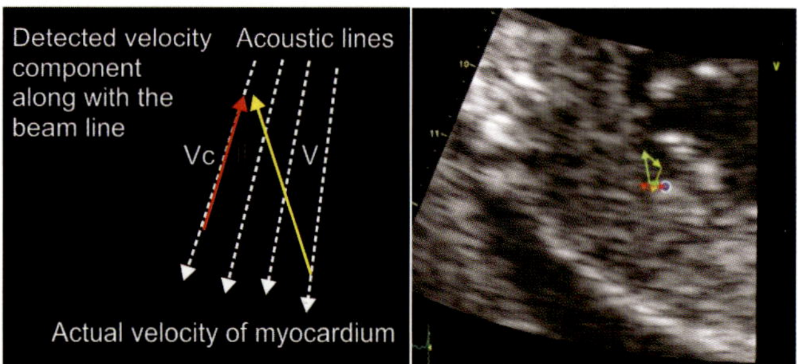


**Figure 7.15B:** Showing why speckle tracking scores over Doppler imaging. Accurate velocity can be obtained by speckle tracking.

advantage of online measurements of velocities and time intervals and an excellent temporal resolution (8 ms).

*Color Doppler myocardial imaging (CDMI):* An imaging technique that provides qualitative or quantitative information about spatial velocities using fast Fournier algorithm of color flow mapping. Peak velocities measured by this technique are about 20–30% lower than that of TDI because these are mean velocities rather than peak values.

*Curved anatomical M-mode TVI:* High resolution semiquantitative technique to study regional tissue velocities and velocity-derived parameters. In M-mode tracing, the derivative of the position vs. time graph of an object is equal to the velocity of the object).

*Acoustic speckle tracking:* Intramural displacement of a natural tissue reflector (speckle or a group of 30–40 pixels called kernel) located in an area of interest on a grayscale image is measured using a phase-sensitive correlation-based speckle tracking approach **(Figure 7.15A to C)**. It is also called two-dimensional (2D) strain imaging. Essentially, it is an automatic tracking of interference patterns from conventional grayscale B-mode images during the cardiac cycle.[12]

Motion and deformation as parameters of cardiac function can be estimated by multiple methods **(Box 7.2)**. But fundamental knowledge is method-independent.

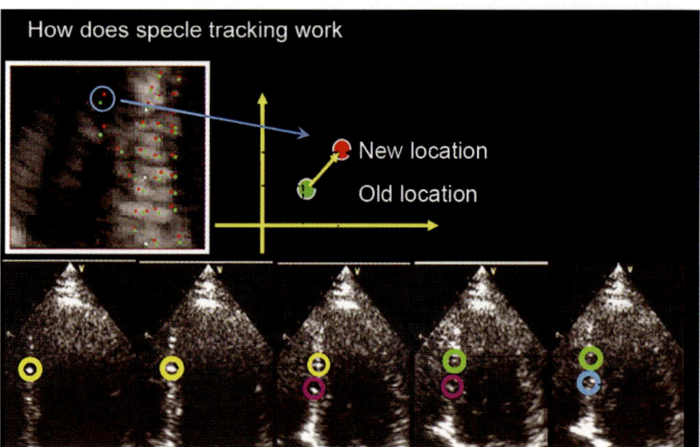


**Figure 7.15C:** Upper panel shows actual motion of the kernel and the lower panel shows how it can be tracked.

**Box 7.2: Various methodology for cardiac funtion**

- Doppler-derived deformation imaging
- Echocardiographic acoustic speckle tracking 2D strain (including velocity vector imaging)
- Echocardiographic acoustic speckle tracking 3D strain
- Sonomicrometry
- Tagged MRI

## CONCEPT OF TISSUE DOPPLER IMAGING

In 1842, an Austrian scientist, Christian Doppler, presented the concept of measuring distance of planets from the earth by using what is now called Doppler effect.[8] A century later, at the University of Osaka, Japan, S Satomura first applied these principles to measure the blood flow velocities in blood vessels.[9] The pioneer of TDI is Karl Isaaz, a French man, who was the first to realize the importance of clinical and diagnostic potentials of TDI.[10] He hypothesized that rate and direction of the heart tissue movement could be obtained by using the tissue Doppler with the assumption that the movement was parallel to the ultrasound beam and within the beam. Movements of myocardial walls include components of low velocity and short duration requiring a high sampling rate. Modifications to the filter settings on pulsed Doppler to image low-velocity, high-intensity myocardial signal rather than the high-velocity, low-intensity signal from blood flow allow tissue velocity estimation. Tissue velocities are nearly one-tenth of the intracardiac flow velocities. Measurement of myocardial tissue motion has created basis for detailed evaluation of systolic and diastolic cardiac function not only in terms of velocity, but also in terms of acceleration, displacement, and deformation variables **(Figure 7.16)**.

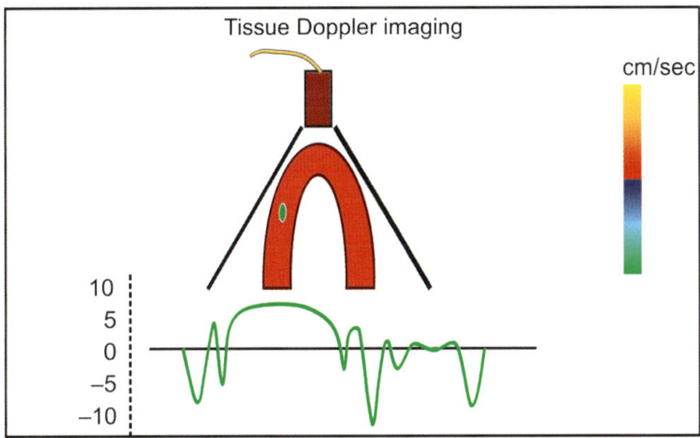


**Figure 7.16:** Concept of tissue Doppler echocardiography. Using a prespecified region for placement of sample volume, a Doppler spectrum is obtained as shown in the figure depicting velocities in various phases of the cardiac cycle with preordained filter settings. Velocities toward the transducer are positive and away from the transducer are negative. Temporal resolution of various waves is due to high frame rates (>100 f/s).

## Labeling of Tissue Velocity Waveforms

1. Two positive waves of myocardial shortening can be recorded in systole. The first positive wave (s'1) occurs as a result of the longitudinal shortening of the myocardial tissue during the phase of isometric contraction. The second wave (s'2) occurs due to LV shortening during LV ejection **(Figure 7.17A to D)**. Two peak velocities in systolic ejection are commonly seen in free wall. These represent functional switchover from subendocardial longitudinal fibers contraction to circumferential fibers shortening during ejection with a variable delay.
2. In healthy subjects, the shortening of the longitudinal fibers predominates over that of the circumferential fibers during early systole, whereas the shortening of the circumferential fibers predominate over that of longitudinal fibers in the ejection phase. However, their relative importance remains ill-defined, and hence, both systolic waves should be measured and mentioned.

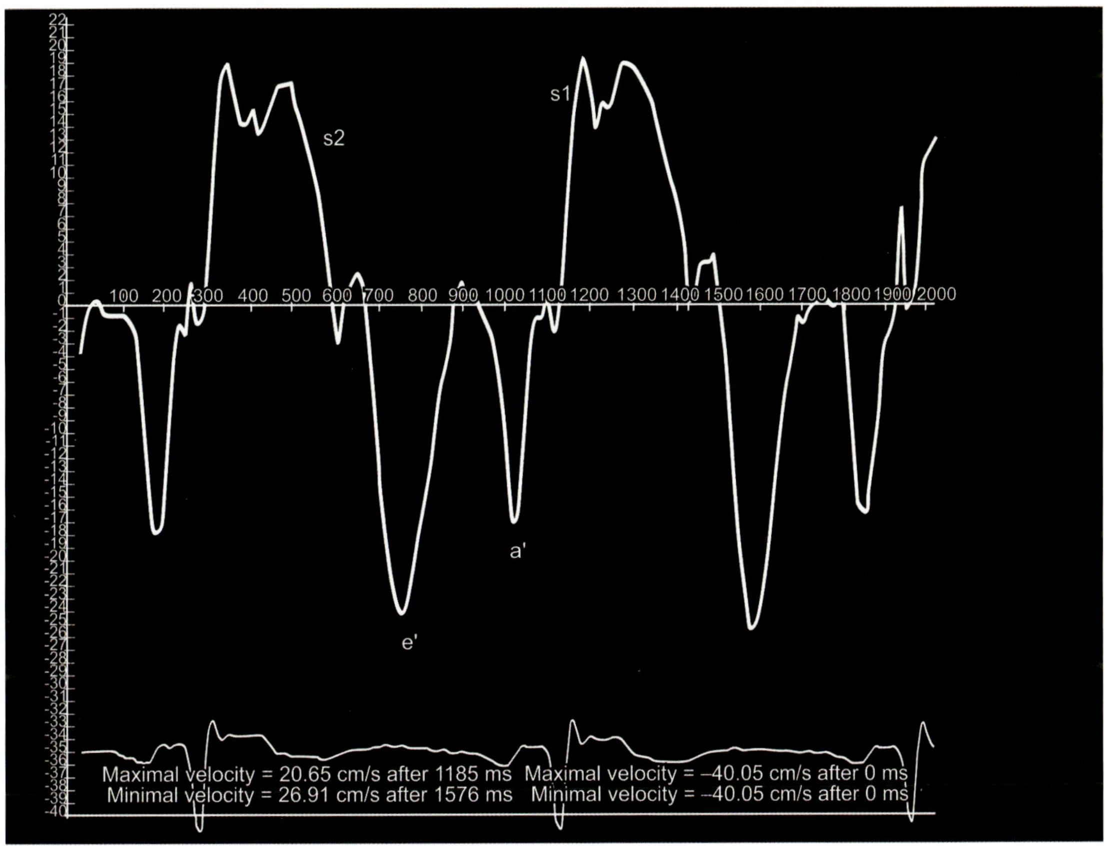


**Figure 7.17A:** Tissue Doppler waveforms s1 and s2 are systolic velocities while e' and a' are early and late diastolic velocities. There are small biphasic velocities in isovolumic phases which are normally not named. s1 represents longitudinal component, while s2 denotes circumferential component of the systolic velocities. Conventionally, tissue velocities are labeled by lower case letters.

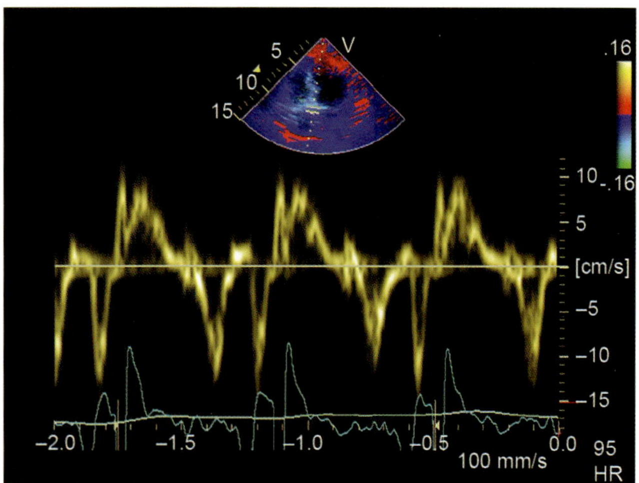


**Figure 7.17B:** Tissue Doppler waveforms of the actual tracing from the medial edge of the mitral annulus). There are two positive (systolic) and two negative (diastolic) waveforms.

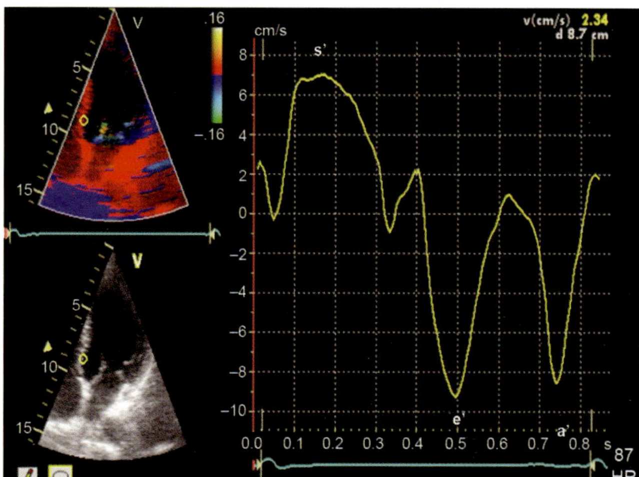


**Figure 7.17D:** Color Doppler myocardial imaging. After acquisition of image containing velocity information, a sample volume of known length is placed (as here at basal inferior septum) and corresponding velocity spectrum is obtained (shown on the right side)

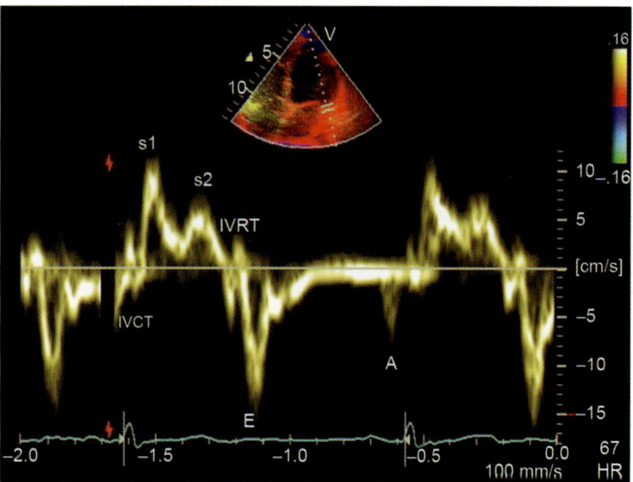


**Figure 7.17C:** Lateral edge mitral annular tissue velocity profile showing two distinct systolic waves (s1 and s2 ) in a healthy young control. It is the s1 which represents contraction of longitudinal fibers that is usually measured.

*Abbreviations:* A, late diastolic velocity; E, early diastolic velocity; IVCT, isovolumetric contraction time; IVRT, isovolumic relaxation time.

Whenever two waves are seen, it is not clear which one should be used. As s'1 corresponds to contraction of subendocardial longitudinal fibers, it is better to use it.

3. Early diastolic velocity which correlates with active relaxation is labeled e'. It is relatively much less load-dependent.[11]
4. Late diastolic velocity which correlates with ventricular stiffness is labeled as a'.[11]
5. There is no consensus on labeling abnormal waves . However, l' wave is that recorded in diastasis.
6. A recoil wave can usually be seen after high velocity movements during isovolumic contraction, relaxation or after early diastolic filling and occurs in a direction opposite to initial movement.
7. The rate of LV pressure decline during isovolumic relaxation (IVR) becomes slower during the development of most forms of cardiovascular disease and also becomes slower during normal aging. Prominent and prolnged IVR phase can be often noticed in diseased states. It may be called ivr'.

## Technical Details

TDI is an assessment of myocardial motion using Doppler ultrasound imaging, often with color coding .The fundamental units are velocity observed from the echocardiographic transducer as a frame of reference.

Most systems have TDI software which automatically brings on tissue velocities once a sample volume is placed in that image after activating the software. The TDI information is embedded in grayscale images that are colored.

1. Velocities are obtained from the selected sample volume (single or multiple point velocity in reference to the position of the transducer) which can be of variable dimension. A sample volume of 2–5 mm is optimum for spectral Doppler while color Doppler myocardial imaging has a wide but well-defined area (6–12 mm) from where velocities can be obtained ex *post-facto.*
2. Tissue velocities are usually less than 25 cm/sec.
3. A high sampling rate is essential for a proper rendering of TVI signals (but introduces noise): too low frame rates result in underestimation (<70 frames/sec). To ensure the optimal signal-to-noise ratio, temporal filtering should be

used with caution (usually 200 frames/sec), governed by the awareness of the interplay between sampling rate and temporal filters.

4. The influence of unfavorable insonation angle may affect tissue Doppler measurements resulting in underestimation of the true myocardial velocities.
5. Default gain settings of 50% saturation should be used to measure velocities accurately. Overgaining results in overestimation of tissue velocities by about 20%. Intervender settings differences also should be noted.
6. In clinical practice, annular velocities are used most often because these are more reproducible **(Figure 7.18)**. Usually, septal or lateral edges of the mitral annulus are interrogated and can be used separately or by averaging the two.[4] Multiple points of the annulus can also be used to enhance accuracy but are cumbersome and are not recommended. The results of averaging mitral annular velocities obtained from the 4 myocardial walls do not differ from the average of using velocities measured at the septal and lateral sites.[12,13]
7. Color Doppler myocardial velocities are obtained ex-post facto and can be obtained from multiple sites either in M-mode or 2D format **(Figure 7.19 to 7.21)**.
8. Color Doppler obtained velocities are 20–30% lesser than the pulsed-wave Doppler velocities but provide mean velocity estimation from several sites Simultaneously.[14]
9. Temporal resolution is maximum in M-mode tissue velocities, followed by pulsed-wave TDI and then color Doppler myocardial imaging **(Figure 7.20B)**.
10. TDI is used for assessing regional longitudinal function. It is possible to obtain radial velocities which are mostly used for pattern reading and understanding myocardial mechanics.
11. Systolic and early diastolic velocities decrease with ageing and hence normal values are age-dependent when used in isolation.[13]
12. Tissue velocities have a base-to-apex gradient and are usually nearly absent close to the apex. Typical annular tissue s' and e' velocities are > 8 cm/sec in healthy subjects while a' is less than e'.
13. Lateral annular velocities are higher than medial annular velocities **(Figure 7.21)**.[13,14]

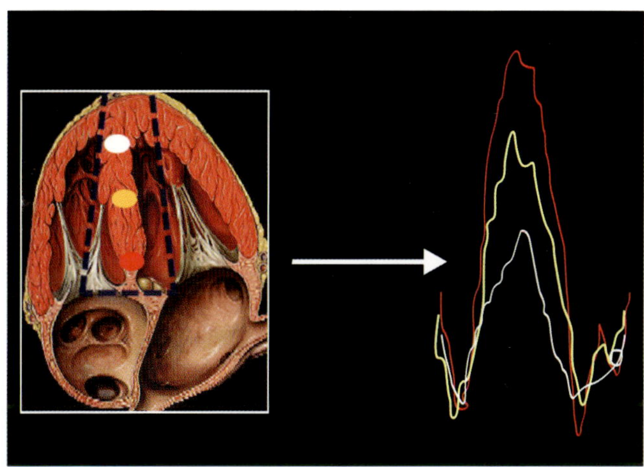

**Figure 7.19A:** Color Doppler myocardial imaging from interventricular septum. Note velocity spectrum derivation from multiple points in a single cardiac cycle. The tissue velocities decrease from base to apex.

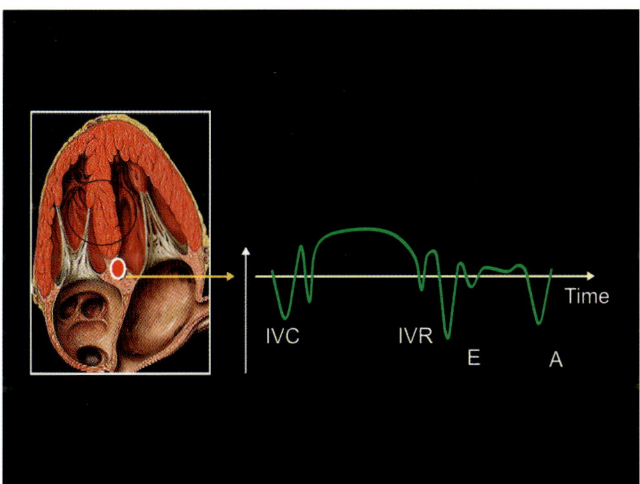


**Figure 7.18:** Spectral pulsed-wave tissue velocities from the medial edge of the mitral annulus. Velocities obtained from here are most stable and commonly used for serial studies. This is because angle of insonation is optimal.
*Abbreviations:* A, late diastolic velocity; E, early diastolic velocity; IVC, isovlumic contraction; IVR, isovolumic relaxation.

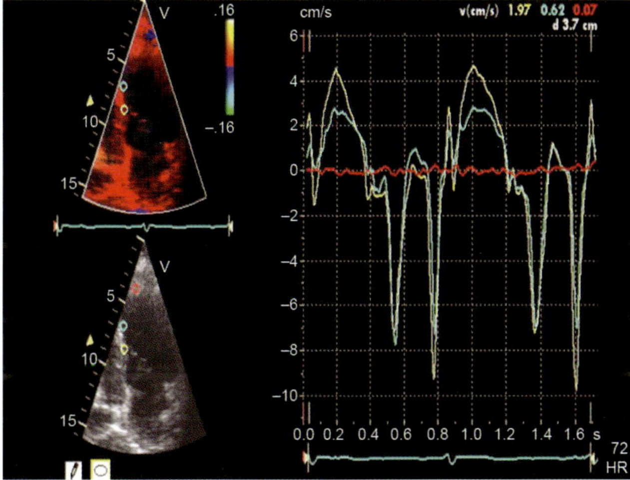


**Figure 7.19B:** Color Doppler myocardial imaging from interventricular septum. Note velocity spectrum derivation from multiple points in a single cardiac cycle. The tissue velocities decrease from base to apex.

**Figure 7.19C:** Right ventricular free wall shows base-to-apex gradient of peak systolic velocities and diastolic velocities in a normal adult.

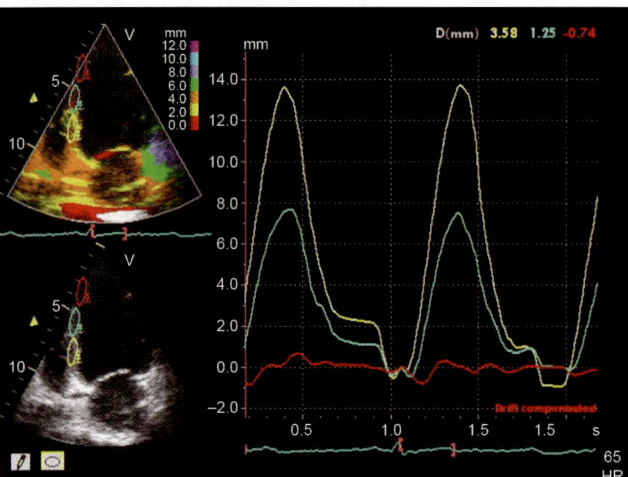


**Figure 7.19D:** Color Doppler displacement imaging of the interventricular septum. Average displacement of a myocardial wall is about 8 mm with a base-to-apex gradient. Note that the apical segment (red curve) is nearly stationary while the basal segment moves a distance of 13.8 mm in systole.

14. Tricuspid annular and right ventricular (RV) free wall velocities are usually higher than mitral annular and LV free wall velocities by about 20–30%.[15]
15. Tissue velocities have greatest utility for estimating subclinical systolic and diastolic dysfunction and prognosis. All waves have implications. Even s′ + e′ have been used for prognosis. High temporal resolution provides information about the behavior of the tissue region over the entire cardiac cycle.[16]

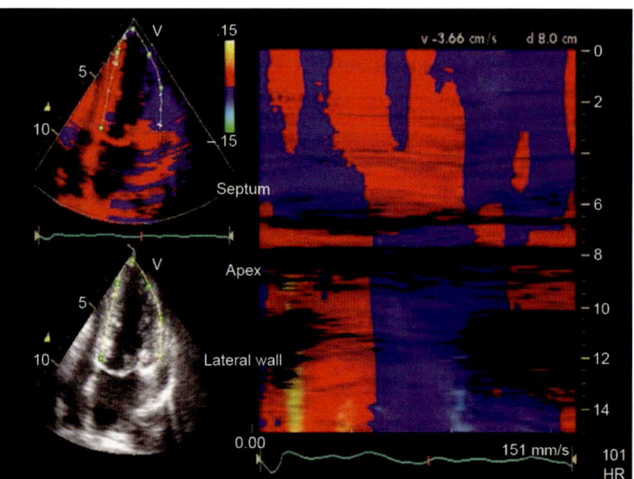


**Figure 7.20A:** M-mode color Doppler myocardial imaging in the apical 4-chamber view of the left ventricle. Bright orange or red color velocities are positive while blue ones are negative. Note lack of any motion at the apex. Also note temporal heterogeneity of the septal wall in this 50-year old female with hypertrophic cardiomyopathy due to myofiber disarray. The walls are traced by curved anatomical M-mode method.

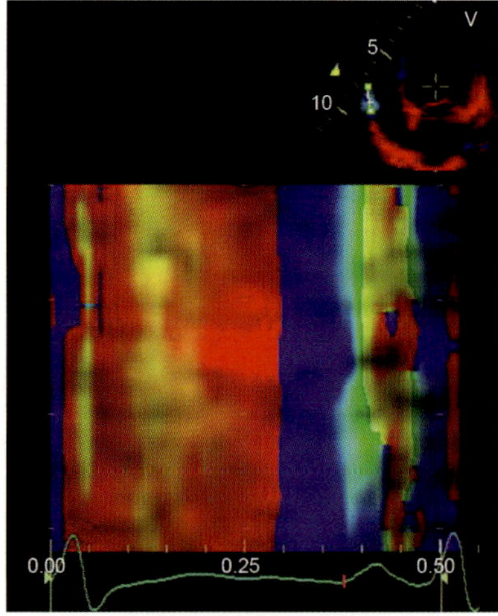


**Figure 7.20B:** M-mode Doppler myocardial imaging of the basal right ventricular free wall. Orange-color are positive velocities while blue are negative velocities. Note the excellent temporal resolution. Positive velocity after early diastolic wave is due to recoil and is normal.

16. The isovolumic myocardial motion variables are of considerable clinical interest since they appear to be early markers of pathological phenomena like ischemia-induced disturbances in myocardial function.[17] Postsystolic prominent positive velocities usually indicate nonspecific myocardial diseased state and are not specific to ischemia **(Figure 7.22)**.

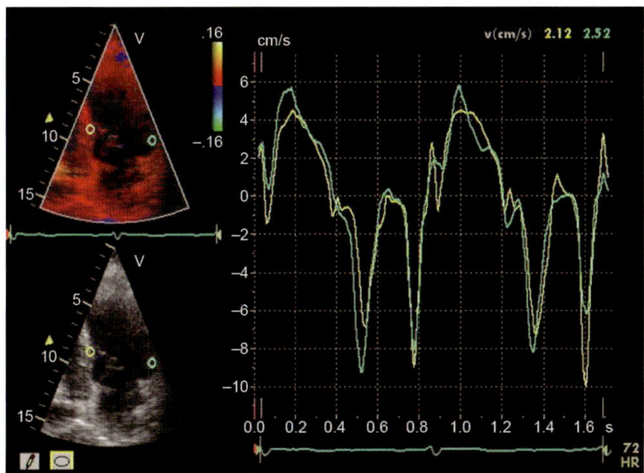


**Figure 7.21:** Color Doppler myocardial velocities from basal septum compared to basal lateral wall. Note the velocities from the lateral wall are higher.

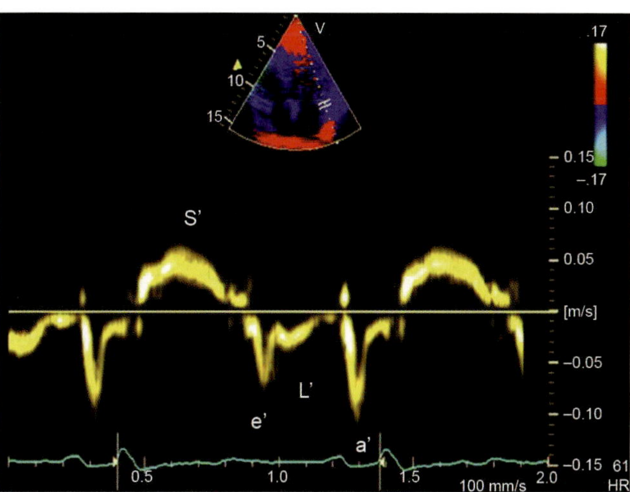


**Figure 7.23:** The TDI of the lateral edge of the mitral annulus. Note prominent L' wave at a heart rate of 61 BPM. L' wave is independent of e' or a' magnitude.

*Abbreviations:* a', late diastolic velocity; e', early diastolic velocity; L', mid-diastolic velocity; S, systolic velocity.

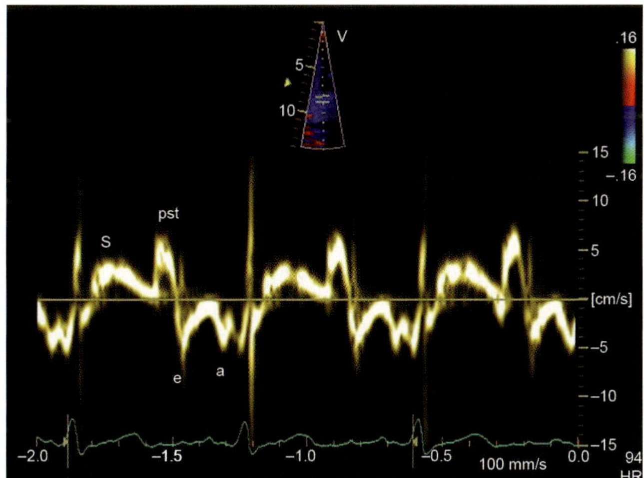


**Figure 7.22:** Tissue Doppler imaging of medial mitral annulus showing prominent postsystolic positive wave (pst). A negative component of similar magnitude is present during isovolumic relaxation. Postsystolic wave indicates nonspecific myopathic process, but ones induced by stress are specific for ischemia.

*Abbreviations:* a', late diastolic velocity; e', early diastolic velocity; S, systolic velocity.

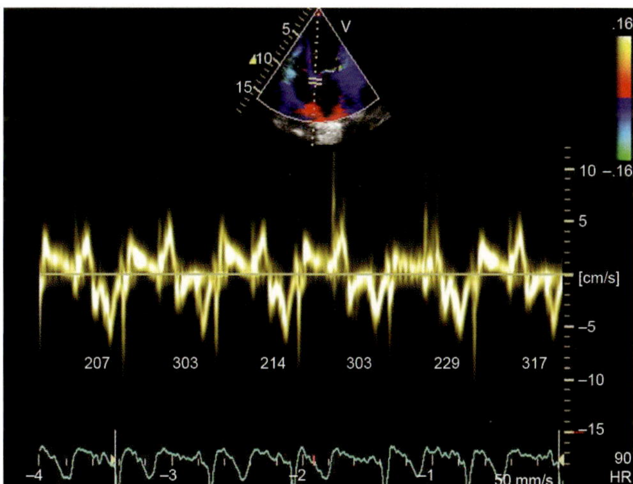


**Figure 7.24A:** Tissue Doppler imaging of the medial edge of the mitral annulus. Note temporal alternans during diastole (tissue diastole in msec is shown in each beat). Also note prominent postsystolic positive wave. Both alternans and positive isovolumic velocities are indicative of advanced myopathic process.

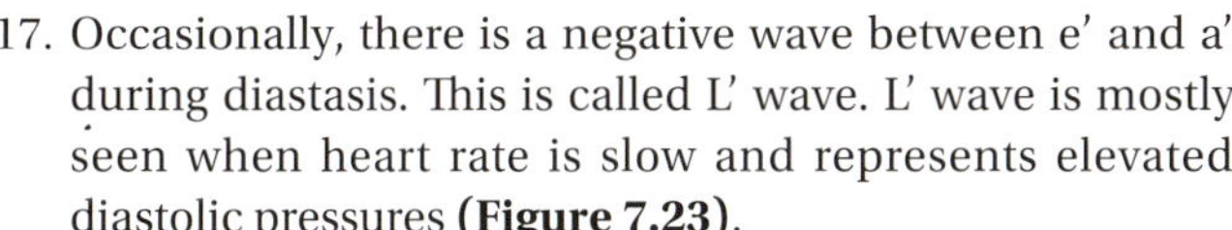
17. Occasionally, there is a negative wave between e' and a' during diastasis. This is called L' wave. L' wave is mostly seen when heart rate is slow and represents elevated diastolic pressures **(Figure 7.23)**.

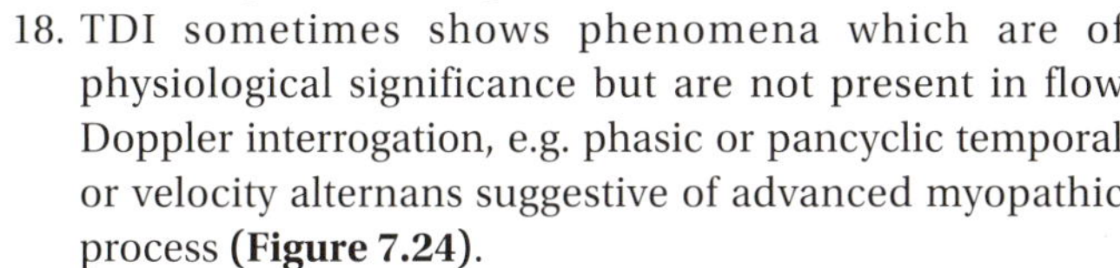
18. TDI sometimes shows phenomena which are of physiological significance but are not present in flow Doppler interrogation, e.g. phasic or pancyclic temporal or velocity alternans suggestive of advanced myopathic process **(Figure 7.24)**.
19. Accurate measurement of myocardial tissues velocities is of considerable clinical interest, since it is accepted that decreased peak systolic and early diastolic velocities indicate failing myocardial function. Attention should be paid to the site and size of sample volume, frames rates, gain, and angle of insonification.[16]
20. Longitudinal systolic dysfunction (s' velocities) might be compensated by an increase of the radial function. Hence, in early disease states, there is no correlation

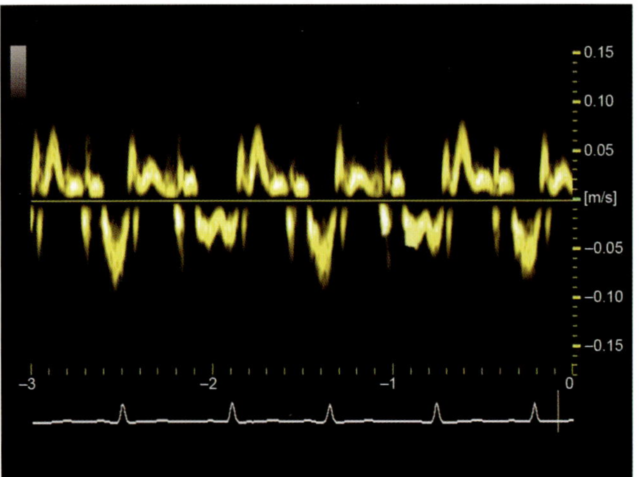


**Figure 7.24B:** Tissue Doppler imaging at mitral annulus shows pancyclic Doppler alternans which usually precedes flow alternans and is more specific than the latter. Note alternation of peak velocities as well as duration of each wave. There is fusion of e' and a' in alternate cardiac cycle due to shortened tissue diastole.

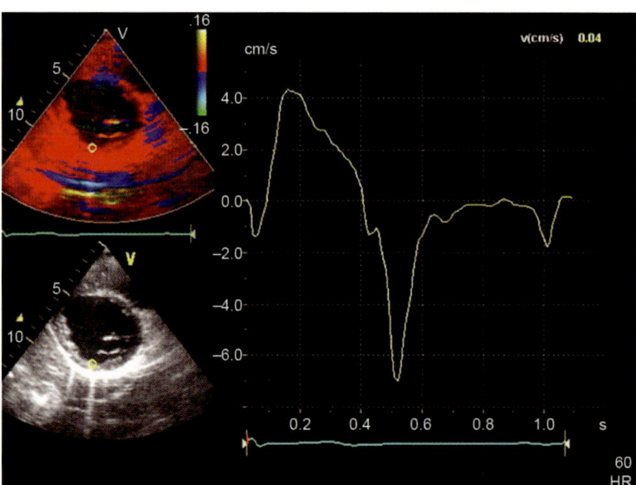


**Figure 7.25:** Myocardial tissue velocities from the posterior wall in short axis.

between systolic velocities and EF and the two provide complementary but different information.

21. Before TDI measurements, it is wise to perform cardiac event marking defining aortic valve opening and closure and mitral valve opening and closure.
22. Age, heart rate and LV dimensions account for between 20% and 70% of the variability seen in LV systolic and diastolic velocities. Instead of relying upon normative data from literature, each center should develop its own normal values.[16]
23. Mitral annular velocity measurement cannot be used in patients with severe mitral annular calcification, prosthetic ring or prosthetic mitral valve.
24. Apical segments cannot be assessed using TDI, because of limited movement of the apex and unfavorable angle of incidence of apical myocardial motion with respect to the transducer position.
25. Although TDI has become synonymous with "velocity measurement", in many cases, it is not the frequency shift (Doppler shift) of the received signal that is measured, but the phase shift (when the received signal arrives). This is used to study cardiac asynchrony and cardiac phase related myocardial performance index (isovolumic phase duration/ejection phase duration) and tissue alternans **(Figure 7.24)**.

## Myocardial Velocities in Short Axis

Myocardial velocities in the short axis are acquired from the posterior wall and the interventricular septum **(Figure 7.25)**. Short-axis TDI implies the possibility of measuring a combination of longitudinal, radial, and circumferential rather than the pure circumferential motion.

1. Posterior wall waves resemble the waveforms of the longitudinal plane with two systolic (s'1 and s'2) and three diastolic waves (IVR, e' and a').
2. The motion of the interventricular septum is more complex as it is shared between the two ventricles. Moreover, there is a hinge point in the septum, proximal to which it moves away from the LV cavity in systole and toward the LV cavity in diastole. The part of the septum distal to it moves in the opposite direction.
3. The tissue velocities in the later part of the septum shows two inward movements in systole, the first (s'1) being due to isometric contraction and the second (s'2) due to ventricular ejection. The s'2 wave in short axis is bigger than in long axis.
4. The diastolic waves show a biphasic wave in early diastole (e') and a wave of atrial contraction (a').
5. The systolic and diastolic waves occur earlier in the septum as compared to the posterior wall and are consistent with the pattern of electrical activation of the septum. This information can be used to detect ventricular preexcitation.[9]
6. The reason for the biphasic motion of the septum in early diastole is not known. It may be due to translational and/or RV influences **(Figure 7.26)**.

## Internal Dependency of Velocities

As systole is coupled with diastole, systolic velocities are related to diastolic tissue velocities. The s' velocity denotes longitudinal systolic function while e' denotes myocardial relaxation. The a' is a reflection of ventricular stiffness.

1. Systolic velocity (s') is positively correlated to the early diastolic velocity (e'). Increased longitudinal contraction is able to improve early diastolic LV filling through the effect of elastic recoil and vice versa.
2. There is a negative correlation between early diastolic (e') and late diastolic (a') velocities except in end-stage disease where both decrease **(Figure 7.27)**.
3. Hence s' and a' are independent predictors of myocardial properties while e' is dependent upon s'.

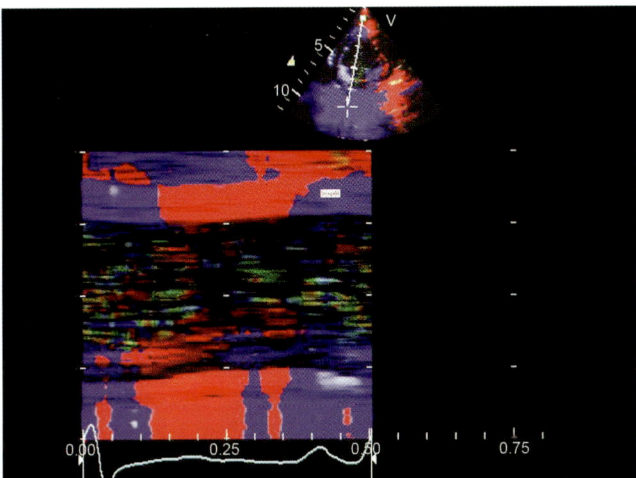


**Figure 7.26:** M-mode depiction of the color-coded tissue velocities of the LV short axis. Note the biphasic motion in the posterior wall in isovolumic phases. Of note is the bidirectional and bilayered pattern of contraction and relaxation in the interventricular septum.
*Abbreviation:* LV, left ventricle.

4. The e'/a' and s' are more robust parameters of abnormal physiology.
5. Limited data exist on isolvolumic phase velocities and their significance at rest. Stress-induced prominent postsystolic positive velocities may be specific markers of ischemia and correlate with extent of perfusion defects. Prominent postsystolic velocities have also been called delayed longitudinal contractions.
6. Regional myocardial tissue velocities, however, represent the net effect of the contractile and elastic properties of the area under investigation and traction and tethering effects from other regions. Tissue motion can be resolved by velocities but difference between active or passive motion cannot be made out. For this myocardial velocity gradient imaging (deformation imaging) is used.
7. The e'/a' ratio increases with increasing physiological stress and exercise in healthy subjects. Abnormal response could signify disease process or aging.
8. The e' is relatively independent of the effect of heart rate, preload and afterload but is affected by age.

The cardiac deformation can also be represented graphically with high temporal resolution when obtained by Doppler method **(Figure 7.28)**: S wave represents the negative deflection occurring during systole with the peak negative deflection representing maximal longitudinal myocardial shortening (or peak systolic strain). With the start of diastole the myocardial fibers start regaining their original length. Graphically, it is represented in three phases: (i) the early, or rapid filling phase (E-wave) followed by (ii) a plateau phase, or diastasis, and finally, (iii) atrial filling (A-wave).

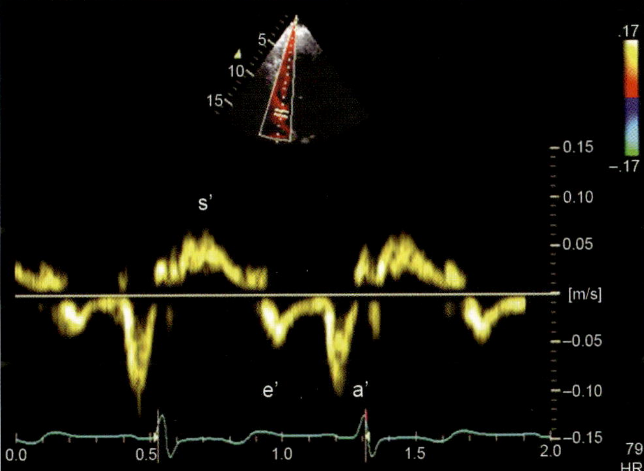


**Figure 7.27:** Septal annular pulsed-wave Doppler tissue velocity pattern in an elderly subject. Both s' and e' are decreased (5–6 cm/sec) while a' is increased (>10 cm/sec). This pattern indicates combined systolic and diastolic dysfunction.
*Abbreviations:* a', late diastolic velocity; e', early diastolic velocity; s', systolic velocity.

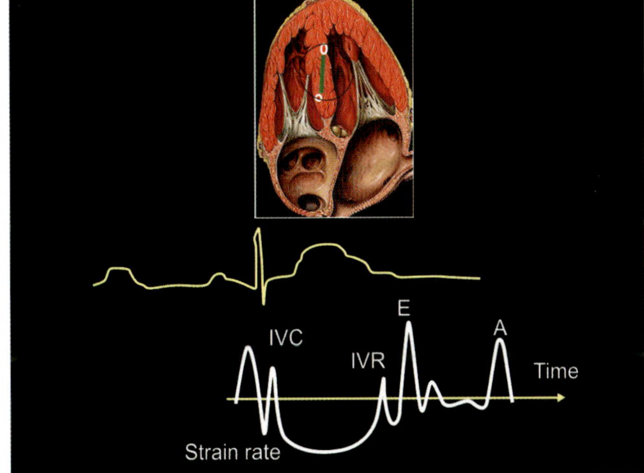


**Figure 7.28:** Strain rate over a fixed segment derived from tissue Doppler method. Lower panel shows various waveforms at frame rate of about 200/sec.
*Abbreviations:* A, late diastolic velocity; E, early diastolic velocity; IVC, isovolumic contraction; IVR, isovolumic relaxation.

There is a definite pattern of electro-mechanical activation with regional inhomogeneity.[18]

9. The speed at which the myocardial deformation occurs is the strain rate and is expressed as unit/sec. Strain rate depicts the change in strain over a period of time **(Figure 7.28)**.[19,20]
10. 2D strain imaging requires high-quality grayscale images[5] with frame rate exceeding 50 f/sec (usually 50–100 frames/sec). Doppler-derived deformation has much greater temporal resolution because of imaging at about 200 frames/sec.[20]
11. To obviate through plane motion, 3D strain estimation has been developed for which the minimum frame rate is 25f/sec.[21] Multibeat acquisition is the preferred way to achieve these frame rates.
12. Deformation parameters can be estimated by multiple methods. But fundamental knowledge is method-independent.
13. Deformation during active contraction is an interaction between contractility (developed force) and the load. Deformation is not a measure of pure contractility.[22]
14. Active contraction occurs only during very early part of systole, but deformation keeps occurring throughout systole and a little beyond.[23]
15. The strain and strain rate subtracts motion due to the effects of neighboring segments.
16. Strain and its rate values are deformation per length and do not need to be corrected for heart size.[24]
17. Deformation parameters depict volume changes of the pressure-volume loop and hence do not provide complete information about the cardiac function.
18. Strain in three dimensions is interrelated, so strain in one direction is representative of regional deformation in more than one direction.[24]
19. Two basic facts to be remembered are as follows: Apex is stationary and the outer boundary of the heart is unchangeable (constant). Action is at the base and within the walls, and the boundary is invariate (the heart has constant volume and outer boundary **(Figure 7.29)**.
20. Isometric function cannot be defined by deformation parameters. However, isometric strain waveforms have clinical applications.
21. Peak velocity and strain rate are early systolic measures, and more closely related to contractility (dP/dT) during active contraction, while displacement and strain are end-systolic measures related to the total stroke volume and EF.
22. Normal myocardium shows the highest strain rate in the first third of the ejection period, whereas the maximal deformation mostly occurs at aortic valve closure (AVC) **(Figure 7.30)**.

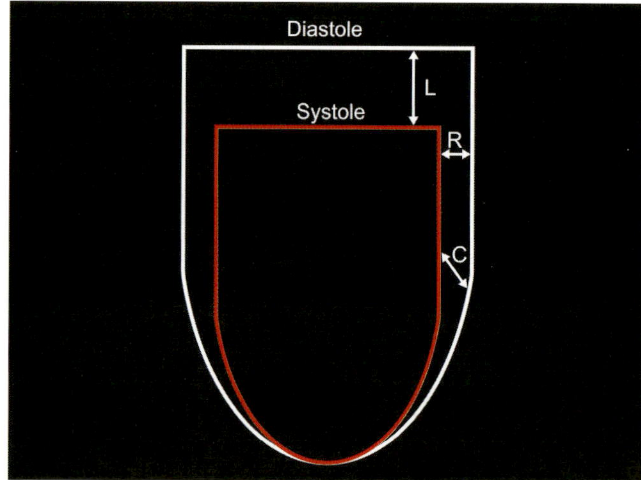


**Figure 7.29:** Depiction of the cavity without walls in diastole and systole. It is the cavity that gets smaller in systole without any change in outer contour (not shown). As the outer contour is constant, longitudinal shortening is coupled with radial thickening, and circumferential shortening.

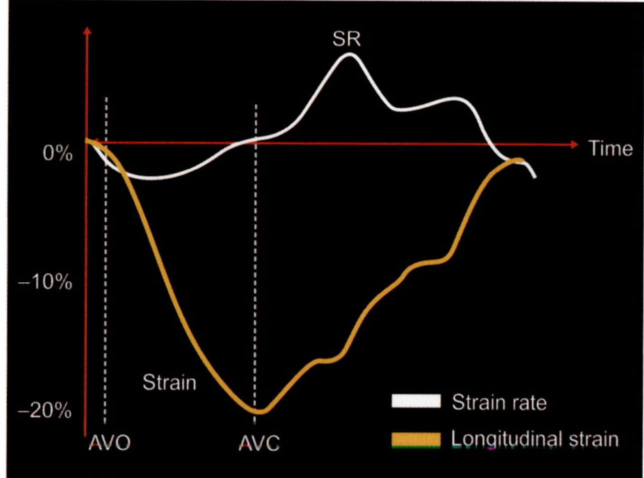


**Figure 7.30:** Diagram showing peaks of strain rate and longitudinal strain with regard to aortic valve closure (AVC). Note early peaking of strain rate.

*Abbreviations:* AVO, aortic valve opening; SR, strain state.

## ACOUSTIC SPECKLE TRACKING

On the basis of the observation that ultrasound images contain many small particles, natural acoustic markers move together with the tissue and can be identified on the adjacent frames. These natural markers are stable acoustic speckles, equally distributed within the myocardium. Each marker can be identified and followed accurately during several consecutive frames.

The new marker location on sequential images is tracked and the local tissue velocity can be calculated as a marker's shift divided by the time between 2 consecutive frames. Changes of the distance between neighboring elements reflect the tissue's contraction or relaxation. Knowing tissue velocity at the previous and current position of the natural acoustic marker and the distance between them, strain rate and strain can be calculated.

It is also called 2D/3D strain imaging. Essentially, it is automatic tracking of interference patterns from conventional grayscale B-mode images during the cardiac cycle.[25] The LV wall is composed of 3 layers of fibers: endocardial layer, mid-layer and epicardial layer. Endocardial and epicardial fibers have longitudinal direction while mid-layer fibers are circumferential. Circumferential strain can be calculated by speckle tracking imaging from the short axis views at all myocardial levels: base, mid-level, and apex. Contraction of longitudinally and circumferentially oriented fibers results in systolic myocardial thickening, which can be characterized by radial strain.

Normally, longitudinal and circumferential endocardial strain is the highest, and epicardial strain is the lowest: epicardial-to-endocardial gradient. Basal strain is the lowest, and apical strain is the highest: base-to-apex gradient.[26] Similar to MRI, acoustic speckle tracking utilizes "Lagrangian strain" which defines motion around a particular point in tissue as it revolves through time and space. Throughout the cardiac cycle, the end-diastolic tissue dimension represents the unstressed initial material length and width. By speckle tracking, normal strains (parallel to the plane of motion) and shear strain (perpendicular to the plane of motion) can be resolved.

The classic example of shear strain is twist or torsional deformation of the left ventricle. Torsion defines the base-to-apex gradient and is the result of myocardial shearing in the circumferential-longitudinal planes such that, when viewed from the apex, the base rotates in an anticlockwise direction. Likewise, the LV apex concomitantly rotates in a clockwise direction. During ejection, LV torsion results in the storage of potential energy into the deformed myofibers. This stored energy is released with the onset of relaxation similar to a spring uncoiling and results in suction forces. These forces are then used for rapid early diastolic restoration.[27]

## STEPS IN OBTAINING TWO-DIMENSIONAL STRAIN

- The 3 levels of the LV short-axis view (basal, middle and apical) and 3 apical views (apical long-axis, 4-chamber and 2-chamber) during 3 consecutive cardiac cycles are acquired in the left lateral decubitus position during a breath hold and digitally stored.
- Care is taken to ensure that the basal short-axis level contains the tip of the mitral valve and that the middle level of the short-axis view contains papillary muscles.
- For the acquisition of the apical short axis view, the transducer position is moved 2 or 3 intercostal spaces more apically to ensure that the view does not contain a papillary muscle with a circular shape.
- The gain and the compression are adjusted to minimize the dropout of the LV endocardial and the epicardial borders.
- The depth and the sector angle are adjusted to include the LV, but the sector size is minimized to achieve a higher frame rate.
- To determine the timing of the cardiac events, the LV inflow and the outflow velocities are recorded using a pulsed-wave Doppler echocardiogram.
- After selecting 1 cardiac cycle with optimal image quality, the endocardial border in the end-systolic frame is manually traced or using automatic function algorithm.
- A region of interest is then drawn to include the entire myocardium.
- The software algorithm automatically segments the LV into 6 equidistant segments and selects the appropriate speckles in the myocardium for tracking.
- The tracking quality is visually evaluated on the 2D images. When the tracking is suboptimal, several attempts are made to adjust the regions of interest.
- Finally, the software automatically generates time-domain LV strain profiles for each of the 6 segments of each view from which the peak strain is measured. The peak strain at each of the 18 segments is determined.
- The level strain is calculated by averaging the segmental values (a maximum of 6 values per level) in the basal, middle, and apical levels.
- The global strain is calculated by averaging the peak strain of the 18 LV segments for each subject.

Following is the description of major strains of the ventricular myocardium.

### Longitudinal Strain

1. Typical global longitudinal strain of the left ventricle is -15% to -25%. This is based upon the assumption that normal mitral annulus systolic excursion is 11–20 mm and the normal length of the base-to-apex left ventricle is 8–9.5 cm.
2. Longitudinal strain increases from base to apex in proportion to the wall stress **(Figure 7.31)**. However, this is not a consistent or universally resolved fact.
3. Abnormality of the longitudinal strain is the earliest sign of myocardial disease including ischemia.[28]
4. Differences in wall stress due to differing wall curvatures between longitudinal, radial, and circumferential axes (by Laplace law) may possibly explain the more frequently observed abnormal systolic longitudinal strain.
5. The high sensitivity of longitudinal strain to detect functional impairment due to subtle ischemia or early

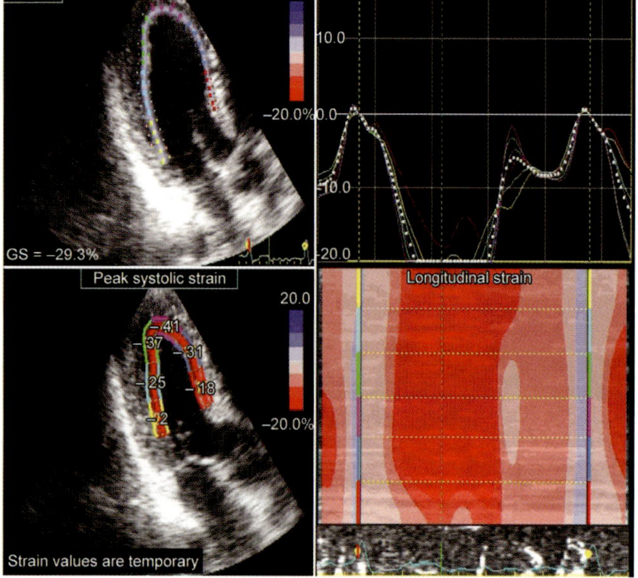


**Figure 7.31:** Two-dimensional longitudinal strain in a modified apical long axis. Note base-to-apex gradient of the anterior septum ( −18, −31, −41) and the posterior wall (−21, −25, −37). *Abbreviations:* APLAX, apical long-axis; AVC, aortic valve closure; GS, global strain.

dysfunction could be also explained by the predominant longitudinal orientation of subendocardial fibers which are more susceptible to ischemia.

6. Longitudinal strain decreases with age,with increasing wall thickness and Obesity.[29] Strain is relatively independent of maturational changes, lending it as a tool for cardiac evaluation across differing ages in pediatric subjects.
7. Speckle-derived strain values are lower than derived by the Doppler method, because the latter has higher temporal resolution. It is also possible because there is greater noise in tissue Doppler method near the peak values.
8. In early stage of disease, radial function acts as a compensatory phenomenon to the decrease in longitudinal deformation to maintain a normal LV ejection fraction. Hence, reduced global longitudinal strain with normal ejection fraction is a subtle sign of dysfunction **(Figure 7.32)**.
9. Different tracking algorithms potentially produce different results. Inter vendor differences could be significant.[30-32] This is the major limitation for prime time use.

## Orthogonal Strain

Circumferential and radial strains represent orthogonalstrains of the myocardium and are obtained from short-axis images **(Figure 7.33)**.

These are affected late in a disease process when the latter becomes transmural.

Three principal strains are interrelated and convey similar information about volume deformation.[26]

## Circumferential Strain

1. Circumferential strain does not reflect circumferential fiber contraction. There would be circumferential shortening even without circumferential fibers.
2. Circumferential strain is mainly the inward movement of mid-wall circumference as the wall thickens **(Figure 7.34)**.
3. The regional circumferential strain may be affected in different ways, depending on the degree of transmural involvement. Subendocardial infarct affects the mid-wall circumferential fibers to a very small extent , if any, with little or no effect on circumferential force.
4. Endocardial circumferential shortening is greater than mid-wall circumferential shortening which is greater than epicardial circumferential shortening. Mean circumferential strain must be taken to mean mid-wall circumferential shortening.
5. Circumferential function plays a pivotal role in maintaining LV structure and tensile strength.
6. Subepicardial organization of collagen structure seems to differ from that in the mid-wall and subendocardial regions accounting for the transmural strain gradients.
7. Circumferential-longitudinal shear, also known as torsion, has been shown to depend strongly on the transmural variation of the helix angle.
8. In patients with early systolic dysfunction or heart failure with normal ejection fraction, longitudinal strain is reduced while circumferential strain remains normal or gets enhanced.

## Radial Strain (Transmural Strain)

Radial strain means wall thickening, but there are no myocardial fibers going in the radial direction **(Figure 7.35)**. Wall thickening is a function of wall shortening to maintain normal muscle volume, as the heart muscle is incompressible. Increased "radial function" (meaning wall thickening) as compensation for decreased longitudinal function actually does not exist, it seems theoretical impossibility.

Clinically, radial strain (time to peak strain) has been used to detect intra-ventricular dyssynchrony **(Figure 7.36)**.[33]

## Velocity Vector Imaging

Velocity vector imaging (VVI) is an echocardiographic method that is based on speckle tracking.[34] In grayscale images, interference by backscattered ultrasound from neighboring structures results in a random, speckled pattern. This gives

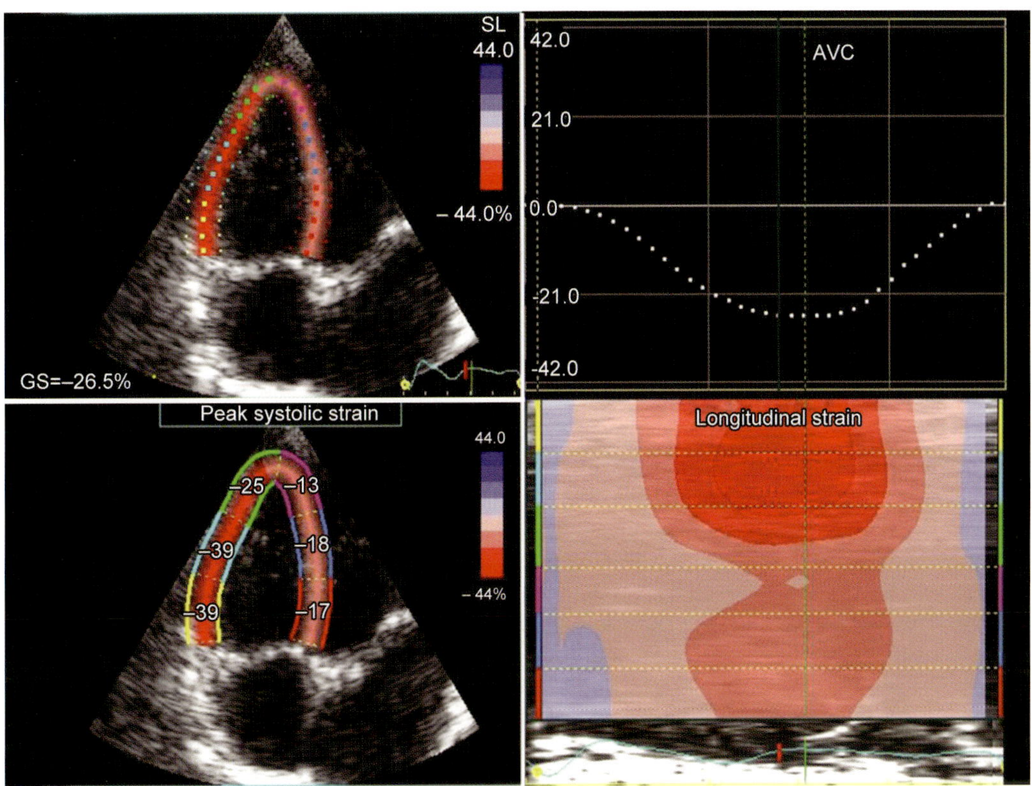


**Figure 7.32:** Right ventricular longitudinal strain by acoustic speckle tracking within the region of interest in apical 4-chamber view in a normal person. Note that the right ventricular free wall has greater longitudinal strain compared to the interventricular septum. *Abbreviations:* AVC, aortic valve closure; GS, global strain; SL, longitudinal strain.

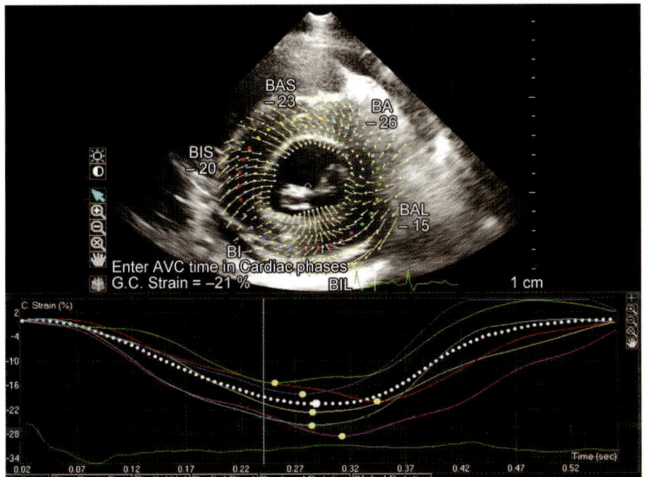


**Figure 7.33:** Vectors of orthogonal strains in short-axis direction. *Abbreviations:* BA, basal anterior; BAL, basal anterolateral; BAS, basal anteroseptal; BI, basal inferior; BIL, basal inferolateral; BIS, basal inferoseptal; AVC, aortic valve closure; GC, global circumferential.

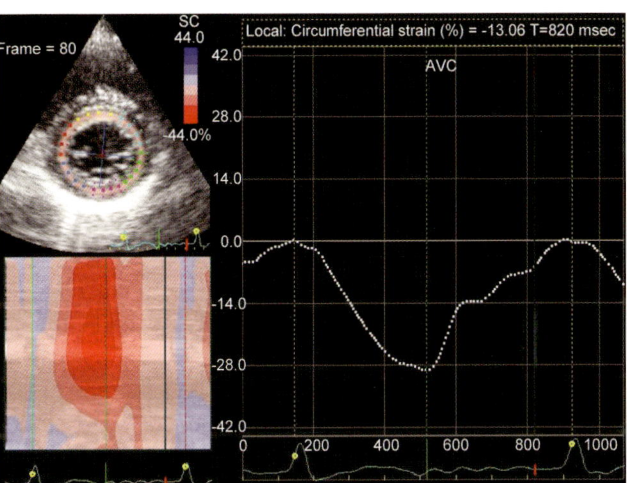


**Figure 7.34:** Short-axis view is used to extract circumferential strain which like longitudinal strain is normally negative and nearly of the same value. Fixed reference point is kept in the center of the cavity from where relative shortening and lengthening in circumferential axis are measured.
*Abbreviations:* AVC, aortic valve closure; SC, circumferential strain.

each small area a unique pattern that remains relatively constant from one frame to the next. With the optimized pattern-matching algorithm, VVI can accurately track these speckles frame by frame, and through reconstructing the deformation and motion, the motion of flow and tissue can be analyzed. The VVI is more precise, self-updating, faster and gives simultaneous information about regional and global ejection fraction. The algorithm works as follows:

1. For each pixel in the image, angle-independent velocity estimation is performed by selecting a search pattern around that pixel in 1 frame and looking for a matching pattern in a search region around that pixel of the following frame.
2. The search pattern is placed at different positions in the search region, and the similarity is measured for the overlapping area.
3. The position, where the highest similarity is found, determines the in-plane frame-to-frame displacement relative to its initial position.
4. A fine grid is automatically positioned within the selected region of interest with an inter-grid point distance of variable size **(Figure 7.37)**.
5. For each frame, the position of each grid point is updated on the basis of the underlying velocity vector.
6. The deformation of the grid follows the deformation of the underlying myocardium.
7. Drifting is compensated for by forcing all grid points to return to their initial positions at the end of the heart cycle **(Figure 7.38)**.
8. Various strains can be estimated from the distance changes between grid points as a function of time **(Figure 7.39)**.

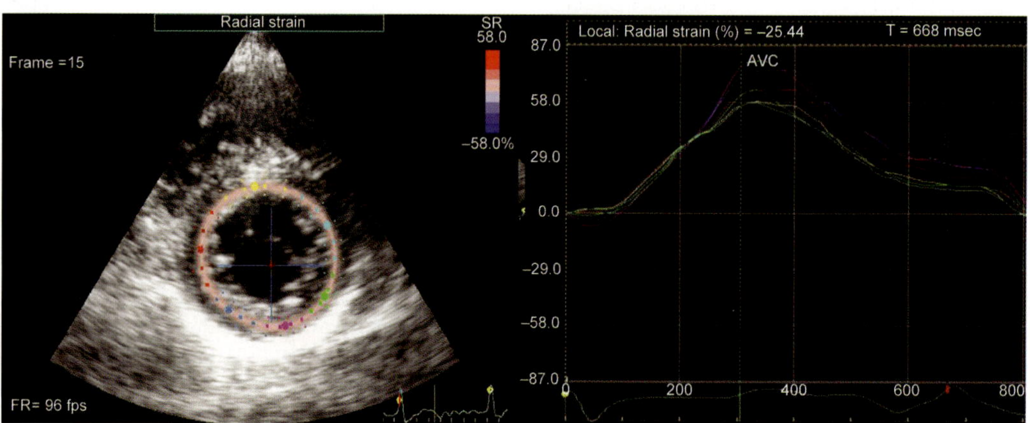


**Figure 7.35:** Short axis at various levels is used to extract radial strain which normally is a positive quantity in systole (thickening) with reference point at the center of the cavity.
*Abbreviation:* AVC, aortic valve closure.

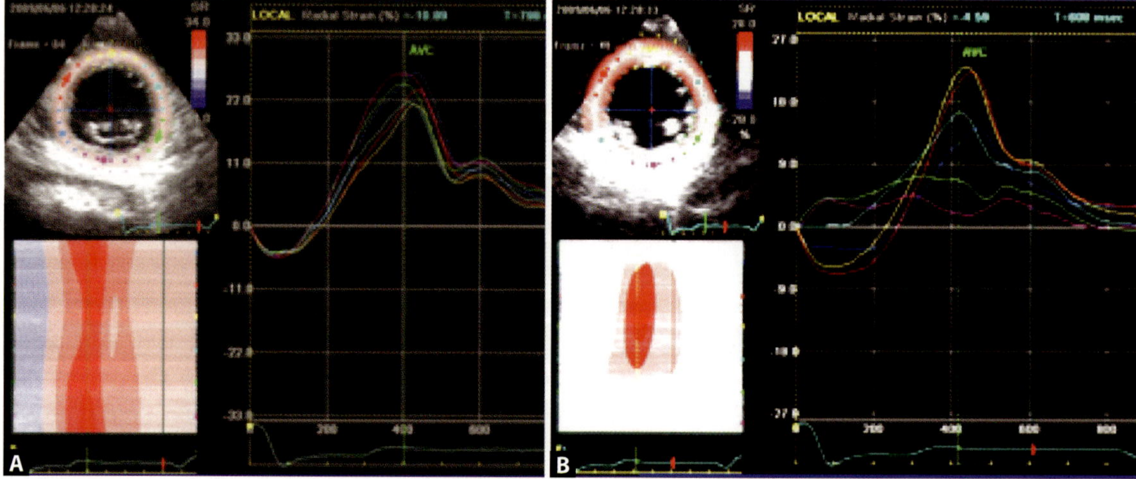


**Figure 7.36A and B:** Left panel shows radial strain waveforms in a patient with heart failure but no intraventricular dyssynchrony. Right panel shows marked dispersion in time to peak radial strain indicating presence of intraventricular dyssynchrony. An anteroposterior segmental peak radial strain delay >130 msec is suggestive of significant intraventricular dyssynchrony[33]
*Abbreviation:* AVC, aortic valve closure.

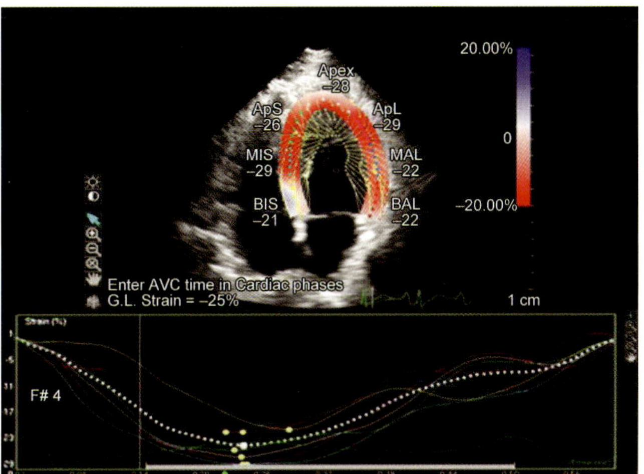


**Figure 7.37:** Longitudinal strain estimation in 4-CV by velocity vector imaging. In early systole, different velocity vectors are depicted.
*Abbreviations:* ApL, apical lateral; ApS, apical septum; AVC, aortic valve closure; BAL, basal anterolateral; BIS, basal inferoseptum; GL, global longitudinal; MAL, mid anterolateral; MIS, mid inferoseptum.

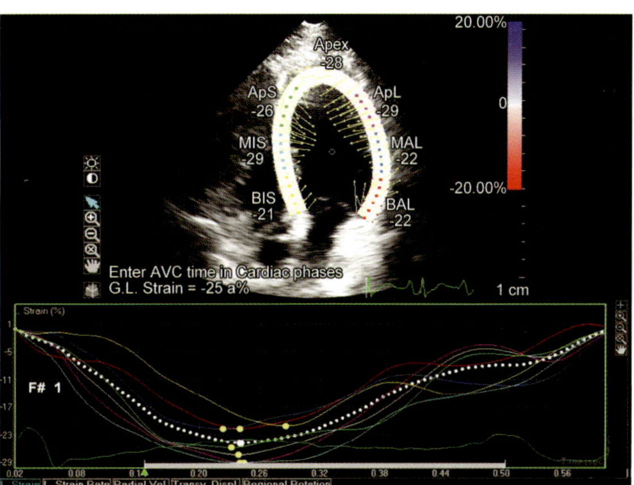


**Figure 7.38:** Velocity vectors shown at end-diastole in apical 4-chamber view.
*Abbreviations:* ApL, apical lateral; ApS, apical septum; AVC, aortic valve closure; BAL, basal anterolateral; BIS, basal inferoseptum; GL, global longitudinal; MAL, mid anterolateral; MIS, mid inferoseptum.

9. Layer-specific strains can be obtained by placing grids in the sub endocardium, mid-wall and subepicardial region. However, this is an area of research with no clear clinical application.

Normal values of various LV peak systolic strains and strain rates aredepicted in **Table 7.2**.

## How to Perform Two-dimensional Strain Imaging?

2D acoustic speckle imaging is a postprocessing technique and is performed on acquired grayscale images in a definite sequence. Frame rates of ≈50–70 are needed to avoid speckle decorrelation, and good image quality is needed for accurate tracking. Translation remains a problem using 2D acquisition methods as error is introduced to strain measurements when the heart swings out of the imaging plane. In addition, out-of-plane motion occurs as the result of rotation and motion of the heart; as a result, only a portion of the real motion can be detected.

1. 2D images of apical 4- and 2-chamber views, as well as the apical long-axis view and the LV parasternal short-axis view (at base, mid and apex) are recorded.
2. Three consecutive cardiac cycle loops are recorded at end expiration.
3. Images are recorded with an acoustic method that provides information frame by frame. The frame rate is kept between 50 f/sec and 100 f/sec. By reducing imaging depth and insonation angle without reducing spatial resolution, frame rate can be optimized.
4. The imaging sector is optimized to complete visualization of the structure under consideration.

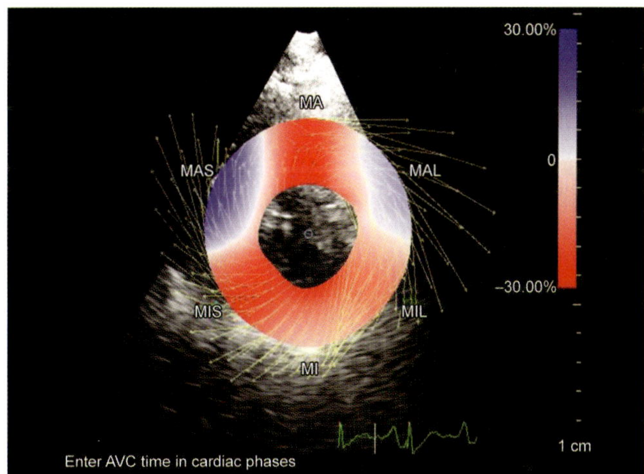


**Figure 7.39:** Velocity vectors seen in short axis of the left ventricle showing circumferential strain. Velocity vectors also suggest possibility of clockwise rotation.
*Abbreviations:* AVC, aortic valve closure; MA, mid anterior; MAL, mid anterolateral; MAS, mid anteroseptum; MI, mid inferior; MIL, mid inferolateral; MIS, mid inferoseptum.

**Table 7.2:** Normal values of various left ventricular peak systolic strains and strain rates

| *Parameter* | *Normal value* |
|---|---|
| Longitudinal strain | –15–25% |
| Longitudinal strain rate | 1.0–1.4 $sec^{-1}$ |
| Radial strain | 50–70% |
| Radial strain rate | 3.1–4.1 $sec^{-1}$ |
| Circumferential strain | –15–30% |
| Area strain | –30 to –50% |

5. The 17-segment LV model of the American Society of Echocardiography is used to analyze regional cardiac function.
6. The long-axis ventricular walls were divided into three levels: base, middle and apical.
7. Using a point-click approach, a number of points are placed along the endocardium or the middle layer of myocardium. The software automatically traces epicardium.
8. The number of points is decided depending on the radian of the endocardium.
9. In apical views, three points are placed: medial edge of the mitral annulus, lateral edge of the mitral annulus, and the apical endocardium **(Figure 7.40)**.
10. The correct tracking of border-zones is visually controlled and manually corrected.
11. Peak-positive or peak-negative strain is extracted from each strain curve. Strain curves and numbers are obtained by off-line analysis.
12. In the VVI analysis, a relatively static reference point is placed at the apical location in the long-axis view and at the center of ventricle in the short-axis view.
13. Segments for which no adequate image quality can be obtained are rejected by the software and excluded from the analysis **(Figure 7.41)**.
14. The region of interest (ROI) is defined by tracing the endocardium in a still frame (default at end systole).
15. The ROI width is set to match the myocardial thickness. This has to be performed manually most often, but automatic function imaging is also gaining ground.
16. Bull's eye map depiction is possible for all types of strain: time-to-peak strain and extracted postsystolic strain **(Figure 7.42 and 7.43)**.
17. 3D strain is less time consuming and provides global longitudinal, radial, circumferential, and area strain from a single pyramidal volume by just tracking the endocardium in systole and diastole.[35]
18. It is crucial that the tracking algorithm is able to track the tissue correctly. Factors that affect the tracking accuracy include image quality, frame rate, and line density.

## EFFECTS OF ISCHEMIA ON REGIONAL DEFORMATION METRICS

Strains and strain rates are homogeneously distributed across the myocardium. The detection of even subtle changes in either measure suggests myocardial dysfunction. In the appropriate patient at rest, subclinical LV systolic dysfunction correlates with the presence of obstructive coronary artery disease (CAD). In response to a flow-limiting stenosis at rest and a nonflow-limiting stenosis during dobutamine infusion, longitudinal and circumferential (but not radial) strain are reduced.[36] Longitudinal and circumferential mechanics are altered earlier than radial mechanics in the ischemic cascade.

- Acute ischemia induces systolic thinning, decreases systolic deformation, and increases postsystolic thickening (PST). These changes are directly related to perfusion.[37]
- With acute total vessel occlusion, systolic deformation is totally ablated and replaced by systolic lengthening (paradoxical strain).
- An acute increase in afterload exaggerates the effects on deformation induced by ischemia, whereas an increase in preload diminishes it.[37]
- Reperfusion restores deformation to near normal, but some early systolic lengthening and PST remain present in the early phase as a result of stunning.
- Late systolic thinning can also occur during ischemia just before the start of PST.[37]

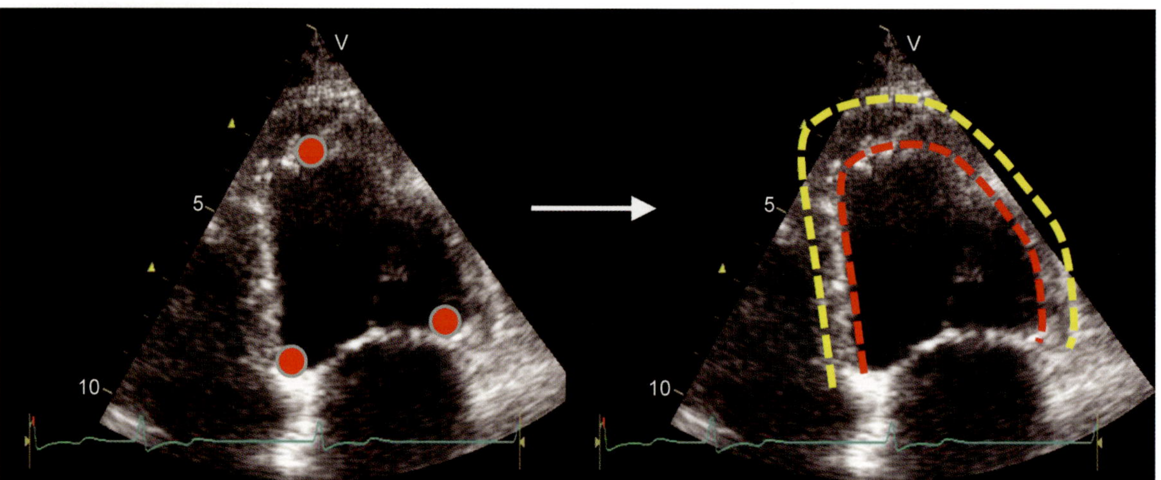


**Figure 7.40:** Point-and-click method to extract longitudinal strain curves in apical views. Marking three points on the endocardium (left panel), generates the region of interest (ROI) which can be manually adjusted, and strain values can be derived after accepting the ROI.

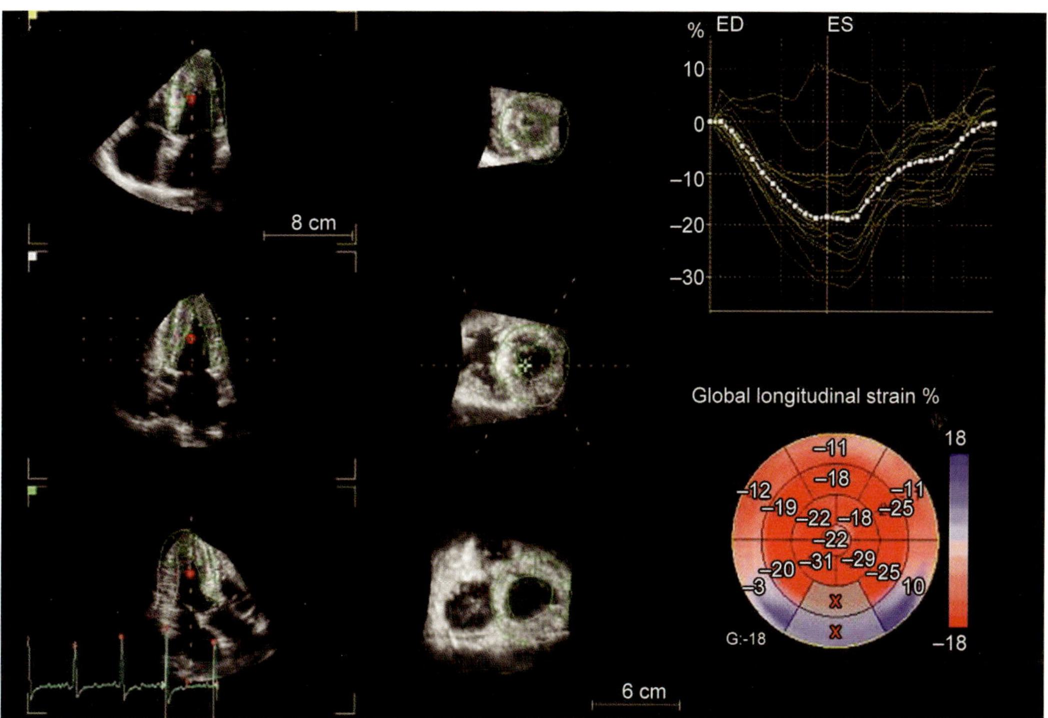


**Figure 7.41:** Three-dimensional strain by acoustic speckle tracking. Bull's eye map is marked "X" in boxes for mid and basal posterior segments because of unacceptable image quality. *Abbreviations:* ED, end-diastole; ES, end-systole.

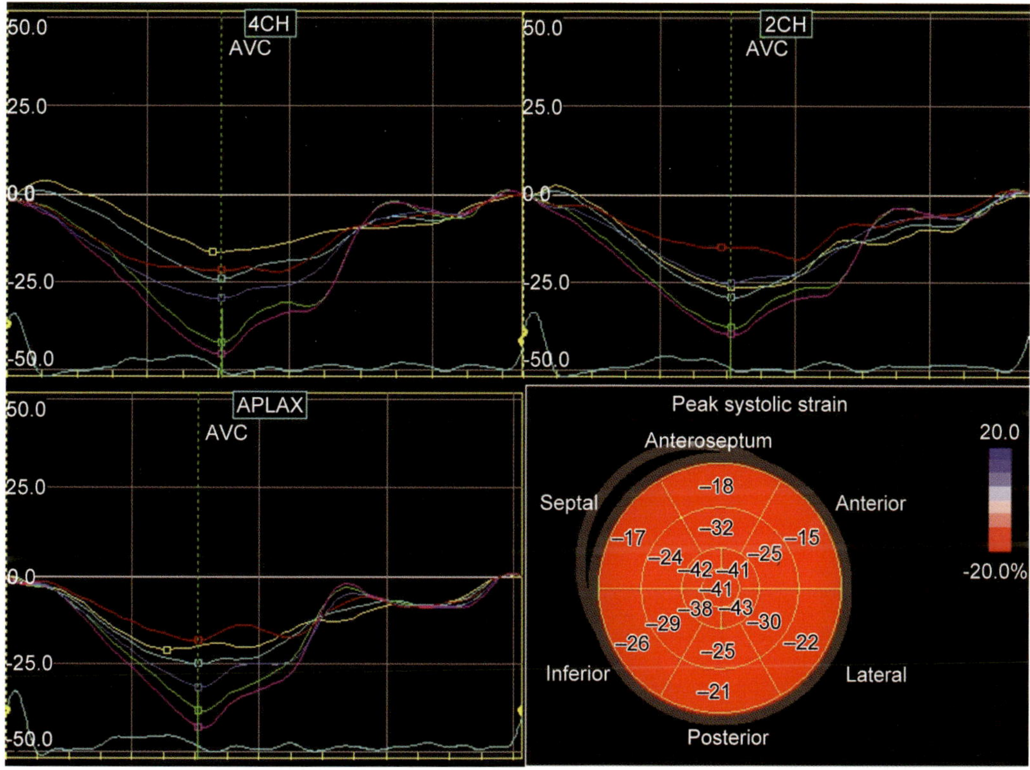


**Figure 7.42:** Bull's eye map showing longitudinal strain in 17-segment model in a normal subject. *Abbreviations:* 2CH, 2-chamber; 4CH, 4-chamber; APLAX, apical long-axis; AVC, aortic valve closure.

- Strain shows a biphasic response to physiological stress and decreases at peak stress due to lower stroke volume as a consequence of higher heart rates.[38-40]

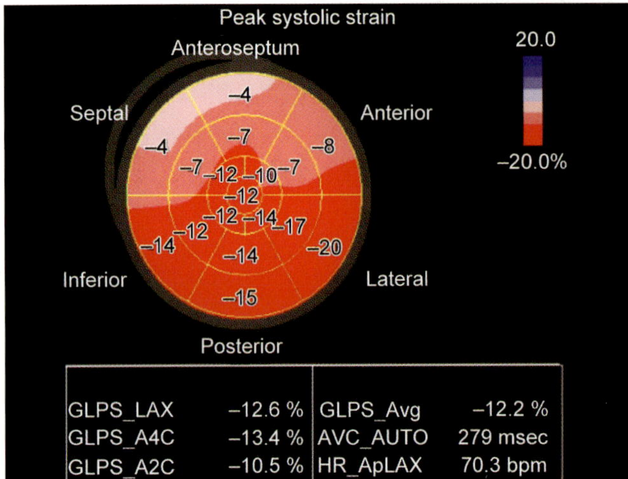


**Figure 7.43:** Bull's eye map of longitudinal strain in a patient with hypertrophic cardiomyopathy and resting intraventricular gradient of 64 mm Hg. Note significantly decreased strain in anterior septum and anterior wall.
*Abbreviations:* A2C, apical 2-chamber; A4C, apical 4-chamber; ApLAX, apical long-axis; AVC, aortic valve closure; Avg, average; GLPS, global longitudinal peak strain; HR, heart rate; LAX, long-axis.

## Early Systolic Longitudinal Lengthening (Paradoxical Longitudinal Systolic Strain)

During isovolumic contraction, there may be a brief systolic lengthening because of contraction of basal circumferential fibers, and this is a normal phenomenon **(Figure 7.44)**.

During the isovolumic contraction phase, segments with reduced rate of force development might demonstrate significant and prolonged systolic lengthening **(Figure 7.45)**:

1. This is possible because of reversible dysfunctionas in ischemia, late activation of the segment due to conduction block, or segmental fibrosis resisting the development of force.
2. Duration of early systolic lengthening may provide incremental value over peak systolic longitudinal strain for the identification of patients with significant systolic dysfunction.[37]
3. Duration of early systolic lengthening has been shown to be a strong and independent predictor of significant CAD.

## Postsystolic Longitudinal Shortening

1. Postsystolic shortening (PSS) means that the segment continues shortening after the AVC, often after a short relaxation giving one or two peaks a systolic and a postsystolic, or a single peak after AVC as shown in **Figure 7.46**.[41]

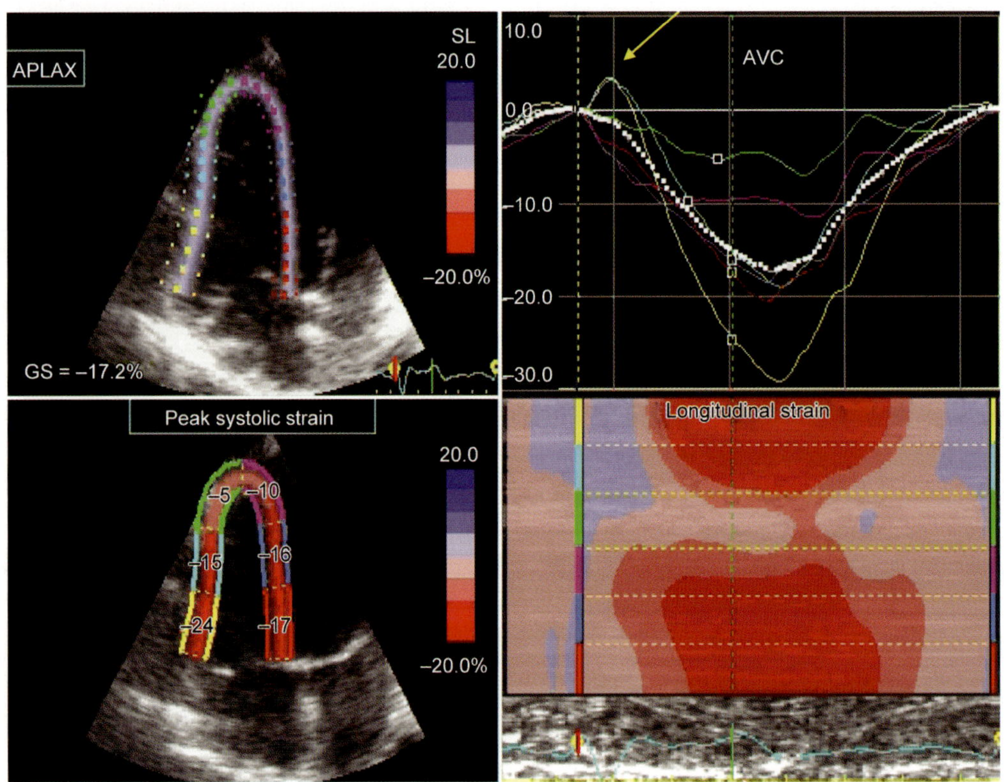


**Figure 7.44:** Two-dimensional longitudinal strain of the right ventricle. Note brief waves (arrow) of longitudinal positive strain for a brief period. *Abbreviations:* APLAX, apical long-axis; AVC, aortic valve closure; GS, global strain.

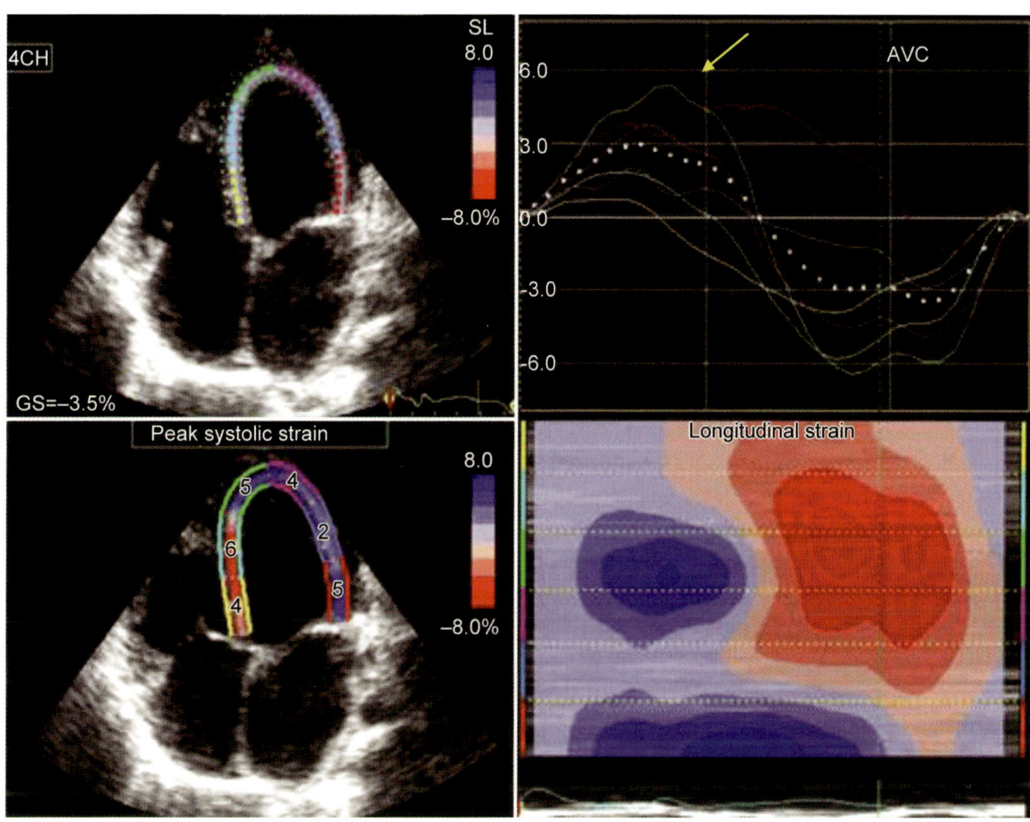


**Figure 7.45:** Two-dimensional longitudinal strain in a patient with idiopathic dilated cardiomyopathy in apical 4-chamber (4CH) view. Arrow points to paradoxical positive strain for nearly half of systole in all the segments.
*Abbreviations:* AVC, aortic valve closure; GS, global strain.

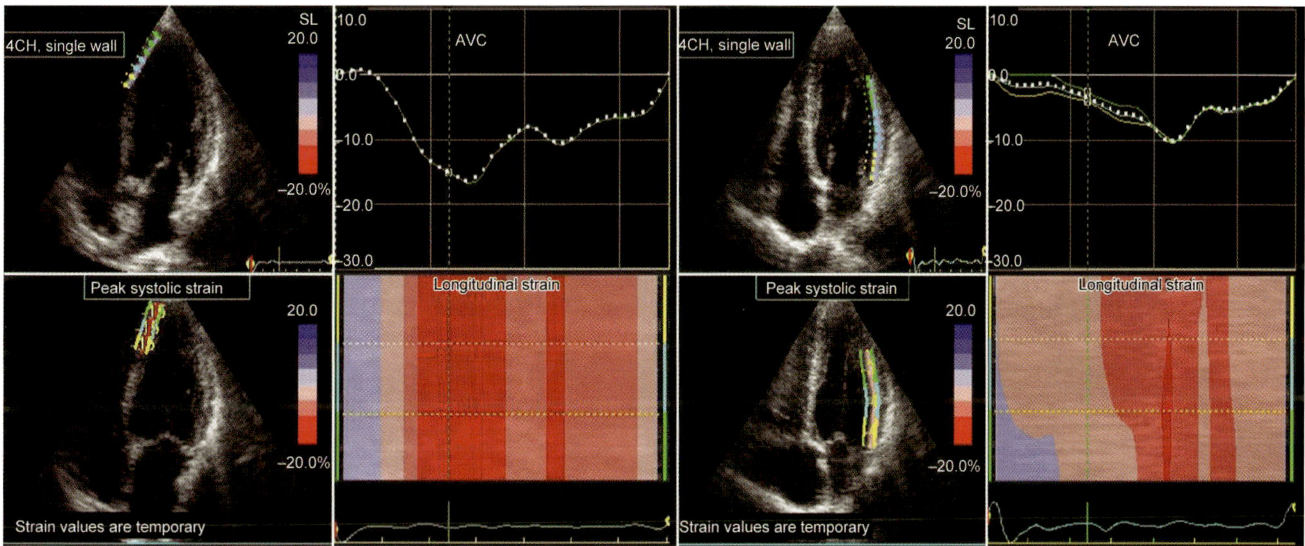


**Figure 7.46:** Left panel shows longitudinal strain from apicoseptal segment and the right panel from the basal and mid-lateral wall. Note markedly reduced end-systolic strain and significant postsystolic strain in the right panel. The patient had critical stenosis of the left circumflex artery.
*Abbreviations:* AVC, aortic valve closure; 4CH, 4-chamber.

2. The definition of shortening as postsystolic is dependent on the location of AVC which can be done by TDI.[41]
3. A small amount of PSS may be present in up to 1/3rd of normal segments but not more than 3%.
4. Pathological strain is concomitant with reduced systolic strain, and higher postsystolic strain (in magnitude), as well as later peak PSS.
5. PSS and PST are to some degree equivalent, because of the incompressibility.
6. Presence of PSS is mainly a measure of inhomogeneity of force development, because of differences in activation, load or contractility, and not as specific marker of ischemia.
7. The new concept of "mechanical dispersion", meaning unequal duration of the shortening phase, seems to be due to variable amount of PSS within the ventricle.
8. Presence of PSS may give rise to asynchrony between walls.
9. Presence of PSS in a segment leads to a delay in the onset of segmental lengthening compared to the normal segments, so the finding is equivalent to the delayed compression/expansion crossover.[41]
10. PSS is mainly the reduced, but prolonged contraction of a segment due to ischemia and/or relative load increase in the early diastolic interaction with normally relaxing segments.[41]
11. Stretch recoil is a mechanism for PSS especially in segments which do not show systolic shortening. Hence, PSS is not always suggestive of viability or ischemia.
12. The degree of this thickening is expressed as the postsystolic index (i.e. postsystolic increment divided by systolic strain.
13. Postsystolic motion is reported in >30% of myocardial segments in normal subjects but can be identified as pathologic, if there is a concomitant reduction of systolic strain, especially if the PST is marked (e.g. index from >25% to 35%).
14. Presence of PST or PSS actually implies that tissue elasticity is preserved, which means that no any important, irreversible fibrosis is present.
15. The PST can also occur in normal myocardium, especially with increased afterload (aortic stenosis, hypertension), myocardial storage diseases, and abnormal activation.[42]

## PARADOXICAL STRAIN PATTERNS

Holosystolic stretching in longitudinal or circumferential plane is an extension of the early systolic lengthening found in diseased states, especially in scarred tissue, dilated cardiomyopathy (indicative of dyssynchrony) **(Figure 7.47)** and in left bundle branch block (septal holosystolic stretch).

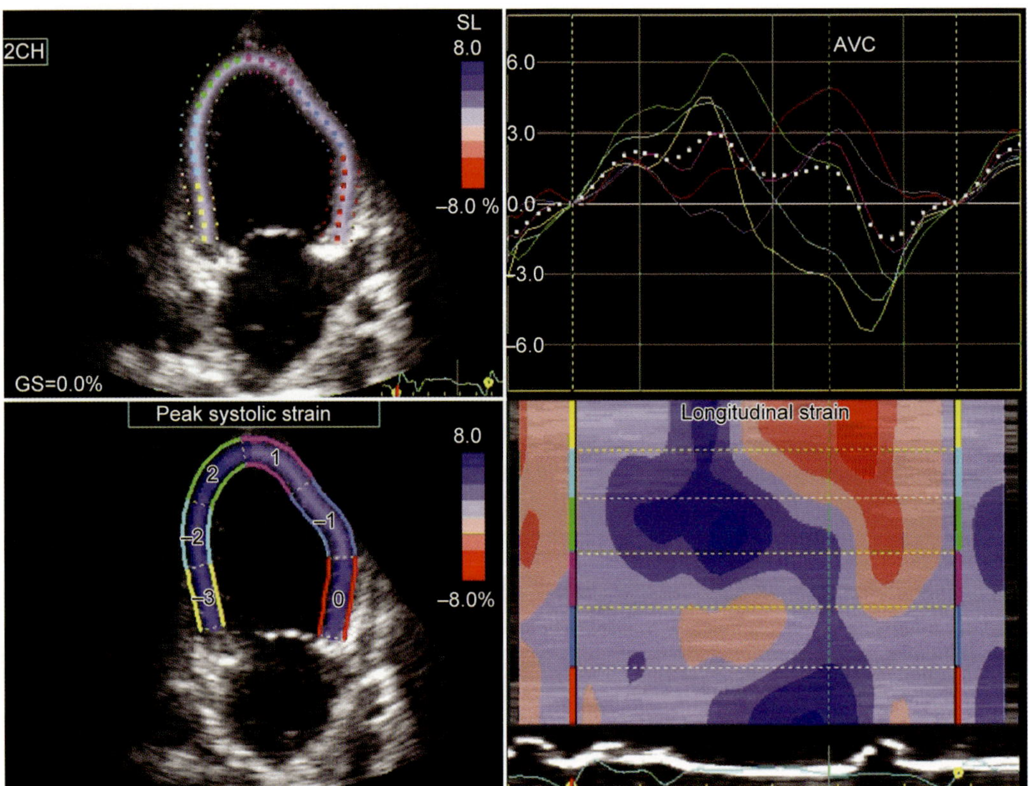


**Figure 7.47:** Holosystolic longitudinal stretch with postsystolic shortening in apical 2-chamber view in a child with dilated cardiomyopathy. *Abbreviations:* 2CH, 2-chamber; AVC, aortic valve closure; GS, global strain.

## Right Ventricular Deformation

The right ventricle has complex geometry with mainly longitudinal/ circumferential fiber orientation in the free wall and minimal radial function due to thin walls. Longitudinal deformation of the RV free wall provides assessment of systolic function **(Figure 7.48 to 7.51)** which does correlate with RV ejection fraction as well as strain estimate by sonomicrometry.[43-45]

1. Apical views are used to obtain RV free wall longitudinal strain.
2. RV free wall longitudinal strain is 5–10% more than the LV free wall.
3. A base-to-apex gradient is also seen but is not a consistent finding.
4. RV free wall deformation assessment is feasible in >90% cases.
5. There is a reasonably good correlation with tissue-Doppler derived strain.
6. Global RV strain,however, has modest correlation with ejection fraction.
7. Significant utility of RV free wall strain lies in assessment of ambiguous conditions like arrhythmogenic dysplasia, noncompaction, pulmonary embolism, Friedrich's ataxia, etc.[45]

## Left Atrial Function by Deformation Imaging

Deformation imaging is a good method for assessing reservoir function of the left atrium.[46-50] The reservoir function (lengthening or increase in volume during ventricular systole) is coupled with longitudinal function of the left ventricle **(Figure 7.52 and 7.53)**. Reduced left atrial diastolic longitudinal strain is an indicator of left atrial dysfunction. However, many conditions are associated with predominant left atrial dysfunction with some decrease in LV longitudinal function.

It may provide incremental information about subclinical atrial pathology like likelihood of developing atrial fibrillation, left atrial thrombus, paroxysmal atrial fibrillation recurrence after ablation, etc. It is still an investigational tool but with great promise **(Figure 7.53)**.

## Mechanical Properties of the Aorta

Understanding the mechanical behavior of the arterial wall and its spatial variations is essential for the study of vascular physiopathology. Although it is generally accepted that the aortic wall gets stiffer along its length, the spatial variations in the mechanical behavior of the aorta are not well understood. Deformation imaging of the aorta aids in understanding the mechanical properties of aorta and may be a great tool in

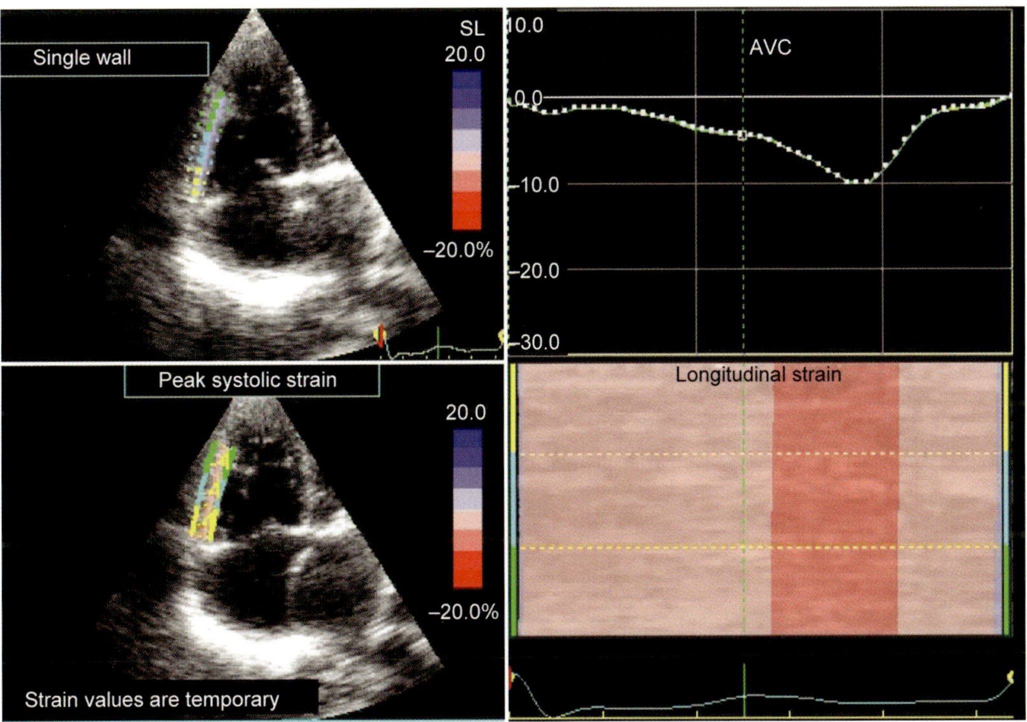


**Figure 7.48:** Right ventricular free wall longitudinal strain in a patient with type I pulmonary hypertension. Note markedly decreased end-systolic strain (–5%) and 50% postsystolic strain. *Abbreviation:* AVC, aortic valve closure; SL, longitudinal strain.

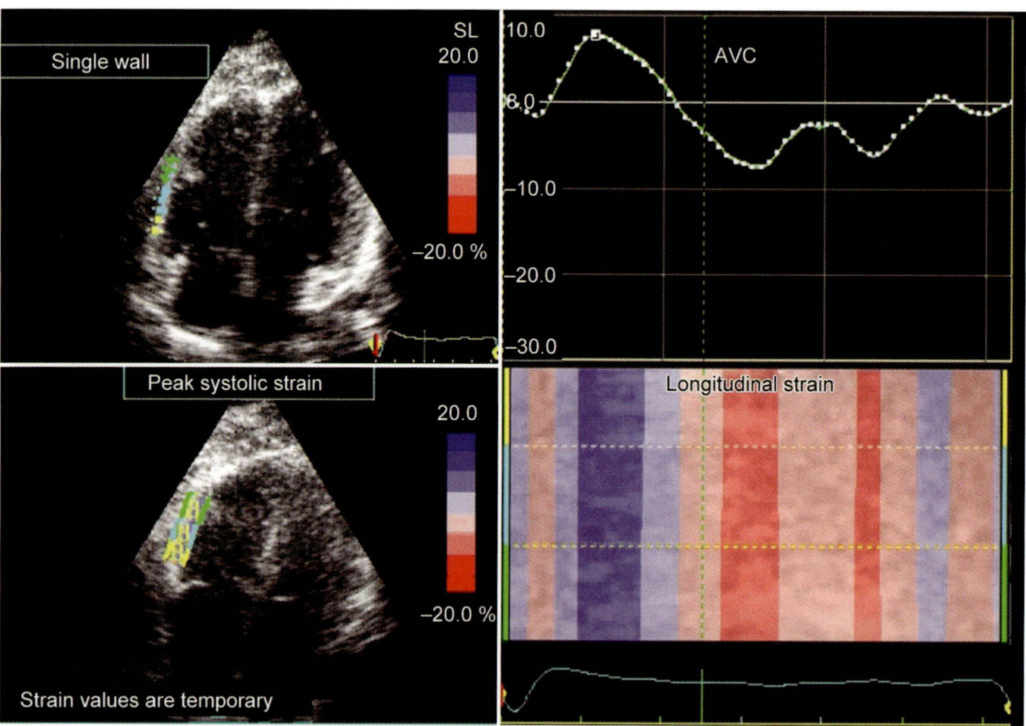


**Figure 7.49:** Right ventricular free wall longitudinal strain in a case of suspected pulmonary embolism. Note early-systolic positive strain (systolic stretching) with markedly reduced end-systolic (–4%) strain and also postsystolic strain. *Abbreviation:* AVC, aortic valve closure; SL, longitudinal strain.

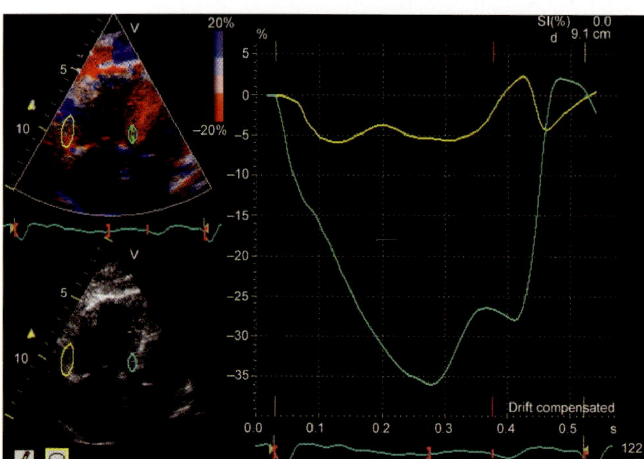


**Figure 7.50:** Comparison of tissue Doppler-derived strain at basal RV free wall (–6%) and the basal septum (–36%) in the same patient as in **Figure 7.34.** Increased basal septal strain may be a compensatory phenomenon.

future **(Figure 7.54)**. The aortic circumferential strain can be measured with 2D strain echocardiography and is a new tool that can be used to directly and easily evaluate aortic stiffness.[51] Normative age-specific data are yet to be reported in adequate numbers. Also through-plane motion remains a major handicap as of now.

## Three-dimensional/Four-dimensional Deformation Imaging

A 3D or four-dimensional (4D) strain is a postprocessing research tool that tracks inherent features in a 3D image called "natural acoustic markers" from frame to frame in three dimensions over time **(Figure 7.55)**. 3D strain uses a tracking algorithm based on frame-to-frame block matching performed in three dimensions. This involves successively searching for a match between 3D patterns found in one 3D frame and in the next. The 3D strain region of interest is automatically generated in the end-systolic frame and is built up from an endocardial and an epicardial mesh. The epicardial mesh is automatically generated from the epicardial mesh used in the LV mass stage. A four- dimensional mapping (three spatial dimensions + time) of myocardial strain-rate would help describe the mechanical properties of the myocardium.

1. 3D strain performs tracking over time in three dimensions, which also means there is no out-of-plane motion issue.
2. It is less time consuming, as it provides global deformation in a quick fashion.
3. This method exclusively provides the area strain which is a combination of longitudinal and circumferential strain. Area strain is superior to any single strain in detecting myocardial function.
4. If more than three segments are rejected because of poor tracking, global strain values will not be calculated.

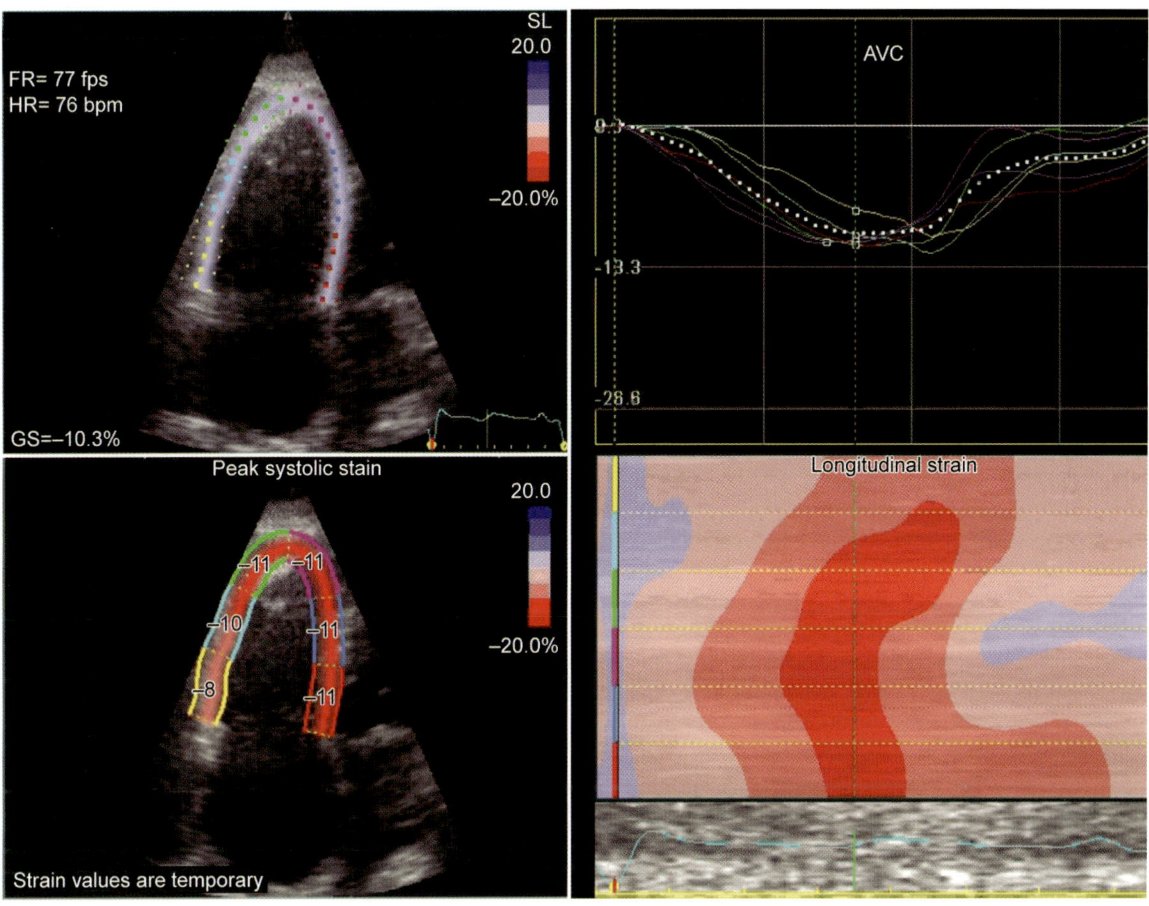


**Figure 7.51:** Reduced global right ventricular (RV) strain with postsystolic strain. Note decrease in RV free wall strain is proportional to that of the interventricular septum.

*Abbreviations:* AVC, aortic valve closure; GS, global strain; SL, longitudinal strain.

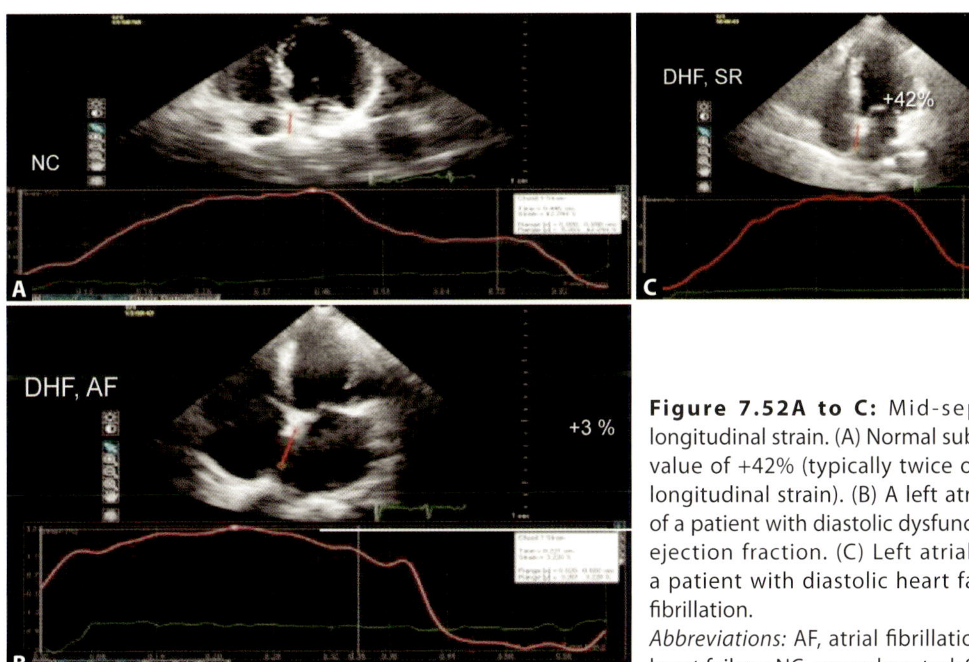


**Figure 7.52A to C:** Mid-septal left atrial longitudinal strain. (A) Normal subject with a strain value of +42% (typically twice of left ventricular longitudinal strain). (B) A left atrial strain (+33%) of a patient with diastolic dysfunction with normal ejection fraction. (C) Left atrial strain (+3%) in a patient with diastolic heart failure with atrial fibrillation.

*Abbreviations:* AF, atrial fibrillation; DHF, diastolic heart failure; NC, normal control; SR, sinus rhythm.

**Figure 7.53A and B:** Left atrial longitudinal strain during ventricular systole (A) and the left ventricular longitudinal strain in 4-chamber view in a patient with heart failure and normal ejection fraction. (B) Reservoir function of the left atrium is markedly reduced (–6% longitudinal strain compared to >+40% in normal subjects). Marked decrease in reservoir function (either with reduced strain or paradoxical shortening) is commonly found in patients with heart failure with or without systolic dysfunction and is an indicator of left atrial dysfunction.
*Abbreviations:* ApL, apical lateral; ApS, apical septum; BAL, basal anterolateral; BIS, basal inferoseptum; MAL, mid anterolateral; MIS, mid inferoseptum.
Please note these segment labels in the first image are erroneous as the speckle tracking software used for measuring left ventricular strain is used here for measuring left atrial strain also.

5. Radial strain is estimated from the area strain assuming that the segment has a constant volume. This way, it is more accurate than the 2D strain method.
6. Strain values in 2D bull's eye map are the peak systolic values, including positive peaks; while in 3D strain, it is the strain values from the end-systolic frame that are used.

## CLINICAL APPLICATIONS OF STRAIN AND STRAIN RATE IMAGING

Technical and vendor-related differences do not allow, at the moment, wide-spread clinical use of strain and strain rate imaging except perhaps the longitudinal strain which is more robust and reproducible and has been used in various clinical situations. Following are the fields wherein strain/strain rate imaging has been used:

1. In CAD to detect ischemia, viability, reperfusion, extent of transmural infarction.
2. To detect subclinical systolic dysfunction in valvular heart disease like asymptomatic aortic stenosis, aortic regurgitation, mitral regurgitation, etc.
3. Detection of intraventricular dyssynchrony.
4. Understanding diastolic dysfunction and heart failure with normal ejection fraction.
5. Incremental value in prognosticating heart failure and ischemic heart disease.

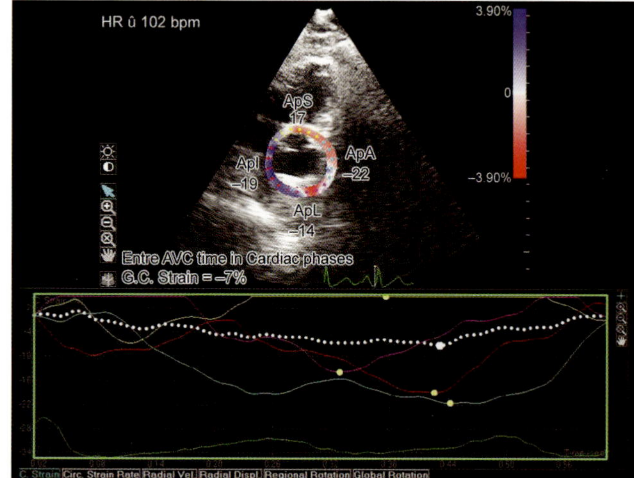


**Figure 7.54:** Circumferential strain of the ascending aorta in a subject with hypertension.
Please ignore the segment labels in this image as they are erroneous.

6. Detecting earliest evidence of cardiotoxicity of chemotherapeutic agents
7. Heart transplant rejection.
8. Study of right ventricular function.
9. Differentiating physiological hypertrophy from the pathological one.
10. Predicting extent of myocardial fibrosis noninvasively.

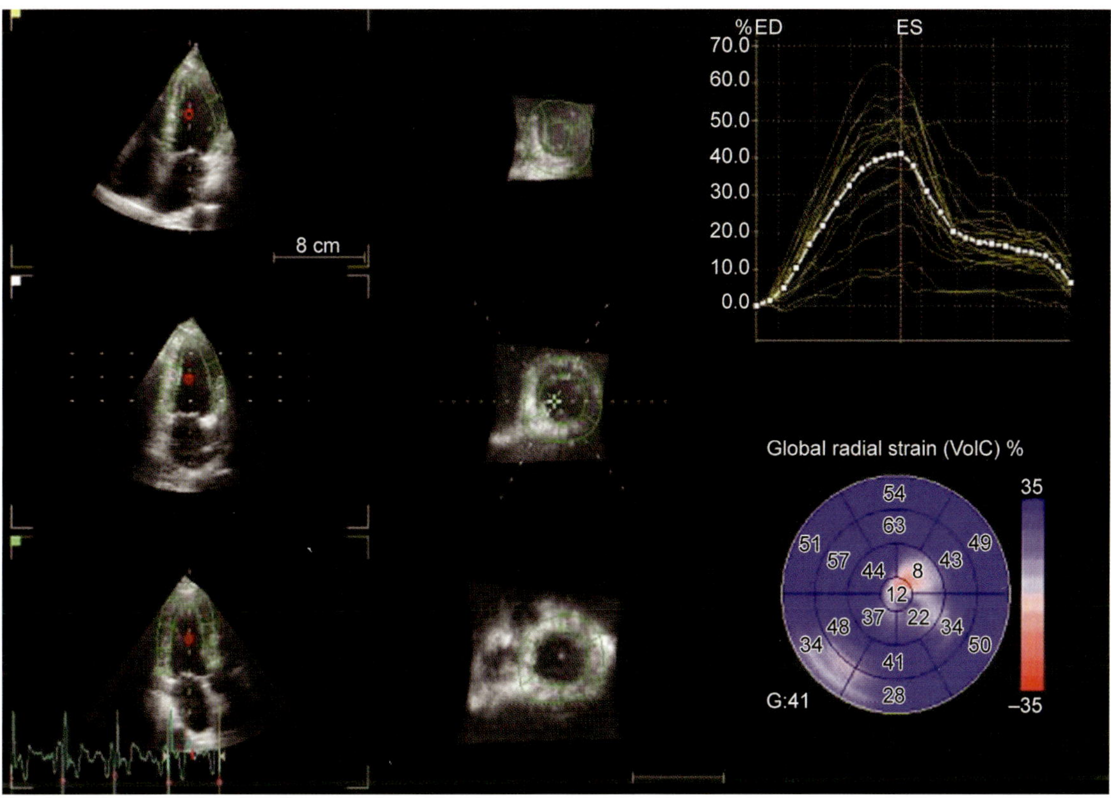


**Figure 7.55:** Three-dimensional (3D) radial strain in a normal subject. All 17 segment-strain curves can be simultaneously shown with the average value (interrupted line) and Bull's eye map. The 3D data-set is sliced to show three apical and three short axis slices, allowing inspection of the tracking of each segment both in apical and short-axis directions.
*Abbreviations:* ED, end-diatsole; ES, end-systole.

## LIMITATIONS

1. 2D/3D speckle tracking echocardiography is generally more smoothed and, therefore, less influenced by artifacts than TDI-derived strain but also less sensitive to detect small regions of pathology.
2. Despite noise reduction by increased smoothing and despite an anticlutter filter, dropout is still problematic, and stationary reverberations are sometimes still tracked or interfered with the frame-by-frame tracking, resulting in drift or incorrect calculation of strain and strain rate.
3. A clear delineation of the endocardial border is also important for a reliable radial and transverse tracking. Since spatial resolution is lower in the transverse direction, tracking perpendicular to the ultrasound beam becomes less robust.
4. At present, the optimal frame rate for speckle tracking seems to be 50–70 frames/sec which is lower compared to TDI: this could result in undersampling, especially in patients with tachycardia.
5. Rapid events during the cardiac cycle (e.g. isovolumic phases) may disappear altogether, and peak strain rate and velocity values may be reduced because of undersampling, especially in isovolumic phases and in early diastole.
6. Higher frame rates could reduce the undersampling problem, although this will result in a reduction of spatial resolution.
7. Speckle-tracking software uses a frame-by-frame approach to follow the myocardial movement and searches each consecutive frame for a speckle pattern closely resembling and in close proximity to the reference frame. With a too low frame rate the speckle pattern could be outside the search area, again resulting in poor tracking. This can be obviated by 3D strain imaging.
8. Optimal tracking of the ROI is not only dependent on optimal image quality, but also on the implemented tracking algorithm. Software programs designed for speckle tracking are relatively new and are subjected to periodical improvements. Different tracking algorithms potentially produce different results.
9. Visualization of the myocardial wall needs to be optimal with a clear delineation of myocardial tissue and extracardiac structures and avoidance of dropout, since this will result in unacceptable ROI tracking and drift.

10. The optimal balance between temporal and spatial resolution is achieved when adjusting the image sector slightly wider than the interrogated wall.
11. Near-field clutter can be reduced with the implementation of dual-focus imaging when artefacts are prominent.
12. For parasternal recordings (for radial and circumferential function on the short axis), small angle recordings are not possible; all myocardial segments need to be in the image field.
13. For any recording, it should be kept in mind that all myocardial segments need to be visualized optimally, since poor tracking of any segment often affects tracking of the adjacent segments.
14. Inaccurate results are obtained near boundaries between different kinds of tissues, and this may limit the utility of 2D strain.

Although the fundamental concept of 2D speckle tracking may be the same, 2 D image tracking ability on a frame-by-frame basis in each of the systems from various vendors is different, resulting in a maximum difference of up to 20% in the feasibility between the 2 vendors. Image quality can affect the tracking feasibility observed in all of the systems from the different vendors (i.e. good image–good tracking, bad image–bad tracking). The tracking ability at medium-range image quality, however, is significantly inferior in some systems compared to the other systems. Therefore, it must be acknowledged that the contribution of image quality to tracking feasibility differs with vendor. The low 2D strain intraclass correlation measured from the same subjects using different systems raises a caution about the clinical application of 2D speckle tracking imaging. Systems from different vendors are not interchangeable when acquiring and analyzing 2D strain data to assess longitudinal changes in the LV function from the same subjects. Although the highest correlations of global longitudinal strain indicates that longitudinal strain is less subject to variation, relatively larger limits of agreement cannot validate whether the observed difference is clinically relevant.

## REFERENCES


1. Smerup M, Nielsen E, Agger P, Frandsen J, Vestergaard-Poulsen P, Andersen J, et al. The three-dimensional arrangement of the myocytes aggregated together within the mammalian ventricular myocardium. Anat Rec (Hoboken). 2009;292:1-11.
2. Takayama Y, Kosta KD, Covell JW. Contribution of laminar myofiber architecture to load-dependent changes in mechanics of LV myocardium. Am J Physiol. 2002;282:H510-20.
3. Hunter PJ, Pullan AJ, Smaill BH. Modeling total heart function. Annu Rev Biomed Eng. 2003;5:147-77.
4. Poveda F, Gil D, Martí E, Andaluz A, Ballester M, Carreras F. Helical structure of the cardiac ventricular anatomy assessed by diffusion tensor magnetic resonance imaging with multi-resolution tractography. Rev Esp Cardiol (Engl Ed). 2013;66(10):782-90.
5. Gao C, Lu K, Ye W, et al. Reconstruction of the architecture of ventricular myocardial fibers in ex vivo human hearts. Heart Surg Forum. 2009; 12(4):E225-9.
6. Munoz-Moreno E, Cardenes R, Frangi AF. Analysis of the helix and transverse angles of the muscle fibers in the myocardium based on Diffusion Tensor Imaging. Conf Proc IEEE Eng Med Biol Soc. 2010;2010:5720-3.
7. Buckberg GD, Hoffman JIE, Coghlan CH, et al.Ventricular structure-function relations in health and disease: Part I. The normal heart. Cardiothorac Surg. 2015;47:587-601.
8. Doppler, CJ (1842). Ueber das farbige Licht der Doppelsterne und einiger anderer Gestirne des Himmels (About the coloured light of the binary stars and some other stars of the heavens). Publisher: Abhandlungen der Königl. Böhm. Gesellschaft der Wissenschaften (V. Folge, Bd. 2, S. 465-482) [Proceedings of the Royal Bohemian Society of Sciences (Part V, Vol 2)]; Prague: 1842 (Reissued 1903).
9. Satomura S. "Ultrasonic Doppler method for the inspection of cardiac function". J Acoust Soc Am. 1957;29(11): 1181-5.
10. Isaaz K, Thompson A, Ethevenot G, Cloez JL, Brembilla B, Pernot C. Doppler echocardiographic measurement of low velocity motion of left ventricular posterior wall. Am J Cardiol. 1989;64:66-75.
11. Nagueh SF, Appleton CP, Gillebert TC, Marino PN, Oh JK, Smiseth OA, et al. A. Recommendations for the evaluation of left ventricular diastolic function by echocardiography. J Am Soc Echocardiogr. 2009;22:107-33.
12. Wierzbowska-Drabik K, Krzeminska-Pakula M, Chrzanowski L, Plewka M, aszyrowski T, Drozdz J, et al. Age-dependency of classic and new parameters of diastolic function. Echocardiography. 2008;25:149-55.
13. Dalen H, Thorstensen A, Vatten LJ, et al. Reference values and distribution of conventional echocardiographic Doppler measures and longitudinal tissue Doppler velocities in a population free from cardiovascular disease. Circ Cardiovasc Imaging. 2010;3(5):614-22.
14. McDicken WN, Sutherland GR, Moran CM, et al. Colour Doppler velocity imaging of the myocardium. Ultrasound Med Biol. 1992;18:651-4.
15. Rudski LG, Lai WW, Afilalo J, Hua L, Handschumacher MD, Chandrasekaran K, et al. Guidelines for the Echocardiographic Assessment of the Right Heart in Adults: A Report from the American Society of Echocardiography. J Am Soc Echocardiogr. 2010;23:685-713.
16. Sengupta PP, Mohan JC, Pandian NG. Tissue Doppler echocardiography: principles and applications. Indian Heart J. 2002;54:368-788.
17. Sengupta PP, Khandheria BK, Korinek J, et al. Biphasic tissue Doppler waveforms during isovolumic phases are associated with asynchronous deformation of subendocardial and subepicardial layers. J Appl Physiol. 2005;99:1104-11.
18. Sengupta PP, Tondato F, Khandheria BK, Belohlavek M, Jahangir A. Electromechanical activation sequence in normal heart. Heart Fail Clin. 2008;4:303-14.
19. Urheim S, Edvardsen T, Torp H, et al. Myocardial strain by Doppler echocardiography: validation of a new method

to quantify regional myocardial function. Circulation. 2000;102:1158-64.

20. Heimdal A, Stylen A, Torp H, et al. Real-time strain rate imaging of the left ventricle by ultrasound. J Am Soc Echocardiogr. 1998;11:1013-9.
21. Yodwut C, Weinert L, Klas B, et al. Effects of frame rate on three-dimensional speckle-tracking-based measurements of myocardial deformation. J Am Soc Echocardiogr. 2012;9:978-85.
22. Edvardsen T, Gerber BL, Garot J, Bluemke DA, Lima JA, Smiseth OA. Quantitative assessment of intrinsic regional myocardial deformation by Doppler strain rate echocardiography in humans: validation against 3-dimensional tagged magnetic resonance imaging. Circulation. 2002;106:50-6.
23. Kaluzynski K, Chen X, Emelianov SY, et al. Strain rate imaging using two-dimensional speckle tracking. IEEE Trans Ultrason Ferroelectr Freq Control. 2001;48:1111-23.
24. D'Hooge J, Heimdal A, Jamal F, Kukulski T, Bijnens B, Rademakers F, et al. Regional strain and strain rate measurements by cardiac ultrasound: principles, implementation and limitations. Eur J Echocardiogr. 2000;1:154-70.
25. Leitman M, Lysyansky P, Sidenko S, Shir V, Peleg E, Binenbaum M, et al. Two-dimensional Strain–A Novel Software for Real-time Quantitative Echocardiographic Assessment of Myocardial Function. J Am Soc Echocardiogr. 2004;17:1021-9.
26. Leitman M, Lysyansky P, Lysyansky M, Friedman Z, Tyomkin V, Fuchs T, et al. Circumferential and longitudinal strain in 3 myocardial layers in normal subjects and in patients with regional left ventricular dysfunction. J Am Soc Echocardiogr. 2010;23(1):64-70.
27. Sengupta PP, Khandheria BK, Narula J. Twist and untwist mechanics of the left ventricle. Heart Fail Clin. 2008;4:315-24.
28. Reisner SA, Lysyansky P, Agmon Y, Mutlak D, Lessick J, Friedman Z. Global longitudinal strain: A novel index of left ventricular systolic function. J Am Soc Echocardogr. 2004;17:630-3.
29. Sun JP, Popovic ZB, Greenberg NL, Xu XF, Asher CR, Stewart WJ, et al. Noninvasive quantification of regional myocardial function using Doppler-derived velocity, displacement, strain rate, and strain in healthy volunteers: effects of aging. J Am Soc Echocardiogr. 2004;17:132-8.
30. Biaggi P, Carasso S, Garceau P, Greutmann M, Gruner C, Tsang W, et al. Comparison of two different speckle tracking software systems: does the method matter? Echocardiography. 2011;28:539-47.
31. Tanaka H, Hara H, Saba S, et al. Prediction of response to cardiac resynchronization therapy by speckle tracking echocardiography using different software approaches. J Am Soc Echocardiogr. 2009;22:677-84.
32. Bansal M, Cho GY, Chan J, Leano R, Haluska BA, Marwick TH. Feasibility and accuracy of different techniques of two-dimensional speckle based strain and validation with harmonic phase magnetic resonance imaging, J Am Soc Echocardiogr. 2008;21:1318-25.
33. Suffoletto MS, Dohi K, Cannesson M, et al. Novel speckle-tracking radial strain from routine black-and-white echocardiographic images to quantify dyssynchrony and predict response to cardiac resynchronization therapy. Circulation. 2006;113:960-8.
34. Azam S, Desjardins CL, Schluchter M, Liner A, Stelzer JE, Yu X, et al. Comparison of velocity vector imaging echocardiography with magnetic resonance imaging in mouse models of cardiomyopathy. Circ Cardiovasc Imaging. 2012;5: 776-81.
35. Mangual JO, De Luca A, Toncelli L, Domenichini F, Galanti G, Pedrizzetti G. Three Dimensional Reconstruction of the Functional Strain-Line Pattern in the Left Ventricle from 3D Echocardiography. Circ Cardiovasc Imaging. 2012;5: 808-9.
36. Reant P, Labrousse L, Lafitte S, Bordachar P, Pillois X, Tariosse L, et al. Experimental validation of circumferential, longitudinal, and radial 2-dimensional strain during dobutamine stress echocardiography in ischemic conditions. J Am Coll Cardiol. 2008;51:149-57.
37. Hoffmann R, Stempel K, Kühl H, Balzer J, Krämer N, Krombach G, et al. Integrated analysis of cardiac tissue structure and function for improved identification of reversible myocardial dysfunction. Coron Artery Dis. 2009;20:21-6.
38. Ishii K, Imai M, Suyama T, Maenaka M, Nagai T, Kawanami M, et al. Exercise-induced post-ischemic left ventricular delayed relaxation or diastolic stunning: is it a reliable marker in detecting coronary artery disease? J Am Coll Cardiol. 2009;53:698-705.
39. Roes SD, Mollema SA, Lamb HJ, van Der Wall EE, de Roos A, Bax JJ. Validation of echocardiographic two-dimensional speckle tracking longitudinal strain imaging for viability assessment in patients with chronic ischemic left ventricular dysfunction and comparison with contrast enhanced magnetic resonance imaging. Am J Cardiol. 2009;104:312-7.
40. Ingul CB, Stoylen A, Slordahl SA, Wiseth R, Burgess M, Marwick TH. Automated analysis of myocardial deformation at dobutamine stress echocardiography: an angiographic validation. J Am Coll Cardiol. 2007;49:1651-9.
41. Lim P, Pasquet A, Gerber B, D'Hondt AM, Vancraeynest D, Guéret P, et al. Is postsystolic shortening a marker of viability in chronic left ventricular ischemic dysfunction? Comparison with late enhancement contrast magnetic resonance imaging. J Am Soc Echocardiogr. 2008;21:452-7.
42. Voigt JU, Lindenmeier G, Exner B, Regenfus M, Werner D, Reulbach U, et al . Incidence and characteristics of segmental postsystolic longitudinal shortening in normal, acutely ischemic, and scarred myocardium. J Am Soc Echocardiogr. 2003;16:415-23.
43. Kossaify A. Echocardiographic Assessment of the Right Ventricle, from the Conventional Approach to Speckle Tracking and Three-Dimensional Imaging, and Insights into the "Right Way" to Explore the Forgotten Chamber. Clin Med Insights Cardiol. 2015; 5;9:65-75.
44. Lipczyńska M, Szymański P, Kumor M, Klisiewicz A, Mazurkiewicz Ł, Hoffman P. Global longitudinal strain may identify preserved systolic function of the systemic right ventricle. Can J Cardiol. 2015;31(6):760-6.
45. Lisi M, Cameli M, Righini FM, Malandrino A, Tacchini D, Focardi M, et al. RV Longitudinal Deformation Correlates With Myocardial Fibrosis in Patients With End-Stage Heart Failure. JACC Cardiovasc Imaging. 2015;8(5):514-22.

46. Leischik R, Littwitz H, Dworrak B, Garg P, Zhu M, Sahn DJ, et al. Echocardiographic Evaluation of Left Atrial Mechanics: Function, History, Novel Techniques, Advantages, and Pitfalls. Biomed Res Int. 2015;2015:765921.
47. Sarvari SI, Haugaa KH, Stokke TM, Ansari HZ, Leren IS, Hegbom F, et al. Strain echocardiographic assessment of left atrial function predicts recurrence of atrial fibrillation. Eur Heart J Cardiovasc Imaging. 2015; Jul 27.
48. Fang NN, Sui DX, Yu JG, Gong HP, Zhong M, Zhang Y, et al. Strain/strain rate imaging of impaired left atrial function in patients with metabolic syndrome. Hypertens Res. 2015; Jul 16.
49. Kowallick JT, Lotz J, Hasenfuß G, et al.. Left atrial physiology and pathophysiology: Role of deformation imaging. World J Cardiol. 2015;7(6):299-305.
50. Miśkowiec D, Karolina K, Michalski BW, Uznańska-Loch B, Kurpesa M, Kasprzak JD, et al. Left Atrial Dysfunction Assessed by Two-Dimensional Speckle Tracking Echocardiography in Patients with Impaired Left Ventricular Ejection Fraction and Sleep-Disordered Breathing. Echocardiography. 2015; Jun 8.
51. Favreau JT, Nguyen BT, Gao I, Yu P, Tao M, Schneiderman J, et al. Murine ultrasound imaging for circumferential strain analyses in the angiotensin II abdominal aortic aneurysm model. J Vasc Surg. 2012; 56(2):462-9.

# Section 2

# Clinical Applications

# Echocardiographic Workup of Chest Pain in the Emergency Department

8
CHAPTER

*Brian Mott, Sanjiv Kaul*

## INTRODUCTION

Chest pain is one of the most common presenting symptoms in emergency departments (ED). The challenge is identifying those patients whose chest pain is cardiac in etiology. The minority of patients (~20%) presenting with chest pain are ultimately diagnosed with acute coronary syndrome (ACS) or acute myocardial infarction (AMI), whereas the majority (55%), have noncardiac causes. Other cardiac conditions besides ACS or AMI make-up approximately 25% of the total patients.[1]

For physicians treating patients with chest pain in the ED, the diagnosis of life-threatening etiologies is crucial. These included ACS/AMI, aortic dissection, pulmonary embolism, tension pneumothorax, pericardial tamponade, and mediastinitis. The usual initial evaluation includes history, physical examination, 12-lead electrocardiogram (ECG), and chest radiography. Troponin enzymes have added greatly to chest pain diagnosis. However, while specific for myocardial cell death when cardiac troponin T is elevated above 0.1 ng·mL-1 at >10 hours from onset of pain, it fails to capture up to 25% of patients with coronary artery disease (CAD).[2]

Even if a patient has known or suspected CAD, the issue in the ED should not be excluding CAD but to exclude an ischemic event. This important distinction seems to be ignored when using noninvasive techniques, such as coronary computed tomography (CT). The sensitivity and specificity of these techniques are often based on whether the patient has a coronary lesion or not. Newer, high sensitivity troponin assays have been developed for earlier diagnosis of cardiac ischemia and with improved prognostic implications,[3] but the specificity of these tests for a clinically significant event remains low.

Even with troponin assays, there remains a window of time between the onset of chest pain and positive biomarker results. In addition, mildly elevated troponin levels can be seen in patients without primary cardiac causes, such as chronic kidney disease, cerebrovascular accidents, pulmonary embolism, chronic obstructive pulmonary disease, direct myocardial trauma, among others.[4] Furthermore, it is important to determine whether myocardial damage, if any, is of clinical and prognostic value. Even in ACS, the size of 'risk area' is of major importance. Hence, echocardiography can have an important additive role in the initial evaluation and diagnosis of chest pain. Given the wide scope of cardiac diagnoses by the echocardiogram, this chapter will focus on primary cardiac causes of chest pain, namely ACS and CAD.

When evaluating a patient with chest pain using echocardiography it is important to keep in mind the cascade of events occurring with progressive myocardial ischemia. While changes in blood flow heterogeneity occur earliest, regional dysfunction precedes ST segment changes,[5,6] which gives echocardiography a distinct advantage in detecting ischemia in those without ST-elevation or other diagnostic ECG changes consistent with ACS.[7] Furthermore, it provides information on the size of risk area or infarcted myocardium, left ventricular (LV) systolic function, presence of LV thrombus, and mechanical complications of AMI, such as papillary muscle, interventricular septal, or cardiac free wall rupture, pericardial effusion, tamponade, or LV pseudoaneurysm.

## CARDIAC CAUSES OF CHEST PAIN

### Understanding Coronary Physiology with Echocardiography

In order to better integrate changes seen on echocardiogram with the clinical presentation and underlying pathophysiology, it is important to briefly review coronary physiology and flow-function relationships in acute myocardial ischemia. Regional function analysis should be dependent on wall thickening assessment. Advantages to measurement of wall thickening over wall motion are that motion is affected by LV loading conditions and relies on a central reference point which can be affected by cardiac translation related to respiration. Additionally, nonfunctioning myocardium can appear to move without thickening, because of wall tethering. Wall thickening measurements rely on identification of the epicardial and endocardial borders. Endocardial borders can be enhanced with harmonic imaging and LV opacification using ultrasound contrast agents.[8]

There are several important points to be made in terms of acute changes in the regional flow–function relation at rest in acute myocardial ischemia: First, epicardial blood flow remains normal despite up to 80–85% reduction in coronary artery luminal diameter, because of coronary autoregulation **(Figure 8.1)**.[9] Therefore, only total or subtotal occlusion of a coronary artery, as caused by an occlusive or nearly occlusive thrombus, results in acute reduction in coronary blood flow and resting ischemia. Second, there is an almost linear relation between reduction in blood flow and wall thickening **(Figure 8.2)**;[10] below 25% of normal flow wall thinning can occur. Therefore, precise and accurate measurement of regional function can reflect even mild reductions in myocardial blood flow (MBF). Third, extensive collaterals can develop with chronic CAD that can maintain regional perfusion at normal or near-normal levels, thus precluding any decline in resting regional function despite total coronary occlusion. Fourth, most wall thickening occurs, because of endocardial thickening **(Figure 8.3)**.[11] Thus, ischemia or infarction located in the inner 20% of the myocardium can result in the abolishment of wall thickening such that lack of wall thickening cannot be used to determine the transmural extent of infarction **(Figure 8.4)**.[12] Fifth, the circumferential extent of abnormal wall thickening overestimates the circumferential extent of infarction because the border zones beyond the infarction have reduced flow (collateral derived) and thus reduced thickening **(Figure 8.5)**.[13] In this regard, perfusion assessment by myocardial contrast echocardiography (MCE) is useful, since it provides estimation of both risk area and collateral flow. Sixth, spontaneous reperfusion can occur in about one-sixth of all AMI resulting in restoration of perfusion without immediate return of function (stunned myocardium) **(Figure 8.6)**.[14] MCE can identify this condition. Finally, in chronic CAD, patients can experience stuttering ischemia (in some instances accompanied by a similar kind of chest pain) that results in repeated episodes of myocardial dysfunction, which after some time, can become prolonged even when resting blood flow is restored.[15] This is a form of repetitive stunning which can also be identified by MCE.

## Prognostic Value of Wall Thickening in Acute Chest Pain

Wall thickening assessment is an important tool, not only in the diagnosis and evaluation of suspected CAD, but also in getting prognostic information. When performed early in the ED evaluation of chest pain, wall thickening on echocardiography predicts both short-term (48 hours) and long-term (up to 2 years) outcome [death, MI, revascularization, unstable angina (UA), and congestive heart failure] **(Figure 8.7)**.[7] Even after accounting for the risk determination by thrombolysis in myocardial infarction (TIMI) score but before traditional serum biomarker results are available from the laboratory, abnormal wall thickening on echocardiography predicts early, intermediate, and late events (death, MI, revascularization, UA).[16] Additionally,

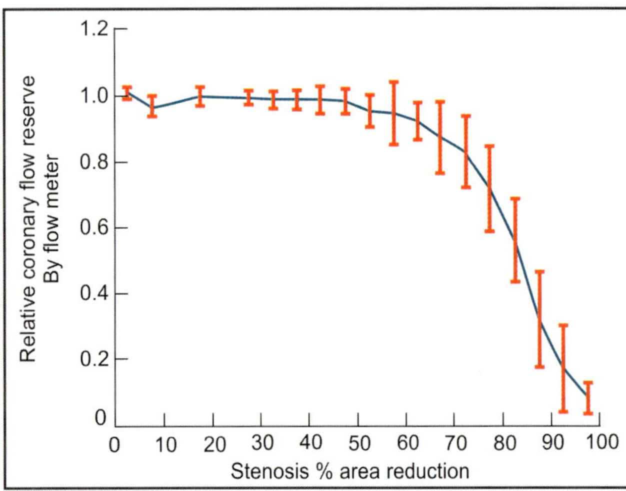


**Figure 8.1:** Relative coronary flow reserve (maximal coronary flow in stenotic artery divided by normal maximal flow in absence of coronary stenosis) is preserved until very severe stenosis. *Source:* Gould KL, Kirkeeide RL, Buchi M. Coronary flow reserve as a physiologic measure of stenosis severity. J Am Coll Cardiol. 1990;15:459-74, with permission.

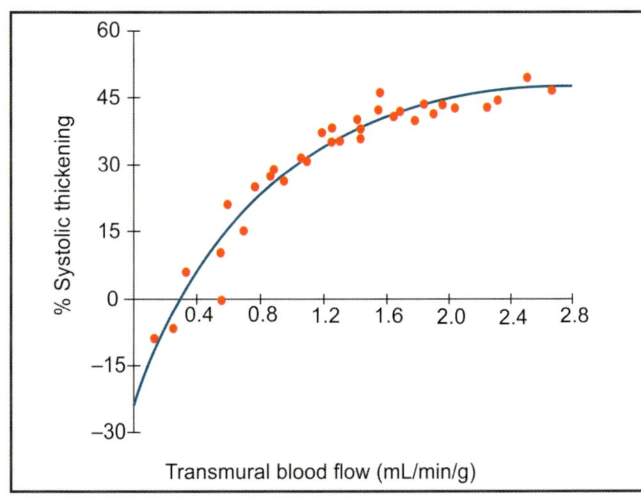


**Figure 8.2:** Relation between regional flow and function. As resting flow decreases below normal levels (1 $mL{\cdot}g^{-1}{\cdot}min^{-1}$, wall thickening decreases proportionally almost in a linear manner. Wall thinning occurs when blood flow is reduced below 0.25 $mL{\cdot}g^{-1}{\cdot}min^{-1}$. *Source:* Kaul S. Echocardiography in coronary artery disease. Curr Probl Cardiol. 1990;15:233-98, with permission.

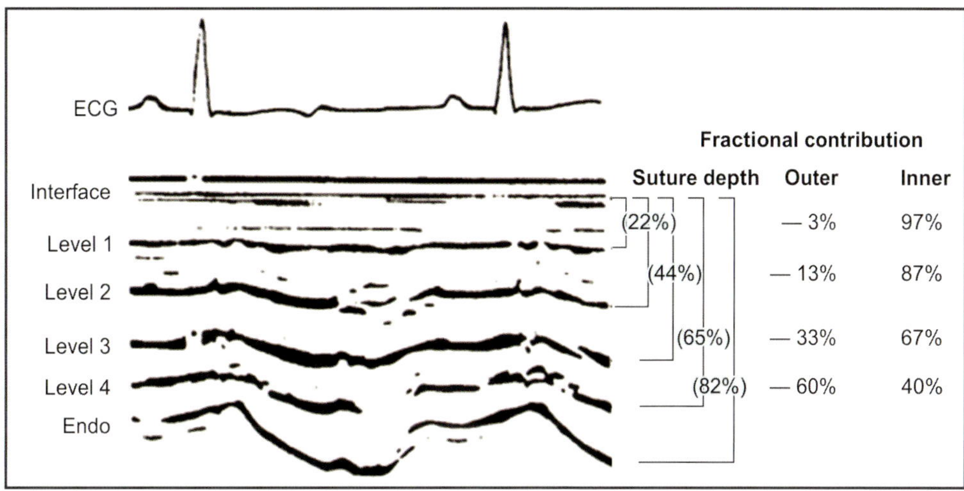


**Figure 8.3:** Contribution of different myocardial layers to wall thickening. Sutures were implanted in different myocardial layers and their excursion noted on M-mode echocardiography. It is evident that two-thirds of wall thickening in systole results from the inner half of the myocardial wall.
*Source:* Myers JH, Stirling MC, Choy M, et al. Direct measurement of inner and outer wall thickening dynamics with epicardial echocardiography. Circulation. 1986;74:164-72, with permission.

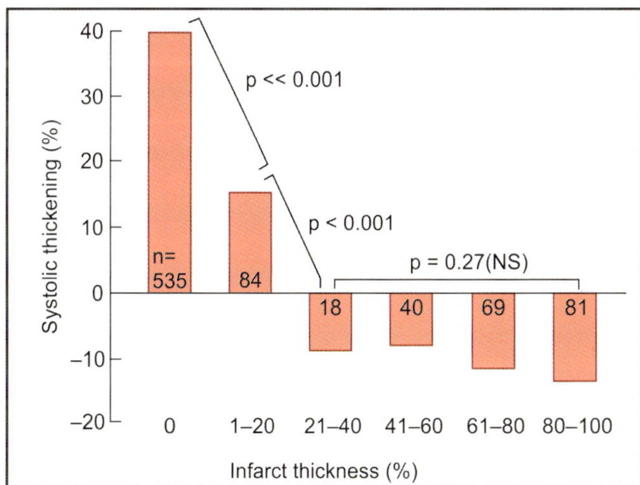


**Figure 8.4:** Relationship between the transmural extent of necrosis and wall thickening in a canine model of coronary occlusion. Wall thickening is reduced when necrosis is limited to <20% of myocardial thickness. Wall thickening is abolished when necrosis exceeds 20% of the myocardial wall.
*Abbreviation:* NS, non-significant.
*Source:* Lieberman AN, Weiss JL, Jugdutt BI, Becker LC, Bulkley BH, Garrison JG, et al. Two-dimensional echocardiography and infarct size: relationship of regional wall motion and thickening to the extent of myocardial infarction in the dog. Circulation. 1981;63:739-46, with permission.

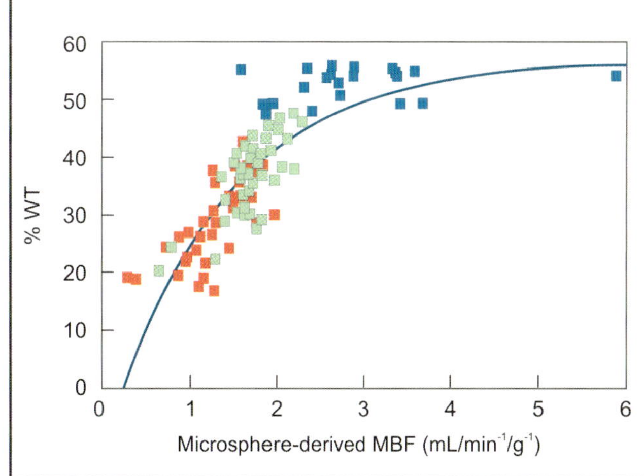


**Figure 8.5:** Flow-function relation in experimental canine model of demand ischemia in the presence of two vessel stenosis where wall thickening and blood flow were increased by dobutamine. Red denotes the central portions of the perfusion defects, green denotes the collateral blood flow-supplied zones, and blue denotes the remote normal myocardium.
Note the similarity to **Figure 8.2** indicating that the flow-function relation during ischemia remains inviolate.
*Abbreviations:* MBF, myocardial blood flow; WT, wall thickening.
*Source:* Leong-Poi H, Coggins MP, Sklenar J, Jayaweera AR, Wang XQ, Kaul S. Role of collateral blood flow in the apparent disparity between the extent of abnormal wall thickening and perfusion defect size during acute myocardial infarction and demand ischemia. J Am Coll Cardiol. 2005;45:565-72, with permission.

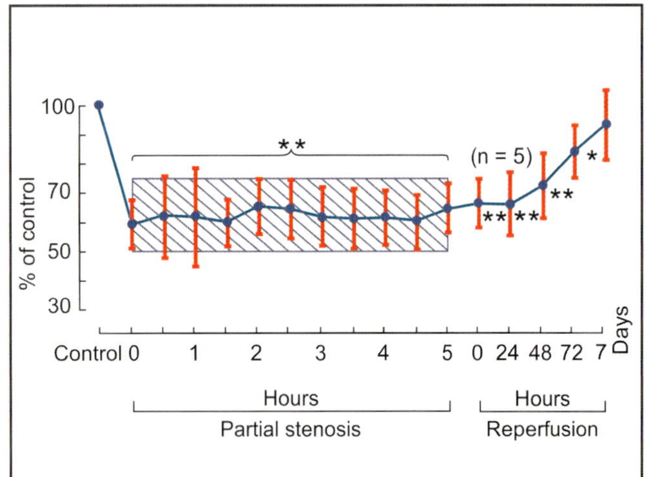


**Figure 8.6:** Changes in systolic wall thickening in the ischemic region during partial coronary stenosis resulting in reduction of regional myocardial blood flow and the reversal of the stenosis in dogs. The cross hatched region represents 25–50% decrease in function. While flow was reduced for 5 hours, it tooks a week for function to completely recover.
*Source:* Matsuzaki M, Gallagher KP, Kemper WS, et al. Sustained regional dysfunction produced by prolonged coronary stenosis: gradual recovery after reperfusion. Circulation. 1983;68:170-82, with permission.

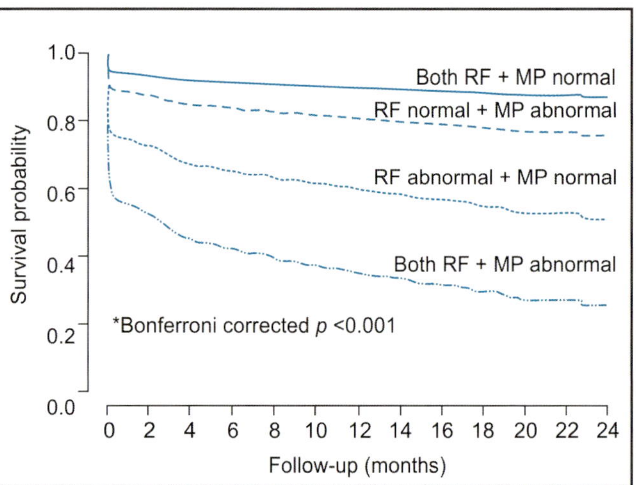


**Figure 8.7:** Survival probabilities for patients with suspected cardiac chest pain and no ST-segment elevation who were evaluated in the emergency department for regional function (RF) and myocardial perfusion (MP) using contrast echocardiography.
*Source:* Rinkevich D, Kaul S, Wang XQ, Tong KL, Belcik T, Kalvaitis S, et al. Regional left ventricular perfusion and function in patients presenting to the emergency department with chest pain and no ST-segment elevation. Eur Heart J. 2005;26:1606-11, with permission.

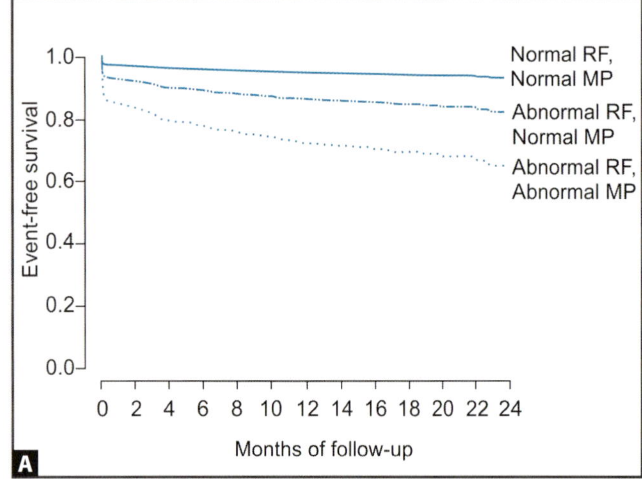


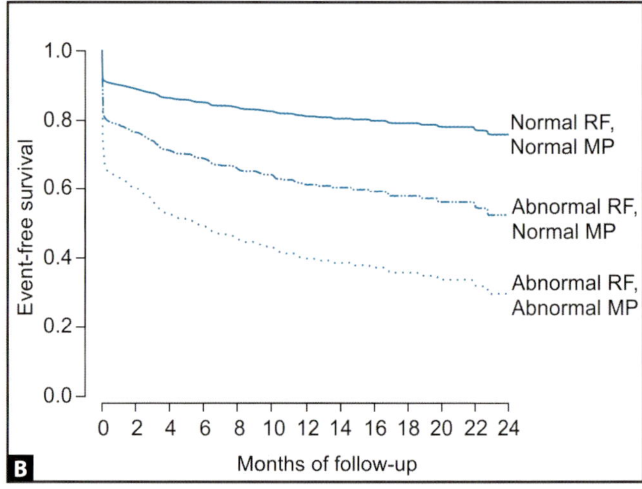


**Figure 8.8A and B:** (A) Event-free survival in patients with a low-risk modified thrombolysis in myocardial infarction score (≤0); (B) Event-free survival in patients with intermediate-risk modified thrombolysis in myocardial infarction score (3 or 4).
*Abbreviations:* MP, myocardial perfusion; RF, regional left ventricular function.
*Source:* Tong KL, Kaul S, Wang XQ, Rinkevich D, Kalvaitis S, Belcik T, et al. Myocardial contrast echocardiography versus thrombolysis in myocardial infarction score in patients presenting to the emergency department with chest pain and a nondiagnostic electrocardiogram. J Am Coll Cardiol. 2005;46:920-7, with permission.

even low-risk patients classified by TIMI score, who could have been discharged from the ED, can be further classified into low-, medium-, and high-risk categories on the basis of wall thickening and regional perfusion assessments. This may assist further in recognition of true low-risk patients and minimize discharging patients at elevated cardiac risk. The same reclassification is true for medium-risk patients on the basis of TIMI score **(Figure 8.8A and B)**.[16]

For wall-thickening analysis, the left ventricle can be divided into individual segments which are scored individually from 1 (normal) to 4 (dyskinetic). The score for the entire left ventricle can then be summed to derive the wall motion score index (WMSI). The larger the WMSI, the greater is the degree and extent of regional dysfunction and the odds of early and late in hospital complications. This relation is true for both patients with AMI [Odds ratio (OR) 2.2/unit] and those without AMI (OR 1.9/unit).[17] This effect remains significant for at least 2 years. There is a significantly lower probability of event-free survival (death, MI, life-threatening arrhythmia, and angina requiring coronary artery bypass surgery or percuatenous coronary intervention) if the WMSI is high; alternatively a normal WMSI indicates a virtually event-free survival.[18,19]

Regional dysfunction resulting from repetitive stunning in patients with severe CAD as well as previous MIs are a potential cause of abnormal wall thickening even in the absence of acute myocardial injury. Notwithstanding that in the above mentioned studies, the index echocardiogram was not compared to a prior one, abnormal wall thickening (acute and chronic) remains important in the prognosis of patients with acute chest pain. If prior echocardiograms are available, they should be directly compared to aid in the diagnosis.

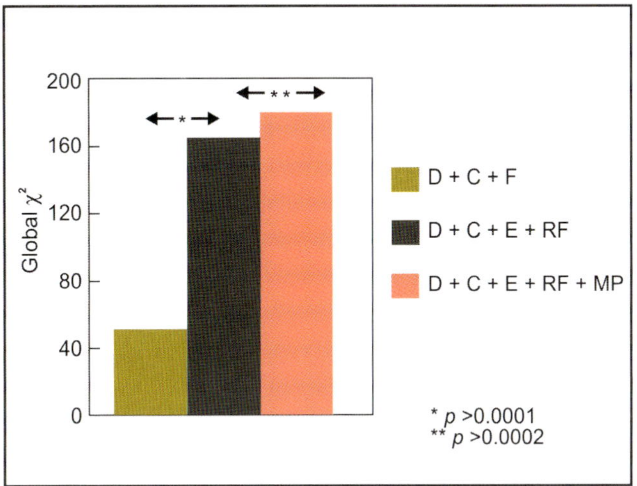


**Figure 8.9:** Incremental value of tests performed for prediction of early events.

*Abbreviations:* C, clinical; D, demographics; E, ECG; RF, regional left ventricle function; MP, myocardial perfusion. P-values as Bonferroni corrected.

*Source:* Rinkevich D, Kaul S, Wang XQ, Tong KL, Belcik T, Kalvaitis S, et al. Regional left ventricular perfusion and function in patients presenting to the emergency department with chest pain and no ST-segment elevation. Eur Heart J. 2005;26:1606-11, with permission.

## Contrast Echocardiography

Contrast-enhanced echocardiography can be used not only to opacify the LV cavity but also to assess myocardial perfusion. Contrast agents consist of small, shelled gas bubbles on the micrometer scale. Several agents have been approved in the United States for LV cavity opacification [Definity (Lantheus Medical), Optison (GE medical), and Lumason (Bracco Diagnostics)]. Lumason is marketed in Asia and Europe as Sonovue. These agents have a similar rheology to erythrocytes allowing them to pass through capillaries just as erythrocytes do.[20-22] Because of this property and since contrast agents remain intravascular, immediate feedback correlating to the perfusion in the myocardial microvasculature can be obtained at the bedside. MCE has contributed to a deeper understanding of coronary physiology. It has also been studied in the setting of chest pain.

In the setting of acute chest pain when all myocardial segments are well seen and wall thickening is normal, myocardial perfusion assessment does not add any additional diagnostic or prognostic information. However, additional diagnostic and prognostic information is provided when myocardial perfusion assessment is added in the presence of abnormal wall thickening. This is classically in patients with spontaneous reperfusion or those with cardiomyopathy or valvular heart disease where regional wall thickening abnormalities are frequent. **Figure 8.9** shows the incremental prognostic value added to clinical, electrocardiographic, and wall-thickening abnormalities when myocardial perfusion was included in patients with chest pain and nondiagnostic ST-T changes in the ED.[7]

There are some caveats to assessing wall thickening. First, it is perhaps the most difficult of all visual echocardiographic assessments even for experienced interpreters, and its quantification has been difficult, because of poor endocardial and epicardial border definition. Adding contrast has greatly enhanced endocardial border definition, but epicardial borders can still be difficult to define. The addition of tissue Doppler imaging and speckle tracking can make the assessment of regional wall function better, particularly in ambiguous cases. Second, it is not always easy to discriminate ischemic-induced wall thickening abnormalities from other causes, such as nonischemic cardiomyopathy that may demonstrate significant heterogeneity in regional function. Third, apart from cases of transmural scar, where the wall is very echogenic and thin, it is not possible to separate acute from chronic ischemia or nontransmural AMI. Therefore, even for experienced interpreters, adding myocardial perfusion assessment can be very helpful.

Another issue that seems to come up in the literature is the notion that echocardiography must be performed during chest pain in order to detect ischemia-induced wall thickening abnormalities. We have performed studies in several thousands of patients in the ED with chest pain and nondiagnostic electrocardiograms up to 6–12 hours after cessation of chest pain and have found that the interval between chest pain and echocardiographic examination does not seem to affect the incidence of wall thickening abnormalities.[18,23] This could be for two reasons: first, ischemia may be silent, and consequently, the absence of chest pain during ACS or AMI may not necessarily denote the absence of ischemia; and second, the myocardium can be stunned for a long time after 30 minutes or more of ischemia. It could also be a combination of these reasons.

We have also performed a cost-benefit analysis of using contrast in patients presenting to the ED with chest pain and a nondiagnostic electrocardiogram. Economic outcome calculations were based on costs estimated from national average Medicare charges adjusted by a cost-charge ratio. On the basis of routine clinical criteria, two-thirds of our patients were admitted to the hospital, whereas one-thirds were discharged directly from the ED. The average cost per patient using this approach was $5,000. Patients with normal MCE results had a very low primary event rate (death, AMI) of 0.6% within 24 hours after presentation, making it relatively safe to discharge patients directly from the ED with a normal MCE result. Hence, if MCE had been used for decision making, 55% of patients would have been discharged directly from the ED and 45% would have been admitted to the hospital. Preventing unnecessary admissions and tests, it would have saved an average of $900 per patient, in addition to reducing their ED stay.[24]

In addition to cost-analysis, we have developed a predictive instrument for risk stratification of patients presenting to the ED with suspected cardiac chest pain and an undifferentiated electrocardiogram using MCE. A risk model was developed in the initial 1,166 patients (cohort 1), and validated in subsequent 720 patients (cohort 2). Any abnormality or ST changes on the electrocardiogram, abnormal wall thickening with normal perfusion, and abnormal wall thickening with abnormal perfusion were found to be significant multivariate predictors in increasing importance for nonfatal AMI or cardiac death. These predictors were then incorporated into a simple risk predictive instrument. The estimate of the probability of concordance for the risk model was 0.82 for cohort 1 and 0.83 for cohort 2. The risk score in both cohorts stratified patients into five distinct risk groups with event rates ranging from 0.3% to 58% (**Figure 8.10**).[25] Thus, echocardiography with MCE performed in the ED can be used very effectively in determining which patients with chest pain can be discharged, which need to be observed, and which need to be admitted to the hospital.

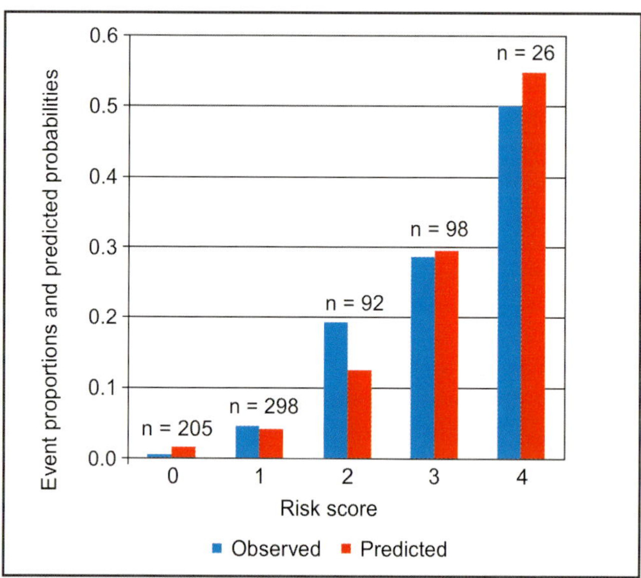


**Figure 8.10:** Proportion of cohort 2 patients with a cardiac event and average of predicted probabilities for a cardiac event based on logistic regression model derived from cohort 1 patients. The numbers above each pair of bars indicate the number of individuals with that risk score.

*Source:* Wei K, Peters D, Belcik T, Kalvaitis S, Womak L, Rinkevich D, et al. A predictive instrument using contrast echocardiography in patients presenting to the emergency department with chest pain and without ST-segment elevation. J Am Soc Echocardiogr. 2010;23:636-42, with permission.

The methodology of MCE is rather straight forward. At steady state, the microbubbles within the myocardium are destroyed with high-energy ultrasound pulse(s), so that there are no microbubbles seen any longer in the myocardium (**Figure 8.11A and B**). As the myocardial tissue fills with microbubbles, the backscatter rapidly reaches a plateau and denotes the volume of blood within the myocardial microvasculature. Because flow constitutes a volume of blood moving at a certain mean velocity, the product of myocardial blood volume and myocardial blood velocity reflects myocardial microvascular flow.[26] While the feared etiology of decreased regional MBF is AMI causing complete lack of capillary filling, reduced myocardial blood volume can also occur from prior AMI with capillary loss or a flow limiting stenosis at rest leading to capillary derecruitment from reduced perfusion pressure. Whereas more sophisticated tools are needed for quantification of MBF with MCE, visual inspection at the bedside can readily identify reduced MBF as etiology of chest pain. At rest, erythrocyte (or microbubble) velocity within the myocardium is 1 mm per second. Since the echocardiographic image elevation (thickness of the ultrasound beam) is about 5 mm, complete microbubble replenishment should occur within 5 seconds (**Figure 8.11A and B**), which in most cases is the first five cardiac cycles (in the absence of bradycardia or tachycardia). If it takes longer it means than MBF is reduced.

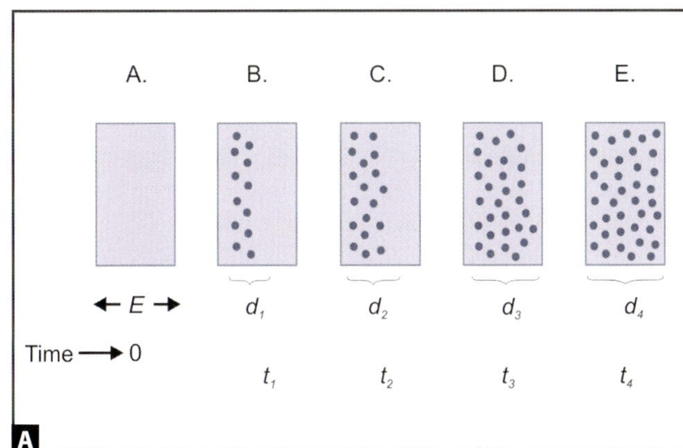


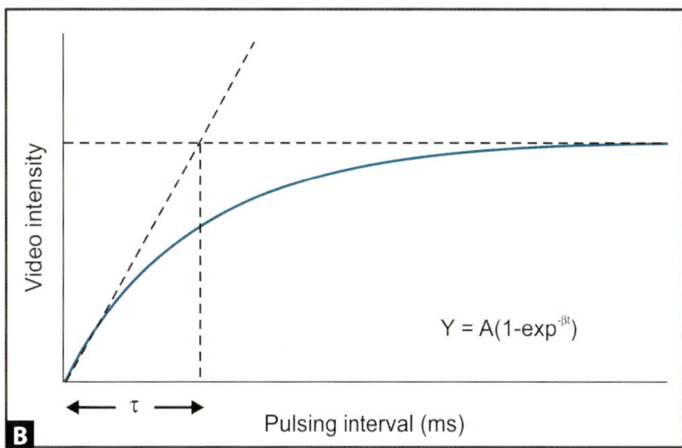


**Figure 8.11A and B:** (A) Replenishment of microbubbles within the ultrasound beam is demonstrated. The elevation (thickness) of the ultrasound beam is represented as E (5 mm). If all the microbubbles in the elevation are destroyed by a single pulse of ultrasound at time $t_0$, then replenishment of the beam elevation will depend on the velocity of microbubbles and the ultrasound pulsing index (PI) τ; (B) A usual replenishment curve after destruction of microbubbles at lengthening pulsing intervals is demonstrated. At longer pulsing intervals the plateau phase can be seen which represents myocardial microvascular blood volume.

*Source:* Wei K, Jayaweera AR, Firoozan S, Linka A, Skyba DM, Kaul S. Quantification of myocardial blood flow with ultrasound-induced destruction of microbubbles administered as a constant venous infusion. Circulation. 1998;97:473-83, with permission.

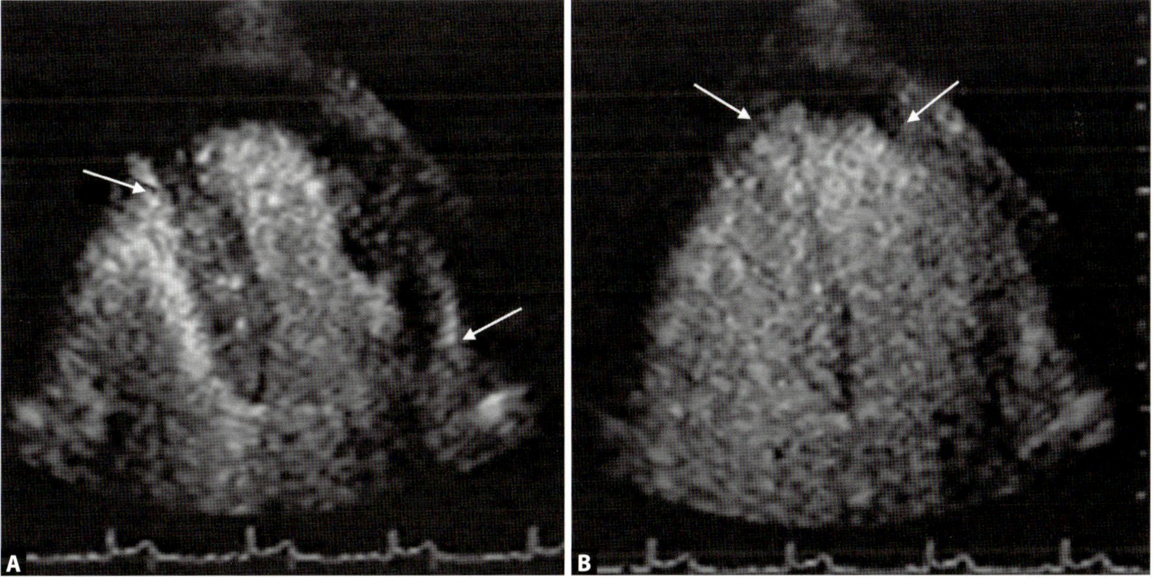


**Figure 8.12A and B:** (A) Risk area (between arrows) at time of coronary occlusion; (B) After reperfusion.

*Source:* Kaul S, Ito H. Microvasculature in acute myocardial ischemia: part II: evolving concepts in pathophysiology, diagnosis, and treatment. Circulation. 2004;109:310-5, with permission.

**Figure 8.12A and B** show a perfusion defect on MCE in a patient presenting to the ED with chest pain and nonspecific ECG changes. The lack of perfusion makes an immediate diagnosis of AMI and also shows that the risk area is large. This patient underwent urgent coronary angiography and angioplasty with stent placement. Immediately thereafter, repeat MCE showed successful reperfusion in all of the previous underperfused areas except for a small region at the apex. Regional function was normal in the erstwhile ischemic area several weeks later. The apex, which demonstrated no reflow, however, continued to be akinetic.

The no-reflow phenomenon in the heart was originally described in a canine model of coronary artery ligation followed by reperfusion. Despite an open infarct-related artery, regions within the myocardium showed low flow which were located exclusively within irreversibly injured myocardium. Consequently, the size of the no-reflow zone approximated the infarct size. Electron microscopy revealed microvascular obstruction because of endothelial cell blebbing, white blood cell infiltration, red blood cell stagnation, and extravascular edema. This process can be accelerated after reperfusion, because of injury from oxygen free radicals.[27,28]

Unlike the experimental setting, however, AMI in the clinical setting is usually caused by an occlusive coronary thrombus which can embolize distally into the myocardium spontaneously, during thrombolytic therapy, or during percutaneous coronary interventions. Necropsy studies have demonstrated the presence of thrombi in the coronary microvasculature from patients who have died of AMI. Thus, early after attempted reperfusion, the no-reflow zone can include regions of the myocardium with microthromboemboli. Vasoactive amines from activated platelets result in microvascular spasm that may further impair regional flow and contribute to the no-reflow phenomenon. Furthermore, inflammation itself can limit flow due to migration of leukocytes into the injured microvasculature.[29-31]

About one-fifth to one-third of AMI patients with TIMI grade 3 flow have evidence of tissue no reflow on the basis of MCE studies. Regions with no reflow show no improvement in regional function over time despite recanalization of the epicardial coronary vessels. These patients also have worse global LV systolic function, malignant ventricular arrhythmias, intractable congestive heart failure from progressive LV remodeling, cardiac rupture, and higher mortality.

Although MCE immediately after reperfusion can provide an accurate assessment of the success of reperfusion, it might underestimate the degree of no reflow because of reactive hyperemia. The degree of reactive hyperemia is influenced by the amount of capillary damage and the degree of residual stenosis in the infarct-related artery. The no-reflow zone also changes dynamically in the first several hours after reperfusion because of vasospasm, myocardial edema, etc.[32-34] Therefore, the ideal time to measure no reflow, in order to determine the extent of myocardial necrosis, is after 48 hours following reperfusion.[35] At that time, dynamic changes in resting tissue perfusion have subsided and the extent of no reflow correlates well with infarct size and denotes a region of irreversible tissue damage.

Collateral MBF is very important in the setting of acute ischemia and can be assessed with MCE. Necrosis does not occur unless MBF is <25% of normal. Collateral vessels develop in response to repeated episodes of silent ischemia in patients with chronic CAD. However, the larger epicardial and interventricular septal collateral vessels seen on angiography usually are not the ones that actually connect to the capillaries within the myocardium. The ones that usually feed capillary beds are present below the endocardium of the heart and are formed from connections between perforating arteries.[36] These vessels are also too small to be seen on coronary angiography. Therefore, angiographic assessment of collateral channels is highly misleading and has led to an underestimation of collateral flow in humans.

Since collateral blood flow is generally less than normal anterograde flow, regions with adequate collateral flow fill later than normal regions do after microbubble destruction on MCE, depending on the magnitude of flow. If they do not fill by 15–20 seconds then flow to the region is markedly reduced, and it is unlikely to be spared from necrosis during coronary occlusion. On the other hand, regions supplied by collateral flow improve function after revascularization even in patients with recent AMI and totally occluded infarct-related arteries. The magnitude of improvement in function is related to the magnitude and spatial extent of collateral flow.

Similar to collateral flow, low flow through an open infarct-related artery can also be assessed using MCE. The myocardium supplied with lower levels of anterograde flow will fill slower than the normal myocardium. If the capillary blood volume is mostly intact (that is, no reflow is limited to a small zone), and the myocardium fills in less than 15–20 seconds then the myocardium is viable and revascularization will result in improvement in function. This has been confirmed in a study of 96 AMI patients imaged on a mean of 5 days post-AMI. If the myocardium did not fill by 10 seconds, it did not recover resting function 84% of the time.[37]

## OTHER CAUSES OF CHEST PAIN

Patients with CAD are not exempted from other causes of chest pain. Often it can be difficult to categorize chest pain into ischemic, pleuritic, musculoskeletal, etc. However, much of the ED evaluations rest on determining severity of chest pain. Life-threatening causes of chest pain include acute aortic dissection, pulmonary embolism, cardiac tamponade, tension pneumothorax, and mediastinitis. Of these, echocardiography can play an important role in identifying the first three. Chest X-ray or CT can be used for other diagnoses, if echocardiography is negative and clinical suspicion is strong.

In patients presenting with typical pleuritic chest pain, about 20% will have pulmonary embolism.[38] However, determining cardiac chest pain from pleuritic pain can be difficult. While CT remains the gold standard for making a diagnosis of pulmonary embolism, direct and indirect signs on echocardiography can also support its diagnosis. It is sometimes possible to directly visualize thrombus in the right ventricle or pulmonary artery **(Videos 8.1 and 8.2)**.[39] Indirect echocardiographic findings to support the diagnosis of pulmonary embolism include right ventricular (RV) dilation, flattening of the interventricular septum from RV pressure overload, RV dysfunction, and McConnell's sign, where RV apex seems to move well despite RV dysfunction **(Video 8.3)**.[40] When taken individually, the sensitivity of these indirect findings for pulmonary embolism is poor[41,42] but together can make a compelling case for pulmonary embolism. One can also gain prognostic value evaluating RV function, with moderately or severely reduced RV systolic dysfunction predicting increased in-hospital mortality.[43]

In patients with both CAD and pulmonary embolism, RV dysfunction on echocardiography can assist in the diagnosis of pulmonary embolism except in those with prior RV infarction or previous open heart surgery. Both sets of patients will demonstrate RV dysfunction in the absence of any other pathology.[44] Therefore, in general, echocardiography provides corroborative evidence of pulmonary embolism and is not the primary imaging modality used for its diagnosis.

Ascending aortic dissection is a life-threatening condition that presents with chest pain. Dissections can infrequently involve the right coronary artery and rarely the left main coronary artery. Echocardiography (transthoracic or transesophageal) can be used as the primary diagnostic modality for making the diagnosis, especially in conjunction with a finding of widened mediastinum on chest X-ray. In the absence of available echocardiography, thoracic CT is an other option for making the diagnosis.

While studies prior to harmonic imaging and high resolution probes reported transthoracic echocardiography sensitivity for aortic dissection at 57–82% and specificity of 65–96%, more recent studies report improved sensitivity at 87% and specificity of 91%.[45] The diagnosis can be made by the presence of two vascular lumens separated by an intimal flap **(Video 8.4)**. Contrast microbubble agents can further enhance the ability to identify separate lumens by highlighting different flow patterns in the lumens and accentuate the intimal flap **(Video 8.5)**.[46]

Even in patients initially suspected to have ascending aortic dissection but, subsequently, found not to have the same, transthoracic echocardiography can identify alternative diagnoses for chest pain in over 40% of patients.[47] Therefore, transthoracic echocardiogram with or without microbubble contrast agents is a useful and rapid evaluation in patients with suspected ascending aortic dissection. If image quality precludes the diagnosis of aortic dissection or if the confidence of the diagnosis is not high enough, transesophageal echocardiography should be performed. In its absence, CT is a better alternative.

Acute pericarditis-related chest pain is usually sharp in character and pleuritic (worse with inspiration). Diffuse ST segment changes on ECG and clinical assessment are the mainstay of diagnosis. However, echocardiography can provide hints of pericarditis. There is sometimes a small pericardial effusion present, but its absence does not rule out pericarditis.

Echocardiography is very valuable for making the diagnosis and providing prognosis in patients with cardiac tamponade. There are several echocardiographic findings of cardiac tamponade that should be used in combination to make a diagnosis. These include fluid in the pericardium that need not be excessive, diastolic collapse of the anterior RV free wall,[48] right atrial inversion lasting into systole,[49] exaggerated inspiratory variation of mitral and tricuspid (and sometimes aortic) flow velocities,[50] paradoxical interventricular septal motion, and protodiastolic inward motion of the posterior LV wall (that coincides with pericardial knock) **(Video 8.6)**.[51]

Many patients with CAD also have valvular diseases which by itself can result in chest pain. Aortic stenosis is a great example where about two-thirds of patients will have exertional chest pain, with only half having significant CAD. In patients with severe aortic stenosis, the presence of wall motion abnormalities is 94% predictive of CAD, while the absence of wall motion abnormalities is insensitive as CAD is found in about half of these patients.[52] In the remaining patients with severe aortic stenosis without CAD, the chest pain may be from LV hypertrophy with high wall stresses and a reduced coronary flow reserve.[53] It is important to identify patients with severe aortic valve disease in the setting of chest pain with or without CAD as their median survival ranges between 2 years and 4.7 years when chest pain is present.[54]

Chest wall trauma can occur as blunt or penetrating injuries. Penetrating traumas usually require immediate surgical consideration. Blunt trauma to the chest can lead to cardiac contusion with regional wall thickening abnormalities. About one-third of patients with severe chest wall trauma will have such abnormalities. Given the anterior location of the RV and its proximity to the chest wall, it is more susceptible to injury than the left ventricle is.[55] Many other etiologies of chest pain resulting from chest wall blunt trauma can be seen on echocardiogram.[56] Contrecoup injuries from thrusting the heart against the spine can result in abnormalities in the posterior wall. Myocardial hematomas can result in increased myocardial echogenicity which can be confirmed on cardiac magnetic resonance imaging.

## SUMMARY

In summary, echocardiography can play a vital role in evaluating chest pain patients in the ED, particularly those in whom a diagnosis has not been established. Using contrast is very helpful for defining LV endocardial borders accurately and assessing myocardial perfusion.[57] A negative comprehensive echocardiogram portends excellent prognosis, and a positive echocardiographic study helps find the putative cause of chest pain and, thus, its management. It is important that the person(s) performing and interpreting the study should be very skilled, particularly in assessing regional function. They also need to be able to perform transesophageal echocardiography when needed. Finally, they should be able to integrate all clinical, electrocardiographic, and other imaging information in order to assist ED physicians in excluding or ruling in life-threatening cardiovascular conditions.

## VIDEO LEGENDS

**Video 8.1:** Right ventricular outflow view in a patient with pulmonary embolism. The arrow denotes thrombus in the right pulmonary artery.

**Video 8.2:** Using direct color comparison, the right ventricular outflow into the main pulmonary artery and its right and left branches can be seen. There is trace pulmonary insufficiency. Again, thrombus can be seen in the right pulmonary artery.

**Video 8.3:** In this modified apical view, the right ventricle is well seen. There is significant right ventricular systolic dysfunction with apical sparing consistent with McConnell's sign in this patient with a large pulmonary embolism seen on CT scan.

**Video 8.4:** A patient with aortic dissection. The abdominal aorta can be seen pulsating with two lumens.

**Video 8.5:** Microbubbles can be used to identify the lumens. The true lumen is seen on top of the false lumen. Microbubbles in the true lumen are constantly flowing without a noticeable flow pulsation. In the false lumen, microbubbles can be seen slowly pulsing into the dissection.

**Video 8.6:** A patient with large pericardial effusion with cardiac tamponade. The entire heart is swinging within the pericardial cavity. Right atrial diastolic collapse can also be appreciated.

## REFERENCES


1. Pope JH, Aufderheide TP, Ruthazer R, Woolard RH, Feldman JA, Beshansky JR, et al. Missed diagnoses of acute cardiac ischemia in the emergency department. N Engl J Med. 2000;342: 1163-70.
2. deFilippi CR, Tocchi M, Parmar RJ, Rosanio S, Abreo G, Potter MA, et al. Cardiac troponin T in chest pain unit patients without ischemic electrocardiographic changes: angiographic correlates and long-term clinical outcomes. JAC. 2000;35:1827-34.
3. Haaf P, Reichlin T, Twerenbold R, Hoeller R, Rubini Gimenez M, Zellweger C, et al. Risk stratification in patients with acute chest pain using three high-sensitivity cardiac troponin assays. Eur Heart J. 2014;35:365-75.
4. Tanindi A, Cemri M. Troponin elevation in conditions other than acute coronary syndromes. Vasc Health Risk Manag. 2011;7:597-603.
5. Leong-Poi H, Rim SJ, Le DE, Fisher NG, Wei K, Kaul S. Perfusion versus function: the ischemic cascade in demand ischemia: implications of single-vessel versus multivessel stenosis. Circulation. 2002;105:987-92.
6. Beller GA. Myocardial perfusion imaging for detection of silent myocardial ischemia. Am J Cardiol. 1988;61:22F-28F.
7. Rinkevich D, Kaul S, Wang XQ, Tong KL, Belcik T, Kalvaitis S, et al. Regional left ventricular perfusion and function in patients presenting to the emergency department with chest pain and no ST-segment elevation. Eur Heart J. 2005;26:1606-11.
8. Lindner JR, Dent JM, Moos SP, et al. Enhancement of left ventricular cavity opacification by harmonic imaging after venous injection of Albunex. Am J Cardiol. 1997;79:1657-62.
9. Gould KL, Kirkeeide RL, Buchi M. Coronary flow reserve as a physiologic measure of stenosis severity. J Am Coll Cardiol. 1990;15:459-74.
10. Kaul, S. Echocardiography in coronary artery disease. Curr Probl Cardiol. 1990;15: 233-98.
11. Myers JH, Stirling MC, Choy M, et al. Direct measurement of inner and outer wall thickening dynamics with epicardial echocardiography. Circulation. 1986;74:164-72.
12. Lieberman AN, Weiss JL, Jugdutt BI, Becker LC, Bulkley BH, Garrison JG, et al. Two-dimensional echocardiography and infarct size: relationship of regional wall motion and thickening to the extent of myocardial infarction in the dog. Circulation. 1981;63:739-46.
13. Leong-Poi H, Coggins MP, Sklenar J, Jayaweera AR, Wang XQ, Kaul S. Role of collateral blood flow in the apparent disparity between the extent of abnormal wall thickening and perfusion defect size during acute myocardial infarction and demand ischemia. J Am Coll Cardiol. 2005;45:565-72.
14. Matsuzaki M, Gallagher KP, Kemper WS, et al. Sustained regional dysfunction produced by prolonged coronary stenosis: gradual recovery after reperfusion. Circulation. 1983;68:170-82.
15. Nicklas JM, Becker LC, Bulkley BH. Effects of repeated brief coronary occlusion on regional left ventricular function and dimension in dogs. Am J Cardiol. 1985;56:473-8.
16. Tong KL, Kaul S, Wang XQ, Rinkevich D, Kalvaitis S, Belcik T, et al. Myocardial contrast echocardiography versus Thrombolysis In Myocardial Infarction score in patients presenting to the emergency department with chest pain and a nondiagnostic electrocardiogram. J Am Coll Cardiol. 2005;46:920-7.
17. Fleischmann KE, Lee TH, Come PC, Goldman L, Cook EF, Caguoia E, et al. Echocardiographic prediction of complications in patients with chest pain. Am J Cardiol. 1997;79:292-8.
18. Sabia P, Abbott RD, Afrookteh A, Keller MW, Touchstone DA, Kaul S. Importance of two-dimensional echocardiographic assessment of left ventricular systolic function in patients presenting to the emergency room with cardiac-related symptoms. Circulation. 1991;84:1615-24.
19. Villanueva FS, Sabia PJ, Afrookteh A, Pollock SG, Hwang LJ, Kaul S. Value and limitations of current methods of evaluating patients presenting to the emergency room with cardiac-related symptoms for determining long-term prognosis. Am J Cardiol. 1992;69:746-50.

20. Keller MW, Segal SS, Kaul S, et al. The behavior of sonicated albumin microbubbles within the microcirculation: a basis for their use during myocardial contrast echocardiography. Circ Res. 1989;65:458-67.
21. Jayaweera AR1, Edwards N, Glasheen WP, Villanueva FS, Abbott RD, Kaul S. In vivo myocardial kinetics of air-filled albumin microbubbles during myocardial contrast echocardiography. Comparison with radiolabeled red blood cells. Circ. Res. 1994;74:1157-65.
22. Lindner JR, Song J, Jayaweera AR, et al. Microvascular rheology of definity microbubbles after intra-arterial and intravenous administration. J Am Soc Echocardiogr. 2002;15(5):396-403.
23. Kalvaitis S, Kaul S, Tong KL, Rinkevich D, Belcik T, Wei K. Effect of time delay on the diagnostic use of contrast echocardiography in patients presenting to the emergency department with chest pain and no S-T segment elevation. J Am Soc Echocardiogr. 2006;19:1488-93.
24. Wyrick JJ, Kalvaitis S, McConnell KJ, Rinkevich D, Kaul S, Wei K. Cost-efficiency of myocardial contrast echocardiography in patients presenting to the emergency department with chest pain of suspected cardiac origin and a nondiagnostic electrocardiogram. Am J Cardiol. 2008;102:649-52.
25. Wei K, Peters D, Belcik T, Kalvaitis S, Womak L, Rinkevich D, et al. A predictive instrument using contrast echocardiography in patients presenting to the emergency department with chest pain and without ST-segment elevation. J Am Soc Echocardiogr. 2010;23:636-42.
26. Wei K, Jayaweera AR, Firoozan S, Linka A, Skyba DM, Kaul S. Quantification of myocardial blood flow with ultrasound-induced destruction of microbubbles administered as a constant venous infusion. Circulation. 1998;97:473-83.
27. Cobb FR, Bache RJ, Rivas F, et al. Local effects of acute cellular injury on regional myocardial blood flow. J Clin Invest. 1976;57:1359-68.
28. Ambrosio G, Weisman HF, Mannisi JA, et al. Progressive impairment of regional myocardial perfusion after initial restoration of postischemic blood flow. Circulation. 1989; 80:1846-61.
29. Sakuma T, Leong-Poi H, Fisher NG, et al. Further insights into the no-reflow phenomenon after primary angioplasty in acute myocardial infarction: the role of microthromboemboli. J Am Soc Echocardiogr. 2003;16:15-21.
30. Sakuma T, Sklenar J, Leong-Poi H, Goodman NC, Glover DK, Kaul S. Molecular imaging identifies regions with microthromboemboli during primary angioplasty in acute coronary thrombosis. J Nucl Med. 2004;45:1194-200.
31. Sakuma T, Sari I, Goodman CN, Lindner JR, Klibanov AL, Kaul S. Simultaneous integrin alphavbeta3 and glycoprotein IIb/IIIa inhibition causes reduction in infarct size in a model of acute coronary thrombosis and primary angioplasty. Cardiovasc Res. 2005;66:552-61.
32. Villanueva FS, Glasheen WP, Sklenar J, et al. Assessment of risk area during coronary occlusion and infarct size after reperfusion with myocardial contrast echocardiography using left and right atrial injections of contrast. Circulation. 1993;88:596-604.
33. Villanueva FS, Glasheen WP, Sklenar J, et al. Characterization of spatial patterns of flow within the reperfused myocardium by myocardial contrast echocardiography. Implications in determining extent of myocardial salvage. Circulation. 1993;88:2596-606.
34. Villanueva FS, Camarano G, Ismail S, Goodman NC, Sklenar J, Kaul S. Coronary reserve abnormalities in the infarcted myocardium. Assessment of myocardial viability immediately versus late after reflow by contrast echocardiography. Circulation. 1996;94:748-54.
35. Sakuma T, Otsuka M, Okimoto T, Fujiwara H, Sumii K, Imazu M, et al. Optimal time for predicting myocardial viability after successful primary angioplasty in acute myocardial infarction: a study using myocardial contrast echocardiography. Am J Cardiol. 2001;87:687-92.
36. Cohen MV. Coronary Collaterals: Clinical and Experimental Observations. Futura Pub. Co; 1985.
37. Vernon S, Kaul S, Powers ER, Camarano G, Gimple LW, Ragosta M. Myocardial viability in patients with chronic coronary artery disease and previous myocardial infarction: comparison of myocardial contrast echocardiography and myocardial perfusion scintigraphy. Am Heart J. 1997;134: 835-40.
38. Hull RD, Raskob GE, Carter CJ, Coates G, Gill GJ, Sackett DL, et al. Pulmonary embolism in outpatients with pleuritic chest pain. Arch Intern Med. 1988;148:838-44.
39. Borloz MP, Frohna WJ, Phillips CA, et al. Emergency department focused bedside echocardiography in massive pulmonary embolism. J Emerg Med. 2011;41:658-60.
40. McConnell MV, Solomon SD, Rayan ME, Come PC, Goldhaber SZ, Lee RT. Regional right ventricular dysfunction detected by echocardiography in acute pulmonary embolism. Am J Cardiol. 1996;78:469-73.
41. Bova C, Greco F, Misuraca G, Serafini O, Crocco F, Greco A, et al. Diagnostic utility of echocardiography in patients with suspected pulmonary embolism. Am J Emerg Med. 2003;21:180-3.
42. Miniati M, Monti S, Pratali L, Di Ricco G, Marini C, Formichi B, et al. Value of transthoracic echocardiography in the diagnosis of pulmonary embolism: results of a prospective study in unselected patients. Am J Med. 2001;110:528-35.
43. Ribeiro A, Lindmarker P, Juhlin-Dannfelt A, et al. Echocardiography Doppler in pulmonary embolism: right ventricular dysfunction as a predictor of mortality rate. Am Heart J. 1997;134:479-87.
44. Yadav H, Unsworth B, Fontana M, Diller GP, Kyriacou A, Baruah R, et al. Selective right ventricular impairment following coronary artery bypass graft surgery. Eur J Cardiothorac Surg. 2010; 37:393-8.
45. Cecconi M, Chirillo F, Costantini C, Iacobone G, Lopez E, Zanoli R, et al. The role of transthoracic echocardiography in the diagnosis and management of acute type A aortic syndrome. Am Heart J. 2012;163:112-8.
46. Evangelista A, Avegliano G, Aguilar R, Cuellar H, Igual A, González-Alujas T, et al. Impact of contrast-enhanced echocardiography on the diagnostic algorithm of acute aortic dissection. Eur Heart J. 2010;31:472-9.
47. Granato JE, Dee P, Gibson RS. Utility of two-dimensional echocardiography in suspected ascending aortic dissection. Am J Cardiol. 1985;56:123-9.

48. Reydel B, Spodick DH. Frequency and significance of chamber collapses during cardiac tamponade. Am Heart J. 1990;119:1160-3.
49. Gillam LD, Guyer DE, Gibson TC, King ME, Marshall JE, Weyman AE. Hydrodynamic compression of the right atrium: a new echocardiographic sign of cardiac tamponade. Circulation. 1983;68:294-301.
50. Picard MH, Sanfilippo AJ, Newell JB, Rodriguez L, Guerrero JL, Weyman AE. Quantitative relation between increased intrapericardial pressure and Doppler flow velocities during experimental cardiac tamponade. J Am Coll Cardiol. 1991;18:234-42.
51. Gibson TC, Grossman W, McLaurin LP, et al. An echocardiographic study of the interventricular septum in constrictive pericarditis. Br Heart J. 1976;38:738-43.
52. Safford RE, Bove AA. Prediction of coronary artery disease by left ventricular regional wall motion abnormalities in patients with stenosis of the aortic valve. Br Heart J. 1987;57:237-41.
53. Julius BK, Spillmann M, Vassalli G, Villari B, Eberli FR, Hess OM. Angina pectoris in patients with aortic stenosis and normal coronary arteries. Mechanisms and pathophysiological concepts. Circulation. 1997;95:892-8.
54. Turina J, Hess O, Sepulcri F, et al. Spontaneous course of aortic valve disease. Eur Heart J. 1987;8:471-83.
55. Weiss RL, Brier JA, O'Connor W, et al. The usefulness of transesophageal echocardiography in diagnosing cardiac contusions. Chest. 1996;109:73-7.
56. Sybrandy KC, Cramer MJM, Burgersdijk C. Diagnosing cardiac contusion: old wisdom and new insights. Heart. 2003;89:485-9.
57. Kaul S, Ito H. Microvasculature in acute myocardial ischemia: part II: evolving concepts in pathophysiology, diagnosis, and treatment. Circulation. 2004;109:310-5.

# Assessment of the Extent of Myocardial Damage

9

CHAPTER

*Vinayak Agrawal*

## INTRODUCTION

Myocardial damage occurs in a variety of pathophysiological states. The most common ones clinically encountered are the ischemia-driven damage or the nonischemic insult as in cardiomyopathies, drug-induced infections, or collateral damage as part of a systemic illness. The extent of myocardial damage affects global cardiac function and prognosis. Equally important is to assess the extent of reversibility of the cardiac dysfunction both of which are closely linked.

Acute coronary syndrome (ACS) necessitates immediate action to identify, alert, diagnose, and treat the occlusive thrombus where time is of the greatest essence. The quote "time is muscle" highlights the impact of myocardial salvage on the expected longevity of life. However, there is a wide variation in accuracy of assessment tools for the extent of myocardial damage, namely cardiac biomarkers, electrocardiogram (ECG), conventional echocardiography, specialized/advanced echocardiographic techniques like contrast echocardiography and strain imaging, nuclear imaging, such as single-photon emission computed tomography (SPECT) and positron-emission tomography (PET), magnetic resonance imaging (MRI), and computed tomography (CT). The following section pertains only to echocardiography and its wide ramifications in assessment of myocardial damage.

## ECHOCARDIOGRAPHY

In 1816, Laennec invented the stethoscope followed almost a decade later in 1902, Willem Einthoven introduced an ECG.[1] Barely 50–60 years back, Edler and Hertz introduced ultrasound transducer which paved the way for the present day echocardiography.[2] There has been an astonishingly rapid strides in the field of echocardiography with progressive introduction of A-mode, M-mode, B-mode, pulsed- and continuous-wave Doppler, transesophageal echocardiography, tissue harmonics, stress echocardiography, contrast perfusion, three-dimensional (3D) echocardiography, and strain imaging. All these techniques have immensely helped in diagnosing myocardial damage and managing the underlying etiologies as well as offer tremendous prognostic information.[3]

### Diagnosing Extent of Myocardial Damage in Acute Coronary Syndrome

Best modality of evaluation in terms of cardiac imaging in acute phase (0–2 days) and subacute phase (3–7 days) of myocardial infarction (MI) is echocardiography and is definitely recommended to be performed as early as possible post-hospitalization preferably within 24–48 hours. Whatever be the underlying etiology leading to myocardial damage, echocardiography offers incremental information far better than any other modality more so, because of its noninvasive, quick, safe, and comprehensive information that it provides.

In the setting of ACS, echocardiography provides an invaluable tool to rapidly establish the diagnosis, the extent of myocardial damage, and its repercussions in the form of the followings:

- Regional wall-motion abnormalities (RWMA) and the coronary artery territories involved **(Video 9.1)**
- Left ventricular (LV) ejection fraction (LVEF)
- Presence of an aneurysm, pseudoaneurysm, or intramural hematoma
- Intracavity clot
- Pulmonary artery hypertension
- Deranged diastolic functions
- Complications of ACS like papillary or chordal rupture with severe mitral regurgitation, ventricular septal rupture, etc.

#### *Regional Wall-motion Abnormalities and Global Left Ventricular Ejection Function*

In the ischemic cascade, RWMA detected on echocardiography appear much before the onset of ECG changes or classical ACS symptoms. In fact, RWMA can be detected within 10–20 seconds of coronary artery occlusion evaluated during transient coronary occlusions while undergoing percutaneous coronary interventions.[4,5]

The RWMA are identified by decreased or absent myocardial systolic thickening. Accompanied adjacent tethering and adverse regional remodeling of left ventricle follow soon after. However, pre-existing RWMA can be seen in conditions like old MI, prior coronary artery bypass surgery and cardiomyopathy. Myocarditis and pericarditis may mimic ACS presentation as well. Hence, echocardiography remains a highly sensitive test albeit with a low specificity. Within 15–30 minutes of complete coronary artery occlusion, ischemic myocardial necrosis begins progressing from the subendocardial to subepicardial region (the wave-front phenomenon). Eventual extent of infarction depends on the rapidity of reperfusion, timely management, and intrinsic recruitment of collaterals which salvages the myocardium at risk. In acute phase of MI, the affected area bulges out due to passive stretching of the ischemic, hypocontractile myocardium and if not treated within time, leads to irreversible infarct expansion and eventual adverse cardiac remodeling.[6,7] Between one-half and one-third of post-infarction patients experience progressive dilatation with distortion of ventricular geometry and secondary mitral regurgitation.

*Wall-motion Analysis*

The RWMA can be assessed either:

- Qualitatively, or
- Quantitatively.

Qualitative method or simply put visually derived "the eyeball" method is the most practical and rapid way of assessment of RWMA and EF and is certainly the most accepted clinical practice tool in rapid triaging units. Furthermore, visually estimated EF has been shown to correlate well with the EF derived using the modified Simpson's method, wall-motion score index (WMSI), atrioventricular plane displacement, and fractional shortening are all established echocardiographic methods for the assessment of LV systolic function.[8]

Wall motion described in accordance with the currently accepted 17-segment model of left ventricle can be graded in each segment.

A semiquantitative wall-motion score can be assigned to each segment to calculate the LV WMSI as the average of the scores of all segments visualized. The following scoring system is recommended:

- Normal or hyperkinetic = 1
- Hypokinetic (reduced thickening) = 2
- Akinetic (absent or negligible thickening, e.g. scar) = 3
- Dyskinetic (systolic thinning or stretching, e.g. aneurysm) = 4.

The sum of all segments is then expressed as WMSI. Prognostic value of WMSI in acute ST-elevation MI[9-12] as well as in non-ST elevation MI[13] has been well established.

*Left Ventricular Volumes and Ejection Fraction*

According to the latest recommendations of the American Society of Echocardiography, LV volumes should be measured from the apical 4- and 2-chamber views aimed at maximizing LV areas, avoiding foreshortening. 3D echocardiography allows more accurate assessment of LV volumes and should be preferred if available. The biplane method of disks (modified Simpson's rule) is the currently recommended two-dimensional (2D) method to assess LVEF. Judicious use of contrast agents improve endocardial border identification when two or more contiguous LV endocardial segments are poorly visualized in apical views, as per published guidelines.[14]

The LVEF is the most commonly understood parameter clinically, which in a simplistic, instant manner conveys the acute as well as long-term prognosis. Accurate assessment of LV volumes and EF is hampered by a number of important limitations like involvement of certain geometric assumptions, load dependency (i.e. both afterload and preload affect it), and influence of heart rate as in increased stroke volume during bradycardia (overestimation of EF) and decreased stroke volume during tachycardia (underestimation of EF). Atrial fibrillation alters LV filling from beat-to-beat depending on the R-R interval. The development of a new, single-beat 3D echocardiography acquisition tends to overcome this limitation for this technique.[15] EF is relatively inefficient in picking up early or subtle signs of subclinical or mild degrees of LV systolic dysfunction.[16] In contrast, global longitudinal strain (GLS) overcomes this and offers the greatest increment in predictive power in patients with EF >35%.[17] Also, the importance of training, retraining and quality control cannot be overemphasized.[18] Clinical impact of EF ≤40% is profound since most outcome studies are linked to the determination and improvement of EF post-therapeutic intervention. Echocardiographically determined EF is marred by poor acoustic windows that allow inadequate visualization of the blood-endocardial interface and introduces errors in measurements, especially in obese patients, patients with chronic obstructive pulmonary disease, and those with crowded ribs. The LVEF using the modified Simpson method could not be accurately determined in 31–38% of patients due to poor image quality. The use of echocardiography contrast has been shown to improve LVEF determination in patients with poor acoustic windows and to reduce interobserver variability.[19] 3D echocardiography **(Figure 9.1)** makes minimal assumptions of LV cavity since the entire LV cavity is captured in the full volume acquisitions, provided the acoustic window is good. The 3D assay has less variability and more accuracy than other echocardiographic methods, when compared with MRI as a reference standard.[20] The LVEF can also be determined by SPECT, MRI, and CT, but

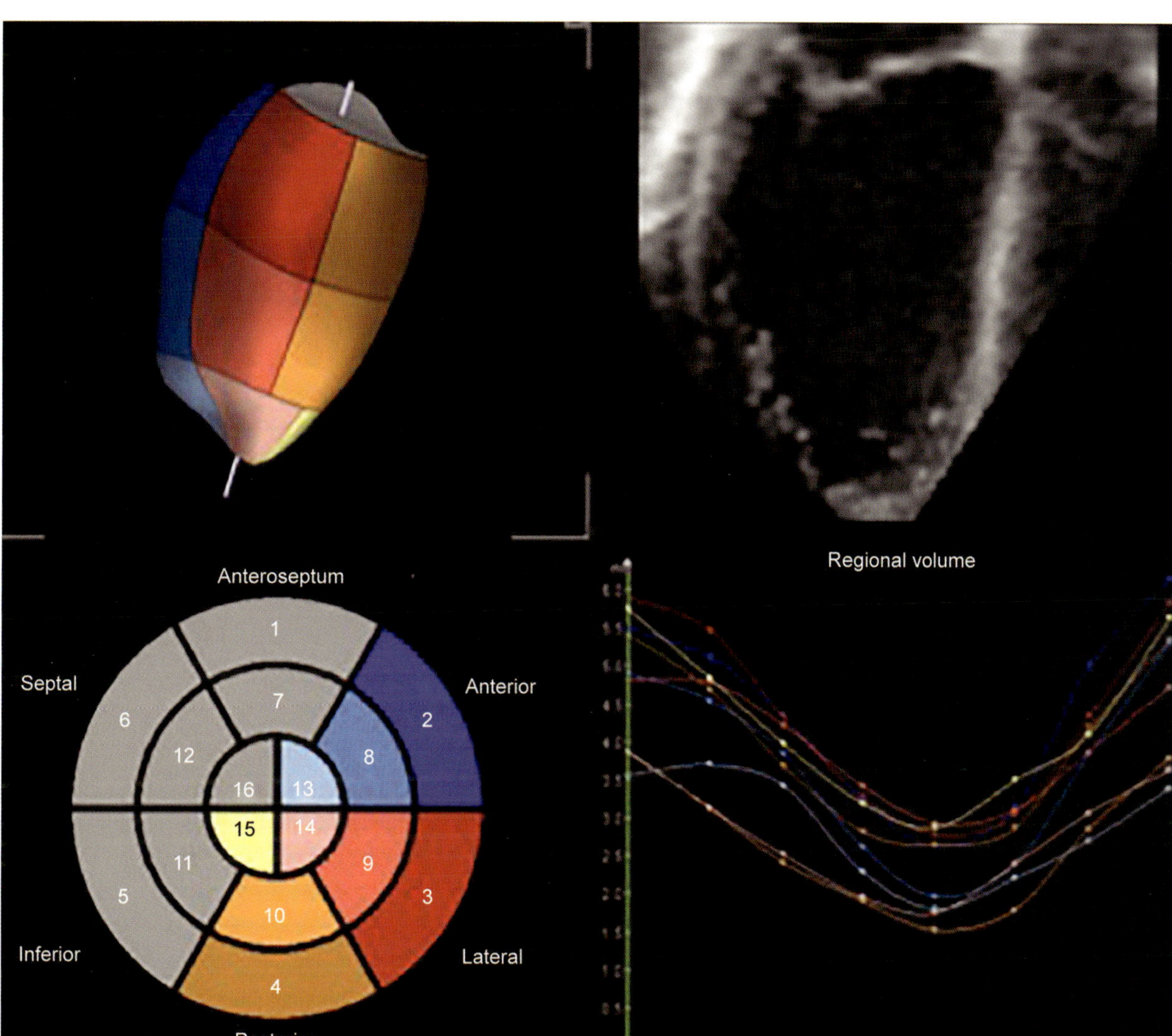


**Figure 9.1:** Three-dimensional echocardiography for estimation of left ventricular volumes and ejection fraction.

echocardiography remains the most widely used, noninvasive, quick, and reliable method for this purpose.

## Myocardial Contrast Echocardiography

Use of myocardial contrast echocardiography (MCE) has traditionally been used for LV opacification and helps in better assessment of cavity size, RWMA, presence of LV clot, pseudoaneurysms or myocardial dissection. However, the MCE best assesses extent of myocardial damage with its prognostic significance. It is an excellent semiquantitative method to evaluate myocardial perfusion, microvascular obstruction (MVO) (akin to "no-reflow" phenomenon on coronary angiography). Absence of myocardial opacification on MCE suggests myocardial necrosis **(Figure 9.2)** while presence suggests salvaged myocardium. The nonopacified myocardial segments on MCE (**Video 9.2**) can help identify nonviable myocardium with higher chances of adverse remodeling in future.[21,22] The role of MCE in patients with ST-elevation MI undergoing primary PCI were assessed using MCE. The group which showed absence of myocardial perfusion defects, fared better with lower WMSI, higher LVEF, with lower combined end-point of death and reinfarction.[23]

## Myocardial Deformation Imaging

Following acute MI, altered global and regional LV function can be further refined and probably more accurately assessed by using longitudinal strain assessed by the 2D speckled-tracking echocardiography (2D-STE) **(Video 9.3)**.

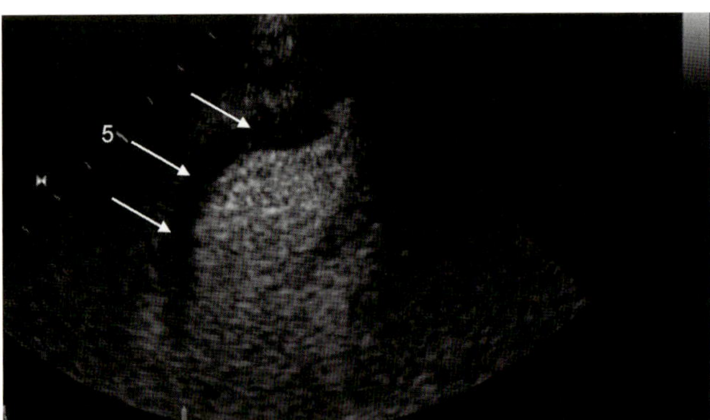

**Figure 9.2:** Myocardial contrast echocardiography showing lack of myocardial perfusion in mid- and distal-septum (arrows).

Unlike tissue-velocity imaging, myocardial deformation imaging is relatively free from the translation motion of the heart as well as tethering artifacts and angle dependence. Transmural extension and the sheer size of the infarct are two of the most important determinants of future adverse cardiovascular events and mortality.[24-26]

GLS is frequently used to quantifying LV function and is more sensitive than LVEF determined by 2D echocardiography.[27-29] Longitudinal strain and its abnormalities are representative of the subendocardial myocardial fibers. Due to the coronary epicardial-to-endocardial gradient across the myocardium, these fibers are least perfused, most vulnerable to ischemia and demonstrate early abnormalities of LV function when compared with LVEF and WMSI in ST-elevation MI patients with mild LV dysfunction. Myocardial post-systolic shortening may also be a marker of ischemic dysfunction **(Figure 9.3)**. Many studies reiterate the reliability of longitudinal strain in identifying ischemic areas and correlates well with extent of wall-thickening, coronary angiographic findings, and ECG changes.[30-32]

As shown in previous but recent studies, reduced regional longitudinal strain on echocardiography correlates well with the delayed enhancement seen on cardiac MRI in accordance with the location (subendocardial, subepicardial, mid-myocardial, and transmural) of the myocardial injury.[33] The association between longitudinal strain measured by 2D-STE with the global and regional transmural extent of myocardial scar as measured by cardiac MRI is well established. In a recent study, a cutoff value of –4.5% for regional strain differentiated between segments with viable myocardium and those with transmural scar tissue with a sensitivity of and specificity of 81% each.[34] Another study suggested it to be a rapid and noninvasive tool for assessment of global myocardial function and transmural extent of necrosis with several far-reaching clinical implications.[35]

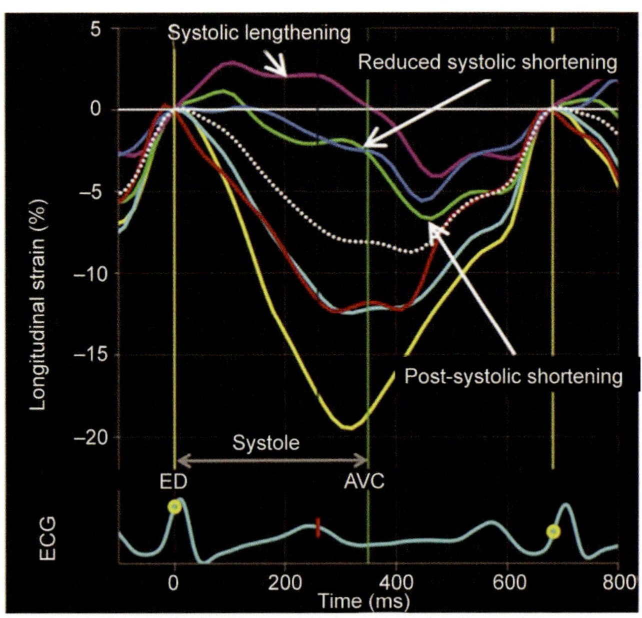


**Figure 9.3:** Speckle-tracking echocardiography showing post-systolic shortening.

*Abbreviations:* AVC, aortic valve closure; ECG, electrocardiogram; ED, end-diastole.

Yet another recent study shows the utility of 2D-STE performed early after an ST-elevation MI as a persistent marker for akinetic segments at 3 months. The GLS correlated significantly with late gadolinium enhancement on cardiac MRI and MVO for final infarct size.[36] The GLS is considered more robust than EF with equivalent prognostic projections.[37,38] The GLS <48 hours post-MI correlates well late recovery of EF.[39] In addition, in patients with suspected ACS without ECG changes or raised cardiac enzymes, myocardial deformation imaging can identify patients at risk early in the triage units and help in quick risk stratification and management.[40] Assessment of layer-specific strain by 2D-STE might also help identify non-ST elevation ACS patients with significant coronary artery disease as the endocardial function (longitudinal fibers) affection is more compared with epicardial function and EF.[41]

Subendocardial infarcts predominantly affect the longitudinal function adversely because the longitudinal LV deformation is determined primarily by the subendocardial fibers. Therefore, radial and circumferential LV deformation remains relatively preserved in subendocardial injury/ischemia. However, with transmural injury, all the myocardial layers are involved resulting in impairment of LV deformation in all directions.[42] For these reasons, impairment of radial and circumferential strain has been used to diagnose transmural infarcts and to predict myocardial viability. However, compared with longitudinal strain, the data is less robust with radial and circumferential strain measurements.

When validated against cardiac MRI, radial and circumferential strain by 2D-STE showed a relatively weak correlation.[43,44]

A radial peak strain cut-off value of 17.2% has been shown to predict viability with a sensitivity of 72% and specificity of 85%,[45] while a GLS cutoff of –10.2% following reperfusion therapy for acute MI, the predicted nonviability with 90.9% sensitivity and 85% specificity.[46]

In another study, a segmental radial strain cutoff of 16.5% and circumferential strain below -11% differentiated nontransmural and transmural infarction with sensitivity of 70% and specificity of 71.2%. Grenne et al. studied 111 patients with suspected non-ST elevation MI in whom echocardiography was performed within an hour of hospital admission. It was found that circumferential strain reliably predicted LVEF, peak cardiac troponin I levels, infarct size and the presence of total coronary occlusion with a cutoff of above -10.0% having 90% sensitivity and 88% specificity for identifying total occlusions.[42]

The rotational mechanics are also impaired in acute MI and correlate with the degree of systolic and diastolic dysfunction.[47-49]

### *Three-dimensional Speckled-tracking Echocardiography*

A major limitation with 2D STE is that it procures only a thin imaging slice of the myocardium at a time and hence cannot compensate for the 'out-of-plane' motion of the myocardium during the cardiac motion leading to suboptimized tracking of the speckles. Short-axis views are affected considerably more in this regard. This explains the relatively less robust data about the accuracy and reproducibility of radial and circumferential strain. The more recently developed 3D-STE promises to offer a potential solution to this problem **(Video 9.4)**. However, presently the temporal and spatial resolution remains a major limitation with 3D-STE which can introduce significant errors in the measurements.[50]

Thus, myocardial strain imaging provides an accurate, quantitative measure of regional as well as global myocardial contractile function sensitive to subtle changes in the myocardial contractility allowing reasonably accurate assessment of the extent of the myocardial damage and prognosis, guiding therapeutic decisions and monitoring response to therapy.

## Left Ventricular Diastolic Function Assessment

Equally important as the systolic function post-MI is the diastolic function. Sheer presence of "restrictive" transmitral filling pattern [peak mitral inflow early diastolic (E) velocity more than double the peak late diastolic (A) velocity with E-wave deceleration time <150 msec] predicts a worse prognosis if associated in low LVEF patients.[51,52] A simple

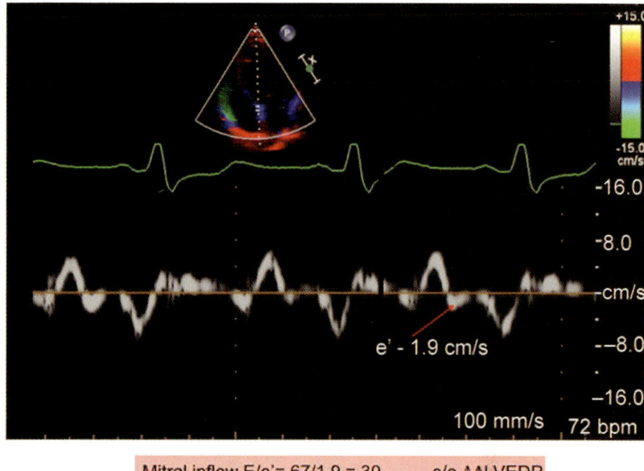


**Figure 9.4:** Markedly reduced mitral annular early diastolic velocity. The ratio of mitral inflow early diastolic velocity to mitral annular early diastolic velocity was 30, suggestive of significantly elevated left ventricular end-diastolic pressure.
*Abbreviations:* E, mitral inflow early diastolic velocity; e', mitral annular early diastolic velocity; LVEDP, left ventricular end-diastolic pressure.

ratio of mitral E to mitral annular early diastolic velocity (e') correlates well with LV end-diastolic pressure. Clearly elevated mitral E/e' (>15) early after MI independently predicts the future occurrence of cardiovascular death and heart failure **(Figure 9.4)**.[53,54] Similarly, increased left atrial size (>32 mL/m$^2$) and elevated pulmonary artery systolic pressure are also adverse prognostic markers in patients with ACS.[55,56]

## SUMMARY

Accurate determination of the extent of MI has tremendous diagnostic, therapeutic and prognostic significance.[57] Despite advances in multimodality imaging, echocardiography still remains the most affordable, rapid, accurate and dependable modality of choice as the first-response tool. Newer advancements like 2D- and 3D-STE are likely to further catapult this versatile modality into the most sought after modality of choice for detection of extent of myocardial damage.

## VIDEO LEGENDS

**Video 9.1:** Extensive regional wall-motion abnormalities in the left anterior descending artery territory with significantly reduced left ventricular ejection fraction. The patient also had pericardial effusion.

**Video 9.2:** Myocardial contrast echocardiography in apical 4-chamber view in a patient with acute myocardial infarction. There is reduced myocardial perfusion of the lateral wall.

**Video 9.3:** Longitudinal strain measurement by 2-dimensional speckle tracking echocardiography.

**Video 9.4:** Three-dimensional speckle-tracking echocardiography.

## REFERENCES

1. Fye WB. A history of the origin, evolution, and impact of electrocardiography. Am J Cardiol. 1994;73:937-49.
2. Edler I, Hertz CH. Use of ultrasonic reflectoscope for the continuous recording of movements of heart walls. Kungl Fysiogr Sallsk Lund Forh.1954;24:40.
3. Allam AH, Thompson RC, Wann L, et al. Atherosclerosis in ancient Egyptian mummies: the Horus study. J Am Coll Cardiol Img. 2011;4:315-27.
4. Hauser AM, Gangadharan V, Ramos RG, et al. Sequence of mechanical, electrocardiographic and clinical effects of repeated coronary artery occlusion in human beings: echocardiographic observations during coronary angioplasty. J Am Coll Cardiol. 1985;5:193.
5. Wohlgelernter D, Cleman M, Highman HA, Fetterman RC, Duncan JS, Zaret BL, et al. Regional myocardial dysfunction during coronary angioplasty: evaluation by two-dimensional echocardiography and 12 lead electrocardiography. J Am Coll Cardiol. 1986;7:1245.
6. Davies MJ. The pathophysiology of acute coronary syndromes. Heart. 2000;83:361-6.
7. Picard MH, Wilkins GT, Ray PA, et al. Natural history of left ventricular size and function after acute myocardial infarction. Assessment and prediction by echocardiographic endocardial surface mapping. Circulation. 1990;82:484-94.
8. Gudmundsson P, Rydberg E, Winter R, et al. Visually estimated left ventricular ejection fraction by echocardiography is closely correlated with formal quantitative methods. Int J Cardiol. 2005;101:209-12.
9. Antman EM, Cohen M, Bernink PJ, McCabe CH, Horacek T, Papuchis G, et al. The TIMI risk score for unstable angina/ non-ST elevation MI: a method for prognostication and therapeutic decision making. JAMA. 2000;284:835-42.
10. Horowitz RS, Morganroth J. Immediate detection of early high-risk patients with acute myocardial infarction using two-dimensional echocardiographic evaluation of left ventricular regional wall motion abnormalities. Am Heart J 1982;103:814-22.
11. Romano S, Dagianti A, Penco M, Varveri A, Biffani E, Fedele F, et al. Usefulness of echocardiography in the prognostic of non-Q-wave myocardial infarction. Am J Cardiol. 2000;86:43G-5.
12. Møller JE, Hillis GS, Oh JK, Reeder GS, Gersh BJ, Pellikka PA. Wall motion score index and ejection fraction for risk stratification after acute myocardial infarction. Am Heart J. 2006;151:419-2.
13. Figueras J, Barrab J A, Evangelista A, Lid RN, Gutierrez L, del Blanco BG, et al. Admission Wall Motion Score and Quantitative ST-Segment Depression in the Assessment of 30-Day Mortality in Patients with First Non–ST-Segment Elevation Acute Coronary Syndromes. J Am Soc Echocardiogr. 2013;26:885-92.
14. Lang RM, Badano LP, Mor-Avi V, Afilalo J, Armstrong A, Ernande L, et al. Recommendations for cardiac chamber quantification by echocardiography in adults: an update from the American Society of Echocardiography and the European Association of Cardiovascular Imaging. J Am Soc Echocardiogr. 2015;28:1-39.
15. Thavendiranathan P, Liu S, Verhaert D, et al. Feasibility, accuracy, and reproducibility of real-time full-volume 3D transthoracic echocardiography to measure LV volumes and systolic function: a fully automated endocardial contouring algorithm in sinus rhythm and atrial fibrillation. JACC Cardiovasc Imaging. 2012;5:239-51.
16. Curtis JP, Sokol SI, Wang Y, et al. The association of left ventricular ejection fraction, mortality, and cause of death in stable outpatients with heart failure. J Am Coll Cardiol. 2003;42:736-42.
17. Stanton T, Leano R, Marwick TH. Prediction of all-cause mortality from global longitudinal speckle strain: comparison with ejection fraction and wall motion scoring. Circ Cardiovasc Imaging. 2009;2:356-64.
18. Johri AM, Picard MH, Newell J, et al. Can a teaching intervention reduce interobserver variability in LVEF assessment: a quality control exercise in the echocardiography lab. JACC Cardiovasc Imaging. 2011;4:821-9.
19. Yu EH, Sloggett CE, Iwanochko RM, et al. Feasibility and accuracy of left ventricular volumes and ejection fraction determination by fundamental, tissue harmonic, and intravenous contrast imaging in difficult-to-image patients. J Am Soc Echocardiogr. 2000;13:216-24.
20. Jenkins C, Bricknell K, Chan J, et al. Comparison of two- and three-dimensional echocardiography with sequential magnetic resonance imaging for evaluating left ventricular volume and ejection fraction over time in patients with healed myocardial infarction. Am J Cardiol. 2007;99:300-6.
21. Ujino K, Hillis GS, Mulvagh SL, et al. Usefulness of real-time intravenous myocardial contrast echocardiography in predicting left ventricular dilation after successfully reperfused acute myocardial infarction. Am J Cardiol. 2005; 96:17-21.
22. Hayat SA, Senior R. Myocardial contrast echocardiography in ST elevation myocardial infarction: ready for prime time? Eur Heart J. 2008;29:299-314.
23. Tomaszuk-Kazberuk A, Sobkowicz B, Dobrzycki S, et al. Perfusion assessed by real-time contrast echocardiography correlates with clinical and echocardiographic parameters in patients with first STEMI treated with PCI – 6-month follow-up. Arch Med Sci. 2010;6:176-82.
24. Pislaru C, Bruce CJ, Anagnostopoulos PC, Allen JL, Seward JB, Pellikka PA, et al. Ultrasound strain imaging of altered myocardial stiffness: stunned versus infarcted reperfused myocardium. Circulation. 2004;109:2905-10.
25. Reffelmann T, Hale SL, Li G, et al. Relationship between no reflow and infarct size as influenced by the duration of ischemia and reperfusion. Am J Physiol Heart Circ Physiol. 2002;282:H766-72.
26. Kim RJ, Wu E, Rafael A, Chen EL, Parker MA, Simonetti O, et al. The use of contrast enhanced magnetic resonance imaging to identify reversible myocardial dysfunction. N Eng J Med. 2000;343:1445-53.
27. Urheim S, Edvardsen T, Torp H, et al. Myocardial strain by Doppler echocardiography. Validation of a new method

to quantify regional myocardial function. Circulation. 2000;102:1158-64.

28. Brown JBS, Jenkins CMS, Marwick TH. Use of myocardial strain to assess global left ventricular function: a comparison with cardiac magnetic resonance and 3-dimensional echocardiography. Am Heart J. 2009;157:102.e1-e5.
29. Sjoli B, Orn S, Grenne B, Vartdal T, Smiseth OA, Edvardsen T, et al. Comparison of left ventricular ejection fraction and left ventricular global strain as determinants of infarct size in patients with acute myocardial infarction. J Am Soc Echocardiogr. 2009;22:1232-8.
30. Gotte MJ, van Rossum AC, Twisk JWR, Kuijer JPA, Marcus JT, Visser CA. Quantification of regional contractile function after infarction: strain analysis superior to wall thickening analysis in discriminating infarct from remote myocardium. J Am Coll Cardiol. 2001;37:808-17.
31. Jamal F, Kukulski T, Sutherland GR, Weidermann F, D'hooge J, Bijnens B, et al. Can changes in systolic longitudinal deformation quantify regional myocardial function after an acute infarction? An ultrasonic strain rate and strain study. J Am Soc Echocardiogr. 2002;15:723-30.
32. Nishikage T, Takeuchi M, Nakai H, et al. Possible link between strain ST-T change on the electrocardiogram and subendocardial dysfunction assessed by two-dimensional speckle-tracking echocardiography. Eur J Echocardiogr 2010;11:451-9.
33. Kansal MM, Panse PM, Abe H, Caracciolo G, Wilansky S, Tajik J, et al. Relationship of contrast-enhanced magnetic resonance imaging-derived intramural scar distribution and speckle tracking echocardiography-derived left ventricular twodimensional strains. Eur J Echocardiogr. 2012;13:152-8.
34. Roes SD, Mollema SA, Lamb HJ, Van der Wall EE, de Roos A, Bax JJ. Validation of echocardiographic two-dimensional speckle tracking longitudinal strain imaging for viability assessment in patients with chronic ischemic left ventricular dysfunction and comparison with contrast-enhanced magnetic resonance imaging. Am J Cardiol. 2009;104:312-7.
35. Cimino S, Canali E, Petronilli V, et al. Global and regional longitudinal strain assessed by two-dimensional speckle tracking echocardiography identifies early myocardial dysfunction and transmural extent of myocardial scar in patients with acute ST elevation myocardial infarction and relatively preserved LV function. Eur Heart J Cardiovasc Imaging. 2013;14:805-11.
36. Bière L, Donal E, Terrien G, Kervio G, Willoteaux S, Furber A, et al. Longitudinal Strain Is a Marker of Microvascular Obstruction and Infarct Size in Patients with Acute ST-Segment Elevation Myocardial Infarction. PLoS ONE. 2014;9:e86959.
37. Stanton T, Leano R, Marwick TH. Prediction of all-cause mortality from global longitudinal speckle strain: comparison with ejection fraction and wall motion scoring. Circ Cardiovasc Imaging. 2009;2:356-64.
38. Dalen H, Thorstensen A, Aase SA, Ingul CB, Torp H, Vatten LJ, et al. Segmental and global longitudinal strain and strain rate based on echocardiography of 1266 healthy individuals: the HUNT study in Norway. Eur J Echocardiogr. 2010;11: 176-83.
39. Mollema SA, Delgado V, Bertini M, Antoni ML, Boersma E, Holman ER, et al. Viability assessment with global left ventricular longitudinal strain predicts recovery of left ventricular function after acute myocardial infarction. Circ Cardiovasc Imaging. 2010;3:15-23.
40. Schroeder J, Hamada S, Gründlinger N, Rubeau T, Altiok E, Ulbrich K, et al. Myocardial deformation by strain echocardiography identifies patients with acute coronary syndrome and non-diagnostic ECG presenting in a chest pain unit: a prospective study of diagnostic accuracy. Clin Res Cardiol. 2016; 105:248-56.
41. Sarvari SI, Haugaa KH, Zahid W, et al. Layer-Specific Quantification of Myocardial Deformation by Strain Echocardiography May Reveal Significant CAD in Patients With Non–ST-Segment Elevation Acute Coronary Syndrome. J Am Coll Cardiol. 2013;6:535-44.
42. Grenne B, Eek C, Sjoli B, et al. Acute coronary occlusion in non-ST-elevation acute coronary syndrome: outcome and early identification by strain echocardiography. Heart. 2010;96:1550-6.
43. Becker M, Hoffmann R, Kühl HP, et al. Analysis of myocardial deformation based on ultrasonic pixel tracking to determine transmurality in chronic myocardial infarction. Eur Heart J. 2006;27:2560-6.
44. Cho GY, Chan J, Leano R, et al. Comparison of two dimensional speckle and tissue velocity based strain and validation with harmonic phase magnetic resonance imaging. Am J Cardiol. 2006;97:1661-6.
45. Becker M, Lenzen A, Ocklenburg C, et al. Myocardial deformation imaging based on ultrasonic pixel tracking to identify reversible myocardial dysfunction. J Am Coll Cardiol. 2008;51:1473-81.
46. Park YH, Kang SJ, Song JK, et al. Prognostic value of longitudinal strain after primary reperfusion therapy in patients with anterior-wall acute myocardial infarction. J Am Soc Echocardiogr. 2008;21:262-7.
47. Becker M, Hoffmann R, Kuhl HP, Grawe H, Katoh M, Kramann R, et al. Analysis of myocardial deformation based on ultrasonic pixel tracking to determine transmurality on chronic myocardial infarction. Eur Heart J. 2006;27:2560-6.
48. Ersbøll MK. Left ventricular global longitudinal strain in acute myocardial infarction—with special reference to neuro-hormonal activation, inhospital heart failure and prognosis. Dan Med J. 2013;60:B4697.
49. Sjøli B, Ørn S, Grenne B, et al. Diagnostic capability and reproducibility of strain by Doppler and by speckle tracking in patients with acute myocardial infarction. JACC Cardiovasc Imaging. 2009;2:24-33.
50. Bière L, Donal E, Terrien G, et al. Longitudinal strain is a marker of microvascular obstruction and infarct size in patients with acute STsegment elevation myocardial infarction. PLoS One. 2014;9:e86959.
51. Yamamoto K, Nishimura RA, Chaliki HP, Appleton CP, Holmes DR Jr, Redfield MM. Determination of left ventricular filling

pressure by Doppler echocardiography in patients with coronary artery disease: critical role of left ventricular systolic function. J Am Coll Cardiol. 1997;30:1819-26.
52. Yodwut C, Weinert L, Klas B, et al. Effects of frame rate on three-dimensional speckle-tracking-based measurements of myocardial deformation. J Am Soc Echocardiogr. 2012; 25:978-85.
53. Meta-Analysis Research Group in Echocardiography (MeRGE) AMI Collaborators. Independent prognostic importance of a restrictive left ventricular filling pattern after myocardial infarction: an individual patient meta-analysis: meta-analysis research group in echocardiography acute myocardial infarction. Circulation. 2008;117:2591-8.
54. Hillis GS, Moller JE, Pellikka PA, Gersh BJ, Wright RS, Ommen SR, et al. Noninvasive estimation of left ventricular filling pressure by E/e′ is a powerful predictor of survival after acute myocardial infarction. J Am Coll Cardiol. 2004;43: 360-7.
55. Kruszewski K, Scott AE, Barclay JL, Small GR, Croal BL, Møller JE, et al. Noninvasive assessment of left ventricular filling pressure after acute myocardial infarction a prospective study of the relative prognostic utility of clinical assessment, echocardiography, and B-type natriuretic peptide. Am Heart J. 2010;159:47-54.
56. Møller JE, Hillis GS, Oh JK, Seward JB, Reeder GS, Wright RS, et al. Left atrial volume: a powerful predictor of survival after acute myocardial infarction. Circulation. 2003;107:2207-12.
57. Møller JE, Hillis GS, Oh JK, et al. Prognostic importance of secondary pulmonary hypertension after acute myocardial infarction. Am J Cardiol. 2005;96:199-203.

# Post-myocardial Infarction Risk Stratification



*G Vijayaraghavan, S Baskaran*

The ability to distinguish reversible from irreversible injury is of critical importance in the management of acute and chronic coronary artery disease (CAD) syndromes. Many subjects with heart failure and underlying CAD have a significant amount of viable but dysfunctional myocardium, wherein the involved myocardial segment retains the ability to contract if perfusion is re-established.[1] Left ventricular (LV) function is the single most important independent predictor of long-term outcomes in patients with CAD. Therapeutic interventions that improve LV function have consistently shown better outcome in terms of reduction in mortality and admission rates for heart failure and improvement in quality of life indicators, including heart failure classifications and exercise capacity.[2-11] Echocardiography helps in the assessment of these parameters and thus plays a vital role in the assessment of CAD and post-myocardial infarction (MI) risk stratification.

## LEFT VENTRICULAR STRUCTURE AND FUNCTION

Depending on the factors such as the extent and reversibility of ischemia, reperfusion therapy, extent of passive myocardial stretch and other factors, there are certain changes take place in the structure and function of the left ventricle following an acute MI. These changes, occurring immediately to over a period of days to weeks, include bulging of the infarcted area, infarct expansion, loss of contractile tissues with hyperkinesia of the distant myocardial areas and eventually dilatation of the left ventricle with resultant mitral regurgitation.

These changes are paralleled by complex set of biochemical and neuroendocrine changes, termed as 'infarct remodeling'.[12] Echocardiography acts as a principal cardiac imaging modality during the acute (0–48 h) and subacute (Day 3–7) phase following acute MI for the assessment of segmental and global LV systolic function, intracavitary thrombus formation, and other mechanical complications of MI. Hence, it is recommended to perform an echocardiography within 24–48 h to provide a post-infarction baseline assessment of function and an additional echo within the first 3 months following an acute MI.[13]

### Postinfarction Remodeling of the Left Ventricle

By progressive increase in systolic and diastolic LV volumes, postinfarction remodeling contributes to an impaired prognosis. During the initial phase of this process, the parallel increase in both end-systolic and end-diastolic-volume increases makes the ejection fraction to be much less affected than volumes alone. Increment of 20% in end-diastolic LV volume from baseline at 6 months after MI strongly correlates with development of clinical heart failure and increased mortality.[14]

### Wall Motion Score Index

Wall motion score index (WMSI) has additional independent prognostic value as to mortality and later hospitalization for heart failure. This is an average of the wall motion score in all LV wall segments, where the score is 1 for normokinesia, 2 for hypokinesia, 3 for akinesia, and 4 for dyskinesia. WMSI is then derived by summing the scores for each segment and dividing by the total number of segments (WMSI of 1 represents normal motion in all segments) **(Figure 10.1)**. WMSI value greater than 1 indicates abnormal wall motion in at least one segment.[15] In case of paradoxical septal motion seen in post-bypass surgery/ ventricular pacing, septal segments may be excluded in both pre- and post-procedural calculations. Both LV ejection fraction (LVEF) and WMSI are strong predictors of all-cause mortality after acute MI. Mortality increases exponentially with decreasing LVEF, whereas it increases linearly with increasing WMSI.[16]

### Strain

Recent developments in the quantification of regional LV myocardial deformation would help in the better post-MI risk stratification. Based on the algorithms which measure the regional deformation of myocardial echo scatterers in several directions [also known as speckle tracking echocardiography (STE) or two dimensional (2D) strain], a global average of

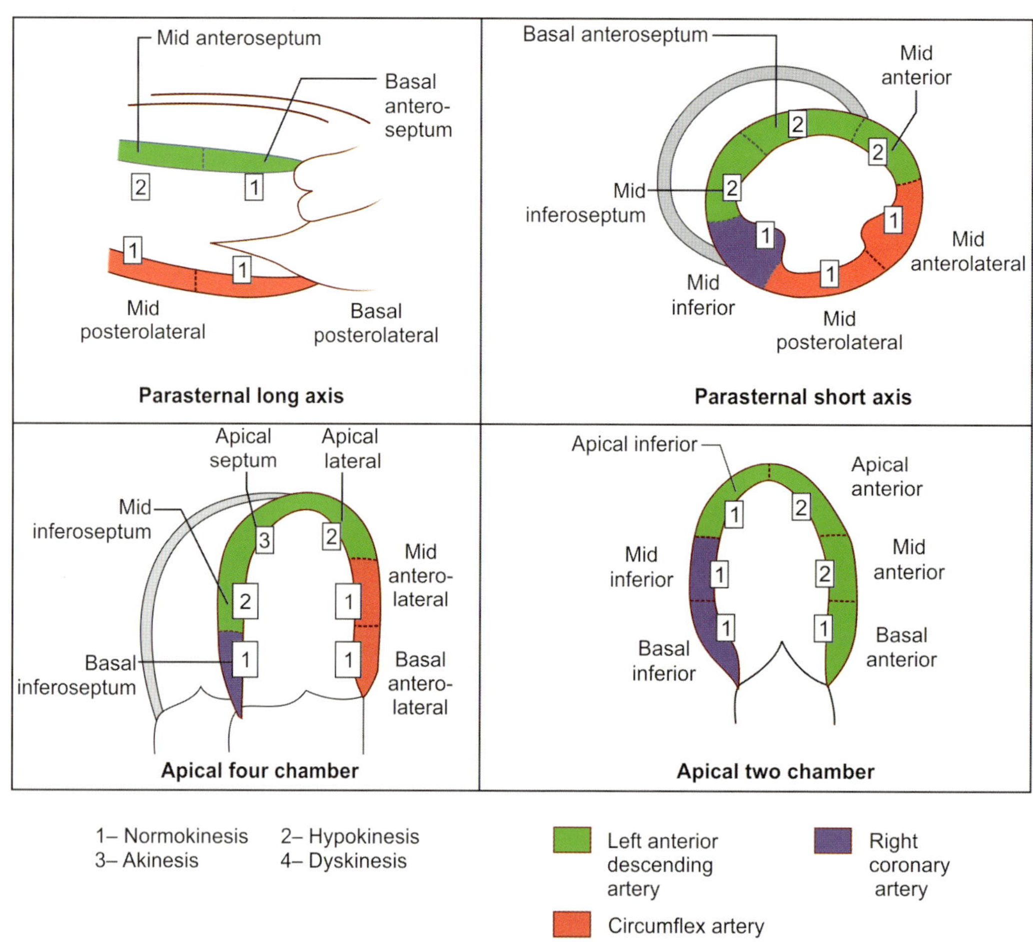


**Figure 10.1:** Demonstration of various segments of LV with wall motion abnormalities and scoring system. *Abbreviation:* LV, left ventricle.

segmental strain can be calculated.[16] The subendocardial fibers, which are responsible for the longitudinal shortening, are the most sensitive to myocardial hypoperfusion and thus, the longitudinal function is affected earliest in the presence of ischemia. Global longitudinal strain (GLS), though more data yet to evolve, has been reported to be better than classic ejection fraction and to be at the same time non-inferior in post-MI risk stratification **(Figure 10.2A to D)**.[17] Speckle tracking with velocity vector imaging (VVI), has shown to be independently associated with increased risk of death or heart failure after acute MI as observed by the VALIANT (VALsartan In Acute myocardial iNfarcTion) echocardiography investigators.[16,17] Absolute GLS early (<48 h) after MI was reported to correlate with the potential for recovery of ejection fraction in future.

## Velocity Vector Imaging[18]

VVI is an angle-independent tool obtained with a modification of the M-Mode principle. VVI analysis helps in the measurement of tissue velocities (S´, E´, A´), 2D-strain and strain rate. VVI analysis with strain measurements in infarcted myocardium assess the global and regional myocardial function accurately, and also differentiates infarcted from non-infarcted segments. Gray-scale frame rate of about 40–50 Hz is suitable for VVI analysis whereas a high or low frame rate would alter the measurements.

## Diastolic Function[19]

Recent develpoment in the understanding of diastolic function as a parameter in the context of management and prognosis after MI, makes it an integral part in the assessment of CAD. The occurence of restrictive transmitral filling pattern [The ratio of early diastolic (E) to late diastolic (A) velocity (E/A ratio) > 2, E-wave deceleration time <150 ms] **(Figure 10.3)** in the presence of impaired ejection fraction has been known to predict poor prognosis. Similarly, shortened transmitral E-wave deceleration time by itself is an

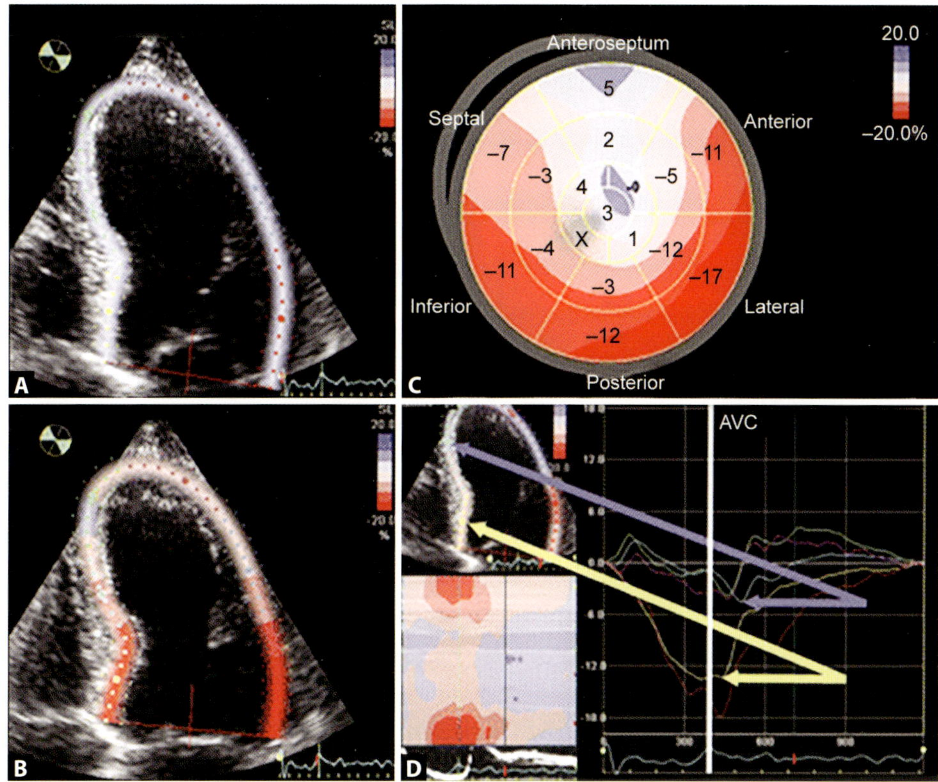


**Figure 10.2A to D:** Determination of regional and global longitudinal strain. (A) End-diastolic and (B) end-systolic frame of four-chamber view from a patient after anterior wall myocardial infarction demonstrating regional longitudinal strain by speckle-tracking, which is color-coded. (C) Bull's eye plot showing regional longitudinal strain from outer to inner circles representing respectively from basal to apical segments of LV, demonstrating grossly reduced mean global longitudinal strain of −5.2%, indicating severely impaired global left ventricular systolic function (normal values for global are 'above' −14%, with a mean of −17%) and bluish areas representing dyskinetic segments with abnormal positive strain. (D) Strain curves obtained with regional longitudinal strain (y-axis) plotted against time (x-axis); the two representative strain curves shown by arrows with color code corresponding to the colored dots on the LV segments; the blue curve demonstrates substantially reduced and delayed peak systolic longitudinal strain of the apical and distal IVS segments.
*Abbreviations:* AVC, aortic valve closure; IVS, interventricular septum; LV, left ventricular.

independent predictor of remodeling process in future. The E/e′ obtained as ratio of peak transmitral E-wave velocity to peak early diastolic mitral annular velocity (e′) at the base of the left ventricle reflects the LV filling pressures, and an elevated E/e′ ratio (typically >15) at baseline (e.g. early after infarction) is a strong independent predictor of mortality and heart failure.

## LEFT ATRIAL ENLARGEMENT

Increased left atrial (LA) size, as measured by a mean LA volume of >32 mL/m$^2$, reflects elevated LA pressure and is associated with adverse prognosis independent of other conventional functional parameters such as LV ejection fraction. In post-MI scenario, such elevation in LA pressures may be due to impaired LV systolic function, impaired diastolic function, or the presence of mitral regurgitation.[13]

## ASSESSMENT OF RIGHT VENTRICULAR FUNCTION

Right ventricular (RV) function is a known predictor of cardiovascular morbidity and mortality in patients with LV dysfunction after MI. Impaired RV function after MI, measured as fractional area shortening of the right ventricle <32%, or tricuspid annular plane systolic excursion (TAPSE) (with a cut-off of ≤14 mm) was predictive of long-term prognosis with regard to mortality and heart failure.[20]

In another study,[21] RV ejection fraction (RVEF) ≤ 37%, TAPSE ≤ 18.5 mm and the peak systolic tricuspid

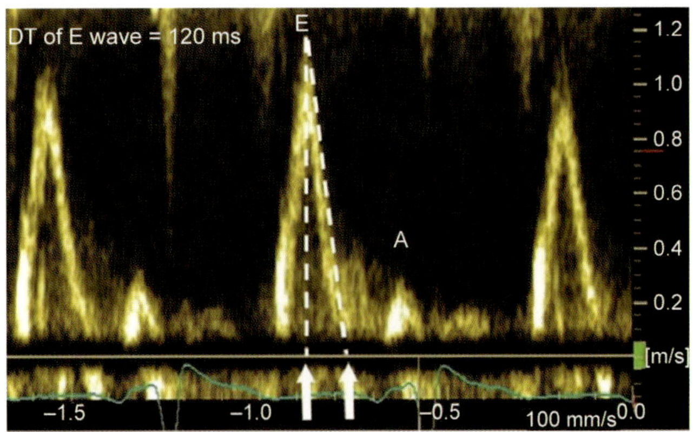


**Figure 10.3**[13]**:** Transmitral Doppler showing a restrictive filling pattern in a patient with recent anterior wall myocardial infarction. *Abbreviations:* A, late diastolic mitral inflow velocity; DT, deceleration time; E, early diastolic mitral inflow velocity.

annular velocity ≤ 9.7 cm/s were independently associated with reduced survival in patients with stable LV dysfunction **(Figure 10.4)**, however patients with recent (<3 months) acute MI were excluded. Among the various RV parameters, the combination of RVEF ≤ 37% and tricuspid annular systolic velocity ≤ 9.7 cm/s was found to be the best predictor of reduced cardiac survival in this group **(Figure 10.5)** and hence the presence of this combination with LV systolic dysfunction after 3 months of MI may be associated with reduced cardiac survival.

The risk of cardiovascular events increased with increasing peak RVWMSI. Stress RVWMSI is an independent predictor of cardiovascular events, independent of LV ischemia and LV function (ejection fraction) and provided incremental prognostic value over rest and conventional stress echocardiographic variables.[22]

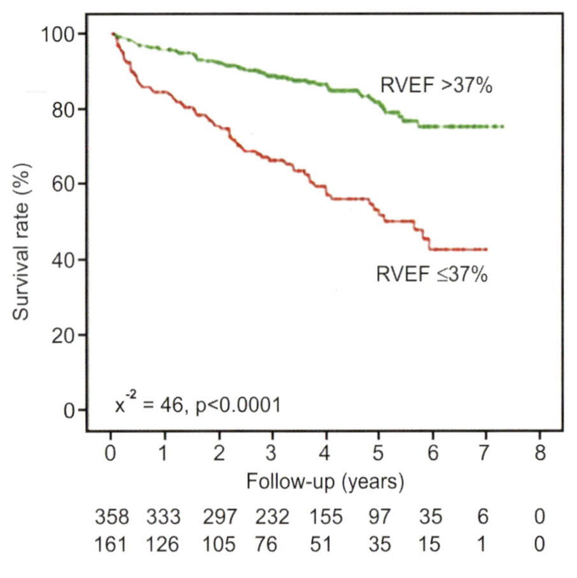


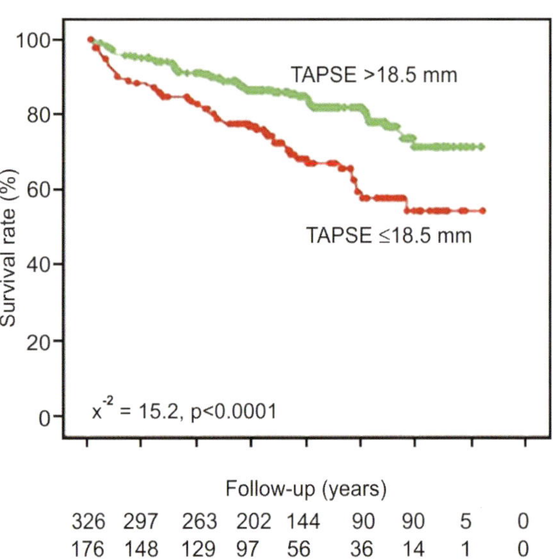


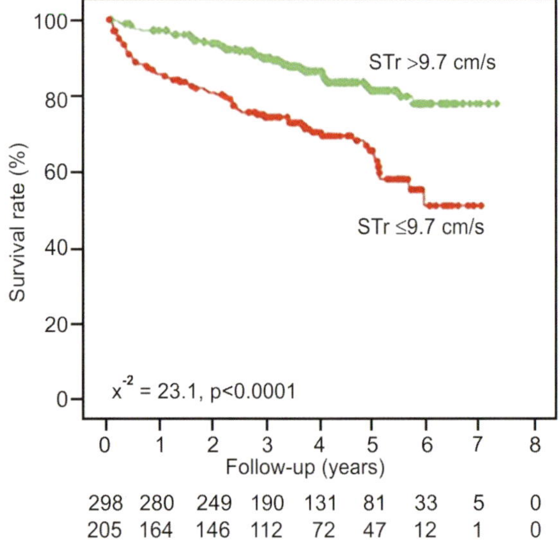


**Figure 10.4:** Survival curves of the study population according to cut-off values of right ventricular ejection fraction, tricuspid annular plane systolic excursion, and peak systolic tricuspid annular velocity (reproduced with permission).[21]
*Abbreviations:* RVEF, right ventricular ejection fraction; STr, peak systolic tricuspid annular velocity; TAPSE, tricuspid annular plane systolic excursion.

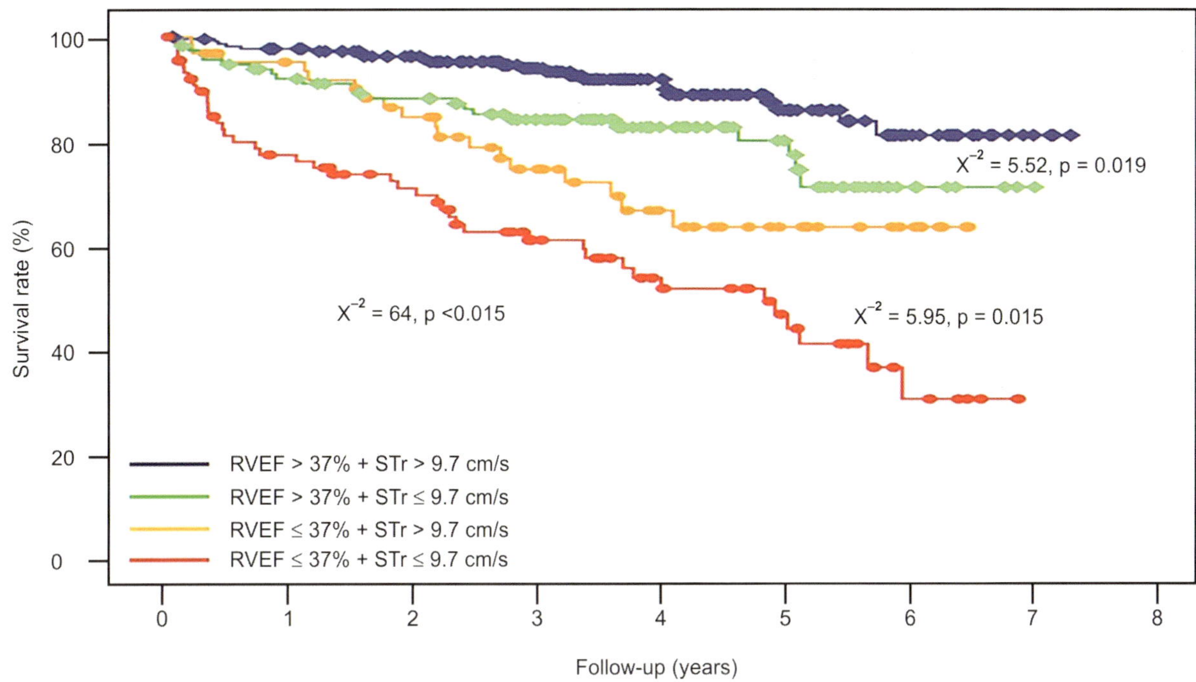


**Figure 10.5:** Survival curves of the study population according to the combination of right ventricular ejection fraction, and peak systolic tricuspid annular velocity (reproduced with permission).[21]
*Abbreviations:* RVEF, right ventricular ejection fraction; STr, peak systolic tricuspid annular velocity.

STE provides objective measures to quantify segmental and global ventricular function independently of angle of incidence, chamber translation, cardiac rotation, and ventricular size **(Figure 10.6A to C)**. Recent study shows that longitudinal RV strain was reduced in patients with old MI in the absence of RV infarction, and the RV strain depends highly on longitudinal LV strain especially in patients with high plasma brain natriuretic peptide levels.[23] These results may indicate that RV dysfunction following MI does not owe fully to excessive afterload but also due to neurohormonal activation, which causing ventricular remodeling response to altered LV wall stress.

### Detection of Microvascular Ischemia[13]

Microvascular ischemia occurs due to the microvascular 'no-reflow' with absence of reperfusion at the tissue level after MI and may go undetected by coronary angiography. This can be demonstrated by the absence of opacification of the affected myocardial segment on contrast echocardiography by injecting intravenous myocardial contrast. Studies have shown that the presence of microvascular no-reflow, as shown by contrast echocardiography as non-opacification of the corresponding segmental myocardium, is a strong predictor of later infarct remodeling.

## GUIDANCE OF REVASCULARIZATION STRATEGIES

### Inducible Ischemia

The presence and the extent of coronary disease and the presence of inducible ischaemia in non-infarcted areas is of the crucial importance in the further risk stratification of MI. This can be assessed by performing one of the imaging stress tests which have a clear advantage over treadmill (Bruce protocol) or bicycle exercise tests in this scenario. Sufficient data are available on the role of both nuclear imaging and stress echocardiography in the assessment of presence, extent and severity of inducible ischemia and of scar and thereby, their contribution to the risk stratification as to cardiac death or re-infarction. MI management guidelines recommend to utilize one of these imaging techniques for this purpose depending on the availability and local expertise. During the sub-acute phase of MI (>48 h), stress tests may be safely performed in clinically stable patients

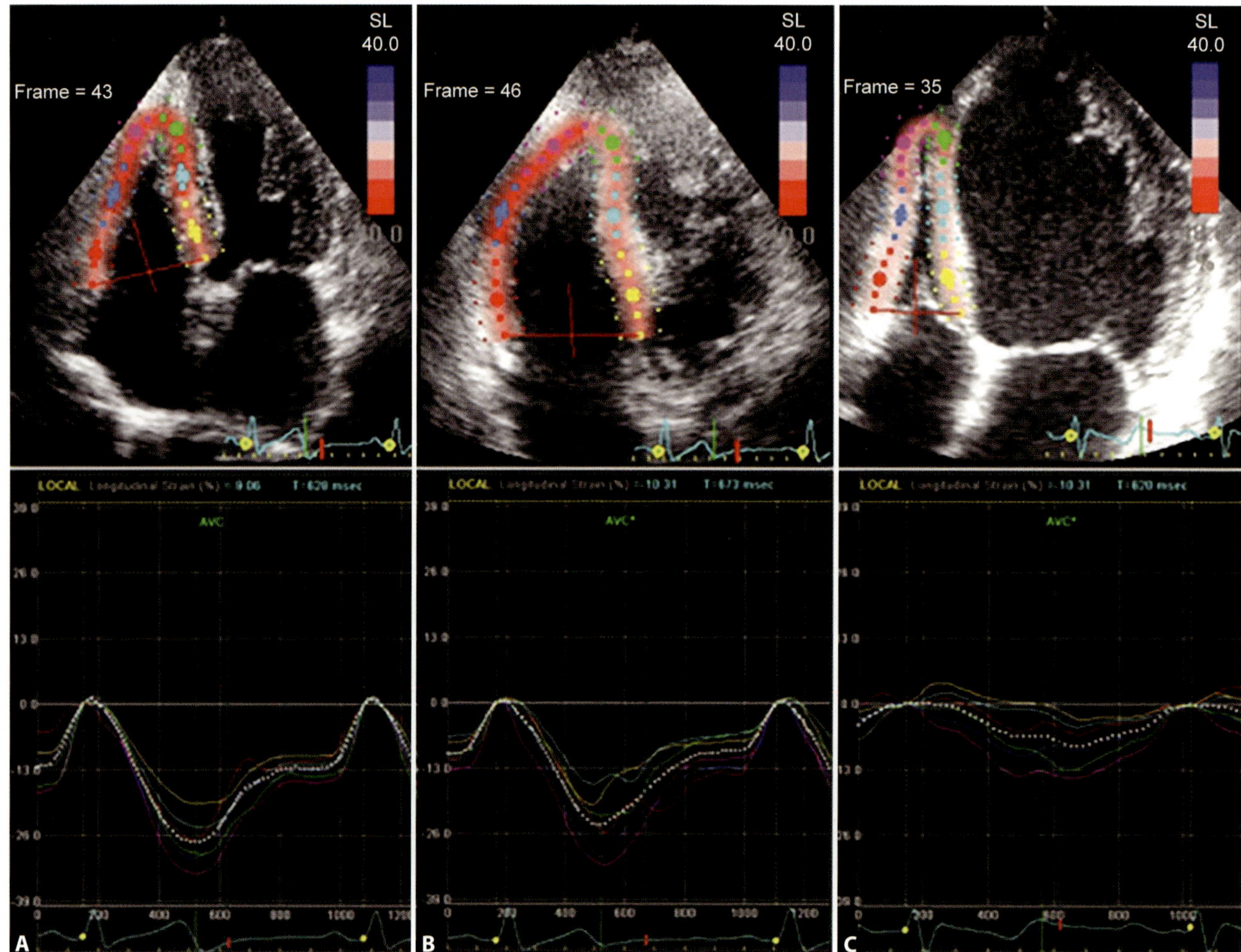


**Figure 10.6A to C[23]:** Examples of right ventricular strain imaging in the apical four-chamber view (top) and corresponding time-strain curves (bottom). (A) A normal subject, (B) A patient with old myocardial infarction (MI) in the territory of left anterior descending artery and low plasma BNP level, and (C) Another patient with old MI in the all 3 coronary artery territories and high plasma BNP level.
*Abbreviations:* BNP, brain natriuretic peptide; SL, longitudinal strain.

and post-MI patients with a negative stress test can be safely discharged early.

## Myocardial Viability (Chapter 17)

### *Reversible Injury*

Within the seconds of onset of severe ischemia, the affected myocardium switches abruptly from predominantly aerobic to anaerobic metabolism. This results in a drastic reduction in the generation of high energy phosphates, namely adenosine triphosphate (ATP) and phosphocreatinine[24] in association with ultrastructural changes identifiable on electron microscopy, ultimately resulting in contractile dysfunction. These changes are entirely reversible if reperfusion is established in 20–40 minutes. The duration of this contractile dysfunction depends on the severity and duration of the ischemic period and clearly, by the occurrence of irreversible injury.

### *Irreversible Injury*

MI follows a distinct pattern of progression from subendocardium to subepicardium. In acute MI, the myofibrillar death begins approximately after 40 minutes and reaches its complete transmural extent in 6–12 hrs for complete infarction of the myocardium at risk.[25] The sequence of inflammatory response in an infarcted myocardium leads to fibrinous exudate inciting connective tissue growth and finally transforming the original site of necrosis into a mature, collagenous, noncontractile scar.

### *Viable Myocardium*

Viable myocardium is defined as one that is dysfunctional due to compromised blood supply, but is likely to recover its contractile function after restoration of adequate perfusion by one of the revascularization methods. In other words, if tissue is viable, it will benefit through improvement in function by restoration of normal blood flow. Myocardial viability provides a definite opportunity to positively influence the patient's prognosis, with an increase in ejection fraction, systolic and diastolic performances, exercise capacity and most importantly, survival. The criteria for myocardial viability are: (1) ability to generate high energy phosphates (ATP and phosphocreatinine), (2) presence of an intact sarcolemma to maintain ionic/electrochemical gradients, and (3) presence of adequate perfusion, both for the delivery of substrates and $O_2$ and for the removal of toxic metabolites.[26,27] In the recent past, two tissue states have been identified that exhibit sustained contractile dysfunction despite meeting the above criteria of viability—stunned and hibernating myocardium.

### *Stunned Myocardium*

Myocardial stunning was a phenomenon first documented by Heyndrickx et al. in the mid 1970s[28] but was not given this label until 1982, when Braunwald and Kloner defined stunned myocardium as tissue which exhibits prolonged contractile dysfunction after a transient ischemic insult and coronary reperfusion.[29] Contractile recovery may take weeks to months despite prompt and complete return of blood flow depending on the duration and severity of ischemia and adequacy of reperfusion. Several hypothesis have been put forward to explain the underlying mechanism of stunning, such as metabolic derangement,[30-37] deleterious effect of oxyradical production on the contractile elements of myocardium[38-43] and the recent concept, abnormal myofilament sensitivity to $Ca^{2+}$ in stunned myocardium.[44,45]

### *Hibernating Myocardium*

As originally defined by Rahimtoola,[46] hibernating myocardium exhibits marked contractile dysfunction as a result of chronic hypoperfusion that will improve or normalize after revascularization. Hibernating myocardium, classically, has adequate residual flow required for the survival of the tissue at rest or at baseline but suffers sustained hypoperfusion during increased demand, especially during tachycardia.[47] In contrast to the extremely reduced perfusion required to induce hibernation in animal studies, human studies suggest that hibernating tissue may have 70–80% of normal coronary flow.[48] Though hibernating myocardium has normal or near normal blood flow at rest, its coronary flow reserve are impaired leading on to recurrent episodes of ischemia at times of increased demand and may eventually produce persistent post-ischemic LV dysfunction.[49] In other words, hibernation results in an apparent chronic reduction in LV function due to the summation of repetitive and cumulative stunning.[50] As per "smart heart" hypothesis,[51] hibernation is viewed as a state of adaptation wherein, there is down-regulation in energy utilization to counterbalance the effects of ischemia at the cost of impaired contractility.[52,53] However, the presence of apoptotic cells and cells with autophagosomes, lysosomes, and vacuoles in the hibernating myocardium has supported an alternative hypothesis of "forced degeneration".[54] Interventions that restore the blood flow to hibernating myocardium may bring back the myocytes to their physiologic function and reprogram the cells to normal expression of key proteins.[55]

## Assessment of Myocardial Viability

Assessment of myocardial viability in a dysfunctional territory prior to revascularization becomes an important component of the decision making process in the management of patients with CAD and heart failure. Based on the available retrospective studies, it is infered that when a viability test is added to clinical and angiographic data as a part of the pre-operative assessment before revascularization, the in-hospital and one-year outcome significantly improves, however more prospective randomized trials are required to strengthen this inference.[56,57] A meta-analysis of viability studies showed (a) a strong correlation between revascularization and improved survival rate in patients with LV dysfunction and evidence of myocardial viability independently of the imaging technique used,[58,59] (b) no benefit of revascularization in the absence of significant viability and (c) higher annual mortality rate in patients with viable myocardium who were treated medically.

Candidates suitable for viability studies are those with the following conditions:

- Depressed LV ejection fraction
- Previous MI
- Previous coronary artery bypass grafts (CABG)
- Congestive heart failure.

As the definition of viability is based on histology, it is practically not feasible to identify accurately the viable myocardium in clinical settings and hence the determination of viability is indirect and depends on the functional response of the myocardial segment to revascularization. This remains a limitation of all clinical studies of viability using non-invasive techniques. Thus, noninvasive methods of viability assessment can only identify tissue that might benefit from revascularization. The assessment of myocardial viability must include an coronary angiogram to determine the potential for revascularization in a given patient. There are various noninvasive imaging modalities available for the assessment of myocardial viability and their utility to predict recovery of global LV function after revascularization is compared in **Table 10.1**.

**Table 10.1:** Comparison of different imaging modalities to predict recovery of global left ventricular function after revascularization[60]

| *Imaging techniques* | | *Sensitivity, mean (95% CI)* | *Specificity, mean (95% CI)* | *PPV, mean (95% CI)* | *NPV, mean (95% CI)* |
|---|---|---|---|---|---|
| Conventional nuclear | $^{99m}$Tc-sestamibi | 71 (51–91) | 40 (18–62) | – | – |
| | SPECT FDG | 86 (79–93) | 93 (88–98) | – | – |
| | $^{201}$Tl rest, reinjection | 84 (79–89) | 70 (64–76) | 97 (92–100) | 93 (86–100) |
| | $^{201}$Tl rest redistribution + FDG | 86 (76–96) | 92 (84–100) | 90 (81–99) | 89 (80–98) |
| | Total | 84 (80–88) | 77 (73–81) | 94 (89–98) | 91 (85–97) |
| Echocardiography | DSE | 76 (71–80) | 81 (77–85) | 84 (77–91) | 91 (85–96) |
| | DSE + strain rate | 67 (55–79) | 89 (81–97) | – | – |
| | End-diastolic wall thickness | 63 (49–77) | 68 (54–82) | – | – |
| | Total | 74 (70–77) | 81 (77–84) | 84 (77–91) | 91 (85–96) |
| PET | FDG | 81 (75–86) | 65 (59–72) | – | – |
| | Total | 81 (75–86) | 65 (59–72) | – | – |

*Abbreviations:* DSE, dobutamine stress echocardiography; FDG, fluorodeoxy-glucose; NPV, negative predictive value; PET, positron emission tomography; PPV, positive predictive value; SPECT, single photon emission computed tomography; Tc, technetium; Tl, thallium.

## *Role of Echocardiography in the Assessment of Viable Myocardium*

Over the years, echocardiography has been used extensively for the assessment of viable myocardium. Echocardiography is readily available, less expensive and has reasonable accuracy to detect the viable myocardium and hence still occupies an important place among the different array of advanced imaging techniques including radionuclide scans. Employing different principles of echocardiography such as 2D resting echocardiography, tissue Doppler imaging (TDI), myocardial contrast echocardiography (MCE), myocardial velocity imaging and pharmacological stress echocardiography, it is often possible to improve the specificity and sensitivity of the myocardial viability studies and to take critical therapeutic decisions, mainly the need for revascularization in a given patient.

### *Resting Echocardiography*

Resting echocardiography gives valuable information such as LV ejection fraction, diastolic performance, regional wall motion abnormalities and global LV function. It also helps to assess whether the myocardium is viable or not based on the assessment of LV wall thickness and the presence of the scar. It has been long recognized that the presence of myocardial thinning detected by echocardiography is a marker of old MI.[61,62] End-diastolic wall thickness (EDWT) > 6 mm has a high sensitivity of 94% but with a low specificity of 48% for predicting recovery of contractile reserve following revascularization **(Figure 10.7)**. However, by combining EDWT > 6 mm and dobutamine stress echocardiography (DSE) (showing improvement in LV regional wall score index), the specificity increases to 77% with a sensitivity of 88%.[63] Scar tissue appears brighter than the normal myocardium and may not necessarily represent non-viability unless the transmural extent of the scar is well established by a three-dimensional (3D) echocardiography.[64]

### *Dobutamine Stress Echocardiography*

The contractile reserve in the dysfunctional, but viable myocardium may be evoked by an appropriate inotropic stimulus such as dobutamine. Infusions of low dose dobutamine (5–10 µg/kg/min) may show improvement in contractility without significant increase in heart rate, in dysfunctional but viable myocardium; this incremental response in contractility is referred to as contractile reserve. Segments without viable myocardium do not exhibit this contractility reserve.[65,66] Abnormal wall motion can be seen either as a lack of hyperdynamic wall motion, relative hypokinesis, or the development of akinesis or dyskinesis in the general distribution of one or more coronary arteries.

#### *Dobutamine Stress Echocardiography Protocol*

Assessment of other causes of cardiac symptoms in addition to ischemic heart disease, such as pericardial effusion, cardiomyopathy, valvular heart disease and aortic dissection by performing a baseline echocardiography before stress echocardiography is recommended. The standard dobutamine stress testing involves a graded dobutamine infusion starting at 5 µg/kg/min and increasing at 5 minutes interval to 10, 20, 30 and 40 µg/kg/min. End-points are achievement of target heart rate (defined as 85% of the age predicted maximum

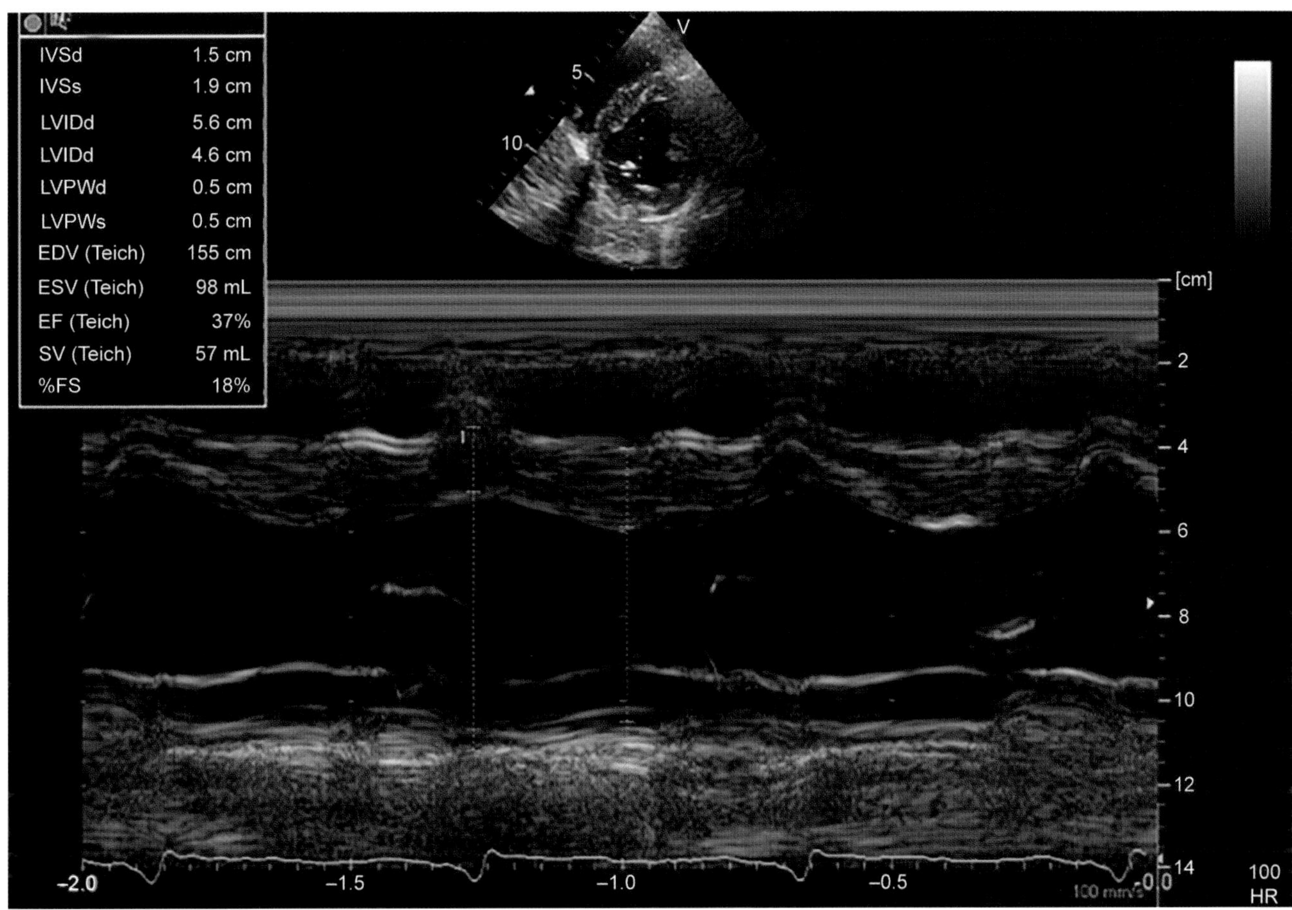


**Figure 10.7:** Parasternal short-axis view of the LV showing concentric hypertrophy and note the inferior wall which is thinned out (EDWT of 6 mm) due to recent inferior wall myocardial infarction (not to be mistaken as asymmetric hypertrophy of hypertrophic cardiomyopathy). *Abbreviations:* IVSd, interventricular septum end diastole; IVSs, interventricular septum end systole; LVIDd, left ventricular internal diameter end diastole; LVPWd, left ventricular posterior wall end diastole; LVPWs, left ventricular posterior wall end systole; EDV, end-diastolic volume; ESV, end-systolic volume; EF, ejection fraction; SV, systolic volume; FS, fractional shortening; LV, left ventricular; EDWT, end-diastolic wall thickness.

heart rate), new or worsening wall motion abnormalities, significant arrythmias, hypotension, severe hypertension and intolerable symptoms. Atropine in divided doses of 0.25 to 0.5 mg to a total dose of 2 mg, may be used as needed to achieve target heart rate. The minimum cumulative dose needed to achieve the desired heart rate effect should be used to avoid central nervous system toxicity of atropine. Patients received atropine at 30 μg/kg/min stage achieved target heart rate more quickly using lower doses of dobutamine and with fewer side effects. Administering high dose dobutamine, in step-wise incremental doses, four different types of responses may be observed[66]: (i) biphasic response—initial improvement in contractility followed by worsening wall motion, suggestive of viable but ischemic myocardium; (ii) direct worsening of wall motion without initial improvement, represents severe ischemia subtended by a critically stenosed artery; (iii) sustained improvement—improvement of wall motion without subsequent deterioration, probably related to subendocardial ischemia; (iv) no change in wall motion during the entire study representing a transmural scar. The predictive value of DSE significantly increases when there is biphasic response.[67,68] The initial improvement in wall motion reflects the recruitment of contractile reserve during low dose dobutamine and hence reflects viability,[69] whereas higher doses lead to sub-endocardial ischemia with worsening of the wall motion abnormality, thus identifying inducible ischemia. Hence, the optimal assessment of hibernating myocardium using DSE includes testing at various doses.

The mean sensitivity and specificity, based on the data from thirty-two studies which employed dobutamine echocardiography (total of 1,090 patients) to predict improvement in regional function after revascularization showed as 82% and 79%, respectively.[65] Seven of these studies, with a total of 254 patients, evaluated improvement in global

LV function after revascularization and showed that the mean LVEF improved from 35% to 43% in patients with viable myocardium whereas it remained unchanged (35% vs. 36%) in those without viable myocardium. Also the improvement in functional status after revascularization, as evidenced by improved New York Heart Association functional class, in patients with viable myocardium is shown in few.[66]

Comparing with various cardiac magnetic resonance imaging (MRI) techniques, which are being increasingly used in the assessment of myocardial viability and ischemia, DSE has equivalent diagnostic performance as that of cardiac MRI. The wall thickness as assessed by cardiac MRI to predict functional recovery has a sensitivity of 95% and a specificity of 41% in comparison with the values of 94% and 48% respectively with DSE.[66] In a Dobutamine MRI, an increased systolic wall thickening of greater than 2 mm during dobutamine infusion was an accurate predictor of functional recovery.[70] Pooled data from various studies on dobutamine MRI showed a mean sensitivity of 73% (range, 50–89%) and a mean specificity of 83% (range, 70–95%).[71]

Dobutamine induced segmental and global functional recovery correlates well with other, more complex imaging techniques, including positron emission tomography (PET) and thallium scintigraphy.[72,73] The ability of DSE to predict the recovery of global LV function after revascularization in comparison with other imaging techniques is depicted in **Table 10.1**.

### *Myocardial Contrast Echocardiography*

MCE utilizes acoustically active gas-filled microbubbles as contrast agent that are smaller than red blood cells (<7μm) and remain within the intravascular space at all times and, consequently, their presence within any myocardial territory denotes the microvascular perfusion within that region. As perfusion is a prerequisite for viability, MCE has been used to assess myocardial viability. It has been shown that these parameters of myocardial perfusion on MCE correlate positively with microvascular density and capillary area and inversely with the extent of fibrosis.[74] In the clinical setting, myocardial perfusion is evaluated qualitatively by MCE and segments are classified as viable if homogeneous contrast intensity is present, whereas the absence of contrast enhancement reflects non-viable myocardium in which necrosis of myocardial cells has resulted in obstruction and collapse of microcirculation.[75]

In a small study,[76] comparing DSE, 201 Tl imaging, and MCE, both 201 Tl imaging and contrast echocardiography showed a high sensitivity and a relatively low specificity for the prediction of improvement in regional function after revascularization, whereas DSE had a lower sensitivity and a relatively high specificity. MCE had a sensitivity of 89% and a specificity of 51%. The lower specificity with MCE is related to the inability to identify sub-endocardial scar tissue, resulting in an over-prediction of recovery of function. Currently, no studies evaluating improvement in symptoms or long-term outcome with MCE are available.

### *Tissue Doppler Imaging*

The use of TDI for the assessment of viability at rest has been limited by its lack of site specificity as the segment of interest may be tethered by neighboring segments. The ability to predict functional recovery using some TDI parameters such as peak systolic velocity, isovolumetric contraction, and time-to-peak systolic velocity has not shown consistent results.[77,78] TDI measurement of pre-ejection velocity, however has been shown to be predictive of viability.[79] Myocardial velocity analysis by TDI at rest and during dobutamine stimulation could allow assessment of myocardial viability.[80-82] A recent study showed that diastolic tissue velocities at rest are enough to differentiate viable form nonviable myocardium although they are affected by age.[83]

### *Strain Rate Imaging*

Sub-endocardial infarcts are more likely to benefit from revascularization as opposed to transmural infarcts. Strain rate imaging is an useful tool to differentiate sub-endocardial infarcts from transmural infarcts.[84] The viability of the given myocardium can be predicted with a sensitivity of 83% and specificity of 84% by demonstrating an increase in peak systolic strain rate by more than 0.23/s from rest to dobutamine stress, using fluorodeoxy-glucose PET.[77,78,85] Analysis of diastolic function by myocardial deformation imaging can be used to assess myocardial viability. Dobutamine stress may demonstrate an increase in early diastolic E-wave and late diastolic A-wave strain rate in a dyssynergic but viable myocardium whereas no significant response in non-viable segments.[86] Furthermore, myocardial deformation imaging done at rest alone is sufficient to determine myocardial viability as shown in few studies.[87]

STE, unlike TDI-based strain, which is largely influenced by the angle between the ultrasound beam and the myocardial wall, tracks frame-to-frame movement of natural acoustic markers or speckles, does not depend on this angle and provides a more reliable assessment of regional myocardial deformation and transmural extent of myocardial necrosis.[88]

Automated function image (AFI) algorithm allows the simultaneous quantification of myocardial strain in various LV segments based on 2D-strain imaging in the form of a "bull's eye" and also provides GLS. GLS obtained by AFI during DSE is a promising objective index to assess myocardial viability in patients who had recent acute MI.[89]

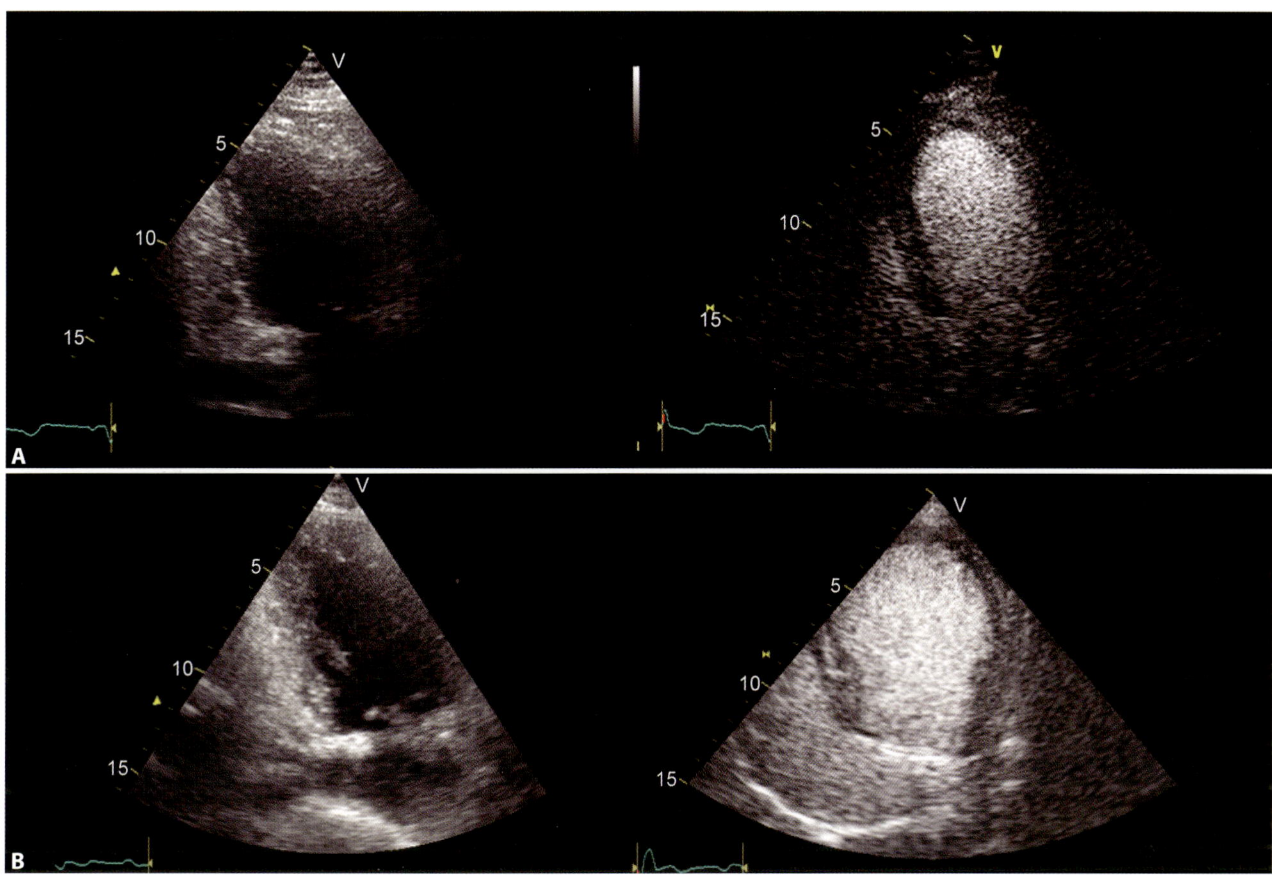


**Figure 10.8A and B:** Left ventricular (LV) contrast echocardiography showing clear delineation of LV wall segments after contrast has filled the LV in a normal subject (A) and in a patient with apical dyskinesia (B).

### *Transesophageal Echocardiography*

The inadequate acoustic windows in patients with large body habitus, significant pulmonary disease, or post-cardiac surgery can be overcome to a great extent by transesophageal echocardiography (TEE), while performing DSE for the assessment of myocardial viability.

Other new echocardiographic techniques are gaining interest in the recent few years to assess the myocardial viability such as 3D echocardiography during dobutamine stress and integrated backscatter analysis. The backscatter analysis is independent of wall motion and is shown to predict contractile reserve in ischemic myocardial damage.[90]

### *Limitations of Echocardiography in the Assessment of Myocardial Viability*

- Results of echocardiography are largely qualitative in nature and dependent on the interpreting physician, hence may lead to inter-operator bias. However, this pitfall would be overcome to an extent with increasing use of objective echocardiographic principles.
- Poor acoustic windows encountered in many patients with large body habitus, significant pulmonary disease or post-cardiac surgery are a major limitation in the assessment of various parameters of echocardiography. Approximately 15% of CAD patients are believed to have inadequate acoustic window.[91] Though TEE may circumvent this, the invasive nature of the procedure may limits its use.
- The endocardial-blood pool interface can be difficult to visualize on 2D echocardiography and may pose a serious limitation in the quantification of wall thickness and ejection fraction. This limitation can be overcome with the use of contrast echocardiography, which would delineate the endocardial-blood pool interface and LV wall segment **(Figure 10.8A and B)**.
- The diagnostic accuracy of DSE is reduced with increasing severity of regional and global LV dysfunction and appears to underestimate the extent of viability.[92,93]

## CONCLUSION

After an MI, cardiac imaging helps in the critical clinical decision making and risk stratification. Echocardiography is widely used in this domain and provides most of the information which help to prognosticate and as well to guide the therapy. Remodeling and heart failure, presence of inducible ischemia, presence of dysfunctional viable myocardium, future risk of adverse events including risk of ventricular arrhythmias, need for anticoagulation, and other questions are mostly addressed by the various tools of echocardiography. Assessment of myocardial viability is critical in the management of patients with CAD and heart failure. The revascularization procedures driven by viability studies have consistently shown favorable cardiovascular outcomes and prognosis. Varios noninvasive methods are available for the assessment of myocardial viability and the knowledge on the advantages and limitations of each technique helps the clinician in better decision making. Despite the advancement in nuclear imaging techniques, echocardiography, due to its versatility, retains its pivotal position among the various methods utilized to assess the myocardial viability and hence post-MI risk stratification.

## REFERENCES


1. Bonow RO, Dilsizian V, Cuocolo A, Bacharach SL. Identification of viable myocardium in patients with chronic coronary artery disease and left ventricular dysfunction. Comparison of thallium scintigraphy with reinjection and PET imaging with 18F-fluorodeoxyglucose. Circulation. 1991;83(1):26-37.
2. Luciani GB, Montalbano G, Casali G, Mazzucco A. Predicting long-term functional results after myocardial revascularization in ischemic cardiomyopathy. J Thorac Cardiovasc Surg. 2000;120:478-89.
3. Alfieri O. Coronary artery bypass grafting for left ventricular dysfunction. Curr Opin Cardiol. 1994;9:658-63.
4. Maddahi J, Schelbert H, Brunken R, Di Carli M. Role of thallium-201 and PET imaging in evaluation of myocardial viability and management of patients with coronary artery disease and left ventricular dysfunction. J Nucl Med. 1994;35:707-15.
5. Di Carli MF, Davidson M, Little R, Khanna S, Mody FV, Brunken RC, et al. Value of metabolic imaging with positron emission tomography for evaluating prognosis in patients with coronary artery disease and left ventricular dysfunction. Am J Cardiol. 1994;73:527-33.
6. Shapira I, Heller I, Pines A, Topilsky M, Isakov A. The impact of myocardial viability as determined by rest-redistribution 201Tl single photon emission CT imaging and the choice of therapy on prognosis in patients with left ventricular dysfunction. J Med. 2000;31:205-14.
7. Chikamori T, Hirose K, Hamada T, Hitomi N, Kitaoka H, Yabe T, et al. Functional recovery after coronary artery bypass grafting in patients with severe left ventricular dysfunction and preserved myocardial viability in the left anterior descending arterial territory as assessed by thallium-201 myocardial perfusion imaging. Jpn Circ J. 1999;63:752-8.
8. Moore RW, Noe S, Carvalho J Jr, Balingit A, Taylor AJ. Rest-distribution 201-Tl single-photon emission CT imaging for determination of myocardial viability: relationship among viability, mode of therapy, and long-term prognosis. Chest. 1999;115:1621-6.
9. Marwick TH, Zuchowski C, Lauer MS, Secknus MA, Williams J, Lytle BW. Functional status and quality of life in patients with heart failure undergoing coronary bypass surgery after assessment of myocardial viability. J Am Coll Cardiol. 1999;33:750-8.
10. Pagano D, Townend JN, Littler WA, Horton R, Camici PG, Bonser RS. Coronary artery bypass surgery as treatment for ischemic heart failure: the predictive value of viability assessment with quantitative positron emission tomography for symptomatic and functional outcome. J Thorac Cardiovasc Surg. 1998;115:791-9.
11. Senior R, Kaul S, Lahiri A. Myocardial viability on echocardiography predicts long-term survival after revascularization in patients with ischemic congestive heart failure. J Am Coll Cardiol. 1999;33:1848-54.
12. Picard MH, Wilkins GT, Ray PA, Weyman AE. Natural history of left ventricular: size and function after acute myocardial infarction. Assessment and prediction by echocardio-graphic endocardial surface mapping. Circulation. 1990;82:484-94.
13. Flachskampf FA, et al. Cardiac imaging after myocardial infarction. Eur Heart J. 2010;32(3):272-83.
14. Bolognese L, Neskovic AN, et al. Left ventricular remodeling after primary coronary angioplasty: patterns of left ventricular dilation and long-term prognostic implications. Circulation. 2002;106:2351-7.
15. Riera JC, et al. Risk stratification after acute myocardial infarction. Rev Esp Cardiol. 2003;56(3):303-13.
16. Piérard LA. Risk stratification after myocardial infarction. JACC. 2010;56(22):1823-5.
17. Bière L, et al. Longitudinal strain is a marker of microvascular obstruction and infarct size in patients with acute ST segment elevation myocardial infarction. PLoS ONE. 2014;9(1):e86959.
18. Thomas Butz, et al. Segment-orientated analysis of two-dimensional strain and strain rate as assessed by velocity vector imaging in patients with acute myocardial infarction. International J Med Sciences.2011;8(2):106-13.
19. Meta-Analysis Research Group in Echocardiography (MeRGE) AMI Collaborators. Independent prognostic importance of a restrictive left ventricular filling pattern after myocardial infarction: an individual patient meta-analysis: meta-analysis research group in echocardiography acute myocardial infarction. Circulation. 2008;117:2591-8.
20. Antoni ML, Roderick WC, Scherptong, Atary JZ, Boersma E, Holman ER, et al. Prognostic value of right ventricular function in patients after acute myocardial infarction treated with primary percutaneous coronary intervention. Circ Cardiovasc Imaging. 2010;3:264-71.
21. de Groote P, Fertin M Ce´line Goe´minne, Petyt G, Peyrot S, Foucher-Hossein C, et al. Right ventricular systolic function for risk stratification in patients with stable left ventricular systolic dysfunction: comparison of radionuclide angiography to echo-Doppler parameters. Eur Heart J. 2012;33: 2672-9.

22. Bangalore S. Role of right ventricular wall motion abnormalities in risk stratification and prognosis of patients referred for stress echocardiography. JACC. 2007;13;50(20):1981-9.
23. Konishi K, Dohi K, Tanimura M, et al. Quantifying longitudinal right ventricular dysfunction in patients with old myocardial infarction by using speckle-tracking strain echocardiography. Cardiovascular Ultrasound. 2013;11:23. doi:10.1186/1476-7120-11-23.
24. Reimer KA, Jennings RB, Tatum AH. Pathobiology of acute myocardial ischemia: metabolic, functional and ultrastructural studies. Am J Cardiol. 1983; 52:72A-81A.
25. Schoen FJ. The heart. In: Cotran RS, Kumar V, Collins T (Eds); Pathologic Basis of Disease. WB Saunders: Philadelphia, 1999; 544-56.
26. Bonow RO. Identification of viable myocardium. Circulation. 1996;94:2674-80.
27. Higgins CB. Prediction of myocardial viability by MRI. Circulation. 1999;99:727-9.
28. Heyndrickx GR, Millard RW, McRitchie RJ, Marako PR, Vatner SF. Regional myocardial functional & electrophysiological alterations after brief coronary artery occlusions in conscious dogs. J Clin Invest. 1975;56:978-85.
29. Braunwald E, Kloner RA. The stunned myocardium: prolonged, post-ischemic ventricular dysfunction. Circulation. 1982;66:1146-9.
30. Reimer KA, Jennings RB, Tatum AH. Pathobiology of acute myocardial ischemia: metabolic, functional and ultrastructural studies. Am J Cardiol. 1983; 52:72A-81A.
31. Puri PS. Correlation between biochemical and contractile changes after myocardial ischemia and revascularization. Recent Adv Stud Cardiac Struct Metab. 1975;7:161-9.
32. Eberli FR, Weinberg EO, Grice WN, Horowitz GL, Apstein CS. Protective effect of increased glycolytic substrate against systolic and diastolic dysfunction and increased coronary resistance from prolonged global underperfusion and reperfusion in isolated rabbit hearts perfused with erythrocyte suspensions. Circ Res. 1991;68:468-81.
33. Owen P, Dennis S, Opie LH. Glucose flux rate regulates onset of ischemic contracture in globally underperfused rat hearts. Circ Res. 1990;66:344-54.
34. Braasch W, Gudbjarnason S, Puri PS, Ravens KG, Bing RJ. Early changes in energy metabolism in the myocardium following acute coronary artery occlusion in anaesthetized dogs. Circ Res. 1968;23:429-38.
35. DeBoer LVW, Ingwall JS, Kloner RA, Braunwald E. Prolonged derangements of canine myocardial purine metabolism after a brief coronary artery occlusion not associated with anatomic evidence of necrosis. Proc Natl Acad Sci. 1980;77: 5471-5.
36. Ellis SG, Henschke CI, Sandor T, Wynne J, Braunwald E, Kloner RA. Time course of functional and biochemical recovery of myocardium salvaged by reperfusion. J Am Coll Cardiol. 1983;1:1047-55.
37. Weiss J, Hiltbrand B. Functional compartmentation of glycolytic versus oxidative metabolism in isolated rabbit heart. J Clin Invest. 1985;82:723-35.
38. Gao WD, Atar D, Backx PH, Marban E. Relationship between intracellular calcium and contractile force in stunned myocardium: direct evidence for decreased myofilament ca2þ responsiveness and altered diastolic function in intact ventricular muscle. Circ Res. 1995;76:1036-48.
39. Van Eyk JE, Powers F, Law W, Larue C, Hodges RS, Solaro RJ. Breakdown and release of myofilament proteins during ischemia and ischemia/reperfusion in rat hearts: identification of degradation products and effects on the PCA-force relation. Circ Res. 1998;82:261-71.
40. Foster DB, Van Eyk JE. In search of the proteins that cause myocardial stunning. Circ Res. 1999;85:470-2.
41. Gao WD, Atar D, Liu Y, Perez NG, Murphy AM, Marban E. Role of troponin I proteolysis in the pathogenesis of stunned myocardium. Circ Res. 1997;80:393-9.
42. McDonough JL, Arrell DK, Van Eyk JE. Troponin I degradation and covalent complex formation accompanies myocardial ischemia/reperfusion injury. Circ Res. 1999;84:9-20.
43. Murphy AM, Kogler H, Georgakopoulos D, McDonough JL, Kass DA, Van Eyk JE, Marban E. Transgenic mouse model of stunned myocardium. Science. 2000; 287:488-91.
44. Li XY, McCay PB, Zughaib M, Jeroudi MO, Triana JF, Bolli R. Demonstration of free radical generation in the "stunned" myocardium in the conscious dog and identification of major differences between conscious and open-chest dogs. J Clin Invest. 1993;92:1025-41.
45. Bolli R, Marban E. Molecular and cellular mechanisms of myocardial stunning. Physiol Rev. 1999;79(2):609-34.
46. Rahimtoola SH. From coronary artery disease to heart failure: role of hibernating myocardium. Am J Cardiol. 1995;75:16e-22e.
47. Shen YT, Vatner SF. Mechanism of impaired myocardial function during progressive coronary stenosis in conscious pigs: hibernation versus stunning? Circ Res. 1995;76(3):479-88.
48. Maes A, Flameng W, Nuyts J, et al. Histological alterations in chronically hypoperfused myocardium: correlation with PET findings. Circulation. vol. 1994;90(2):735-45.
49. Vanoverschelde JLJ, Wijns W, Depre C, et al. Mechanisms of chronic regional postischemic dysfunction in humans: new insights from the study of noninfarcted collateral-dependent myocardium. Circulation. 1993;87(5):1513-23.
50. Homans DC, Laxson DD, Sublett E, Lindstrom P, Bache RJ. Cumulative deterioration of myocardial function after repeated episodes of exercise-induced ischemia. Am J Physiol—Heart Circulat Physiol. 1989;256(5):H1462-H71.
51. Redwood SR, Ferrari R, Marber MS. Myocardial hibernation and stunning: from physiological principles to clinical practice. Heart. 1998;80(3):218-22.
52. Depre C, Vatner SF. Cardioprotection in stunned and hibernating myocardium. Heart Failure Reviews. 2007;12(3-4):307-17.
53. Depre C, Kim SJ, John AS, et al. Program of cell survival underlying human and experimental hibernating myocardium. Circ Res. 2004;95(4):433-40.
54. Slezak J, Tribulova N, Okruhlicova L, et al. Hibernating myocardium: pathophysiology, diagnosis, and treatment. Can J Physiol Pharmacol. 2009;87(4):252-65.
55. Kelly RF, Sluiter W, McFalls EO. Hibernating myocardium: Is the program to survive a pathway to failure? Circ Res. 2008;102(1):3-5.
56. Haas F, Haehnel CJ, Picker W, Nekolla S, Martinoff S, Meisner H, Schwaiger M. Preoperative positron emission tomographic

viability assessment and perioperative and postoperative risk in patients with advanced ischemic heart disease. J Am Coll Cardiol. 1997;30:1693-700.
57. Tarakji KG, Brunken R, McCarthy PM, Al-Chekakie MO, Abdel-Latif A, Pothier CE, et al. Myocardial viability testing and the effect of early intervention in patients with advanced left ventricular systolic dysfunction. Circulation. 2006;113:230-7.
58. Allman KC, Shaw LJ, Hachamovitch R, Udelson JE. Myocardial viability testing and impact of revascularization on prognosis in patients with coronary artery disease and left ventricular dysfunction: a meta-analysis. J Am Coll Cardiol. 2002;39:1151-8.
59. MacDonald Bourque J, Hasselblad V, Velazquez EJ, Borges-Neto S, O'Connor CM. Revascularization in patients with coronary artery disease, left ventricular dysfunction, and viability: a meta-analysis. Am Heart J. 2003;146:621-7.
60. Camici PG, Prasad SK, Rimoldi OE. Stunning, hibernation, and assessment of myocardial viability. Circulation. 2008;117:103-14.
61. Rasmussen S, Corya BC, Feigenbaum H, Knoebel SB. Detection of myocardial scar tissue by M-mode echocardiography. Circulation. 1978;57:230-7.
62. Siu SCB, Weyman AE. Left ventricle III: coronary artery disease—clinical manifestations and complications. In: Anonymous Principles and Practice of Echocardiography, 2nd edition. Baltimore: Lea & Febiger, 1994:656-86.
63. Cwajg J, Cwajg E, Nagueh S, et al. End-diastolic wall thickness as a predictor of recovery of function in myocardial hibernation: Relation to rest-redistribution Tl-201 tomography and dobutamine stress echocardiography. J Am Coll Cardiol. 2000;35(5):1152-61.
64. Montant P, Chenot F, Goffinet C, et al. Detection and quantification of myocardial scars by contrast-enhanced 3D echocardiography. Circ Cardiovasc Imaging. 2010;3:415-23.
65. Bax JJ, Poldermans D, Elhendy A, Boersma E, Rahimtoola SH. Sensitivity, specificity, and predictive accuracies of various noninvasive techniques for detecting hibernating myocardium. Curr Probl Cardiol. 2001;26:142-86.
66. Schinkel AFL, Poldermans D, Hendy A, Bax JJ. Assessment of myocardial viability in patients with heart failure. J Nucl Med. 2007;48:1135-46.
67. Cornel JH, Bax JJ, Elhendy A, et al. Biphasic response to dobutamine predicts improvement of global left ventricular function after surgical revascularization in patients with stable coronary artery disease: implications of time course of recovery on diagnostic accuracy. J Am Coll Cardiol. 1998;31(5):1002.
68. Afridi I, Kleiman NS, Raizner AE, Zoghbi WA. Dobutamine echocardiography in myocardial hibernation. Optimal dose and accuracy in predicting recovery of ventricular function after coronary angioplasty. Circulation. 1995;91(3):663.
69. Sawada SG, Lewis SJ, Foltz J, et al. Usefulness of rest and low-dose dobutamine wall motion scores in predicting survival and benefit from revascularization in patients with ischemic cardiomyopathy. Am J Cardiol. 2002;89(7):811.
70. Baer FM, Voth E, Schneider CA, Theissen P, Schicha H, Sechtem U. Comparison of low-dose dobutamine-gradient-echo magnetic resonance imaging and positron emission tomography with [18F]fluorodeoxyglucose in patients with chronic coronary artery disease: a functional and morphological approach to the detection of residual myocardial viability. Circulation. 1995;91:1006-15.
71. Kim RJ, Fieno DS, Parrish TB, et al. Relationship of MRI delayed contrast enhancement to irreversible injury, infarct age, and contractile function. Circulation. 1999;100:1992-2002.
72. Perrone-Filardi P, Pace L, Prastaro M, et al. Dobutamine echocardiography predicts improvement of hypoperfused dysfunctional myocardium after revascularization in patients with coronary artery disease. Circulation. 1995;91(10):2556-65.
73. Haque T, Furukawa T, Takahashi M, Kinoshita M. Identification of hibernating myocardium by dobutamine stress echocardiography: comparison with thallium-201 reinjection imaging. Am Heart J. 1995;130(3):553-63.
74. Shimoni S, Frangogiannis NG, Aggeli CJ, et al. Microvascular structural correlates of myocardial contrast echocardiography in patients with coronary artery disease and left ventricular dysfunction: implications for the assessment of myocardial hibernation. Circulation. 2002;106:950-6.
75. Ragosta M, Camarano G, Kaul S, Powers ER, Sarembok IJ, Gimple LV. Microvascular integrity indicates myocellular viability in patients with recent myocardial infarction: new insights using myocardial contrast echocardiography. Circulation. 1994;89:2562-9.
76. Nagueh SF, Vaduganathan P, Ali N, et al. Identification of hibernating myocardium: comparative accuracy of myocardial contrast echocardiography, rest-redistribution thallium-201 tomography and dobutamine echocardiography. J Am Coll Cardiol. 1997;29:985-93.
77. Hanekom L, Jenkins C, Jeffries L, et al. Incremental value of strain rate analysis as an adjunct to wall-motion scoring for assessment of myocardial viability by dobutamine echocardiography: a follow-up study after revascularization. Circulation. 2005;112(25):3892-900.
78. Hoffmann R, Altiok E, Nowak B, et al. Strain rate measurement by Doppler echocardiography allows improved assessment of myocardial viability in patients with depressed left ventricular function. J Am Coll Cardiol. 2002;39(3): 443-9.
79. McLean DS, Anadiotis AV, Lerakis S. Role of echocardiography in the assessment of myocardial viability. Am J Med Sci. 2009;337(5):349-54.
80. Bountioukos M, Schinkel AFL, Bax JJ, et al. Pulsed wave tissue Doppler quantification of systolic and diastolic function of viable and nonviable myocardium in patients with ischemic cardiomyopathy. Am Heart J. 2004;148(6):1079-84.
81. Yang HS, Kang SJ, Song JK, et al. Diagnosis of viable myocardium using velocity data of Doppler myocardial imaging: comparison with positron emission tomography. J Am Soc Echocard. 2004;17(9):933-40.
82. Rambaldi R, Poldermans D, Bax JJ, et al. Doppler tissue velocity sampling improves diagnostic accuracy during dobutamine stress echocardiography for the assessment of viable myocardium in patients with severe left ventricular dysfunction. Eur Heart J. 2000;21(13):1091-8.
83. Bountioukos M, Schinkel AFL, Bax JJ, et al. Pulsed wave tissue Doppler imaging for the quantification of contractile reserve

in stunned, hibernating, and scarred myocardium. Heart. 2004;90(5):506-10.
84. Chan J, Hanekom L, Wong C, Leano R, Cho GY, Marwick TH. Differentiation of subendocardial and transmural infarction using two-dimensional strain rate imaging to assess short-axis and long-axis myocardial function. J Am Coll Cardiol. 2006;48(10):2026-33.
85. Fujimoto H, Honma H, Ohno T, Mizuno K, Kumita S. Longitudinal Doppler strain measurement for assessment of damaged and/or hibernating myocardium by dobutamine stress echocardiography in patients with old myocardial infarction. J Cardiol. 2010;55(3):309-16.
86. Hoffmann R, Altiok E, Nowak B, et al. Strain rate analysis allows detection of differences in diastolic function between viable and nonviable myocardial segments. J Am Soc Echocard. 2005;18(4):330-5.
87. Hoffmann R. Tissue Doppler and innovative myocardial deformation imaging techniques for assessment of myocardial viability. Current Opinion in Cardiology. 2006;21(5):438-42.
88. Adel Shabana, Ayman El-Menyar. Myocardial viability: what we knew and what is new. Cardiol Res Prac. 2012;2012:1-13.
89. Hyodo E, Tamita K, Tokuda T, et al. Validity of automated global longitudinal strain measurements with low-dose dobutamine stress echocardiography for the assessment of myocardial viability after acute myocardial infarction: comparison with delayed enhancement and microvascular obstruction by cardiac magnetic resonance imaging. J Am Coll Cardiol. 2014;63(12_S):. doi:10.1016/S0735-1097(14)61245-6.
90. Pasquet A, D'Hondt AM, Melin JA, Vanoverschelde JLJ. Relation of ultrasonic tissue characterization with integrated backscatter to contractile reserve in chronic left ventricular ischemic dysfunction. Am J Cardiol.1998;81(1):68-74.
91. Kasprzak JD, Paelinck B, Ten Cate FJ, Vletter WB, de Jong N, Poldermans D, et al. Comparison of native and contrast-enhanced harmonic echocardiography for visualization of left ventricular endocardial border. Am J Cardiol. 1999;83:211-7.
92. Pagano D, Bonser RS, Townend JN, Ordoubadi F, Lorenzoni R, Camici PG. Predictive value of dobutamine echocardiography and positron emission tomography in identifying hibernating myocardium in patients with postischemic heart failure. Heart 1998;79:281-8.
93. Wiggers H, Nielsen TT, Bottcher M, Egeblad H, Botker HE. Positron emission tomography and low- dose dobutamine echocardiography in the prediction of post revascularization improvement in left ventricular function and exercise parameters. Am Heart J. 2000;140:928-36.

# Mechanical Complications of Acute Myocardial Infarction



*Sanjay Mittal, Vivek Jain*

## INTRODUCTION

Acute myocardial infarction (AMI) remains a leading cause of morbidity and mortality worldwide. In hospital, mortality among patient with AMI is primarily due to circulatory failure from severe left ventricular (LV) dysfunction or from one of the complication of myocardial infarction (MI). Complications of AMI occurs in a time-dependent manner, and it can be directly related to the anatomy of the coronary artery blood supply. Complications may occur due to ischemic or injured tissue and therefore may begin within 20 minutes of the onset of MI, when myocardial tissue injury begins. The complications may be broadly classified as follows:

- Mechanical
- Electrical or arrhythmic
- Ischemic
- Embolic
- Inflammatory, e.g. pericarditis.

Mechanical complications of AMI are some of the deadliest cardiac conditions and are associated with very high mortality rates. It is difficult to assess the true incidence of these complications as both clinical and autopsy series differ considerably, though they are thought to be responsible for about 15% of all AMI deaths. In general, patients at increased risk include elderly women, first AMI, and hypertension. Mechanical complications can be subdivided into two basic categories: the acute phase complications and the chronic phase complications. The acute phase usually involves rupture of damaged myocardium. This can take the form of rupture of the ventricular free wall, the interventricular septum, or a papillary muscle. The chronic phase usually involves formation of a ventricular aneurysm. This results in either a true aneurysm or a pseudoaneurysm. Thus, the mechanical complications of AMI broadly include the following:

- Acute mechanical complications of AMI:
  - Ventricular septal rupture (VSR)
  - Ventricular free-wall rupture
  - Papillary muscle rupture (PMR).
- Chronic mechanical complications of AMI:
  - LV aneurysm
  - LV pseudoaneurysm
  - LV thrombus.

This chapter discusses how to detect, diagnose, and treat each of these entities.

## ACUTE MECHANICAL COMPLICATIONS OF ACUTE MYOCARDIAL INFARCTION

### Ventricular Septal Rupture

Post-MI ventricular rupture is an infrequent but serious complication of MI. VSR occurred in 1–2% of patient after AMI in the pre-thrombolytic era and 0.2–0.34% in the post-thrombolytic era.[1] VSR complicating MI was first described at autopsy by Latham. One of the first antemortem diagnoses of postinfarction VSR was made by Brunn in 1923. Sager in 1934 established specific clinical criteria for diagnosis and stressed the association of postinfarction VSR with coronary artery disease (CAD). In 1957, Cooley et al. reported the successful surgical repair of postinfarction VSR in a patient 9 weeks after the diagnosis of septal rupture.[2-5]

Septal blood supply comes from branches of the left anterior descending coronary artery, the posterior descending branch of the right coronary artery, or the circumflex artery when it is dominant. Infarction associated with a VSR is usually transmural and extensive. About 60% of VSRs occur with infarction of the anterior wall, 40% with infarction of the posterior or inferior wall. Posterior VSR may be accompanied by mitral valve insufficiency secondary to papillary muscle infarction or dysfunction. Patients with VSR usually show complete coronary artery occlusion with little or no collateral flow. Sometimes, multiple septal perforations occur. These may occur simultaneously or within several days of each other.[6]

Patients with a ruptured septum usually present with the abrupt onset of hemodynamic compromise characterized by hypotension and failure usually 3–8 days after a massive MI. Rarely, VSR may occurs as early as 24 hours and as late as 2 weeks after the index MI. There is a new, harsh, loud, and holosystolic murmur that is best heard at the lower left sternal border with occasionally wide spread radiation. Clinically, murmur could be confused with mitral regurgitation (MR) as it is heard best at the apex.[7-9]

In this situation of hemodynamic compromise, the diagnosis is established by echocardiography with color-flow imaging. It is a highly sensitive tool for diagnosing and characterizing VSR. Smyllie et al. have shown a diagnostic accuracy of 95% for pulsed and continuous-wave Doppler and 100% for color-flow Doppler. It is useful to define the site, size, and hemodynamic consequence of the ventricular septal defect.[10,11] As an echocardiologist, it is important to suspect a VSR in patients with large transmural infarcts, especially at the apex. As VSRs usually happen at a junction of akinetic and hyperkinetic segments, same should be evaluated cautiously. Off-axis views may be very useful to localize the defect. Defect size varies from millimeters to several centimeters, and size directly influences the extent of left-to-right shunting and clinical risk. A basal VSR is best visualized in the parasternal long axis with medial angulation, apical long-axis, and subcostal long-axis views. An apical VSR is best visualized in the apical 4-chamber view. **Figure 11.1** shows various common locations of VSR in relation to ventricular septum. Locations 1–3 are common after inferior wall infarct, whereas the locations 3–5 are common after anterior wall MI.

The ventricular septum should be scanned in multiple standard and nonstandard two-dimensional (2D) echocardiographic imaging planes concurrently with Doppler color-flow mapping. Multiple nonstandard apical planes, variants of the standard apical 4-chamber view, should be used extensively. Anterior angulation of the transducer from the apical position with the aorta in view allows visualization of the anterior ventricular septum. Posterior angulation of the transducer to the inferobasal plane allows visualization of the posterior ventricular septum. In the posterobasal plane, the echo beam exits through the basal walls of both ventricles, and the atria are not visualized. Counterclockwise rotation of the transducer, from the standard apical 4-chamber position to apical 2-chamber and apical long-axis views, enables visualization of the entire ventricular septum from base to apex. In addition, standard and nonstandard subcostal views of the septum should be obtained. The apical septum should be interrogated with multiple angulations to ensure that unusually situated defects do not go undetected.

A VSR is diagnosed when turbulent blood flow signals occur moving from the left into the right ventricle through an area of discontinuity in the ventricular septum or across an apparently intact ventricular septum. **Figure 11.2A** shows an apicoanterior VSR in an off-axis view; however, the confirmation is only after you see the color flow from left to right (**Figure 11.2B and Videos 11.1A to C**).

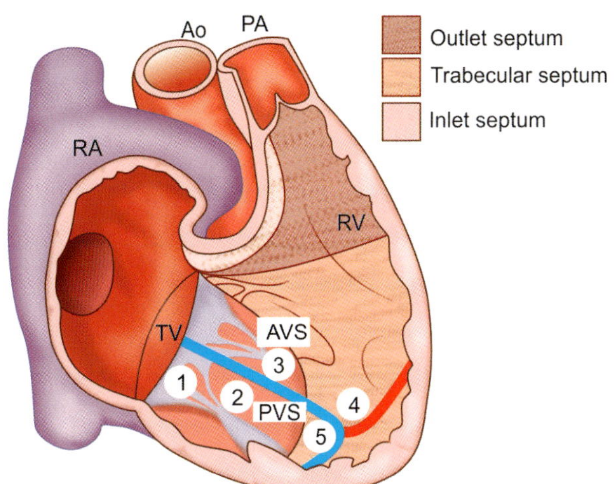


**Figure 11.1:** J-shaped zone lies between the anterior and posterior inlet septum and apically the trabecular septum. Common ventricular septal rupture locations are numbered as 1, posterior basal septum; 2, posterior mid septum; 3, anterior mid septum; 4, anterior apical septum; and 5, posterior apical septum. *Abbreviations:* Ao, aorta; AVS, anterior ventricular septum; PA, pulmonary artery; PVS, posterior ventricular septum; RA, right atrium; RV, right ventricle; TV, tricuspid valve.

Turbulent blood flow in the right ventricle adjacent to the septum and flow signal acceleration and convergence (defined as a localized area of increased velocity and/or aliasing) along the LV side of the septum should alert the echocardiographer to the possibility of a VSR in that region. Once a suspicious area is detected, the transducer should be manipulated to determine the precise origin of the abnormal flow signals. The maximum color jet width at the LV side of the defect should be measured in multiple planes as a measure of VSR size **(Videos 11.1B and C, Video 11.2B)**. When multiple jets are detected, individual jet widths should be added. VSRs should be assessed for site and size of the defect. It should be determined whether the defect is in apical mid or basal septum, and whether it is located anteriorly or posteriorly. The description helps the surgeon understand the anatomy for repair purposes. **Videos 11.1A to C** depict an apical anterior VSR in a patient with anterior wall MI, whereas **Videos 11.2A and B** show a mid-posterior VSR in a patient with inferoposterior infarct.

Abnormal flow signals can be assessed to characterize the timing and direction of shunt flow in each phase of the cardiac cycle by color-guided M-mode and/or pulsed- or continuous-wave Doppler rather than by 2D color Doppler, because of the high update rate of the former techniques. Aligning the cursor as parallel to the direction of the VSR jet as possible, continuous-wave Doppler signals of the maximum

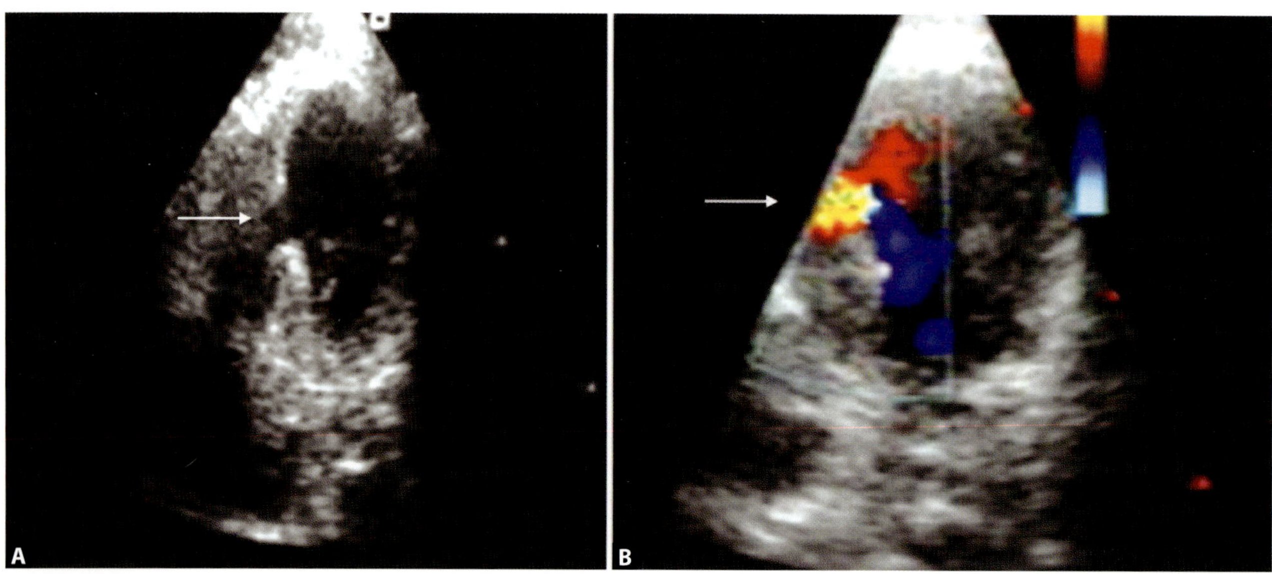


**Figure 11.2A and B:** (A) Off-axis apical view showing anterior interventricular septum with a breach in continuity of the ventricular septum (indicated by arrow). Not all cases are so clearly demarcated. (B) Color flow through the ventricular septal rupture seen from left-to-right (arrow). The flow convergence is on the left of the septum and turbulence on the right **(Videos 11.1A to C)**.

velocity in systole should be obtained. The pressure gradient between left and right ventricles should be calculated, which when subtracted from systemic cuff blood pressure can give an estimated right ventricular systolic pressure. Detailed LV wall motion analysis should be performed to assess the extent of myocardial injury. We should be cautious while estimating LV ejection fraction as it is usually an overestimation owing to the fact that LV is decompressing into a low pressure chamber (the right ventricle). Another important prognostic factor is function of the right ventricle, and knowledge of right ventricular function is important in surgical decision making. In some cases, transesophageal echocardiography (TEE) may help in determining the extent of the defect. Not all patients are anatomically suitable for transcatheter closure. The exact position of the defect, its anatomy (simple vs complex), and its size affect the likelihood of successful deployment and subsequent stability of a percutaneously implanted device. Consequently, careful assessment by 2D/three-dimensional transthoracic echocardiography (TTE) or TEE is important in patient selection.

## Ventricular Free-wall Rupture

Acute or subacute myocardial rupture is a serious and invariably fatal complication of MI. Rupture of the free wall of the infarcted ventricle is a relatively common finding in patients dying with an AMI. Several large studies have found cardiac rupture in 14–26% of such patients. The incidence is much lower when all patients with AMI are considered. According to the U.S. National Registry of Myocardial Infarction published data on 350,755 patients in 1996 the incidence of cardiac rupture was less than 1%; this is consistent with a 0.85% incidence of tamponade in a review of over 100,000 patients treated with fibrinolytic therapy.[12-15] Cardiac rupture was responsible for 7.3% of all deaths and for 12.1% among those receiving a fibrinolytic agent. Death from rupture occurred earlier among patients receiving a fibrinolytic agent, often within 24 hours of drug administration.

Myocardial rupture occurs within the first 5 days after MI in about one-half of cases and within 2 weeks in over 90% of cases. Free-wall myocardial rupture could be early phase (<72 hours) or late phase (>4 days) ruptures. Early rupture is characterized by an abrupt slit-like tear in the infarcted myocardium, with a preference for anterior infarction sites whereas late rupture is characterized by the presence of infarct expansion, with no preferential infarction site. Myocardial rupture more frequently involves the left ventricle than the right ventricle and rarely involves the atria. The infarct commonly affects the anterior and lateral walls of the left ventricle near the junction of the infarcted and normal myocardium.[16-19]

Rupture is usually a dramatic clinical presentation with sudden hemodynamic compromise, shock, and death. It is thus rare to be able to record an echo during a free wall rupture; however, suspicion of impending rupture should come to mind in large transmural infarcts (>20% of myocardium) with tracts or crypts seen burrowing into the myocardium.[20] Incomplete/subacute rupture of the LV free

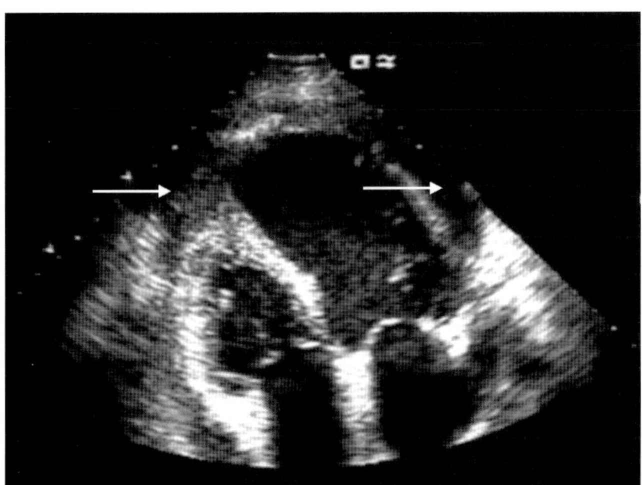

**Figure 11.3:** Apical 4-chamber view showing a rent at the apex with circumferential pericardial collection (right arrow) with echogenic specks and layered thrombus (left arrow) at the apex.

wall can occur when organized thrombus and the pericardium seal the ventricular perforation **(Figure 11.3)**. This condition can progress to frank rupture with cardiac tamponade and hemodynamic compromise. Alternatively, it may progress to formation of a false aneurysm walled off by pericardial tissue and communicating with the left ventricle through the perforation or to formation of a LV diverticulum.

The diagnosis is made clinically with confirmation from TTE. The most frequent echocardiographic finding in the case of LV free-wall rupture is a localized pericardial effusion overlying the infarcted akinetic area. A finding of pericardial effusion of 5 mm during diastole and layered thrombus within the pericardial space are highly sensitive for detection of free-wall rupture. Other signs include echogenic "specks" within the effusion and visible wall defects.[21,22]

In subacute and chronic free-wall ruptures, the rent in the myocardium is sealed by fibrosis and organized clots. The situation is then called as pseudoaneurysm of LV and is discussed subsequently.

## Mitral Papillary Muscle Rupture

Presence of MR is a predictor of poor prognosis in the setting of CAD. An MR of mild-to-moderate nature is common among patients with AMI, occurring in 13–45% patient.[23,24] The causes of MR after AMI include ischemic papillary muscle displacement (previously known as papillary muscle dysfunction),[25] LV dilatation or true aneurysm, and papillary muscle or chordal rupture. Papillary muscle rupture is a life-threatening complication of AMI that accounts for approximately 5% of deaths in these patients. It usually occurs 2–7 days after the infarct. The rupture may be partial (occurring at one of the muscle heads) or complete. Because of differences in blood supply, rupture of the posteromedial papillary muscle occurs 6–12 times more frequently than rupture of the anterolateral papillary muscle. The posteromedial papillary muscle is supplied with blood from the posterior descending artery, while the anterolateral papillary muscle has a dual blood supply from the left anterior descending and left circumflex arteries.[26] Papillary muscle rupture occurs in both ST elevation and non-ST elevation infarcts. Most patients have relatively small areas of necrosis with poor collaterals, and up to 50% have single vessel disease.[8,27,28] An autopsy study of 22 patients with postinfarction PMR found that 82% occurred in patients with a first MI.[29]

PMR presents with sudden torrential regurgitation of blood into a noncompliant left atrium leading to elevation of left atrial pressures resulting in pulmonary edema. The clinical manifestations of PMR include the acute onset of hypotension and pulmonary edema with a hyperactive precordium and a mid, late, or holosystolic murmur that may radiate to the axilla or the base of the heart suggesting acute MR.

The diagnostic test of choice is 2D echocardiography with Doppler and color-flow imaging. The first report of PMR diagnosed by 2D echocardiography appeared in 1981 and many other reports followed in which color-Doppler echocardiography had been used to assess the condition. The first report of PMR diagnosis by TEE was made in 1985. PMR could be diagnosed in most patients, but not in all patients, by the use of TTE or TEE alone. For PMR after AMI, the diagnostic sensitivity of TTE is about 52% and of TEE up to 92%. On TTE, PMR can be visualized as a fluttering structure in relation to the posteromedial papillary muscle that is usually affected. **Figure 11.4** shows a classic case of prolapsed anterior mitral leaflet with ruptured papillary muscle attached to it (**Videos 11.3 and 11.4A and B**).

Many a times, the ruptured part of the papillary muscle is not directly visible. In such situations, indirect evidences of PMR should be assessed. Indirect evidences include presence of a prolapsed mitral valve, dyskinesis as a sign of an MI, presence of significant MR jet using pulsed-wave Doppler and eccentric MR jet into the left atrium on color-Doppler echo. **Video 11.4A** shows the eccentric MR jet in a patient with PMR. Advantage of color Doppler is that it helps in quick visualization of the mitral insufficiency and distinguishes PMR from VSR. We have to be cautious while evaluating color Doppler in patients with acute MI with severe MR as the color flow jet of MR could be undervisualized. Many factors could be responsible for this phenomenon: low LV systolic function due to MI leading to low LV systolic pressure, rapid rise of left atrial pressure as left atrium is noncompliant and small, large MR orifice leading

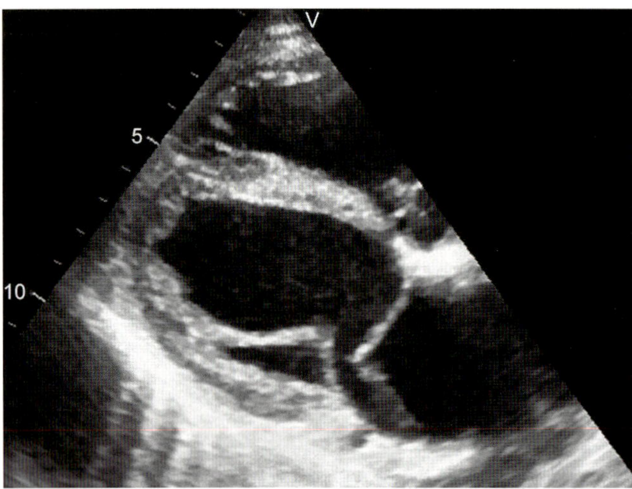


**Figure 11.4:** Parasternal long-axis view of a patient with posterior wall infarct showing flail anterior mitral leaflet. Note the upturned tip of the anterior mitral leaflet into the left atrium. Ruptured head of the papillary muscle is seen attached to the anterior mitral leaflet tip in the left atrium **(Videos 11.3, 11.4A and B)**.

to equalization of LV and left atrial pressures during late systole. When taking into account, the clinical situation of the patients after MI, with newly developing systolic murmur and acute clinical deterioration, these indirect signs make the diagnosis of PMR or VSR very likely. By combining TEE and TTE, the diagnostic sensitivity could be improved to 100%. **Videos 11.4A and B** demonstrate the power of TEE in clearly delineating the anatomic defect and MR severity in patients with PMR.

## CHRONIC MECHANICAL COMPLICATIONS OF ACUTE MYOCARDIAL INFARCTION

### Left Ventricular Aneurysm

LV aneurysm is a complication of transmural MI which can lead to serious morbidity and subsequently death. Patients with apical transmural MI are at higher risk for aneurysm formation, followed by those with posterior-basal infarcts. LV aneurysm is most common in patients who do not receive reperfusion therapy and occurs in up to 10–30% of cases.

Approximately, 70–85% of LV aneurysms are located in the anterior or apical walls due to total occlusion of the left anterior descending coronary artery with absence of collateralization. Only 10–15% involves the inferior-basal walls due to right coronary artery occlusion. Lateral aneurysms secondary to left circumflex occlusion is very rare. Among patients with multivessel disease, aneurysms are uncommon if there is extensive collateralization or a non-occluded left anterior descending artery.[30-33]

#### *Acute Aneurysm*

Acute development of a large LV aneurysm can result in severe congestive heart failure and even cardiogenic shock. These are usually dyskinetic, i.e expands during systole. This expansion wastes contractile energy generated by normal myocardium and puts the entire ventricle at a mechanical disadvantage.

#### *Chronic Aneurysms*

Chronic aneurysms occur more than 6 weeks after MI and are less compliant than acute aneurysms and rarely expand during systole. Patient can present with heart failure, ventricular arrhythmias, and systemic embolism. Echocardiography is the gold standard and accurately identifies the aneurysmal segment. LV aneurysm as seen on 2D echocardiography is defined as a distinct break in the geometry of the LV contour that is present in both diastole and systole with replacement of necrotic myocardium by fibrous scar tissue, demonstrating dyskinetic or akinetic motion.[34] It may also demonstrate the presence of a mural thrombus. Additionally, echocardiography is useful in differentiating true aneurysms from pseudoaneurysms. Generally, a true aneurysm has a relatively wide mouth communicating with the aneurysmal cavity compared with a narrow neck that is seen in pseudoaneurysm.[35] This results in a fairly board gradual opening to the aneurysm as opposed to a distinct shelf like opening. **Figure 11.5** shows apical 4-chamber view of a patient with anteroapical infarct with apical aneurysm **(Video 11.5)**. Compare this with **Figure 11.6** which is an example of large apical pseudoaneurysm **(Video 11.6)**. Please note the relatively narrow neck of the pseudoaneurysm in **Figure 11.6**.

There are several echocardiographic features that should be recorded if aneurysm resection is contemplated. The traditional indications for resection of ventricular aneurysm are intractable heart failure and less commonly for control of arrhythmias. Mechanically, the aneurysm acts as a dead space reservoir with no ability to eject blood from its diastolic volume. The remaining myocardial walls may move normally; however, the aneurysmal cavity serves as a second output for ejection and thus compromises stroke volume. When contemplating aneurysm resection, it is essential to ensure that the basal portions of the cardiac wall have normal function. This can be accomplished by calculating ejection fraction of only the basal half of the left ventricle. A simplified method to evaluate basal function is to calculate basal fractional shortening or fractional area change using a 2D short-axis view at the base of the heart. Generally, if basal function is normal and the basal half ejection fraction or fractional shortening is greater than 35% or 18% , respectively, then aneurysm resection is more likely to be of clinical benefit. If there is more extensive proximal septal involvement and

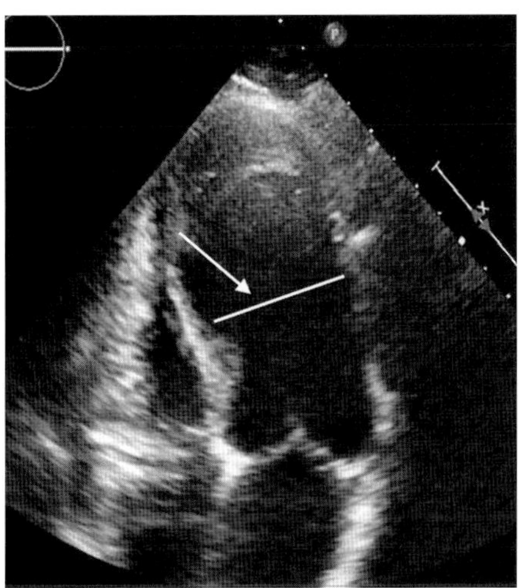

**Figure 11.5:** Apical 4-chamber view in a patient with extensive anterior wall myocardial infarction showing distorted contour of the left ventricular apex even during diastole. The neck of the aneurysm is wide (marked by an arrow) **(Video 11.5)**. Apical thrombus is also seen.

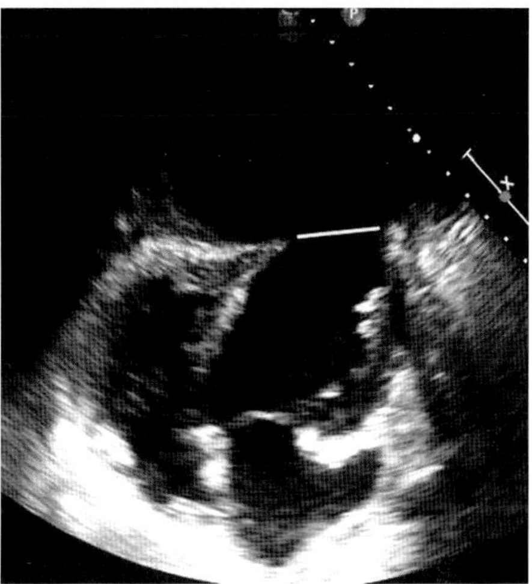

**Figure 11.6:** Apical 4-chamber view in a patient with anterior wall myocardial infarction showing a large apical pseudoaneurysm. Note the narrow neck and the large aneurysm which has ill-defined margins **(Video 11.6)**.

the basal half ejection fraction is pathologically decreased, traditional aneurysmectomy may not result in the significant relief of congestive heart failure.[36]

More recently, other approaches have been taken to control heart failure in patients with ventricular aneurysm. These have included reduction myoplasty and Dor's myoplasty. In the reduction myoplasty, a large segment of the aneurysmal wall is resected, resulting in immediate remodeling of the left ventricle. In the Dor's myoplasty, an intraventricular patch is placed that exclude a wall. The advantage of the Dor's myoplasty is that the aneurysm portion of the ventricular septum can also be excluded from the functional LV cavity. Echocardiography can play a valuable role in assessing feasibility of either of these approaches by determining the degree to which an aneurysm is located in the anterior septum and apex (which is more favorable for Dor's myoplasty) and determining the function of the residual myocardium. After Dor's myoplasty, it is not uncommon to see small degrees of residual flow into the apical dead space created by the intraventricular patch.[37]

## Left Ventricular Pseudoaneurysm

A pseudoaneurysm, or false aneurysm, develops after an AMI that is complicated by a ventricular free-wall rupture that is contained by localized pericardial adhesions. In rare instances, a pseudoaneurysm can actually occur within the ventricular septum rather than along the free wall. It is important to recognize a pseudoaneurysm because the likelihood of spontaneous rupture is high. Unlike a true aneurysm in which the wall consists of dense fibrous tissue with excellent tensile strength, the wall of a pseudoaneurysm is composed of organizing thrombus and varying portions of the epicardium. Pathologically, it is the sequela of myocardial rupture with hemorrhage into the pericardial space, which then becomes locally compressive. Local tamponade occurs, preventing further hemorrhage into pericardium. Over time, the intrapericardial thrombus organizes, creating a wall to the pseudoaneurysm, however, with poor structural integrity. As such, it is at risk of spontaneous rupture, which is generally a fatal event.

Pseudoaneurysm can be separated from true aneurysms by several characteristics. Separation of true from pseudoaneurysm in the proximal posterior wall is often problematic. **Video 11.7** shows an example of posterior wall pseudoaneurysm with to and fro blood flow into the sac. **Video 11.6** is an example of large apical pseudoaneurysm with tell-tale features of narrow neck, shelf-like projection, large aneurysm layered with clot. The pseudoaneurysms usually have narrow opening to the aneurysm with an overhanging shelf-like edge. Traditionally, it is thought that if the size of the opening to the LV cavity is less than that of the maximal dimension of the aneurysm, the defect is more likely to be a pseudoaneurysm. As the pseudoaneurysm is composed of both a free aneurysmal cavity and the organizing hematoma, its true size is often under-represented on echocardiography, because the organized hematoma has a soft tissue density similar to that of many surrounding structures. It is therefore not uncommon to have the situation of a large pericardiac mass on chest radiography or computed tomographic scan in the presence of what appears to be a modest size pseudoaneurysmal cavity detected with echocardiography. This phenomenon also makes it more difficult to assess the ratio of the size of the opening to the LV cavity to the actual aneurysm size, because only the blood filled aspects of the pseudoaneurysm may be easily visualized. Pseudoaneurysm at the base of the heart, most commonly after inferior MI, may be difficult to separate from a true aneurysm. In this location, they may have a wider mouth than is traditionally taught and be difficult to distinguish from a true aneurysm. Their true nature is often only confirmed at the time of surgical inspection or autopsy.[38-40]

## Left Ventricular Thrombus

Chronic thrombus formation is not an infrequent sequela of MI. It is substantially more common after larger anterior MI, especially with involvement of the apex, than after inferior MI. Before the lytic and urgent interventional era, LV thrombus occurred in 25–40% of patient after the first anteroapical MI. With the advent of lytic therapy, there has been a decline in this prevalence; however, thrombus formation is still seen after lytic therapy even with concurrent heparinization. The major risk of LV thrombus is of subsequent embolization with stroke or major organ loss. The likelihood of embolic events is greater in the first 2 weeks after the acute event and tapers off over the 6 weeks after MI. After this time, there is presumed endothelialization of the thrombus with reduction in its embolic potential. There are several characteristics of ventricular thrombus that should be noted echocardiographically. These include not only size but also whether it is laminar thrombus forming a layer along the akinetic wall **(Figure 11.5)** or whether it is pedunculated and/or protruding into the ventricle **(Figure 11.7)**. Thrombi may be mobile. Mobility tends to be seen in fresher rather than chronic thrombi. Both a pedunculated character and mobility confer a greater likelihood of embolization with embolic rates reported as high as 40% when both mobility and protrusion into the cavity are noted. On occasion, fresh thrombi take on a cyst appearance. This is due to a combination of factors, including varying degrees of maturity of the clot and results in acoustic boundaries between relatively fresh and more organized regions. This results in a relative echolucency to the center of the thrombus. **Video 11.5** shows large apical clot with central zone of lucency suggesting a process of dissolution of clot.[40-42]

When seen in the presence of a wall-motion abnormality in which thrombus would be expected, it is important to reorganized this as such rather than make the diagnosis of presumed cyst or tumor. In addition to frank thrombus formation, when using newer generation, high frequency transducers, spontaneous contrast is occasionally noted in the LV cavity. This typically will be seen immediately in the area of a regional wall-motion abnormality. The etiology of the spontaneous contrast is presumably stagnant blood in the region of an aneurysmal dilation. Color-flow imaging at low velocities can also demonstrate abnormal swirling patterns of blood.

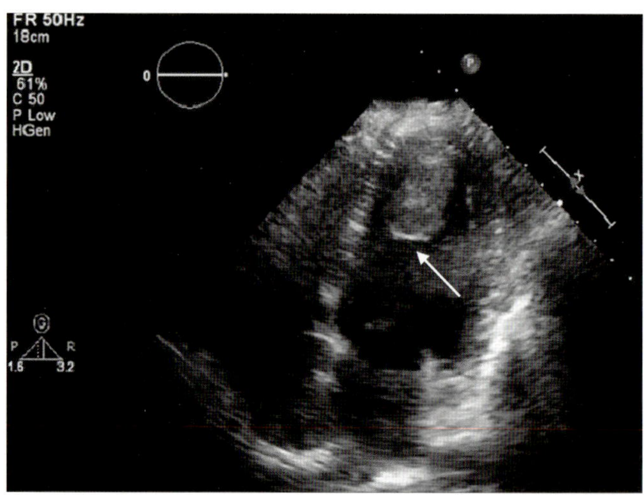


**Figure 11.7:** Apical four-chamber view in a patient with anterior wall myocardial infarction with large pedunculated left ventricular apical clot (arrow).

Occasionally, either the vague nature of a thrombus or technical limitation in the examination render it difficult to either exclude or confirm the presence of ventricular thrombus. The use of higher frequency showed focus transducers can often the certain higher quality imaging in the apex and resolve the dilemma. An additional echocardiographic tool to further evaluate the presence or absence of thrombus is the use of intravenous contrast. Using the newer generation perfluorocarbon-based agents, which pass into the LV cavity, it is possible to fully opacify the LV apex. In doing so, one may then detected true fixed filling defect in the apex and thereby confirm the presence of ventricular thrombus.[43,44]

## CONCLUSION

Mechanical complications of AMI are life-threatening. Acute complications like rupture of the LV free wall, rupture of the interventricular septum, the development of severe MR and chronic complications like LV aneurysm, pseudoaneurysm, and mural thrombi. The diagnosis is markedly facilitated by a heightened index of suspicion. Thus, a new murmur or evidence of hypoperfusion or severe acute decompensated heart failure in the presence of preserved or relatively preserved LV systolic function should raise the possibility of a mechanical complication. The diagnosis can invariably be made using 2D TTE. It is important to clinically suspect, look for and diagnose the possible complications on echocardiography. Echocardiography should be done with great caution as a missed diagnosis could cost a life. Since each of these can lead to cardiogenic shock and death, therapy is most helpful if initiated emergently. Early surgical intervention is the definitive treatment and should be considered when there is a reasonable likelihood of survival. Insertion of an intra-aortic balloon pump may support the patient prior to surgery.

## VIDEO LEGENDS

**Video 11.1:** An example of a ventricular septal rupture. The patient presented 6 days after anterior wall myocardial infarction with shortness of breath. (A) Apical 4-chamber view showing a rent in the apical ventricular septum suggestive of ventricular septal rupture. There is also a large serpentine clot floating in the right atrium. This is likely an embolized clot from deep vein thrombosis in the legs. (B) Color flow through the apical ventricular septal rupture. Note the flow acceleration on the left ventricular side and the turbulent jet on the right ventricular side of the defect. The location is clearly apical. (C) Short-axis view showing left-to-right shunt though the ventricular septal rupture. Note the shunt is located in anterior septum and therefore this was an apicoanterior ventricular septal rupture.

**Video 11.2:** Another example of a ventricular septal rupture in a patient with inferior-posterior wall infarct who had presented with cardiogenic shock. (A) Modified apical longitudinal view shows a breach in the mid-ventricular septum. (B) Subcostal long-axis view with color showing left-to-right shunt through mid-posterior septum. This is an example of mid-posterior ventricular septal rupture.

**Video 11.3:** Parasternal long-axis view in a patient with posterior wall infarct. Note the wall motion defect in mid posterior wall along with flail A2 scallop of the anterior mitral leaflet. The fragment of the ruptured papillary muscle head is seen attached to the tip of the anterior mitral leaflet and is freely moving in and out of the left atrium.

**Video 11.4:** Transesophageal echocardiography in the same patient as in Video 11.3. (A) Lower esophageal view shows eccentric severe mitral regurgitation directed posteriorly. (B) Flail A1, A2 scallops of the anterior mitral leaflet with ruptured head of papillary muscle seen attached to it. Fragments of ruptured chordae are also seen at the tip of the posterior mitral leaflet. Transesophageal echocardiography is much better in detection and evaluation of papillary muscle rupture.

**Video 11.5:** Apical 4-chamber view in a patient with large anterior wall infarct showing apical dyskinetic aneurysm. The aneurysm is seen to expand during systole. There is large layered clot attached to the aneurysm. One can notice the central portion of the clot is echolucent as compared to the periphery. This central echolucency is a marker of dissolving clot as commonly observed in patients on anticoagulants.

**Video 11.6:** Zoomed apical 4-chamber view in a patient with anteroapical infarction showing a large apical pseudoaneurysm with a shelf-like structure at its origin. Note the relatively narrow neck of opening and large aneurysmal cavity, which is partially layered with clot. Spontaneous echo contrast is seen in the aneurysm as swirling smoke.

**Video 11.7:** Parasternal long-axis view in a patient with posterior wall infarct showing scarred posterior wall with a rupture. There is a pericardial collection posteriorly, which has contained the rupture. The color flow shows to and fro blood movement into the pseudoaneurysm.

## REFERENCES


1. Topez O, Taylor AL. Interventriculer septal rupture complicating acute myocardial infarction from pathophysiologig feature of the role of invasive and noninvasive diagnostic modalities in current management.
2. Latham PM. Lectures on Subjects Connected with Clinical Medicine Comprising Diseases of the Heart. London: Longman Rees; 1845.
3. Brunn F. Diagnosis of acquired rupture of the ventricular septum of the heart. Wien Arch Inn Med. 1923;6:533.
4. Sager R. Coronary thrombosis: perforation of the infarcted interventricular septum. Arch Intern Med. 1934;53:140.
5. Cooley DA, Belmonte BA, Zeis LB, et al. Surgical repair of ruptured interventricular septum following acute myocardial infarction. Surgery. 1957;41:930-7.
6. Koh AS, Loh YJ, Lim YP, et al. Ventricular septal rupture following acute myocardial infarction. Acta Cardiol. 2011;66:225-30.
7. Garshaw BS, Granger CB, Bunbaum Y, et al. Risk factors in angiographic patterns and outcome in patient with ventricular septal defect complicating acute myocardial infarction. GUSTO l Investigators. Circulation. 2000;101;2732.
8. Reeder GS. Identification and treatment of complications of myocardial infarction. Mayo Clin Proc. 1995;70:880.
9. Pasternak RC, Braunwald E, Sobel BE. Acute myocardial infarction. In: Braunwald EB (ed): Heart Disease, 4th edition. Philadelphia: Saunders; 1992. p. 200.
10. Smyllie J, Dawkins K, Conway N, et al. Diagnosis of ventricular septal rupture after myocardial infarction: value of colour flow mapping. Br Heart J. 1989;62:260-7.
11. Obarski TP, Rogers PJ, Debeats DL, et al. Assessment of postinfarction ventricular septal ruptures by transesophageal Doppler Ecchocardiography. J Am Soc Echocardiogr. 1995;8;728-34.
12. Stevenson WG, Linssen GC, Havenith MG, et al. The spectrum of death after myocardial infarction: a necropsy study. Am Heart J. 1989;118:1182.
13. Pohjola-Sintonen S, Muller JE, Stone PH, et al. Ventricular septal and free wall rupture complicating acute myocardial infarction: experience in the Multicenter Investigation of Limitation of Infarct Size. Am Heart J. 1989;117:809.
14. Becker RC, Gore JM, Lambrew C, et al. A composite view of cardiac rupture in the United States National Registry of Myocardial Infarction. J Am Coll Cardiol. 1996;27:1321.

15. Patel MR, Meine TJ, Lindblad L, et al. Cardiac tamponade in the fibrinolytic era: analysis of >100,000 patients with ST-segment elevation myocardial infarction. Am Heart J. 2006; 151:316.
16. Figueras J, Alcalde O, Barrabés JA, et al. Changes in hospital mortality rates in 425 patients with acute ST-elevation myocardial infarction and cardiac rupture over a 30-year period. Circulation. 2008;118:2783.
17. Becker RC, Hochman JS, Cannon CP, et al. Fatal cardiac rupture among patients treated with thrombolytic agents and adjunctive thrombin antagonists: observations from the Thrombolysis and Thrombin Inhibition in Myocardial Infarction 9 Study. J Am Coll Cardiol. 1999;33:479.
18. Moreno R, López-Sendón J, García E, et al. Primary angioplasty reduces the risk of left ventricular free wall rupture compared with thrombolysis in patients with acute myocardial infarction. J Am Coll Cardiol. 2002;39:598.
19. Mann JM, Roberts WC. Rupture of the left ventricular free wall during acute myocardial infarction: analysis of 138 necropsy patients and comparison with 50 necropsy patients with acute myocardial infarction without rupture. Am J Cardiol. 1988; 62:847.
20. Figueras J, Cortadellas J, Soler-Soler J. Left ventricular free wall rupture: clinical presentation and management. Heart. 2000;83:499.
21. McMullan MH, Maples MD, Kilgore TL, et al. Surgical experience with left ventricular free wall rupture. Ann Thorac Surg. 2001;71:1894-8.
22. Raitt MH, Kraft CD, Gardner CJ, et al. Subacute ventricular free wall rupture complicating acute myocardial infarction. Am Heart J. 1993;126: 946-55.
23. Barzilai B, Gessler C, Prez JE, et al. Significance of Doppler detected mitral regurgitation in acute myocardial infarction. Am J Cardiol. 1988;61:220-3.
24. Lehmann KG, Fransis CK, Dodge HT, et al. Mitral regurgitation in early myocardial infarction: incidence, clinical detection and prognosis implications. TIMI study group. Ann Intern Med. 1992;117;10-7.
25. Wei JY, Hutchins GM, Bulkey BH. Papillary muscle rupture in fatel acute myocardial infarction: a potentially treatable form of cardiogenic shock. Ann Int Med. 1979;90:149-152.
26. Voci P Bilotta F, Caretta Q, et al. Papillary muscle perfusion pattern: a hypothesis for ischemic papillary muscle dysfunction. Circulation. 1995;1714-8.
27. Purcaro A, Costantini C, Ciampani N, et al. Diagnostic criteria and management of subacute ventricular free wall rupture complicating acute myocardial infarction. Am J Cardiol. 1997; 80:397.
28. Lavie CJ, Gersh BJ. Mechanical and electrical complications of acute myocardial infarction. Mayo Clin Proc. 1990; 65:709.
29. David TE. Techniques and results of mitral valve repair for ischemic mitral regurgitation. J Card Surg. 1994; 9:274.
30. Nagle RE, Williams DO. Proceedings: Natural history of ventricular aneurysm without surgical treatment. Br Heart J. 1974;36:1037.
31. Dubnow MH, Burchell HB, Titus JL. Postinfarction ventricular aneurysm. A clinicomorphologic and electrocardiographic study of 80 cases. Am Heart J. 1965;70:753.
32. Rao G, Zikria EA, Miller WH, et al. Experience with sixty consecutive ventricular aneurysm resections. Circulation. 1974;50:II149.
33. Gorlin R, Klein MD, Sullivan JM. Prospective correlative study of ventricular aneurysm. Mechanistic concept and clinical recognition. Am J Med. 1967;42:512.
34. Rueda B, Panidis IP, Gonzales R, et al. Left ventricular pseudoaneurysm: detection and postoperative follow-up by color Doppler echocardiography. Am Heart J. 1990;120:990-2.
35. Hironaka E, Kojima S, Hongo M, et al. Echocardiographic diagnosis of subepicardial aneurysm ruptured into the right ventricle after inferior myocardial infarction. J Am Soc Echocardiogr. 1997;10:192-6.
36. Ryan T, Petrovic O, Armstrong WF,et al. Quantitative two-dimensional echocardiographic assessment of patient undergoing left ventricular aneurysmectomy. Am Heart J. 1986;111:714-20.
37. Sabia P, Abbott RD, Afrookteh A, Keller MW, Touchstone DA, Kaul S. Importence of two-dimensional echocardiographic assessment of left ventricular systolic function in patient presenting to the emergency room with cardiac releted symptoms. Circulation. 1991;84615-24.
38. Frances C, Romero A, Grady D. Left ventricular pseudo-aneurysm. J Am Coll Cardiol. 1998;32:557.
39. Yeo TC, Malouf JF, Oh JK, et al. Clinical profile and outcome in 52 patients with cardiac pseudoaneurysm. Ann Intern Med. 1998;128:299.
40. al-Saadon K, Walley VM, Green M, et al. Angiographic diagnosis of true and false LV aneurysms after inferior wall myocardial infarction. Cathet Cardiovasc Diagn. 1995;35:266.
41. Visser CA, Kan G, Meltzer RS, et al. Embolic potential of left ventricular thrombus after myocardial infarction: a two-dimensional echocardiographic study of 119 patients. J Am Coll Cardiol. 1985; 5:1276.
42. Asinger RW, Mikell FL, Elsperger J, et al. Incidence of left-ventricular thrombosis after acute transmural myocardial infarction. Serial evaluation by two-dimensional echocardiography. N Engl J Med. 1981; 305:297.
43. Keren A, Goldberg S, Gottlieb S, et al. Natural history of left ventricular thrombi: their appearance and resolution in the posthospitalization period of acute myocardial infarction. J Am Coll Cardiol. 1990;15:790.
44. Weinreich DJ, Burke JF, Pauletto FJ. Left ventricular mural thrombi complicating acute myocardial infarction. Long-term follow-up with serial echocardiography. Ann Intern Med. 1984;100:789.

# Cardiac Rupture Following Acute Myocardial Infarction: Role of Three-dimensional Transesophageal Echocardiography in Transcatheter Repair

12
CHAPTER

*Amrita Kushal, Itzhak Kronzon*

## INTRODUCTION

Three-dimensional (3D) transesophageal echocardiography (TEE) is a rapidly advancing technology, with its potential uses growing in routine clinical evaluations as well as in both surgical and interventional procedures. This chapter explores the role of 3D TEE in the evaluation of cardiac rupture following acute myocardial infarction and in its transcatheter repair.

## THREE-DIMENSIONAL ECHOCARDIOGRAPHY *VS* TWO-DIMENSIONAL ECHOCARDIOGRAPHY

Piezoelectric crystals move in a predictable way when placed in an electrical field. These predictable vibrations generate sound waves, which are the basis of echocardiography. Two-dimensional (2D) transducers have piezoelectric elements arranged in a linear array, while 3D transducers have piezoelectric elements arranged in a 2D matrix.[1] The latter allows acquisition of a pyramidal dataset necessary for accurate volume assessment. This pyramidal dataset also allows for generation of 2D slices from essentially any plane via cropping. The infinitely variable cropping planes can be used for customizable and precise imaging, including the more standard 2D views (e.g. apical four-chamber or short-axis views).

3D echocardiography may further be classified into a real-time mode and electrocardiographic-gated (ECG-gated) multiple-beat mode. The real-time mode obtains multiple pyramidal datasets per second in a single heartbeat. This minimizes artifacts resulting from rhythm disturbances or respiratory motion but compromises temporal and spatial resolution.[2] There are newer 3D probes, however, that allow real-time imaging with acceptable temporal and spatial resolution. The ECG-gated multiple-beat mode acquires multiple narrow volumes of data over several heartbeats (2–7 beats), which are combined to form a single volumetric dataset. This mode, however, is susceptible to generation of artifacts, because of respiratory motion and, when present, abnormal heart rhythms.

3D echocardiography, including real-time 3D TEE, is utilized in the evaluation of and guiding repair of cardiac rupture following an acute myocardial infarction.

## CARDIAC RUPTURE FOLLOWING ACUTE MYOCARDIAL INFARCTION AND THE ROLE OF THREE-DIMENSIONAL TRANSESOPHAGEAL ECHOCARDIOGRAPHY IN TRANSCATHETER REPAIR

There are three major types of cardiac rupture following an acute myocardial infarction: ventricular septal rupture (VSR), ventricular free wall rupture, and acute papillary muscle rupture. Though incidence of these have decreased since the advent of reperfusion therapies, each of these complications carries a high mortality rate and are typically managed surgically. Recently, transcatheter interventions have offered a less invasive alternative to surgery for repair of cardiac rupture. Both postinfarction VSR and pseudoaneurysm complicating free wall rupture have been repaired successfully by transcatheter approaches. Though transcatheter repair of papillary muscle rupture has not yet been reported, early reports of successful transcatheter mitral valve replacement[3,4] suggest a promising future for less invasive papillary muscle rupture repair options.

3D TEE plays an integral role during various stages in transcatheter repair of cardiac rupture. Preprocedurally, it is essential in localizing the defect and detailing the anatomy of the defect, both for technical considerations and appropriate device selection. Intraprocedurally, it is complementary to existing fluoroscopy for catheter guidance and assessing successful device deployment.

## Ventricular Septal Rupture

Post-myocardial infarction VSR most often occurs 3–5 days following acute myocardial infarction, usually in patients who did not receive reperfusion therapy.[5] In patients who receive thrombolysis, it usually occurs within 24 hours.[5] Pathogenetically, it is caused by neutrophilic infiltration of the necrotic area, followed by apoptosis and release of lytic enzymes causing disintegration of the necrotic myocardium.[5] The resulting VSR may be simple (usually in anterior infarctions) or complex (usually in inferior infarctions); a simple VSR has a relatively "straight" path, while a complex VSR is associated with a serpiginous tract.[5] This may account for the increased risk of mortality in patients with inferobasal VSRs.[6] Postinfarction VSR incidence is roughly equal in both anterior or inferior infarctions.[7] Prior to reperfusion therapy, overall incidence was 1–3%.[7] Incidence has decreased with both thrombolytic therapy (approximately 0.2–0.4%) and with percutaneous coronary intervention (approximately 0.2–0.5%), although mortality remains high at 20–87%.[6,7] Urgent repair is indicated, and despite it, high mortality is expected;[8] there are reports of inpatient mortality of 45% in those treated with surgery.[7] Unrepaired VSR has had a long-term quoted mortality of 90% without significant change in mortality in the more recent years.[7]

Current guidelines for patients with ST-elevation myocardial infarction complicated by VSR recommend emergent surgical repair given the high-associated mortality, even in hemodynamically stable patients.[6] Transcatheter repair is mentioned as a possible alternative or adjunct, but data are limited, and it is, therefore, not further expanded on.

Surgical repair techniques utilize different approaches on the basis of location of the defect.[9] For anterior defects **(Figure 12.1)**, an incision is made at the left ventricular apex through the infarcted muscle, and the margins of the infarcted muscle are delineated.[9] The VSR is located and a custom-sized patch is stitched to noninfarcted septal tissue and to noninfarcted tissue on the anterolateral wall. For posterior defects **(Figure 12.2)**, an incision is made in the inferior wall and a triangular-shaped patch is stitched to the mitral annulus, the posterior wall, and to a healthy part of the septum. Because the posterior wall is infarcted, these stitches must be anchored with full-thickness bites to the pericardium or on felt applied to the epicardium.[9] The ventriculotomy is closed with stitches or strips of bovine pericardium. Complications of surgical repair include repair failure, late recurrence of shunt, free wall rupture, papillary muscle rupture, ventricular arrhythmia, stroke, and cardiogenic shock.

Transcatheter approaches to closure of VSRs can also vary, as the defects can be closed by a variety of closure devices on the basis of the actual size and dimensions of the defect[10] **(Figure 12.3)**. Essentially, in the arteriovenous technique[11] **(Figure 12.4)**, a wire is passed from a femoral artery, through the aortic valve, the left ventricle, and through the VSR to the right ventricle. It is then advanced and anchored into the pulmonary artery. A snare wire is inserted into a central vein and is advanced through the right heart into the pulmonary artery. This snare wire "catches" the existing arterial wire in the pulmonary artery and pulls it out to the venous access site, exteriorizing it to the selected central vein. This leaves a single, continuous arteriovenous wire "rail" **(Figure 12.4 and 12.5)**. A closure device is loaded through a delivery sheath on the venous side of the continuous wire circuit. It is passed through the VSR, and the left disk is slowly deployed once the device tip reaches the left ventricle. The whole system (sheath, device, wire) is pulled back from the venous side to approximate the left disk against the septum. The right disk is then deployed by retracting the venous delivery sheath over

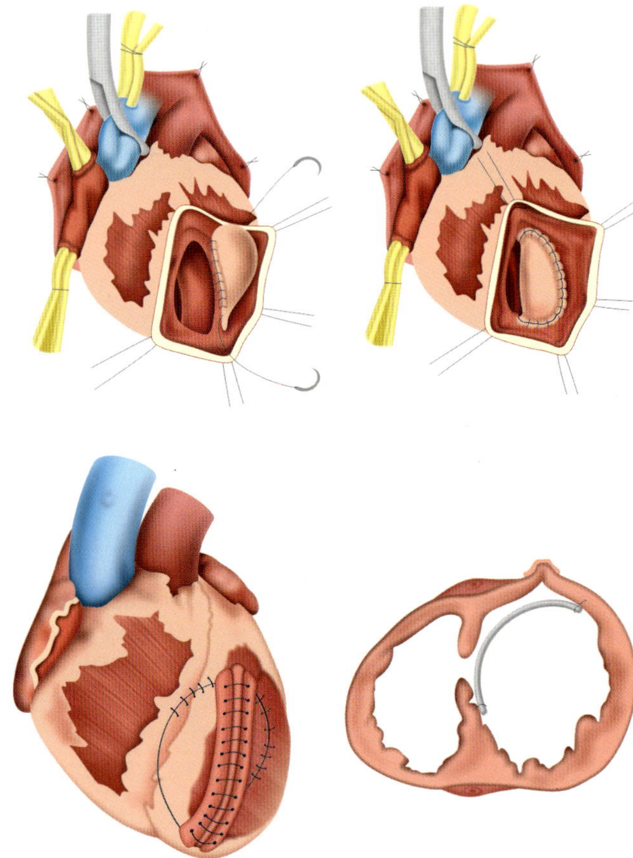

**Figure 12.1:** Repair of anterior ventricular septal defect by endocardial patch with infarct exclusion. Pericardial patch is sutured to septum first then to lateral wall.
David TE, Dale L, Sun Z. Postinfarction ventricular septal rupture: repair by endocardial patch with infarct exclusion. J Thorac Card Surg. 1995;10(5):1315-22. *With permission from Elsevier.*

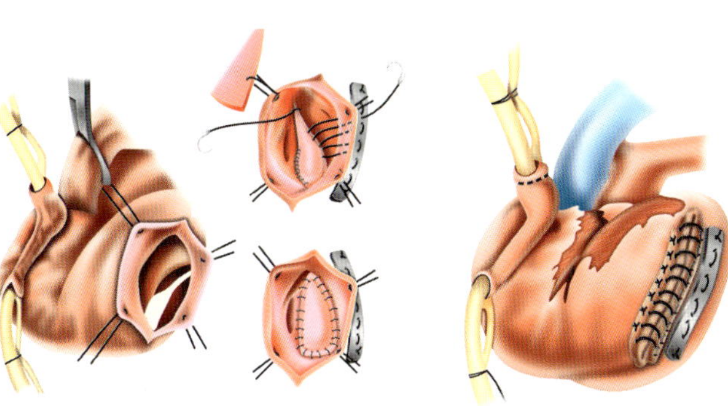

**Figure 12.2:** Repair of posterior ventricular septal defect by endocardial patch with infarct exclusion. Pericardial patch is sutured to mitral annulus, septum, and posterior wall.
David TE, Dale L, Sun Z. Postinfarction ventricular septal rupture: repair by endocardial patch with infarct exclusion. J Thorac Card Surg. 1995;10(5):1315-22. *With permission from Elsevier.*

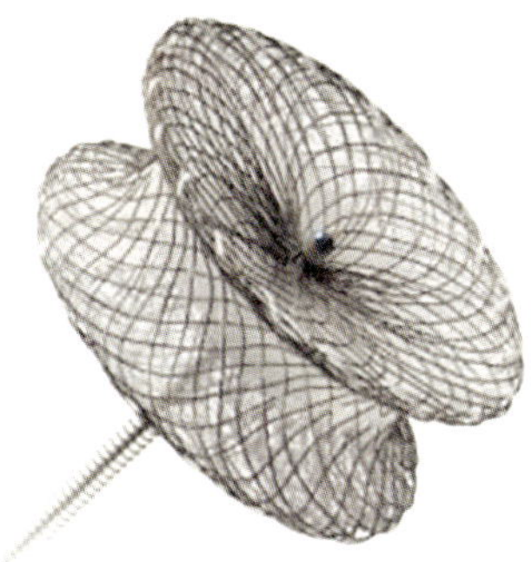

**Figure 12.3:** Amplatzer muscular ventricular septal supture occluder: An example of a closure device.
Image reproduced, *With permission from St. Jude Medical 2012.*

the cable. Positioning of the device and the complete closure of the defect are confirmed by angiography and Doppler echocardiography. In the venovenous technique, a wire is advanced from a femoral vein to the right atrium, through a patent foramen ovale or atrial trans-septal puncture, to left atrium and then left ventricle.[12] The VSR is crossed. A snare wire from a different central vein (e.g. internal jugular vein) is used to exteriorize the femoral venous wire to the second central venous access point, creating a continuous venovenous wire "rail" **(Figure 12.6)**. The remainder of the process is similar to the described arteriovenous technique. In the retrograde[13] approach, a wire is advanced from the femoral artery, through the aortic valve, to the left ventricle. The VSR is crossed and the device is deployed first on right ventricular side while a second, left-sided disk, is positioned in a retrograde fashion. The retrograde approach is usually not considered first-line, because of the greater potential damage to femoral arteries from the use of large catheters in the femoral arteries.[11,13]

Complications of transcatheter VSR repair include residual shunting, enlargement of the defects, left ventricular rupture during implantation, device dislodgement, valvular dysfunction, cardiac tamponade, vascular access complications, ventricular arrhythmia, and clot formation with embolic phenomena, including stroke.

There are currently no randomized trials comparing outcomes of transcatheter postinfarction VSR repair with traditional surgical repair, and prospective trials are limited; most studies are case-control trials. Nonetheless, recent reports suggest that transcatheter VSR closure may in fact be noninferior to surgical repair.[14,15] Thiele et al. presented a small prospective trial evaluating transcatheter VSR repair immediately following an acute myocardial infarction in 29 patients, with a median time from VSR occurrence to repair of one day.[16] During VSR occlusion, echocardiography was performed for device guidance and VSR visualization.[16] Similar to studies of surgical repair, overall mortality remained high, attributed to either disease severity or possible suboptimal interventional closure techniques.[16] Zhu et al. reported another small prospective trial evaluating postinfarction transcatheter VSR repair, with a median time to repair of 18 days, with significantly lower in-hospital mortality of approximately 15%.[8] Further outcomes of transcatheter postinfarction VSR closure must be followed in the forthcoming years with larger studies, as this approach would provide a therapeutic option that would obviate both the need for open heart surgery and suturing into necrotic material, amongst offering other potential benefits.[17]

## Ventricular Free Wall Rupture

The majority of ventricular free wall ruptures occur within the first week after myocardial infarction.[18] Its pathophysiology is likely similar to that of VSR, with the underlying mechanism being disintegration of infarcted myocardium. Other contributing mechanisms may include small perforations in areas of softening or a plasmin-mediated collagen breakdown causing an abrupt tear or erosion in the infarcted myocardium.[18] The variation in the underlying mechanism may explain why the advent of tissue-plasminogen activator may both decrease (by minimizing or halting myocardial infarction) or increase (via plasmin-mediated collagen breakdown) the risk for ventricular free wall rupture. In fact, early thrombolytic therapy appears to be associated with decreased risk of ventricular free wall rupture, but delayed use (>11 hours after infarction) may increase risk.[18] Primary angioplasty is associated with a decreased risk of ventricular

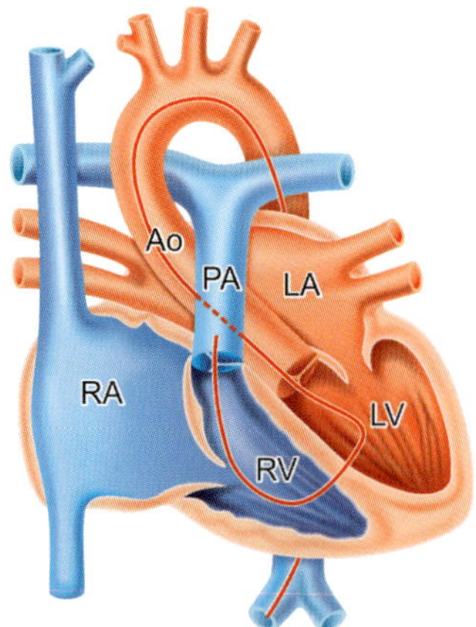


1. A wire (red) is passed from a femoral artery, through the aortic valve, the LV, and through the VSR to the RV. It is advanced and anchored into the PA.

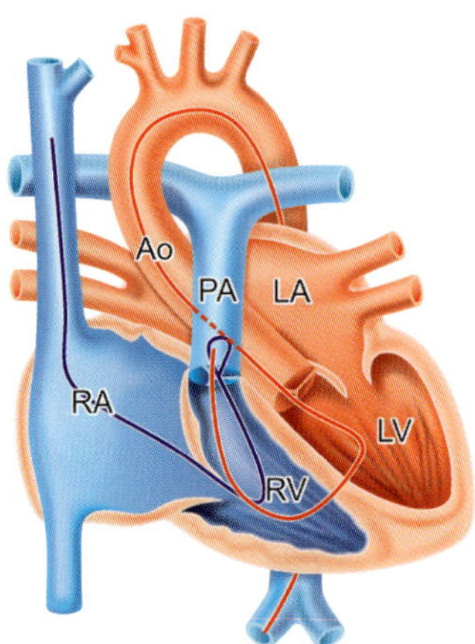


2. A snare wire (blue) is inserted into a central vein and advanced through the right heart into the PA, around the existing arterial wire in the PA.

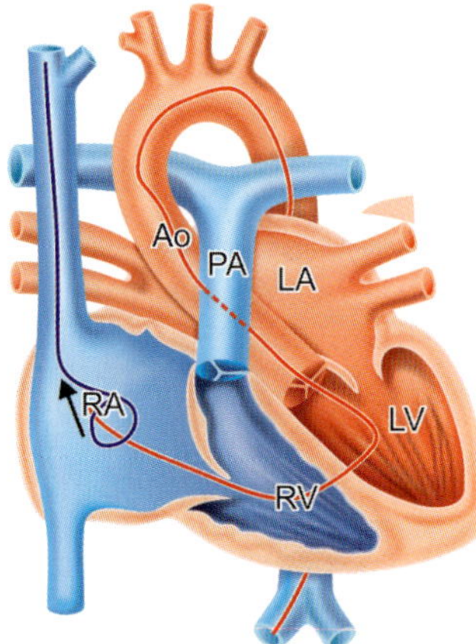


3. The snare wire "catches" the arterial wire in the PA and pulls it out to the venous access site. This leaves a single, continuous arteriovenous wire "rail".

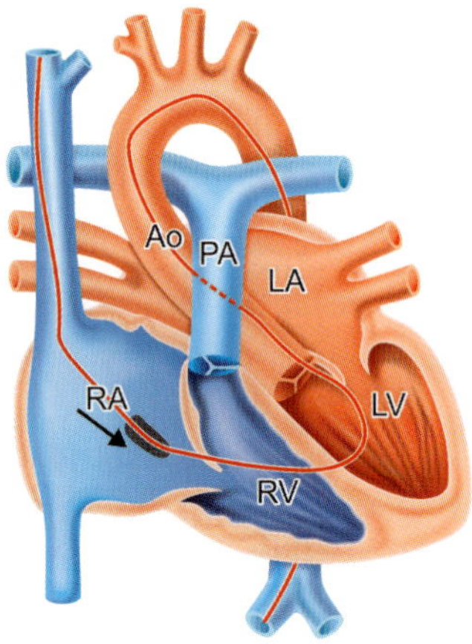


4. A closure device (gray) is loaded through a delivery sheath on the venous side of the continuous wire circuit.

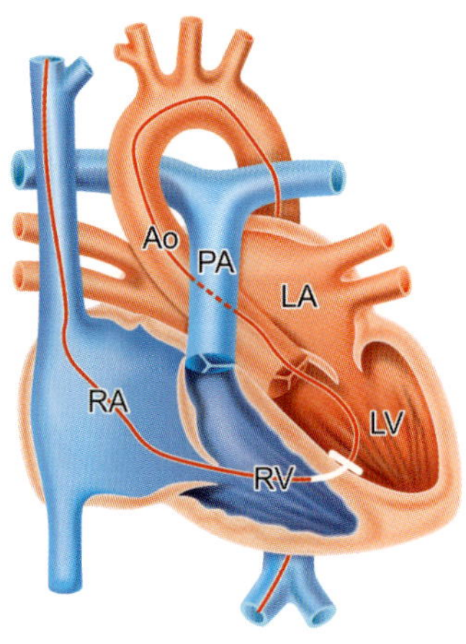


5. The closure device is passed through the VSR. In the LV, the left disk is deployed. The whole system (sheath, device, wire) is pulled back from the venous side to approximate the left

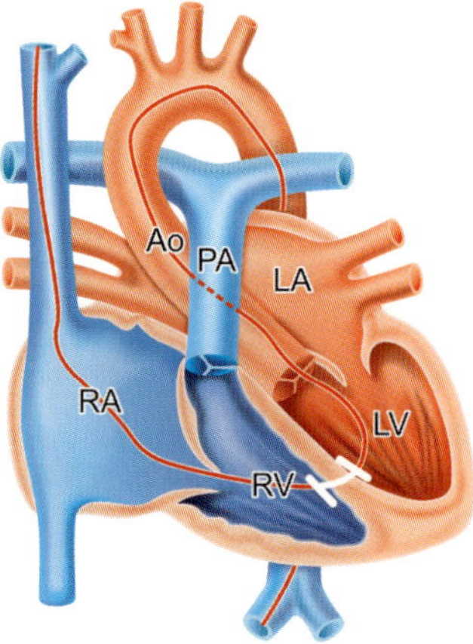


6. The right disk is then deployed by retracting the venous delivery sheath over the cable.

**Figure 12.4:** Schematic of transcatheter ventricular septal defect closure, arteriovenous technique.
*Abbreviations:* Ao, aorta; LA, left atrium; LV, left ventricle; PA, pulmonary artery; RA, right atrium; RV, right ventricle; VSR, ventricular septal rupture.
Base cardiac diagram modified from Pediatric Pulmonology, Caldwell RL, Congenital heart disease: A diagramatic atlas, Liss, Inc., 1988, October 2005, *With permission from John Wiley and Sons.*

free wall rupture. Overall incidence of free wall rupture is approximately 0.8–6.2%, and it is a common cause of death after myocardial infarction, especially within the first 24 hours and in patients receiving thrombolytic therapy.[18] Ventricular free wall rupture is the most common form of cardiac rupture and due to the high mortality, incidence in pathological specimens is likely much higher. Most ruptures occur anterolaterally at the mid-papillary level, as the muscle fiber arrangement and high mechanical stress in this area predispose to rupture.[18] Although long-term survival of free wall rupture without surgical repair has been reported,[18] mortality approaches 60% and emergent surgery should be considered in all cases.[6]

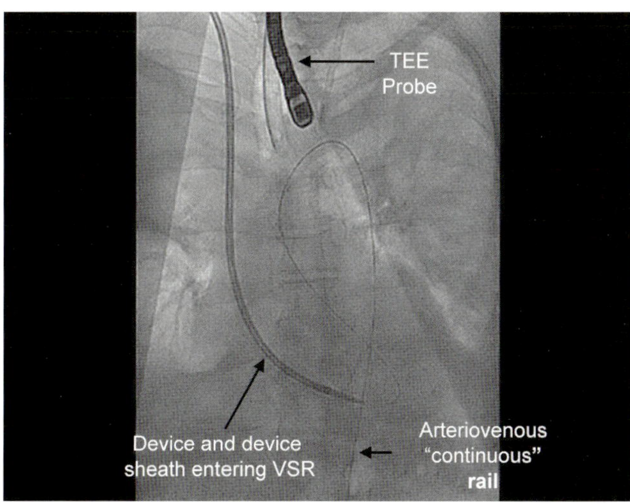


**Figure 12.5:** Fluoroscopic image of arteriovenous "rail" in transcatheter ventricular septal defect closure.
*Abbreviations:* TEE, transesophageal echocardiography; VSR, ventricular septal rupture.

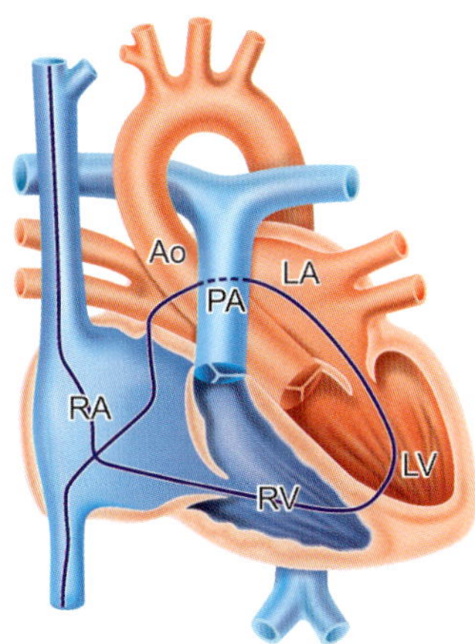


**Figure 12.6:** Diagram of venovenous "rail" in transcatheter ventricular septal defect closure. A femoral venous wire exteriorized to a second central venous access point creating a continuous venovenous "rail" as shown.
*Abbreviations:* Ao, aorta; LA, left atrium; LV, left ventricle; PA, pulmonary artery; RA, right atrium; RV, right ventricle.
Base cardiac diagram modified from Pediatric Pulmonology, Caldwell RL, Congenital heart disease: A diagramatic atlas, Liss, Inc., 1988, October 2005, *With permission from John Wiley and Sons.*

Despite surgery, postoperative mortality ranges from 23 to 35.7%.[19] A ventricular free wall rupture which does not lead to bleeding and tamponade may be contained in the pericardium, resulting in a pseudoaneurysm; it usually occurs in about one-third of cases.[18] The resulting pseudoaneurysm typically has a narrow neck and is not surrounded by any myocardium as a true aneurysm is. Because the pericardium is not a reliable tissue for containment, pseudoaneurysms are also at risk of rupturing. Untreated pseudoaneurysms may also cause cardiac compression and distal embolization from clot formation within their cavity. As with VSR repair, transcatheter approaches may play a significant role in the repair of ventricular free wall ruptures, specifically pseudoaneurysms, especially in candidates with high surgical risk. Data, again, are limited to a few case reports and even fewer case series.

In surgical closure, essentially, the pseudoaneurysm is resected, and defect is closed. Closure techniques can vary on the basis of the size of the aneurysm or chronicity. For small, wide-based aneurysms, closure may be completed with linear closure or small plication,[20] while large aneurysms can be closed with patches. For chronic pseudoaneurysms, the pseudoaneurysm may be directly closed and its fibrotic edges reinforced with teflon felt;[19] for acute cases, synthetic pericardial patches may be used to cover the defect due to friable, necrotic myocardium.[19]

In transcatheter closure techniques,[21] pseudoaneurysms may be repaired with closure devices (similar to the ones used for VSR closures), fibrin glue, and/or with thrombin-coated coil embolization. Devices can be implanted at the pseudoaneurysm orifice via a few approaches.

In a transapical approach **(Figure 12.7)**, the left ventricle is punctured percutaneously and a catheter and wire is passed through left ventricle into the pseudoaneurysm orifice, over which a delivery system is deployed. Alternatively, the pseudoaneurysm can also be punctured directly and the wire advanced through the pseudoaneurysm into the left ventricular cavity. A snare wire inserted through the femoral artery is used to exteriorize the wire in the left ventricle to the femoral artery, providing a continuous supporting rail between the anterior chest incision and the femoral artery.[21] The delivery sheath and device are then advanced from the arterial side into the pseudoaneurysm for retrograde delivery of the closure device. Alternatively, the snare wire may be used to exteriorize the system to the femoral vein via a femoral vein insertion and an atrial trans-septal puncture **(Figure 12.8)**. The delivery sheath and device in this case are advanced from the pseudoaneurysm side.

In closures using coil embolization, the neck of the defect is engaged and embolization coils are deployed into the pseudoaneurysm.[22] The coils are thrombin-coated, thus inducing clot formation in the pseudoaneurysm. Fibrin glue can also be injected into the pseudoaneurysm and the narrow neck opening closed with a closure technique as described. Coil embolization may be technically easier but may not be suitable for large pseudoaneurysms and may result in incomplete closure.[22] Septal occluder devices may require careful consideration in cases of posterobasal pseudoaneurysms and may be technically more challenging

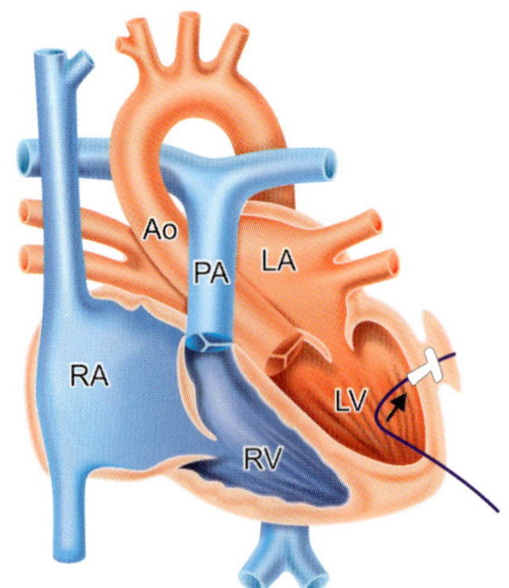


**Figure 12.7:** Diagram of transcatheter pseudoaneurysm closure, using a transapical puncture. The LV is puncture percutaneously and a wire (blue) is passed through left ventricle into the pseudoaneurysm orifice, over which a delivery system and device (gray) is deployed (arrow).
*Abbreviations:* Ao, aorta; LA, left atrium; LV, left ventricle; PA, pulmonary artery; RA, right atrium; RV, right ventricle.
Base cardiac diagram modified from Pediatric Pulmonology, Caldwell RL, Congenital heart disease: A diagramatic atlas, Liss, Inc., 1988, October 2005, *With permission from John Wiley and Sons.*

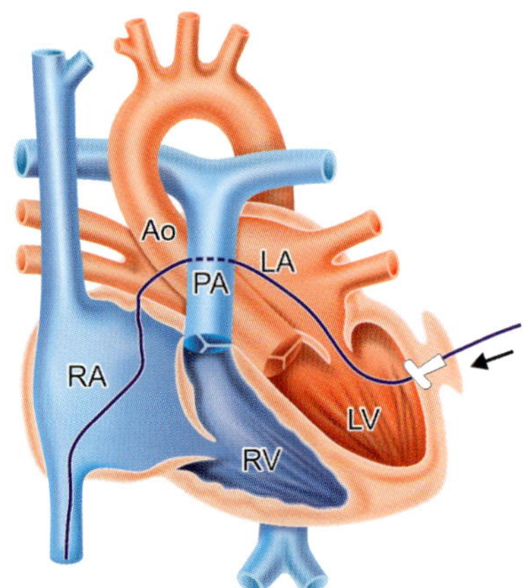


**Figure 12.8:** Diagram of transcatheter pseudoaneurysm closure, using a direct pseudoaneurysm puncture. Continuous supporting rail (blue) between the anterior chest incision into the pseudoaneurysm and the femoral vein, via an atrial transseptal puncture. The delivery sheath and device (gray) are advanced from the pseudoaneurysm side (arrow).
*Abbreviations:* Ao, aorta; LA, left atrium; LV, left ventricle; PA, pulmonary artery; RA, right atrium; RV, right ventricle.
Base cardiac diagram modified from Pediatric Pulmonology, Caldwell RL, Congenital heart disease: A diagramatic atlas, Liss, Inc., 1988, October 2005, *With permission from John Wiley and Sons.*

with greater potential for coronary or valvular damage but may result in more complete closure.[22]

In all of the described approaches, transapical or direct pseudoaneurysm puncture sites are closed with a closure device.

Potential complications of the procedure include incomplete closure, left ventricular rupture, device migration, stroke and embolic phenomenon, vascular access complications, ventricular arrhythmia, coronary artery compression, and myocardial infarction.

Dudiy et al., from our laboratory, reported 7 patients who underwent transcatheter pseudoaneurysm repair, two of which were following a myocardial infarction.[21] TEE was used in all patients, and real-time 3D TEE was used in 5 of the 7 patients. Closure was successful in all 7 patients, however, 1 patient had early device dislodgment twice and needed 2 additional transcatheter closures. Patients were followed for a mean of 18 months. Aside from the early device migrations, there were no other reported complications.[21] Kumar et al. reviewed 8 patients with pseudoaneurysm who also underwent transcatheter closure, either with occluder devices or embolization coils. All 8 patients survived, but follow-up was only for 6 months.[22] One patient had device-related occlusion of the left circumflex artery causing an acute myocardial infarction/ventricular fibrillation, treated successfully with bare metal stents to the left circumflex artery. Given the lack of adequate data, larger studies with longer follow-up are required to clearly define the outcomes, safety, and potential benefits of transcatheter closure of postinfarction pseudoaneurysms.

## Role of Three-dimensional Transesophageal Echocardiography

3D TEE plays a significant role in guiding the above described procedures for transcatheter repair of cardiac rupture.

Both transthoracic and transesophageal echocardiographic imaging are essential for initial diagnostic assessment. 3D echocardiography can better characterize the anatomical defect of ventricular septal and free wall rupture, both preprocedurally and intraprocedurally. It permits visualization of the defect in an "en face" view, which is not achievable via other real-time echocardiographic imaging techniques **(Figure 12.9)**.[17] Identifying the exact location of the rupture is essential in determining the stability of the closure device, because certain locations may not be amenable to transcatheter repair, or perhaps may be prone to certain complications (e.g. mitral and/or tricuspid

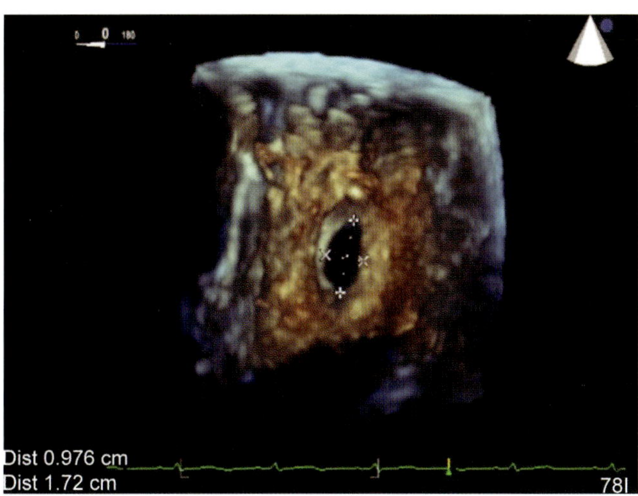


**Figure 12.9:** Three-dimensional transesophageal echocardiographic image of an "En face" view of a ventricular septal rupture.

regurgitation).[5] Despite concerns about image quality, in a small study, Chen et al. showed that the images from real-time 3D TEE had findings comparable to surgical and 2D images for VSR characterization, thus offering a way to evaluate the lesion intraoperatively without prolonging examination time.[23]

By characterizing the size and nature of the defect, 3D TEE also plays a key part in selecting the most optimal device and approach. Incorrect size selection predisposes to significant complications, including device migration or closure failure if a device is too small, or local compression, lesion expansion, or fatal rupture if a device is too large.

Intraprocedural 3D TEE also allows continuous visualization of the catheters, allowing safer device manipulation **(Figure 12.10 to 12.12)**.[24] Minimizing attempts to pass catheters through the defect may be important in preventing expansion of the size of the rupture due to the fragile nature of the surrounding necrotic tissue.[5] It may also decrease the dependence on fluoroscopy for guidance of the catheters, thereby potentially reducing both radiation exposure and contrast use.[17] Furthermore, during the procedure, continuous imaging with real-time 3D TEE enables identification of exact location of remnant shunts and/or of suboptimal device expansion. It is possible that real-time 3D TEE guidance may help prevent, or detect and adequately address some of the previously listed complications of the transcatheter repairs, such as valve damage. However, the role of intraprocedural TEE in reducing complications is currently speculative and has not yet been proven.

Limitations to 3D echocardiography include the aforementioned compromise of spatial and temporal resolution in real-time 3D images, which is improving as technology advances. Other limitations include cost, need for general anesthesia for longer cases, and specialized training required to gather accurate anatomical information from the acquired images. It may also require two operators, one manipulating the probe and the other manipulating the machine.[17]

## OTHER IMAGING MODALITIES AND FUTURE DIRECTIONS

Intracardiac echocardiography, computed tomography (CT), and both echocardiographic and CT fusion imaging are other imaging modalities being evaluated for their roles in guiding transcatheter procedures.

Though intracardiac echocardiography can obtain 3D images with a very narrow field of view, its limited resolution and very high cost associated with disposable probes have prevented its widespread use. It also requires an additional central venous access point.

Cardiac CT imaging and real-time CT imaging is also establishing a role in transcatheter cardiac interventions. In addition to providing 3D images, it has the benefits of giving coronary anatomical assessment which can be helpful in patients with coexisting coronary disease (e.g. for identifying ideal candidates for transcatheter interventions to minimize damage to neighboring epicardial vessels). The use of real-time CT has been limited, perhaps due to its high cost, significant radiation exposure, and need for contrast use, though these may be minimized as technology and software advance.

The general concept of fusion imaging consists of overlaying a CT or TEE image on top of a real-time fluoroscopic image. There is specialized software that has the ability to allow such image acquisition. Both TEE and CT fusion with fluoroscopy show great potential in transcatheter procedures. CT fusion involves fusion of a preprocedure contrast-enhanced CT image, intraprocedural noncontrast-enhanced CT-like image, and "real-time" fluoroscopic images.[25] The anatomic area of interest is marked on the preprocerdural contrast-enhanced CT image. A noncontrast-enhanced CT-like image is repeated on the fluoroscopic/angiographic system, and the resulting 3D dataset is registered to the preprocedural CT image.[25] This registration is used to overlay the initially marked area of interest onto the fluoroscopic image.[25] The fusion process is not done in real-time but is usually completed over the course of several minutes.

A similar fusion system is available for echocardiography, though the fusion of 3D TEE with fluoroscopy occurs in real-time. The TEE probe is detected by X-ray and the echocardiographic images are merged with fluoroscopy. The image orientation follows the C-arm position, so both

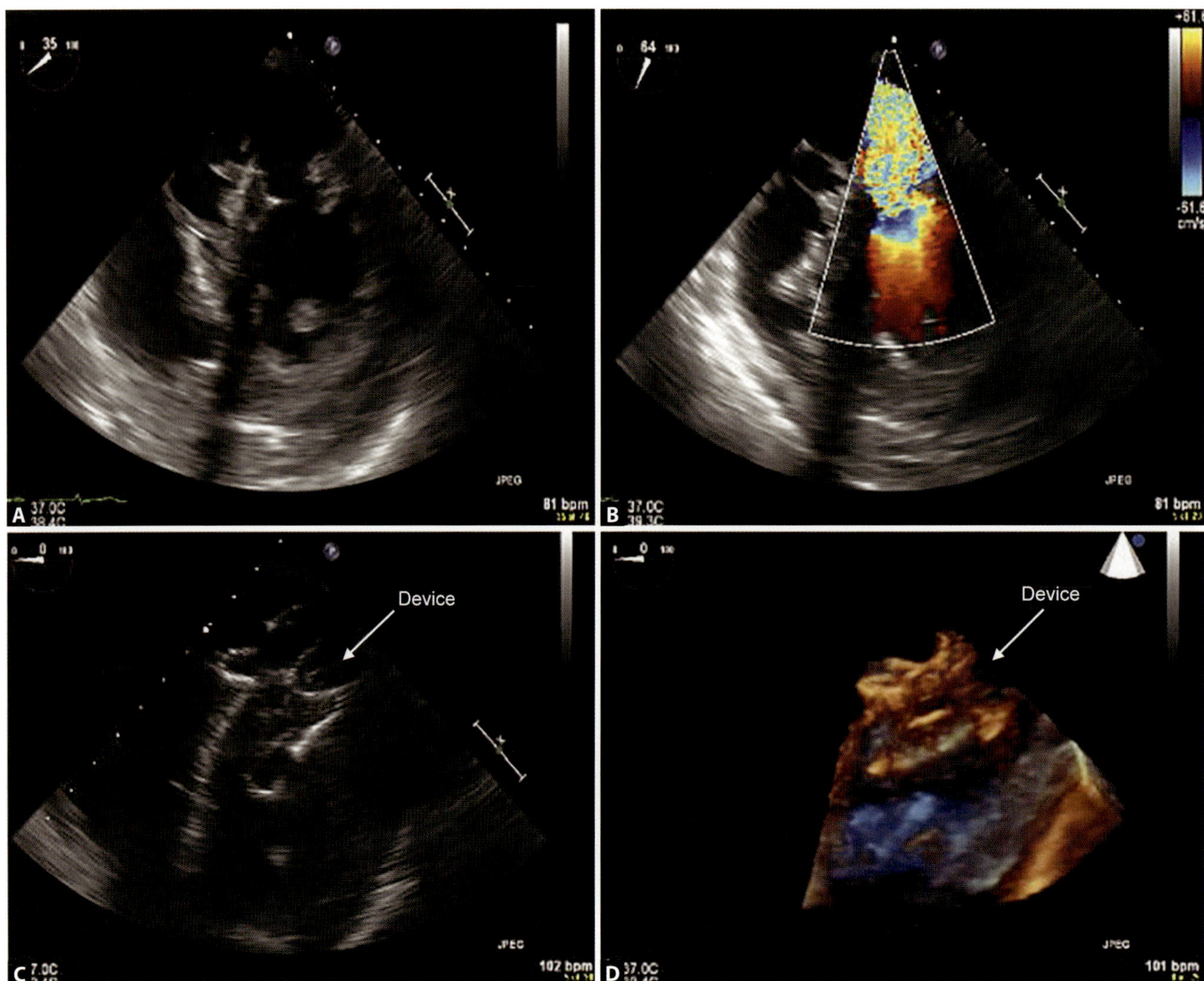


**Figure 12.10A to D:** Images from a transcatheter VSR repair, using a closure device. (A) 2D TEE image showing a communication between the right and left ventricle. (B) 2D TEE image with Doppler showing flow between the right and left ventricle via the VSR. (C) 2D TEE image showing deployed closure device. (D) 3D TEE image showing deployed closure device.
*Abbreviations:* 2D, two-dimensional; 3D, three-dimensional; TEE, transesophageal echocardiography; VSR, ventricular septal rupture.

images move synchronously. Simultaneous, unmerged echocardiographic views are displayed in real time as well. Areas of interest are marked on echocardiographic images and appear in the fluoroscopic and the fused images.

## CONCLUSION

As the demand for less invasive procedures increases, transcatheter alternatives to previously strictly surgical interventions are likely to continue to evolve. Transcatheter approaches for cardiac rupture repair may offer not only less invasive options obviating the need for cardiac bypass, but hopefully, more effective ones, as they preclude the need to stitch into friable tissue. Such procedures may also be associated with shorter length-of-stay, increased patient comfort, and subsequent decreased morbidity and mortality. 3D TEE provides valuable guidance to transcatheter repairs and may become standard of care as an adjunct during these procedures.

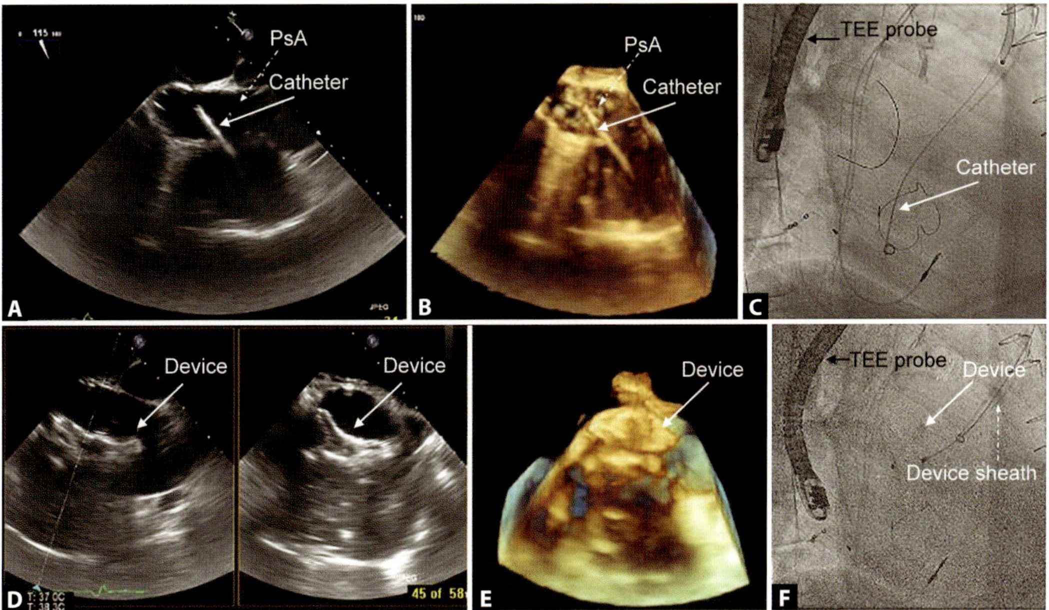


**Figure 12.11A to F:** Images from a transcatheter pseudoaneurysm (PsA) repair, using a closure device. (A to C) Compare images of the catheter engaging the PsA cavity in different imaging modalities. (D to F) Compare images of a deployed closure device at the PsA orifice in different imaging modalities. Panels A, D: two-dimensional transesophageal echocardiography (TEE); Panels B, E: three-dimensional TEE; Panel C, F, fluoroscopy.

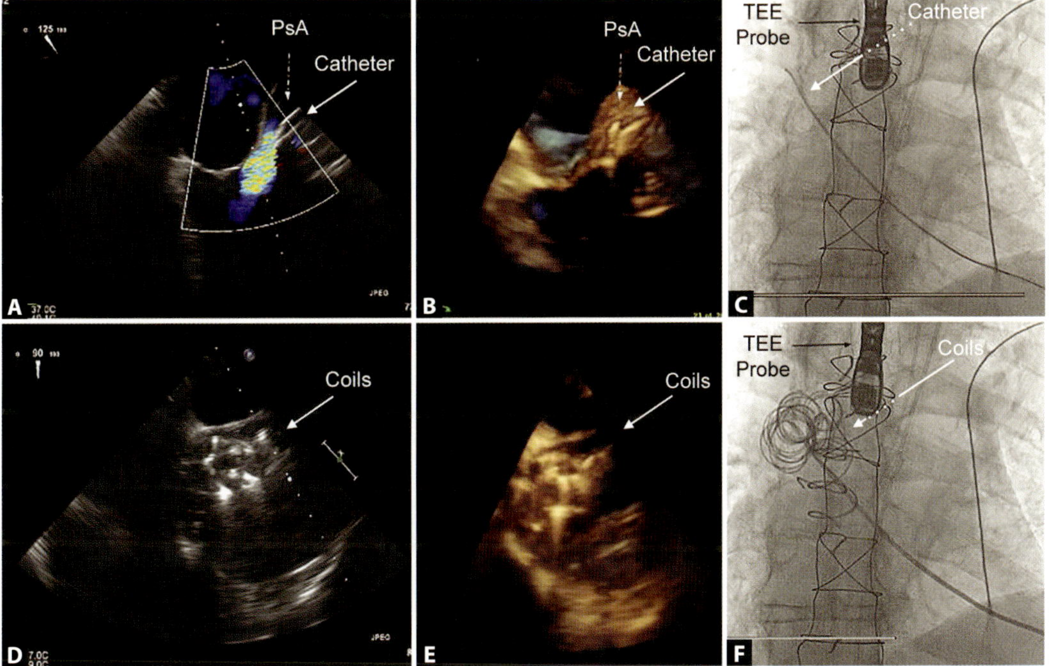


**Figure 12.12A to F:** Images from a transcatheter PsA repair, using coil embolization. (A to C) Compare images of the catheter engaging the PsA cavity in different imaging modalities. (D to F) Compare images of coils deployed in the PsA in different imaging modalities. Panels A, D: two-dimensional transesophageal echocardiography (TEE); Panels B, E: three-dimensional TEE; Panel C, F, fluoroscopy.

## REFERENCES


1. Armstrong WF, Ryan T Feigenbaum H. Feigenbaum's Echocardiography, 7th edition. Lippincott Williams and Wilkins; 2010.
2. Lang RM, Badano LP, Tsang W, Adams DH, Agricola E, Buck T, et al. American Society of Echocardiography; European Association of Echocardiography. EAE/ASE recommendations for image acquisition and display using three-dimensional echocardiography. Eur Heart J Cardiovasc Imaging. 2012; 13(1):1-46.
3. Lutter G, Lozonschi L, Ebner A, Gallo S, Marin y Kall C, Missov E, et al. First-in-human off-pump transcatheter mitral valve replacement. JACC Cardiovasc Interv. 2014;7(9):1077-8.
4. Cheung A, Webb J, Verheye S, et al. Short-term results of transapical transcatheter mitral valve implantation for mitral regurgitation. J Am Coll Cardiol. 2014;64(17):1814-9.
5. Birnbaum Y, Fishbein MC, Blanche C, et al. Ventricular septal rupture after acute myocardial infarction. N Engl J Med. 2002;347(18):1426-32.
6. O'Gara PT, Kushner FG, Ascheim DD, Casey DE Jr, Chung MK, de Lemos JA, et al. American College of Cardiology Foundation/American Heart Association Task Force on Practice Guidelines. 2013 ACCF/AHA guideline for the management of ST-elevation myocardial infarction: a report of the American College of Cardiology Foundation/American Heart Association Task Force on Practice Guidelines. Circulation. 2013;127(4):e362-425.
7. Moreyra AE, Huang MS, Wilson AC, Deng Y, Cosgrove NM, Kostis JB. MIDAS Study Group (MIDAS 13). Trends in incidence and mortality rates of ventricular septal rupture during acute myocardial infarction. Am J Cardiol. 2010;106(8):1095-100.
8. Zhu XY, Qin YW, Han YL, Zhang DZ, Wang P, Liu YF, et al. Long-term efficacy of transcatheter closure of ventricular septal defect in combination with percutaneous coronary intervention in patients with ventricular septal defect complicating acute myocardial infarction: a multicentre study. Euro Intervention. 2013;8(11):1270-6.
9. David TE, Dale L, Sun Z. Postinfarction ventricular septal rupture: repair by endocardial patch with infarct exclusion. J Thorac Cardiovasc Surg. 1995;110(5):1315-22.
10. Amplatzer Muscular VSD Occluder: A Patient's Guide to the Non-surgical closure of a muscular ventricular septal defect. St. Jude Medical Product Manual; 2012.
11. Amin Z, Cao QL, Hijazi ZM. Closure of muscular ventricular septal defects: transcatheter and hybrid techniques. Catheter Cardiovasc Interv. 2008;72(1):102-11
12. Caldwell RL. Congenital heart disease: A diagrammatic atlas. Charles E Mullins, David C Mayer (Eds). New York: Alan R. Liss, Inc., Pediatr. Pulmonol. 1989;7:190.
13. Retzer EM, Dill KE, Shah AP. Novel transcatheter closure of an iatrogenic perimembranous ventricular septal defect. Catheter Cardiovasc Interv; 2014.
14. Kronzon I, Ruiz CE, Perk G. Guidance of post myocardial infarction ventricular septal defect and pseudoaneurysm closure. Curr Cardiol Rep. 2014;16(3):456.
15. Sathananthan J, Ruygrok P. Evolution in the management of postinfarct ventricular septal defects from surgical to percutaneous approach: a single-center experience. J Invasive Cardiol. 2013;25(7):339-43.
16. Thiele H, Kaulfersch C, Daehnert I, Schoenauer M, Eitel I, Borger M, et al. Immediate primary transcatheter closure of postinfarction ventricular septal defects. Eur Heart J. 2009;30(1):81-8.
17. Perk G, Lang RM, Garcia-Fernandez MA, Lodato J, Sugeng L, Lopez J, et al. Use of real time three-dimensional trans-esophageal echocardiography in intracardiac catheter based interventions. J Am Soc Echocardiogr. 2009;22(8):865-82.
18. Birnbaum Y, Chamoun AJ, Anzuini A, Lick SD, Ahmad M, Uretsky BF. Ventricular free wall rupture following acute myocardial infarction. Coron Artery Dis. 2003;14(6): 463-70.
19. Villanueva C, Milder D, Manganas C. Ruptured left ventricular false aneurysm following acute myocardial infarction: case report and review of the literature. Heart Lung Circ. 2014 Aug 4. pii: S1443-9506(14)00627-1. doi: 10.1016/j.hlc.2014.07.069. [Epub ahead of print] PubMed PMID: 25150648.
20. Chen X, Qiu ZB, Xu M, Liu LL, Jiang YS, Wang LM. Surgery for left ventricular aneurysm after myocardial infarction: techniques selection and results assessment. Chin Med J (Engl). 2012;125(24):4373-9.
21. Dudiy Y, Jelnin V, Einhorn BN, Kronzon I, Cohen HA, Ruiz CE. Percutaneous closure of left ventricular pseudoaneurysm. Circ Cardiovasc Interv. 2011;4(4):322-6.
22. Kumar PV, Alli O, Bjarnason H, Hagler DJ, Sundt TM, Rihal CS. Percutaneous therapeutic approaches to closure of cardiac pseudoaneurysms. Catheter Cardiovasc Interv. 2012; 80(4):687-99.
23. Chen FL, Hsiung MC, Nanda N, Hsieh KS, Chou MC. Real time three-dimensional echocardiography in assessing ventricular septal defects: an echocardiographic-surgical correlative study. Echocardiography. 2006;23(7):562-8.
24. Halpern DG, Perk G, Ruiz C, Marino N, Kronzon I. Percutaneous closure of a post-myocardial infarction ventricular septal defect guided by real-time three-dimensional echocardiography. Eur J Echocardiogr. 2009;10(4):569-71.
25. Krishnaswamy A, Tuzcu EM, Kapadia SR. Integration of MDCT and fluoroscopy using C-arm computed tomography to guide structural cardiac interventions in the cardiac catheterization laboratory. Catheter Cardiovasc Interv; 2014.

# Stress Echocardiography for Detection of Myocardial Ischemia and Guiding Treatment in Stable Coronary Artery Disease

13
CHAPTER

*Rahul Mehrotra, Ravi R Kasliwal*

## INTRODUCTION

The noninvasive diagnosis of obstructive coronary artery disease (CAD) rests on the demonstration of stress-induced myocardial ischemia. Echocardiography is one of the most commonly utilized imaging modalities for this purpose. Since its first use three decades ago, stress echocardiography has steadily gained in popularity and has undergone extensive evaluation in different patient subsets and populations for diagnosis and prognostication of patients with suspected or known CAD. Owing to the inherent advantages associated with the modality of echocardiography (its noninvasive nature, lack of ionizing radiation, portability, and ease of use), it can be easily combined with the stress modalities (exercise as well as pharmacological agents) in a variety of clinical settings. The result is available immediately and at almost no discomfort to the patient. In recent times, the advances in imaging with the use of harmonics and injection of ultrasound contrast have led to improvements in detection of endocardial excursion, thereby resulting in enhanced diagnostic accuracy. Incorporation of deformation imaging and three-dimensional (3D) echocardiography has added an altogether new dimension to the performance and interpretation of stress echocardiography. Besides these advances and its excellent diagnostic accuracy and prognostic power, it remains one of the most cost effective methods compared to other imaging modalities for the purpose of diagnosis and risk stratification of patients with known or suspected CAD.

Stress echocardiography can be used to answer several questions in a patient of known or suspected CAD. It is generally not recommended to be used in asymptomatic patients with low pretest probability of CAD as a routine screening test.[1] In certain situations, however, stress echocardiography may be warranted even in asymptomatic patients. These include patients who undergo computed tomographic coronary angiography and are found to have high coronary calcium score (typically >400 Agatston units), or shown to have borderline significant coronary stenosis (50–70% luminal narrowing), or are found to have elevated or rising in cardiac biomarker levels in absence of any other evidence of an acute coronary event, or in whom a screening exercise electrocardiography (ECG) reveals intermediate to high Duke score. Before cardiac stress testing is advised in patients without known CAD, an estimate of the likelihood of presence of CAD should be made. This is known as pretest probability and can be determined using several clinical parameters (age, gender, symptoms, risk factors for CAD, prior history of myocardial infarction (MI), presence of ECG changes, etc.). Several algorithms are also available, which help in estimation of pretest probability of CAD in a given patient. This is also a useful approach in interpretation of the results of stress test after it has been performed.[2-4] In general, cardiac stress testing is not useful in patients with low-pretest probability of CAD and should not be performed.

The common indications for performing stress echocardiography are as follows:

- For patients with known CAD
  - Patients with a history of previous MI.
  - Patients with recent low-risk acute coronary syndrome, planned to undergo conservative management.
  - In patients with angiographically proven CAD to determine physiological significance of stenosis.
  - Previously stable patients of chronic angina with change in symptomatic status.
  - Previously revascularized patients who become symptomatic.
  - For assessment of myocardial viability.
- For patients with suspected CAD
  - When stress ECG is not interpretable or likely to be false-positive (e.g. resting nonspecific ST/T wave changes on ECG, in middle-aged women, left bundle-branch block (LBBB) or pre-excitation on ECG and presence of left ventricular hypertrophy (LVH) with strain pattern on ECG.
  - When stress ECG cannot be performed as the patient is unable to exercise (e.g. orthopedic, neurological, or psychological reasons). Pharmacological stress test should be performed in such cases.

  - When stress ECG has been performed and is likely to be false-positive or there is intermediate probability of CAD based on Duke treadmill score.
  - In patients with typical symptoms and intermediate to high pretest probability of CAD.
  - In patients without typical angina but with dyspnea on exertion to determine the cause.
- Risk stratification of patients going in for major noncardiac surgery.

## METHODOLOGY OF STRESS ECHOCARDIOGRAPHY

As mentioned earlier, stress echocardiography includes using a stressing modality-either with the use of exercise or pharmacological agents (like dobutamine or dipyridamole) and imaging by echocardiography. The fundamental principle behind stress echocardiography is comparison of images acquired at rest, before stress, to the images at peak stress for detection of stress-induced regional wall motion abnormalities (RWMA) **(Videos 13.1 and 13.2)**. Pharmacological stress echocardiography also entails imaging at every stage of increasing dose and late into recovery thereby offering a unique opportunity for detection of early wall-motion abnormalities and for use in viability testing. In addition, recovery images are also useful for detection of ischemia in some patients with LVH in whom dobutamine-induced reduction in LV cavity size reduces wall stress and masks ischemia. In such patients, impairment of contractility does not occur at peak dobutamine dose but becomes easily apparent during recovery phase **(Video 13.3)**.

The pathophysiology of stress-induced myocardial ischemia due to stress, demand supply mismatch due to coronary stenosis, and the effects of progressive ischemia on ECG, echocardiographically determined diastolic and systolic function and its interpretation have been dealt with elsewhere in the book. The current chapter essentially focuses on the clinical significance of stress echocardiography in patients of chronic angina.

## CLINICAL UTILITY OF STRESS ECHOCARDIOGRAPHY

Stress echocardiography is useful in detection of myocardial ischemia and prognostication of patients with chronic angina. Before we compare stress echocardiography with other modalities, which can be used in a patient with chronic stable angina like stress ECG and stress myocardial perfusion imaging, it would be pertinent to point out certain unique features of stress echocardiography where it cannot be compared to other modalities at all.

Stress ECG does not help in detection of resting wall motion abnormalities or previous MI in a given patient as the ECG is notoriously unreliable in this respect. Apart from detection of stress-induced myocardial ischemia, the use of echocardiography provides additional information about the presence and extent of RWMA, LV systolic and diastolic function, valvular abnormalities, pulmonary pressures, etc. at rest and at peak-stress, which are of immense help in guiding patient management. Sometimes, the incidental detection of RWMA, significant valvular disease, pericardial disease (effusion or constriction), elevated pulmonary artery systolic pressure, congenital anomalies (like atrial septal defects), cardiomyopathies or aortic dissection on resting imaging obviate the need for performing the stress test and avoiding serious potential complications. It may thus diagnose the clinical problem responsible for the patients' symptoms and guide proper management. These advantages are not available even with perfusion imaging. Besides, the clinical safety, rapidity, repeatability and lack of ionizing radiation are other advantages of stress echocardiography.

### Stress Echocardiography for Detection of Myocardial Ischemia

Diagnostic accuracy of stress tests is determined by comparing it with the "gold standard" for diagnosis of coronary artery disease-coronary angiography. The accuracy thus depends on the ability to detect angiographically significant coronary artery disease, defined as presence of plaques with diameter stenosis of at least 50–70%. This approach has several limitations. The fundamental problem is the fact that it is comparison of a physiological techniques with an anatomic index of coronary disease. It is not only the severity of the stenosis but also numerous other factors which determine that physiological significance of the stenosis and whether the given lesion/lesions will produce myocardial ischemia upon stress. These include the stenosis length, site, and presence, adequacy or absence of collateral flow.[5] Another key factor is the use of different cutoffs for defining angiographic severity of the disease in different studies.[6] The sensitivity of detection of the disease at stress echocardiography is likely to be higher when higher cutoff is used for defining the disease at angiography. In contrast, a lower cut-off will adversely affect sensitivity though specificity may improve.

In general, stress echocardiography compares well with other modalities for detection of myocardial ischemia in patients with chronic angina. Large volume of data is available comparing the various stress tests in different scenarios and patient subsets. It should be pointed out that all modalities differ in the diagnostic accuracy for detection of myocardial ischemia in different patient subsets. Therefore, the comparisons of diagnostic accuracy should be made keeping in mind this fact. Having said that, in general the sensitivity and specificity of stress ECG based on a number of studies is in the range of 63–68% and 74–77% respectively.[7] Stress echocardiography is known to have significantly higher diagnostic accuracy in comparison to this. The difference is much more pronounced if data of patients with LVH[8] or data in women[9] is compared.

The overall diagnostic accuracy of stress perfusion imaging is comparable to that of stress echocardiography (80–84%) with a higher sensitivity (80–88% vs. 86–98%) but lower specificity (77–82% vs. 36–71%)[10-13] of stress perfusion imaging for detection of myocardial ischemia.

Stress magnetic resonance imaging (MRI) on the other hand has been shown to be superior to both, nuclear stress testing and stress echo-cardiography with a sensitivity of 90%, specificity of 81% and overall diagnostic accuracy of 87%.[14]

## *Adjunctive Techniques*

It is worth pointing out that most of this data is based on segmental wall-motion analysis alone and is from the time period before the advent of certain adjunctive techniques of echocardiography. The advent of techniques like the use of coronary flow reserve assessment, contrast imaging, triplane imaging using 3D echocardiography, tissue velocity and strain measurement has added a new dimension to the utility of stress echocardiography in detection of myocardial ischemia. For example, it is feasible to visualize blood flow in left anterior descending artery in the anterior interventricular groove and measure coronary flow reserve following intravenous infusion of adenosine or dipyridamole. Combining this with wall-motion analysis has been shown to improve the sensitivity and overall diagnostic accuracy of stress echocardiography for detection of coronary artery disease, particularly when the disease is less severe.[13,15] Similarly, the use of ultrasound contrast improves endocardial visualization, thereby resulting in better visualization of wall-motion abnormalities and improved diagnostic accuracy of the test.[16] Since it is useful in patients with poor acoustic windows, the use of LV cavity contrast is recommended by the American Society of Echocardiography in stress echocardiography, whenever 2 or more LV myocardial segments are not clearly visualized.[17] Ultrasound contrast also permits assessment of myocardial perfusion, not otherwise feasible with conventional echocardiography. The value of myocardial contrast perfusion imaging for detection of coronary artery disease is discussed in greater detail in the subsequent chapter.

The interpretation of wall-motion abnormalities developing during stress testing depends on the expertise of the observer and thus is quite subjective. Several techniques for objective assessment of myocardial contractile function, such as tissue velocity and strain imaging have been developed to overcome this limitation. Initial studies utilized myocardial tissue velocity as the measure of myocardial function. While these studies showed some promise,[18-20] tissue velocity was not found to be much reliable because it only measured velocity of the myocardium relative to the transducer and not true myocardial deformation. In comparison, strain imaging measures actual myocardial deformation and has therefore become the modality of choice for assessing myocardial contractile function. Strain imaging can be either Doppler-based or gray-scale-based, which is also called speckle-tracking echocardiography. Both forms of strain imaging can be combined with stress echocardiography, and with both forms of stress (i.e. exercise or pharmacological). Doppler-based strain imaging has high frame rate which makes it suitable for peak-stress imaging but it has several limitations such as angle dependency, poor signal-to-noise ratio and is also technically more demanding. Speckle tracking echocardiography overcomes these limitations but is dependent on good quality gray-scale images.

Several different strain parameters have been used for assessment of inducible myocardial ischemia. Of these, reduced peak systolic strain with or without increased post-systolic shortening has been the most commonly studied measurement. Voigt et al. studied 44 patients with known or suspected coronary artery disease.[21,22] They found that the ratio of postsystolic strain to peak strain was the most predictive of inducible ischemia. A cut-off of 35% yielded 82% sensitivity and 85% specificity for detection of significant coronary stenosis, as compared to 81% and 82% respectively for wall-motion analysis.[4] Ingul et al. evaluated a strategy of automated deformation analysis in 197 patients undergoing dobutamine echocardiography.[23] It was found that both peak-systolic strain rate and end-systolic strain had much higher sensitivity for detection of inducible ischemia as compared to wall-motion analysis alone (~87%, ~87% and 75% respectively). Several other systolic phase parameters, including LV torsion, have also been shown to be useful for detection of myocardial ischemia.[24]

Apart from the systolic phase abnormalities, diastolic phase strain parameters have also been evaluated for detection of myocardial ischemia. Early diastolic relaxation is an active, energy-demanding process and is therefore highly susceptible to myocardial ischemia. Accordingly, impairment of early myocardial relaxation is the first functional abnormality to develop with the onset of myocardial ischemia. On strain imaging, it can be identified either as reduced early diastolic untwist rate or as impaired decay of end-systolic strain. In a recent study involving 162 patients with stable effort angina, the extent of strain decay during the first third of diastole was measured and quantified as strain imaging diastolic index.[25] Not only was this parameter found to be highly accurate for detection of inducible ischemia, it was also observed that the impairment of diastolic decay of strain persisted for several minutes after cessation of stress. A cutoff value of 0.74 for the ratio of pre- and 5 minutes post-exercise strain imaging diastolic index was found to have 97% and a specificity of 93% for detection of significant coronary stenosis. From imaging stand-point, such 'diastolic stunning' offers a great advantage, particularly after exercise stress, as it greatly minimizes the impact of delay in poststress image acquisition on the sensitivity of the test.

The relative diagnostic accuracy of the Doppler-based and the gray scale-based strain imaging for detection of myocardial ischemia has also been evaluated. Hanekom et al. compared the two modalities in 150 patients undergoing dobutamine echocardiography and coronary angiography.[26] It was found that both these techniques had comparable diagnostic accuracy for detection of coronary stenosis in the anterior circulation (i.e. in the left anterior descending coronary artery). However, when the stenosis was located in the posterior circulation, Doppler-based strain was much more accurate than the gray-scale based strain.[27]

The above data suggest that incorporation of strain imaging in routine stress echocardiography has the potential to improve the diagnostic accuracy of the test and reduce intra- and interobserver variability. However, it must be noted that segmental strain analysis still has considerable variability which limits its widespread use in routine clinical practice.

One of the fundamental requirements for accurate determination of stress induced myocardial ischemia by stress echocardiography is to capture several images of the LV, from different windows, immediately post stress (within 90 seconds). The wall-motion abnormalities produced resolve if there is any delay in capturing the images. This is one of the key technical factors in optimal performance of exercise stress echocardiography. With the advent of matrix array 3D transducers, it is now possible to capture the entire LV volume from apical imaging, obviating the need to move the transducer for capturing different views and also avoiding foreshortening. The other advantage is that there is no need of separate transducers for capturing two-dimensional (2D) images, 3D images and Doppler data. The new generation transducers are capable of all these functions and allow capturing good quality images very quickly at high frame rates. It is thus, less dependent on operator skills and experience.[28] It has also been shown to be very useful in conjunction with dobutamine stress echocardiography and saves lot of time and effort of the echocardiographer.[29,30] The incorporation of these techniques in routine stress echocardiography will likely result in better diagnostic accuracy but more studies with different subsets are needed before the actual incremental value of these techniques can be determined.

The diagnostic accuracy of stress tests also depends on several other variables like the acoustic window, female gender, expertise of the operator, the extent, distribution and severity of CAD, etc. We therefore discuss the diagnostic accuracy of stress echocardiography in light of all these factors.

## *Stress Echocardiography in Women*

It has been well known that women with chest pain are a technically challenging group. They generally have smaller stature with small heart size and due to breast tissue, are not easy to image by nuclear scintigraphy. Also, women more commonly have ST segment T-wave changes in ECG that interfere with performance and interpretation of exercise electrocardiography tracings. Young and middle-aged women also have lesser prevalence and extent of CAD as compared to men. Hormonal influences are also responsible for occurrence of false positive ECG changes following exercise stress testing.[31] For all these reasons, stress echocardiography has been shown to be more accurate than exercise ECG in women. In a study involving only women, exercise echocardiography had much higher specificity (80% vs. 64%) and diagnostic accuracy (81% vs. 64%) for detection of CAD as compared to exercise ECG.[32] It was also shown in this study that since the use of stress echocardiography helped avoid unnecessary coronary angiography, it also proved to be the most cost-effective approach to diagnose CAD in women.

## *Factors Influencing the Accuracy of Stress Echocardiography*

*Technical factors:* Accurate interpretation of stress-induced wall-motion abnormalities depends of several factors inherent in the technique itself. For example, RWMA confined only to the lateral wall of LV may be missed or incorrectly labeled because lateral wall is aligned parallel to the ultrasound beam in apical views. As such, the interpretation should be based on use of harmonic imaging, analyzing wall motion in multiple views and by adjusting lateral gain setting. As discussed previously, the use of contrast for LV opacification (LVO) is also very useful in this scenario.[33,34]

Similarly, the performing physician should be well aware of the fact that in some patients, the presence of membranous septum may falsely give an impression of apparent RWMA in the basal inferoseptal region. This should also be resolved by corroborating in different views. Basal segment of the inferior wall may also often appear to be hypokinetic owing to tethering due to the mitral valve and also may not be adequately visualized due to shadowing by papillary muscles. This may result in false-positive results.

Inadequate performance of stress and resulting in false negative result is a frequently encountered problem in clinical practice. Stress-induced wall-motion abnormalities are produced only on performing significant, sustained myocardial ischemia by adequate level of stress. This is based on the concept of ischemic cascade, according to which, wall-motion abnormalities appear after reduction in perfusion and ECG changes appear even later than that.[35] The type of stressor also determines the level of workload achieved. Since upright exercise results in greater increase in cardiac workload and hence stress, as compared to bicycle ergometry or dobutamine-stress echocardiography, exercise echocardiography is generally the preferred modality if the patient is able to exercise optimally.[36] Also, during pharmacological stress testing, use of antianginal therapy like beta-blockers and dose-limiting side effects of the stress agents (dobutamine), may compromise ability to develop significant ischemia and thus adversely affect the sensitivity of the test.[37] In some situations where pharmacological stress testing is a better option (for example, when viability is also to be determined), atropine injection should be added when target heart rate cannot be achieved otherwise.[38]

The skill, expertise, and the level of competence of the person performing and interpreting stress echocardiograms is also a key factor determining the accuracy of the results, since it is a subjective observer-dependent technique. As discussed above, incorporation of techniques like strain imaging is useful in this regard. Also, several simple methods like regular upgradation of training, development of adherence protocols, joint reading sessions for interpretation of the results, help in ensuring greater degree of accuracy and less variability in the results.[39,40]

*Patient-related factors:* Imaging by echocardiography is critically dependent on availability of good images, which depends on presence of good acoustic windows. This becomes very important in case of stress echocardiography where images with good endocardial definition of the entire LV have to be acquired at high-heart rates.

Poor image quality thus significantly compromises accuracy and the reproducibility of the stress echocardiography, particularly for the assessment of the extent of the disease.[41] Common reasons like obesity, pulmonary disease and chest deformities are responsible for sub-optimal images in almost one-third of the patients.[42] The LVO with the use of contrast is a useful adjunct in some of these cases.

The presence of underlying disease states like LVH, resting RWMA, LBBB pattern, and pacemaker rhythm significantly alters the accuracy of stress echocardiography. An LVH with small LV cavity size can produce both false-positive and false-negative results.[43,44] Resting wall-motion abnormalities make it difficult to interpret the development of stress-induced abnormalities in different segments accurately and sensitively. Perfusion imaging has been shown to be the best option in these patients.[45] Rhythm abnormalities like LBBB or pacemaker also make interpretation of RWMA difficult for the same reason. In a large meta-analysis of around 50 studies involving stress echocardiography and stress perfusion imaging, stress echocardiography emerged as the most specific technique with highest accuracy (84%) as compared to stress ECG and stress perfusion imaging.[46] Pharmacological stress echocardiography with dobutamine is superior to exercise stress echocardiography in this regard.

## Stress Echocardiography for Prognostication

Stress echocardiography provides useful prognostic information in patients with stable CAD in addition to detecting myocardial ischemia. The prognostic information provided by stress echocardiography is incremental to the information available from the patient's clinical examination, resting ECG, exercise ECG, and resting LV systolic function determined by echocardiography.[47]

In addition, the prognostic power of stress echocardiography (both exercise and dobutamine) is comparable to nuclear imaging using the same stress modality. For example, in patients who cannot exercise, a positive-dobutamine stress echocardiogram and a positive nuclear stress test are associated with a similar annual cardiac mortality rate of 2.5%.[48] Apart from the status of positivity, other variables like presence of resting RWMA, wall-motion score index (WMSI) at maximal stress, change in LV ejection fraction with exercise and LV end-systolic volume at maximal stress further add to the prognostic power of a positive stress echocardiogram.[49-51]

Just as in resting echocardiogram, LV volume and ejection fraction changes at peak stress are powerful predictors of future cardiovascular events. In a study of more than 2000 patients of at least 65 years of age, it was demonstrated that lack of reduction of LV end-systolic volume, increase in LV end-systolic volume at peak stress, and failure to increase or subnormal peak exercise LV ejection fraction are independent predictors of cardiac death or nonfatal MI.[52] In another large study involving more than 5000 patients subjected to stress echocardiography, exercise WMSI was shown to be the strongest predictor of cardiac events over a mean follow-up of 3.2 years.[53] The WMSI is a useful objective tool for prognosis. The greater the WMSI, greater is the risk.

# SUMMARY

In clinical practice, when faced with patients of stable CAD, the purpose of management is to detect the presence of myocardial ischemia, assess the severity, determine the risk of future cardiac events and decide upon the need of myocardial revascularization in spite of optimal medical therapy. All this needs to be done keeping in mind the safety of the patient, feasibility and in a cost-effective manner. Stress echocardiography can do all this quite effectively and guide the clinician in decision making. The inherent advantages of echocardiography like safety, portability, ease of use, less cost and less demanding infrastructure needs, widespread availability as compared to other imaging tools like MRI and nuclear scanning, along with robust data, make it the best option for comprehensive assessment of patients of stable CAD. The use of adjunctive techniques like contrast, 3D, and deformation imaging are likely to further improve the utility and accuracy of this technique.

## VIDEO LEGENDS

**Video 13.1:** Dobutamine stress echocardiography showing significant inducible ischemia in left anterior descending artery territory. Compared with the baseline image (upper left), there is impairment of contractility in the septal and apical segments at low-dose itself (upper right) which becomes much more apparent at peak-dose dobutamine (lower left).

**Video 13.2:** Apical two-chamber view from the same patient as in Video 13.1. Inducible ischemia is easily apparent in the anterior wall and apex. Basal and mid-inferior wall is akinetic at baseline itself which is suggestive of previous infarct.

**Video 13.3:** Significance of recovery images in assessment of myocardial ischemia. In this patient, because of significant left ventricular hypertrophy and reduction in left ventricular cavity size with dobutamine, inducible ischemia is not apparent at peak-dose (lower left) but becomes glaring during recovery phase (lower right).

## REFERENCES


1. Douglas PS, Garcia MJ, Haines DE, et al. ACCF/ASE/AHA/ASNC/HFSA/HRS/SCAI/SCCM/SCCT/SCMR 2011 appropriate use criteria for echocardiography. A Report of the American College of Cardiology Foundation Appropriate use Criteria Task Force, American Society of Echocardiography, American Heart Association, American Society of Nuclear Cardiology, Heart Failure Society of America, Heart Rhythm Society, Society for Cardiovascular Angiography and Interventions, Society of Critical Care Medicine, Society of Cardiovascular Computed Tomography, and Society for Cardiovascular Magnetic Resonance Endorsed by the American College of Chest Physicians. J Am Coll Cardiol. 2011;57:1126-66.
2. McCully RB, Roger VL, Mahoney DW, et al. Outcome after normal exercise echocardiography and predictors of subsequent cardiac events: Follow-up of 1,325 patients. J Am Coll Cardiol. 1998;31:144-9.
3. Pryor DB, Harrell FE Jr, Lee KL, et al. Estimating the likelihood of significant coronary artery disease. Am J Med. 1983;75:771-80.
4. Gibbons RJ. ACC/AHA 2002 guideline update for the management of patients with chronic stable angina--summary article: A report of the American College of Cardiology/American Heart Association Task Force on Practice Guidelines (Committee on the Management of Patients with Chronic Stable Angina). Circulation. 2003;107:149-58.
5. Gould KL. Percent coronary stenosis: battered gold standard, pernicious relic or clinical practicality? J Am Coll Cardiol. 1988;11:886-8.
6. Baptista J, Arnese M, Roelandt JR, et al. Quantitative coronary angiography in the estimation of the functional significance of coronary stenosis: correlations with dobutamine-atropine stress test. J Am Coll Cardiol. 1994;23:1434-9.
7. Garber AM, Solomon NA. Cost-effectiveness of alternative test strategies for the diagnosis of coronary artery disease. Ann Intern Med. 1999;130:719-28.
8. Marwick TH, Torelli J, Harjai K, et al. Influence of left ventricular hypertrophy on detection of coronary artery disease using exercise echocardiography. J Am Coll Cardiol. 1995;26:1180-6.
9. Marwick TH, Anderson T, Williams MJ, et al. Exercise echocardiography is an accurate and cost-efficient technique for detection of coronary artery disease in women. J Am Coll Cardiol. 1995;26:335-41.
10. Fragasso G, Lu C, Dabrowski P, Pagnotta P, Sheiban I, Chierchia SL. Comparison of stress/rest myocardial perfusion tomography, dipyridamole and dobutamine stress echocardiography for the detection of coronary disease in hypertensive patients with chest pain and positive exercise test. J Am Coll Cardiol. 1999;34:441-7.
11. Kim C, Kwok YS, Heagerty P, et al. Pharmacologic stress testing for coronary disease diagnosis: a meta-analysis. Am Heart J. 2001;142:934-44.
12. Fleischmann KE, Hunink MG, Kuntz KM, et al. Exercise echocardiography or exercise spect imaging? A meta-analysis of diagnostic test performance. JAMA. 1998;280:913-20.
13. Marwick T, Willemart B, D'Hondt AM, et al. Selection of the optimal nonexercise stress for the evaluation of ischemic regional myocardial dysfunction and malperfusion. Comparison of dobutamine and adenosine using echocardiography and 99mTc-MIBI single photon emission computed tomography. Circulation. 1993;87:345-54.
14. Arnold JR, Karamitsos TD, Pegg TJ, et al. Adenosine stress myocardial contrast echocardiography for the detection of coronary artery disease: a comparison with coronary angiography and cardiac magnetic resonance. JACC Cardiovasc Imaging. 2010;3:934-43.
15. Gaibazzi N, Rigo F, Reverberi C. Detection of coronary artery disease by combined assessment of wall motion, myocardial perfusion and coronary flow reserve: a multiparametric contrast stress-echocardiography study. J Am Soc Echocardiogr. 2010;23:1242-50.
16. Plana JC, Mikati IA, Dokainish H, et al. A randomized cross-over study for evaluation of the effect of image optimization with contrast on the diagnostic accuracy of dobutamine

echocardiography in coronary artery disease the optimize trial. JACC Cardiovasc Imaging. 2008;1:145-52.

17. Pellikka PA, Nagueh SF, Elhendy AA, et al. American Society of Echocardiography recommendations for performance, interpretation, and application of stress echocardiography. J Am Soc Echocardiogr. 2007;20:1021-41.
18. Fathi R, Cain P, Nakatani S, et al. Effect of tissue Doppler on the accuracy of novice and expert interpreters of dobutamine echocardiography. Am J Cardiol. 2001;88:400-5.
19. Cain P, Baglin T, Case C, Spicer D, Short L, Marwick TH. Application of tissue Doppler to interpretation of dobutamine echocardiography and comparison with quantitative coronary angiography. Am J Cardiol. 2001;87:525-31.
20. Cain P, Short L, Baglin T, Case C, Bosch HG, Marwick TH. Development of a fully quantitative approach to the interpretation of stress echocardiography using radial and longitudinal myocardial velocities. J Am Soc Echocardiogr. 2002;15:759-67.
21. Voigt JU, Exner B, Schmiedehausen K, et al. Strain-rate imaging during dobutamine stress echocardiography provides objective evidence of inducible ischemia. Circulation. 2003;107:2120-6.
22. Voigt JU, Nixdorff U, Bogdan R, et al. Comparison of deformation imaging and velocity imaging for detecting regional inducible ischaemia during dobutamine stress echocardiography. Eur Heart J. 2004;25:1517-25.
23. Ingul CB, Stoylen A, Slordahl SA, Wiseth R, Burgess M, Marwick TH. Automated analysis of myocardial deformation at dobutamine stress echocardiography: An angiographic validation. J Am Coll Cardiol. 2007;49:1651-9.
24. Bansal M, Leano RL, Marwick TH. Clinical assessment of left ventricular systolic torsion: Effects of myocardial infarction and ischemia. J Am Soc Echocardiogr. 2008;21:887-94.
25. Ishii K, Imai M, Suyama T, et al. Exercise-induced post-ischemic left ventricular delayed relaxation or diastolic stunning: Is it a reliable marker in detecting coronary artery disease? J Am Coll Cardiol. 2009;53:698-705.
26. Hanekom L, Cho GY, Leano R, et al. Comparison of two-dimensional speckle and tissue Doppler strain measurement during dobutamine stress echocardiography: an angiographic correlation. Eur Heart J. 2007;28:1765-72.
27. Voigt JU, Arnold MF, Karlsson M, et al. Assessment of regional longitudinal myocardial strain rate derived from doppler myocardial imaging indexes in normal and infarcted myocardium. J Am Soc Echocardiogr. 2000;13:588-98.
28. Abusaid GH, Ahmad M. Real time three-dimensional stress echocardiography advantages and limitations. Echocardiography. 2012;29:200-6.
29. Hanekom L, Jenkins C, Jeffries L, et al. Incremental value of strain rate analysis as an adjunct to wall-motion scoring for assessment of myocardial viability by dobutamine echocardiography: a follow-up study after revascularization. Circulation. 2005;112:3892-900.
30. Eroglu E, D'Hooge J, Herbots L, et al. Comparison of real-time tri-plane and conventional 2D dobutamine stress echocardiography for the assessment of coronary artery disease. Eur Heart J. 2006;27:1719-24.
31. Bokhari S, Bergmann SR. The effect of estrogen compared to estrogen plus progesterone on the exercise electrocardiogram. J Am Coll Cardiol. 2002;40:1092-6.
32. Marwick TH, Anderson T, Williams MJ, et al. Exercise echocardiography is an accurate and cost-efficient technique for detection of coronary artery disease in women. J Am Coll Cardiol. 1995;26:335-41.
33. Hoffmann R, Marwick TH, Poldermans D, et al. Refinements in stress echocardiographic techniques improve inter-institutional agreement in interpretation of dobutamine stress echocardiograms. Eur Heart J. 2002;23:821-9.
34. Dolan MS, Riad K, El-Shafei A, et al. Effect of intravenous contrast for left ventricular opacification and border definition on sensitivity and specificity of dobutamine stress echocardiography compared with coronary angiography in technically difficult patients. Am Heart J. 2001;142: 908-15.
35. Nesto RW, Kowalchuk GJ. The ischemic cascade: temporal sequence of hemodynamic, electrocardiographic and symptomatic expressions of ischemia. Am J Cardiol. 1987;59: 23C-30C.
36. Marwick TH, D'Hondt AM, Mairesse GH, et al. Comparative ability of dobutamine and exercise stress in inducing myocardial ischaemia in active patients. Br Heart J. 1994;72:31-8.
37. Marwick T, D'Hondt AM, Baudhuin T, et al. Optimal use of dobutamine stress for the detection and evaluation of coronary artery disease: combination with echocardiography or scintigraphy, or both? J Am Coll Cardiol 1993;22:159-67.
38. Fioretti PM, Poldermans D, Salustri A, et al. Atropine increases the accuracy of dobutamine stress echocardiography in patients taking beta-blockers. Eur Heart J. 1994;15:355-60.
39. Varga A, Picano E, Dodi C, Barbieri A, Pratali L, Gaddi O. Madness and method in stress echo reading. Eur Heart J. 1999;20:1271-5.
40. Hoffmann R, Lethen H, Marwick T, et al. Standardized guidelines for the interpretation of dobutamine echocardiography reduce interinstitutional variance in interpretation. Am J Cardiol. 1998; 82:1520-4.
41. Hoffmann R, Lethen H, Marwick T, et al. Analysis of interinstitutional observer agreement in interpretation of dobutamine stress echocardiograms. J Am Coll Cardiol. 1996;27:330-6.
42. Marwick TH, Nemec JJ, Pashkow FJ, et al. Accuracy and limitations of exercise echocardiography in a routine clinical setting. J Am Coll Cardiol. 1992;19:74-81.
43. Fragasso G, Lu C, Dabrowski P, Pagnotta P, Sheiban I, Chierchia SL. Comparison of stress/rest myocardial perfusion tomography, dipyridamole and dobutamine stress echocardiography for the detection of coronary disease in hypertensive patients with chest pain and positive exercise test. J Am Coll Cardiol. 1999;34:441-7.
44. Secknus MA, Niedermaier ON, Lauer MS, et al. Diagnostic and prognostic implications of left ventricular cavity obliteration response to dobutamine echocardiography. Am J Cardiol. 1998;81:1318-22.
45. Quinones MA, Verani MS, Haichin RM, Mahmarian JJ, Suarez J, Zoghbi WA. Exercise echocardiography versus 201Tl single-photon emission computed tomography in evaluation of coronary artery disease. Analysis of 292 patients. Circulation. 1992;85:1026-31.
46. Biagini E, Shaw LJ, Poldermans D, et al. Accuracy of non-invasive techniques for diagnosis of coronary artery disease

and prediction of cardiac events in patients with left bundle branch block: a meta-analysis. Eur J Nucl Med Mol Imaging. 2006;33:1442-51.
47. Bouzas-Mosquera A, Peteiro J, Alvarez-Garcia N, et al. Prediction of mortality and major cardiac events by exercise echocardiography in patients with normal exercise electrocardiographic testing. J Am Coll Cardiol. 2009;53: 1981-990.
48. Schinkel AF, Bax JJ, Elhendy A, et al. Long-term prognostic value of dobutamine stress echocardiography compared with myocardial perfusion scanning in patients unable to perform exercise tests. Am J Med. 2004;117:1-9.
49. McCully RB, Roger VL, Mahoney DW, et al. Outcome after normal exercise echocardiography and predictors of subsequent cardiac events: Follow-up of 1,325 patients. J Am Coll Cardiol. 1998;31:144-9.
50. Chuah SC, Pellikka PA, Roger VL, et al. Role of dobutamine stress echocardiography in predicting outcome in 860 patients with known or suspected coronary artery disease. Circulation. 1998;97:1474-80.
51. Shaw LJ, Vasey C, Sawada S, et al. Impact of gender on risk stratification by exercise and dobutamine stress echocardiography: Long-term mortality in 4234 women and 6898 men. Eur Heart J. 2005;26:447-56.
52. Arruda AM, Das MK, Roger VL, Klarich KW, Mahoney DW, Pellikka PA. Prognostic value of exercise echocardiography in 2,632 patients ≥65 years of age. J Am Coll Cardiol. 2001;37: 1036-41.
53. Arruda-Olson AM, Juracan EM, Mahoney DW, McCully RB, Roger VL, Pellikka PA. Prognostic value of exercise echocardiography in 5,798 patients: Is there a gender difference? J Am Coll Cardiol. 2002;39:625-31.

# Use of Contrast in Ischemic Heart Disease

14
CHAPTER

*Nitin J Burkule*

## HOW TO PERFORM THE CONTRAST LEFT VENTRICULAR CAVITY OPACIFICATION?

For contrast, echocardiography patients need intravenous (IV) access, and it is generally the main obstacle in most of the busy echo-laboratories. Whenever echocardiographer feels the need of contrast after initial assessment of the patient, the availability of a trained nurse to quickly introduce IV cannula, prepare and inject contrast, is the key for establishing a successful contrast echocardiography program.

The high-end echocardiography machine generally have presets for contrast left ventricular (LV) cavity opacification (LVO) and also for myocardial contrast echocardiography (MCE). The mechanical index (MI) is set at 0.3– 0.6 for LVO. The dynamic range can be kept modest for LVO (40–60 dB), but wider range is required for MCE. The depth and sector width should encompass only the ventricles. The focus is generally kept at mitral level. At low MI, the LV structural details are not quite well visualized because of low power and penetration of ultrasound beam. The gains are adjusted to visualize only the epicardium.[1,2]

The ultrasound contrast is prepared with the diluent as per the manufacturer's instruction manual. Approximately 0.2–0.5 mL of contrast bolus is injected IV followed by gentle flushing with 5–10 mL of saline till the contrast is seen in right ventricular cavity when the flushing is stopped.[2]

Larger bolus of contrast and/or rapid flushing leads to higher quantity of contrast in the LV cavity leading to shadowing in lower half of the image. One has to wait for partial destruction of the contrast till uniform LVO is seen. Less quantity of contrast bolus or higher destruction of contrast by higher MI imaging or prolonged insonation by continuous imaging leads to swirling defect in LV cavity. In this case, additional small bolus of IV contrast or lowering of MI is required.

An optimal imaging window period of 2–3 minutes with uniform LVO is generally available by above technique which is sufficient to take LV apical 4-chamber, 2-chamber and apical long-axis views and basal, mid, and apical parasternal short-axis views **(Figure 14.1A and B)**. All 6 views are carefully evaluated by looking one segment at a time for endocardial excursion and myocardial thickening.

To circumvent the apical contrast destruction the focus can be set near the apex. Any rib shadowing, if cannot be avoided, should be maneuvered to go through center of the LV cavity to allow unhindered viewing of all regional wall motion.[3]

## WHY DO WE NEED LEFT VENTRICULAR CAVITY OPACIFICATION IN CLINICAL PRACTICE?

The objective of echocardiography in patients with ischemic heart disease (IHD) is variable depending on the clinical presentation. The contrast echocardiography helps in every stage of evaluation of IHD.

In patient with symptoms suggestive of IHD, it is invaluable to detect resting regional wall motion abnormality (RWMA). The RWMA may be due to the followings:

- Old or evolving transmural or subendocardial infarction
- Critical resting ischemia with hibernation or repetitive stunning
- Transient, stress-induced due to hemodynamically significant coronary lesion.

LVO by contrast is indicated, if there is poor endocardial visualization of at least two consecutive segments of the left ventricle.[1,3] The sustained and uniform opacification of LV cavity almost universally enhances the endocardial delineation of all LV wall segments thereby increasing the diagnostic information available to the clinician rapidly and in a cost-effective way.[1,5] The LVO clearly improves the interpreters' confidence to assess LV systolic function over and above the routine harmonic imaging.[6,7] The low MI imaging preserves the epicardial echoes, and contrast LVO clearly delineates endocardial border, thereby clearly demarcating the myocardial boundaries in all the LV wall segments. This has multiple benefits in echo imaging of IHD. It helps for echocardiographer's confidence in appreciating regional wall

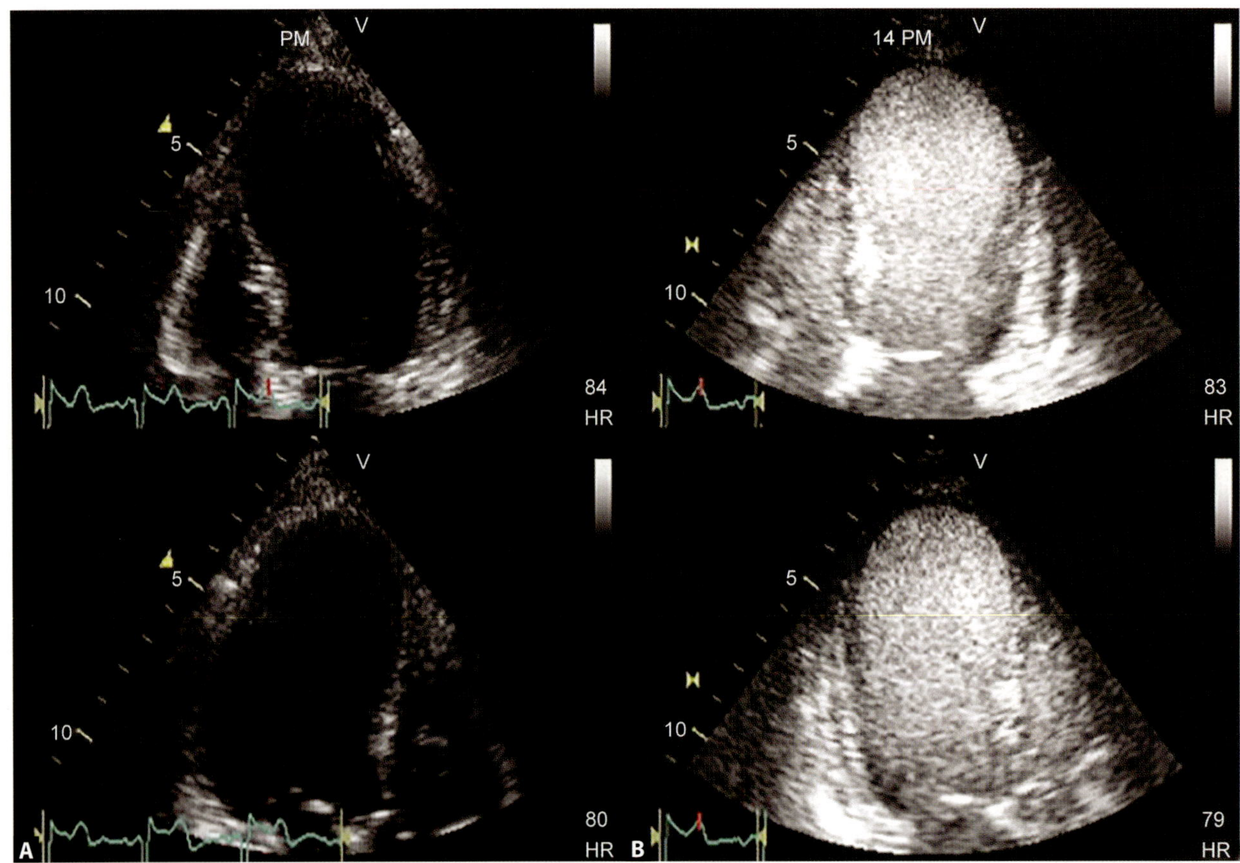


**Figure 14.1A and B:** Uniform opacification of left ventricular cavity on contrast imaging. Compared to harmonic images (A) the contrast left ventricular cavity opacification (B) shows clear endocardial visualization of all the left ventricular segments.

thickness, thickening and regional wall motion both at rest or at peak stress **(Figure 14.2A and B and Video 14.1)**.[1]

The contrast LVO clearly shows stress-induced regional wall motion and thickening abnormality or stress induced regional thinning or LV dilatation **(Figure 14.3A to D and Videos 14.2A to E)**. It improves reproducibility in the quantitative analysis of LV function, both at rest and during stress, and diagnostic accuracy of the stress echo.[8-10] It also reduces the physical effort and time taken in acquisition of diagnostic quality rest and peak stress images, perfectly aligned to long-axis of the left ventricle, during exercise echo.[3]

Suboptimal, nondiagnostic stress-echo images are seen in up to 20–30% of stress echo studies. The interobserver and interinstitutional agreement on RWMA in suboptimal stress echo studies reduces considerably.[11,12] The use of contrast LVO in exercise echo improves interobserver agreement and considerably reduces the number of nondiagnostic stress echo studies. The OPTIMIZE trial compared dobutamine stress echo (DSE) with and without contrast LVO in the same group of patients. The contrast LVO improved the diagnostic confidence of the reader and improved the sensitivity of DSE in patients with suboptimal echo images.[13] The use of contrast during DSE, in patients with poor echo window, has shown to improve the sensitivity, specificity and accuracy of the test equal to the non-contrast DSE in patients with good echo window.[14]

The wall thickness in akinetic territories can be accurately measured with contrast LVO **(Figure 14.4)**. An akinetic segment with end-diastolic thickness of 6 mm or more suggests nontransmural infarct (hence highly likely to be viable), while a segment with thickness 4 mm or less suggests transmural infarct (hence highly likely to be nonviable); however, exceptions do exist.[15]

The ease of appreciating LV segmental thickness and thickening is useful in early triage of patients presenting to emergency department with chest pain.[16,17] The presence of RWMA, however subtle it may be, is confidently diagnosed by contrast LVO. The presence of or absence of RWMA

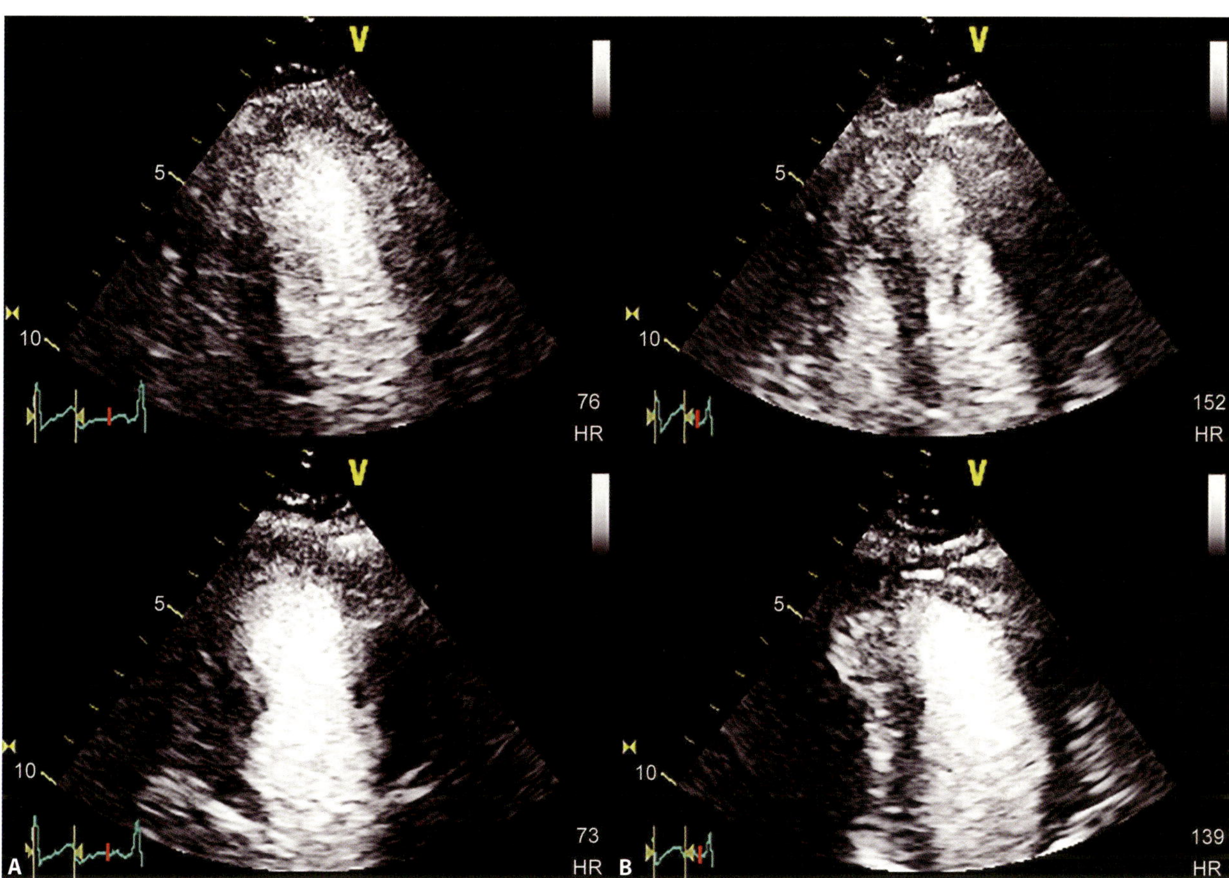


**Figure 14.2A and B:** Normal exercise stress echo images. End systolic frames of rest (A) and peak stress (B) left ventricular apical 4-chamber (upper panel) and 2-chamber (lower panel) images with contrast left ventricular cavity opacification. **(Video 14.1)**

can help to rapidly risk stratify these patients, better than Thrombolysis In Myocardial Infarction score, while awaiting the troponin results.[18] Patients with RWMA at presentation are more likely to have adverse cardiac events like acute myocardial infarctions, unstable angina, congestive heart failure, or revascularization within 48 hours of presentation.[19]

## Illustrative Case 1

***A 45-year-old male without known coronary risk factors presented to emergency department with chest pain and normal electrocardiogram (ECG). While the troponin reports were awaited, a bedside two-dimensional (2D) echo was done which showed good quality images with normal LV function and no RWMA. However, due to typical nature of chest pain, the echocardiographer decided to use contrast LVO to pick up any subtle RWMA. To his surprise, there was distinct akinesia of LV apical cap which was missed due to apical clutter. This helped triage the patient rapidly to invasive strategy without waiting for troponin results*** **(Figure 14.5A to D, Videos 14.3A to D)**.

In non-contrast 2D echocardiography, often the trabecular edges are mistaken for endocardial border while planimetering for LV volumes by Simpson's method. The clear border detection of compact myocardium by LVO, distinct from the trabeculae, helps in measuring more accurate and reproducible LV volumes by Simpson's method. It reduces interobserver and inter-study variability in LV volume measurements **(Figure 14.6A and B)**.[1,20] The LV volumes measured by 2D or three-dimensional (3D) LVO are larger than noncontrast 2D echocardiography and more close to gold standard cardiac magnetic resonance imaging (MRI).[1,21] This is useful in a spectrum of clinical situations like confirming preclinical, borderline LV dysfunction at one end and determination of exact LV ejection fraction (LVEF) and LV volumes for indications of implantable cardioverter defibrillator or cardiac resynchronization therapy implantation at the other end.

During contrast LVO imaging in intensive care unit (ICU), occasionally one may stumble upon an unsuspected

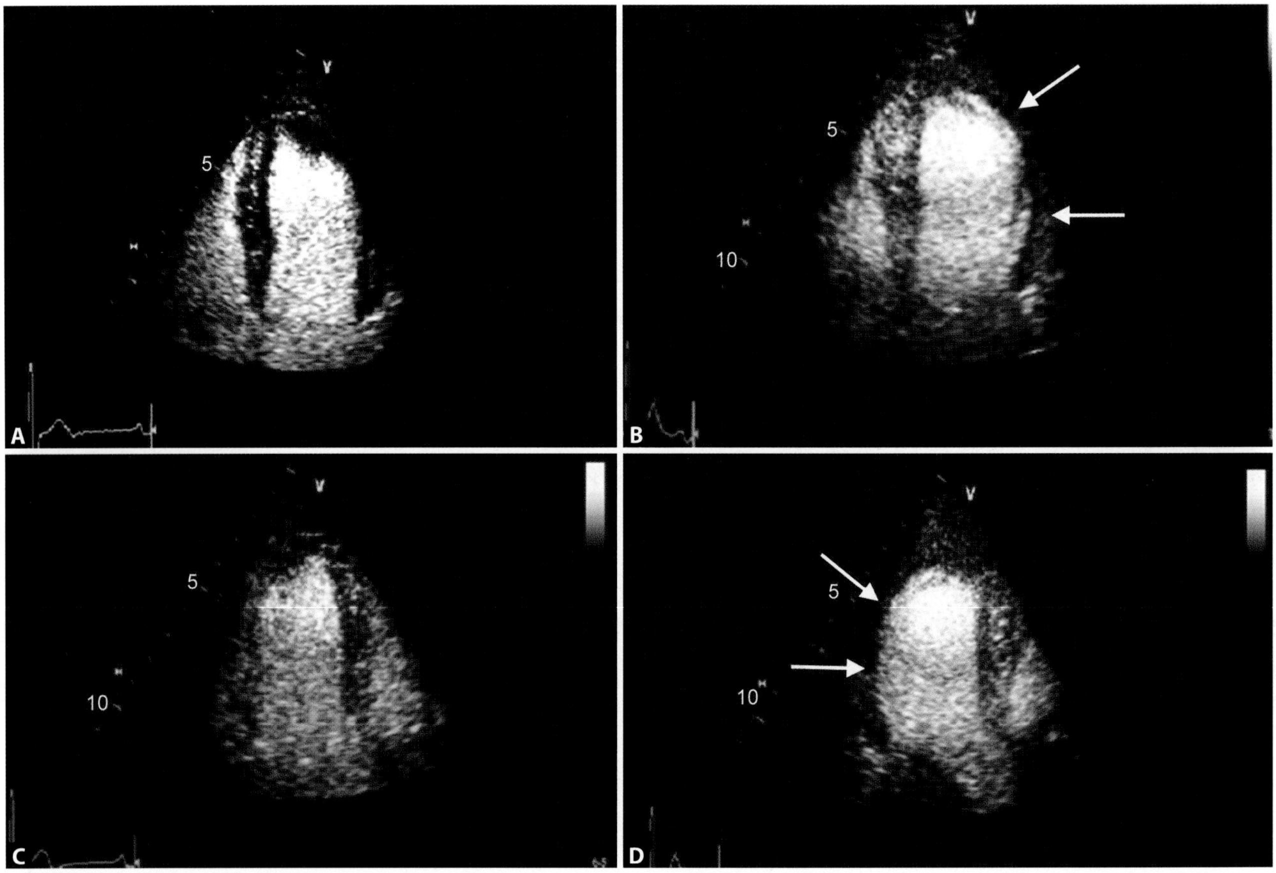

**Figure 14.3A to D:** Abnormal exercise stress echo with stress induced akinesia of postero-lateral wall [left circumflex territory]. End systolic frames with contrast left ventricular cavity opacification of (A) 4-chamber rest (C) Apical long-axis rest (B) 4-chamber peak stress and (D) Apical long-axis peak stress images. Note thinning and bulging of posterolateral wall (arrows). **(Videos 14.2A to E)**

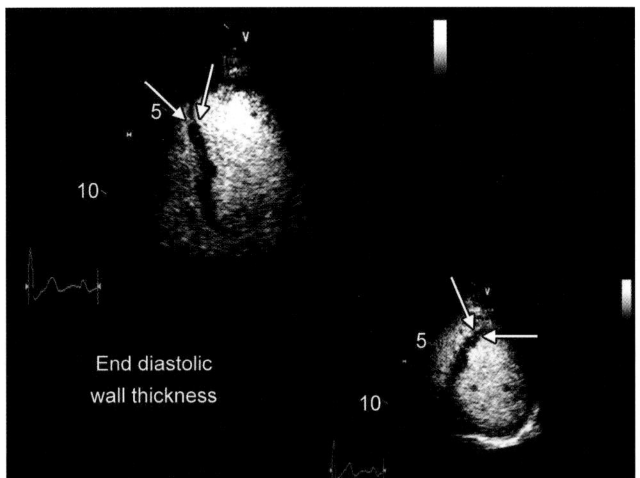


**Figure 14.4:** Clear visualization of myocardial wall boundaries helping in correct measurement of end diastolic wall thickness for viability.

complication of myocardial infarction, such as LV aneurysm, pseudoaneurysm or myocardial rupture which may have far reaching clinical implications.[1,22] The LVO clearly delineates LV apical territory where the imaging clarity is poor due to apical clutter of near-field artifact. Unsuspected LV apical clots in LV apical infarction are more often visualized and confidently diagnosed by LVO with high interobserver agreement **(Figure 14.7 and Video 14.4)**.[1,23,24] Pseudoaneurysms are better demarcated by LVO so also the layered clots in true aneurysms.

## *Illustrative Case 2*

***A 58-year-male with history of acute anterior wall myocardial infarction following bee stings from a perturbed beehive received primary percutaneous coronary intervention (PCI) and dual antiplatelet maintenance treatment for drug eluting stent. A routine 2D echo after 1 month from the episode showed a distinct LV apical clot. It is not unusual to detect unsuspected LV apical***

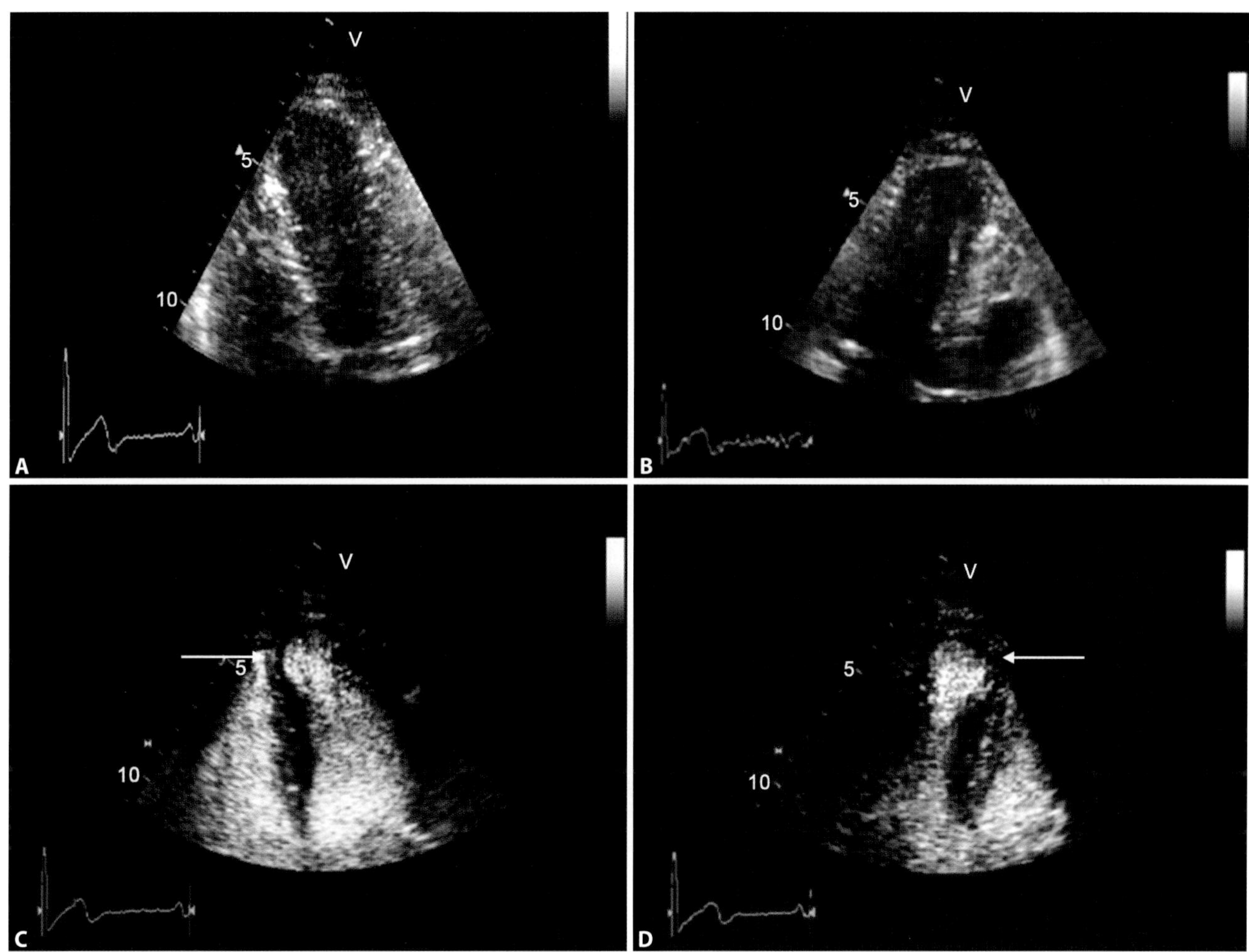


**Figure 14.5A to D:** A patient with chest pain (A) Noncontrast harmonic 2D 4-chamber and (B) Apical long-axis views do not show any regional wall motion abnormality. (C) Contrast left ventricular cavity opacification in apical 4-chamber and (D) Apical long-axis views show apical septal akinesia (arrows). **(Videos 14.3A to D)**

***clot on routine follow-up 2D echo study of patients with apical infarction, if contrast LVO is utilized. This has important management implications. He was anticoagulated with warfarin and shifted to single antiplatelet (clopidogrel) for next 3 months. The reduction in size or complete resolution of clot can be monitored with confidence and accuracy by repeat contrast LVO*** **(Figure 14.8A and B and Videos 14.5A and B)**.

## Illustrative Case 3

***A 58-year-old male with history of thrombolyzed anterior wall myocardial infarction one month back, referred for 2D echo for LVEF assessment. Contrast LVO was used for accurate LVEF estimation. During LVO study, off axis long-axis views and apical short-axis views, showed a pseudoaneurysm which was completely missed on standard noncontrast 2D echo imaging*** **(Figure 14.9A to C and Videos 14.6A to C)**.

Patient with atypical symptoms and abnormal ST/T changes in ECG may be referred for echocardiography to differentiate between IHD and hypertrophic cardiomyopathy (HCM). The apical clutter precludes the confident diagnosis of apical HCM. The contrast LVO gives clear visualization of apical hypertrophy with apical cavity systolic obliteration.[1] With LVO, the myocardial thickness can be measured in almost all LV wall segments. Hence, the diagnosis of noncontiguous variants of HCM (hypertrophy restricted to few segments) is more feasible than routine harmonic 2D echo.

## Illustrative Case 4

***A 45-year-old male referred in emergency from a diagnostic center for abnormal ECG which was recorded for life***

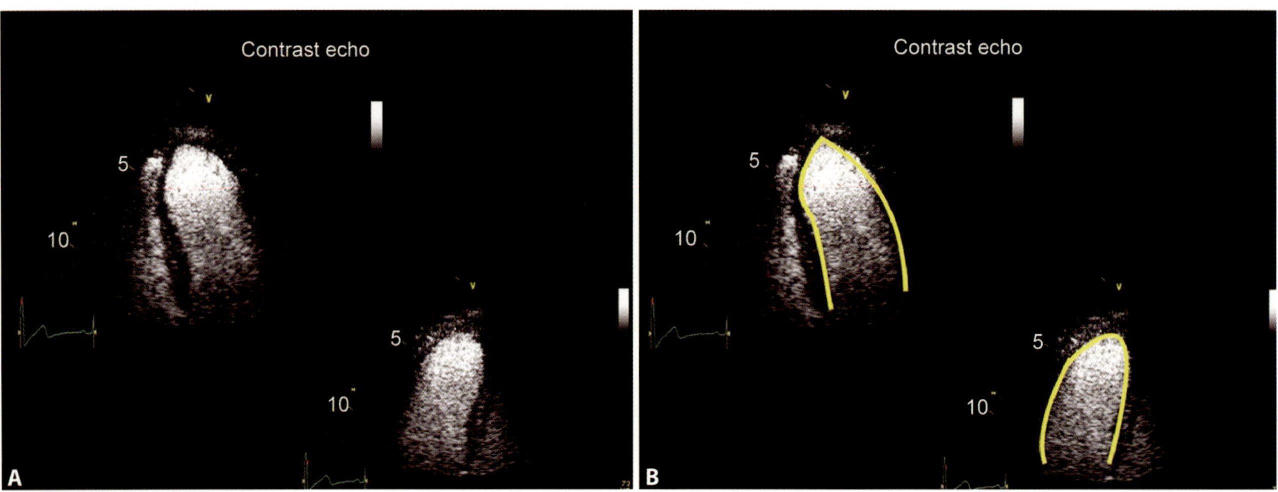


**Figure 14.6A and B:** (A) Clear visualization of tissue-blood interface of compact myocardium (B) correct marking of endocardial border gives reliable and reproducible left ventricle volume measurements by Simpson's method.

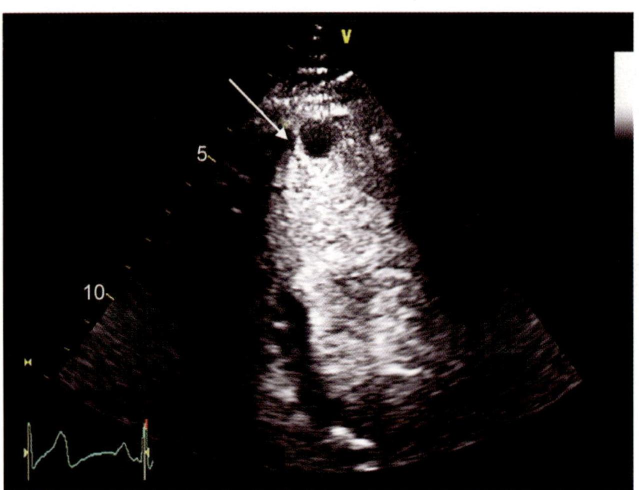


**Figure 14.7:** Left ventricle apical clot on contrast left ventricular cavity opacification (arrow). **(Video 14.4)**

***insurance policy. The ECG showed precordial lead deep symmetric T-wave inversions. It was wrongly interpreted as non-ST segment elevation myocardial infarction (NSTEMI) by casualty officer due to inconsistent history given by the worried and frightened patient and was channelized to rapid invasive management plan. Coronary angiography revealed nonobstructive 50% plaque in a large diagonal, and laboratory reports showed normal troponins. 2D echo done post-cath showed apical hypertrophy with apical cavity systolic obliteration leading to the obvious diagnosis of apical variant of HCM. However, a contrast LVO showed apical displacement of large papillary muscle, a benign abnormality, which was later confirmed on cardiac MRI*** **(Figure 14.10A and B and Videos 14.7A and B)**.

The greater benefit of contrast LVO is seen in more sicker patients admitted to ICUs. These patients are often on mechanical ventilators with chest bandages and drains and are cumbersome to be turned to left lateral position and hence provide limited and poor echo window. In these patients, contrast LVO gives diagnostic quality images equivalent to transesophageal echo images rapidly and noninvasively.[25] Clinician can take confident decisions on the basis of the LV function data and enhanced Doppler signals by LVO and can avoid unnecessary downstream diagnostic tests. The use of contrast LVO in ICU patients have clearly shown to have incremental value over conventional echo, leading to change in patient management plan, reducing invasive tests and ultimately leading to cost saving.[26]

### *Illustrative Case 5*

***A 50-year-old male patient admitted in emergency for road-traffic accident. He was intubated on arrival due to cerebral contusions and obtunded sensorium. After two days, his sedation was withdrawn, and he was put on weaning mode (continuous positive airway pressure). On becoming awake patient became severely agitated, tachycardic and had fall in blood pressure. The intensivist started noradrenalin and hiked the dose rapidly due to persistent hypotension. The ECG on monitor showed acute ST elevation. The emergency bedside echo showed nondiagnostic poor quality images. Use of bedside contrast LVO clearly showed apical ballooning (Takotsubo cardiomyopathy) and hypovolemia. Just rapidly infusing***

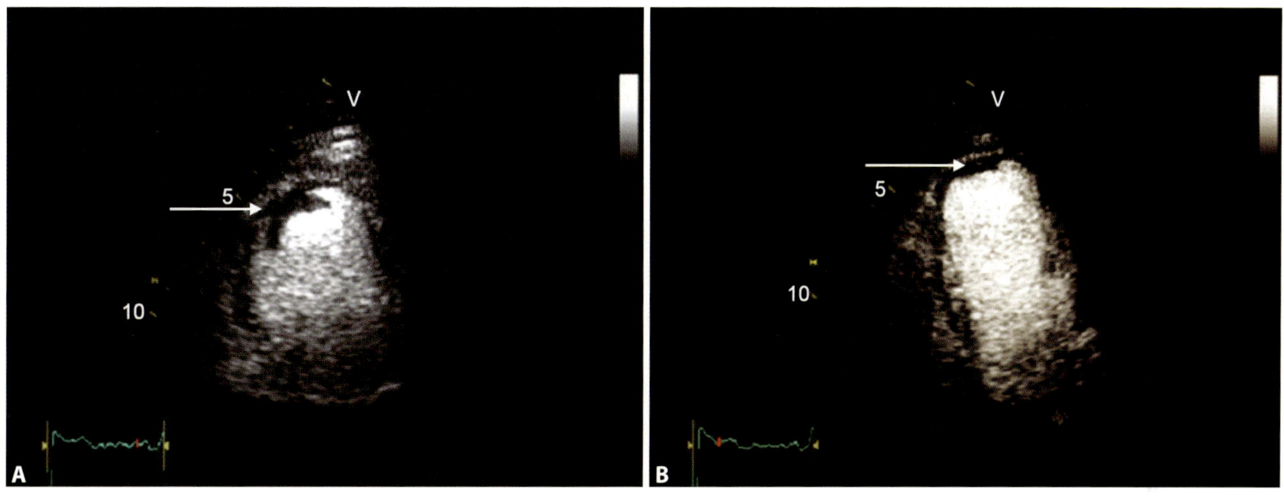


**Figure 14.8A and B:** (A) Left ventricular apical clot (arrow). (B) Minimal residual layer of clot after 2 weeks of anticoagulation (arrow). **(Videos 14.5A and B)**

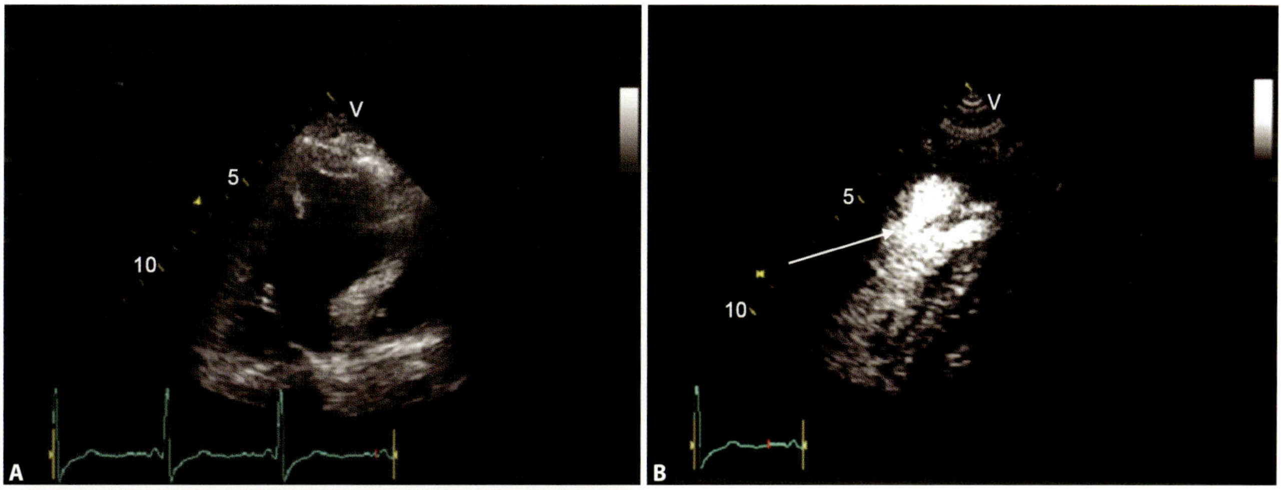

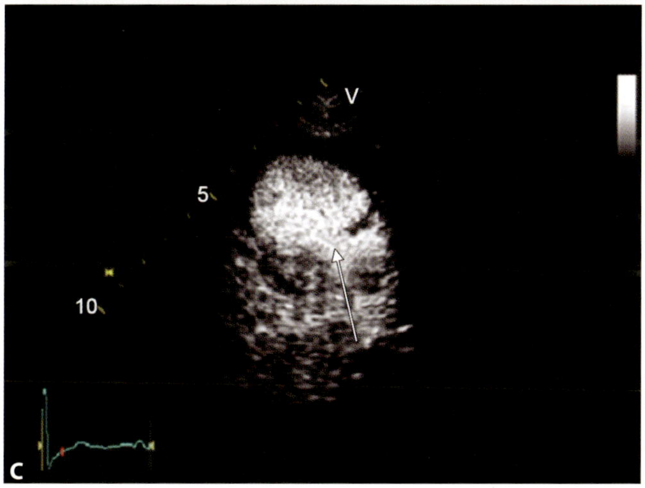

**Figure 14.9A to C:** Left ventricular pseudoaneurysm. (A) Apical long-axis noncontrast 2D harmonic image does not show the pseudoaneurysm. (B) Apical long-axis contrast left ventricular cavity opacification and (C) apical short-axis contrast left ventricular cavity opacification clearly delineate the pseudoaneurysm and the contained rupture (arrow). **(Videos 14.6A to C)**

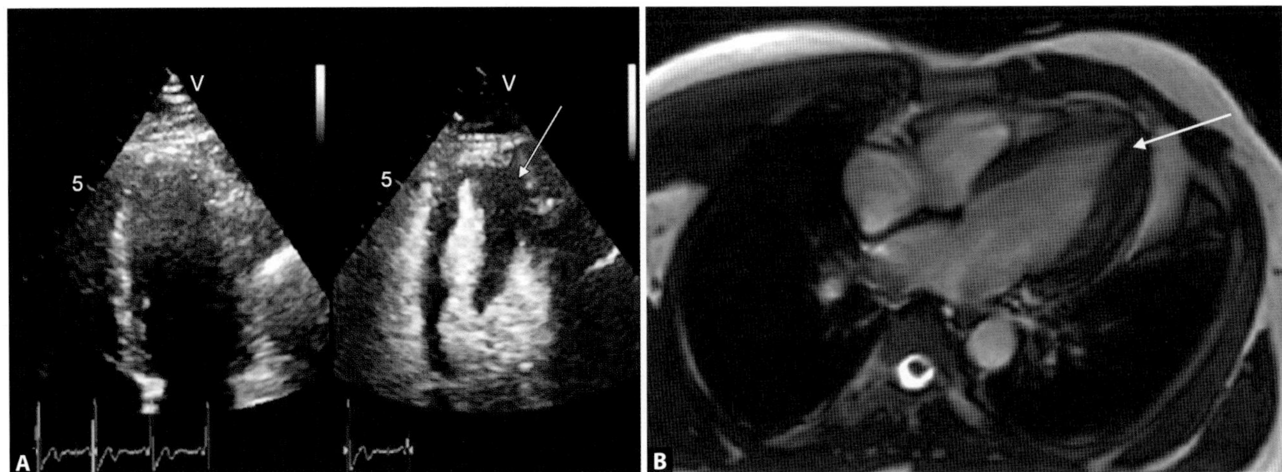

**Figure 14.10A and B:** (A) The contrast left ventricular cavity opacification (right panel) clearly shows apical displacement of papillary muscle (arrow) not visualized on noncontrast two-dimensional harmonic imaging (left panel). (B) Apical displacement of papillary muscle confirmed on cardiac magnetic resonance imaging (arrow). **(Videos 14.7A and B)**

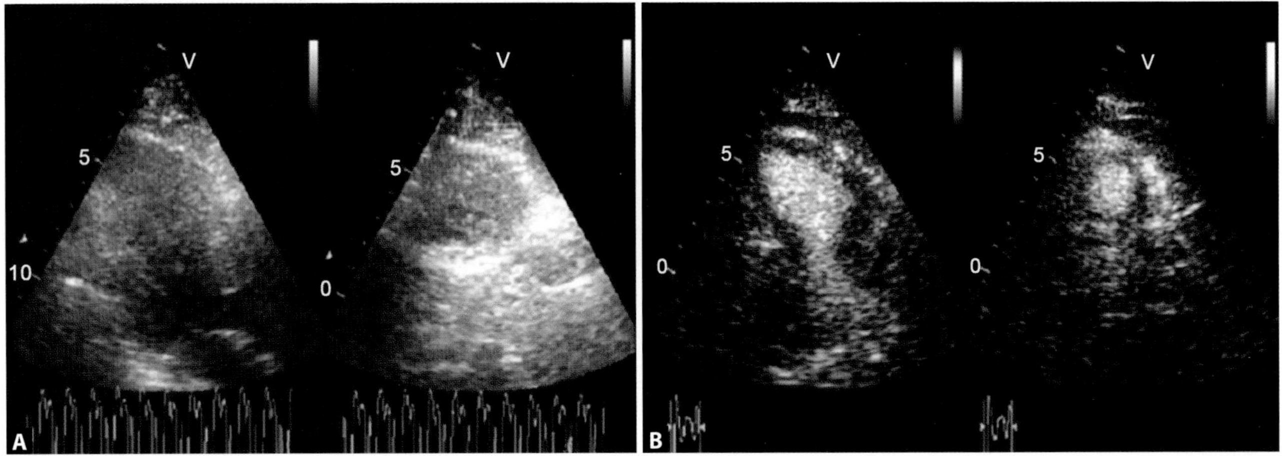

**Figure 14.11A and B:** Stress cardiomyopathy in a patient of road-traffic accident admitted in intensive care unit and on high dose noradrenaline. (A) Nondiagnostic bedside two-dimensional (2D) echo image on noncontrast 2D harmonic imaging. (B) Bedside contrast left ventricular cavity opacification clearly shows left ventricular apical ballooning and hypovolemia. **(Videos 14.8A and B)**

***fluid, withdrawal of noradrenalin and administration of IV β blockers normalized the ECG ST changes and rapidly normalized the hemodynamics. The LV function completely recovered during the hospitalization*** **(Figure 14.11A and B, Videos 14.8A and B).**

## *Illustrative Case 6*

***A 60-year-old male patient underwent coronary artery bypass graft (CABG) surgery with 5 grafts with left anterior descending (LAD) endarterectomy for severe triple vessel coronary disease. On second postoperative day, patient had sustained ventricular tachycardia (received DC cardioversion) and hypotension. The bedside 2D echo was necessary for crucial information of LV function and RWMA to detect graft closure. However, the echo image quality was poor and echo window access was limited due to chest tubes, dressings, and mechanical ventilation. A quick bedside LVO showed significantly hypovolemic and hypercontractile LV ruling out any graft dysfunction. Rapid IV fluid administration and withdrawal of inotropes salvaged the situation*** **(Figure 14.12A and B and Videos 14.9A and B).**

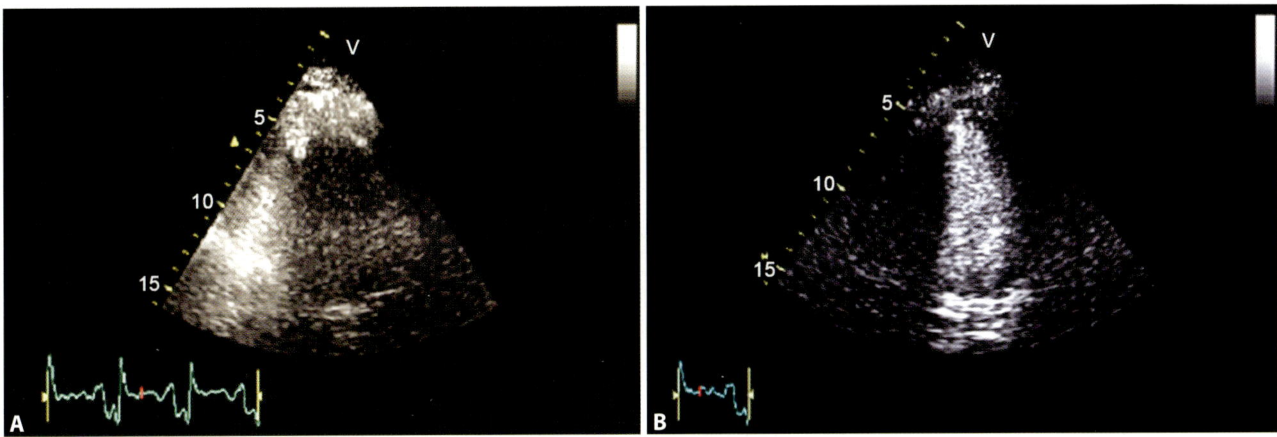


**Figure 14.12A and B:** Post-coronary bypass patient with hemodynamic instability. (A) Nondiagnostic bedside two-dimensional echo image on harmonic imaging. (B) Bedside contrast left ventricular cavity opacification clearly shows all left ventricle wall segments and hypovolemic left ventricle cavity. **(Videos 14.9A and B)**

## HOW TO USE CONTRAST FOR MYOCARDIAL PERFUSION ASSESSMENT?

Basic principles of visualizing myocardial contrast both at rest and peak vasodilatory stress are discussed further:[1,27]

1. Prevent destruction of contrast bubbles so that sufficient quantity is retained in myocardium. This is achieved by imaging with very low MI (0.06) continuously in real time (real-time MCE) or imaging at intermittent higher MI (0.1) end-systolic frames using an ECG trigger positioned at end of T-wave.
2. Enhancing the nonlinear signals from microbubbles in second harmonics and suppressing the myocardial tissue signal by various amplitude and/or phase modulated pulse sequences or by power Doppler. These algorithms are copyrighted MCE presets of different echo machine vendors.

For vasodilatory stress MCE, the contrast is injected as continuous infusion at 1-2 mL/minute at a concentration prescribed by the manufacturers (e.g. Sonovue is prepared at a dilution of 5 mL per ampule). The steady state is achieved within 1-2 minutes. The rate of infusion is adjusted for each patient in such a way that a uniform LVO is achieved, and there is no shadowing (excess concentration) or swirling (less concentration). The rapidity of myocardial contrast opacification is observed qualitatively after a short pulse of high MI frame, both at rest and during IV infusion of adenosine (140 µg/kg/minute for 3 minutes). The high MI frame should be of sufficient power to make entire myocardium jet black by destroying all the microbubbles in the myocardium. In presence of normal myocardial blood flow the myocardium shows peak contrast opacificationin 4-5 seconds (4-5 beats) at rest but in 1-2 seconds (1-2 beats) at peak coronary vasodilatation by adenosine. Any delay in myocardial opacificationon vasodilatory stress and/or distinct subendocardial filling defects suggest poor coronary flow reserve and hence significant coronary stenosis.[28] The whole stress test is over in just 3-5 minutes, however, with very transient chest discomfort to patient due to adenosine.

The elaborate infusion protocol is not needed for visualizing perfusion for viability in the culprit coronary territory after primary PCI or thrombolysis. A single bolus of 0.5 mL of Sonovue can be chased from right ventricular to LV cavity and then to target myocardial opacification by using end-systolic triggered imaging.

## WHY DO WE NEED MYOCARDIAL CONTRAST ECHOCARDIOGRAPHY?

In an echo laboratory with established contrast echo program, the need of MCE is not infrequent. The most common and technically an easy indication is to evaluate for myocardial salvage in early period after primary PCI or thrombolysis in ST elevation myocardial infarction (STEMI). Generally, the myocardial thickness is preserved due to post-reperfusion tissue edema and hence myocardial perfusion is easy to visualize. A salvaged myocardium will have reflow at microvasculature level and MCE will show homogeneous myocardial opacification in infarct territory **(Figure 14.13)**. Absence of MCE opacification (no reflow at microvasculature level) in infarct territory suggests myocardial necrosis, while uniform MCE opacification suggests salvage of myocardium.[29,30] The presence or absence of MCE opacification can predict LV remodeling and adverse cardiac outcome post-reperfusion in STEMI.

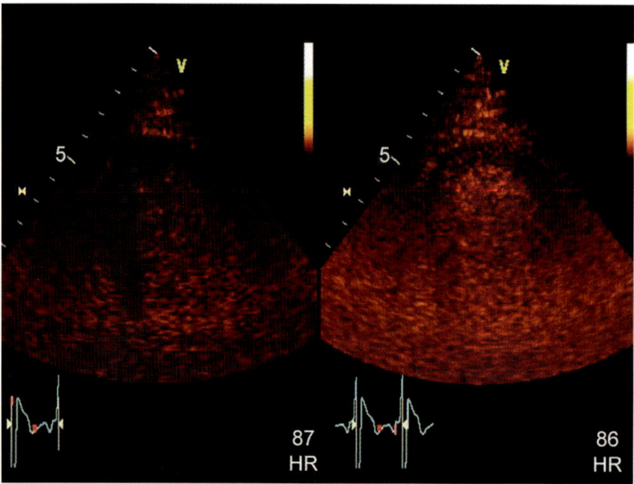


**Figure 14.13:** Postprimary percutaneous coronary intervention myocardial contrast echocardiography for myocardial perfusion in left anterior descending territory after IV bolus of contrast. After left ventricle cavity opacification (left panel) within 9 seconds, the entire left anterior descending territory shows uniform myocardial opacification (right panel) suggesting salvaged myocardium.

### *Illustrative Case 7*

***A 35-year-old male, chronic smoker, presented with anterior wall STEMI outside window period (>12 hours). During primary PCI, after stent deployment in LAD, patient had transient no reflow which recovered after intracoronary administration of vasodilators and tirofiban. The bedside MCE performed after 48 hours showed uniform myocardial opacification suggesting viability despite late presentation and transient no reflow during PCI. The RWMA and LV function completely recovered at 2 weeks follow-up*** **(Figure 14.14A to C and Videos 14.10A to D).**

### *Illustrative Case 8*

***An 80-year-old gentleman with history of previous CABG 10 years back presented to peripheral nursing home with typical resting chest pain and ST elevation in V1–V4 and aVR and ST depression in II, III and aVF suggesting proximal LAD occlusion. He received heparin and antiplatelets and transferred to tertiary care after 24 hours, by which time, he was symptom free and***

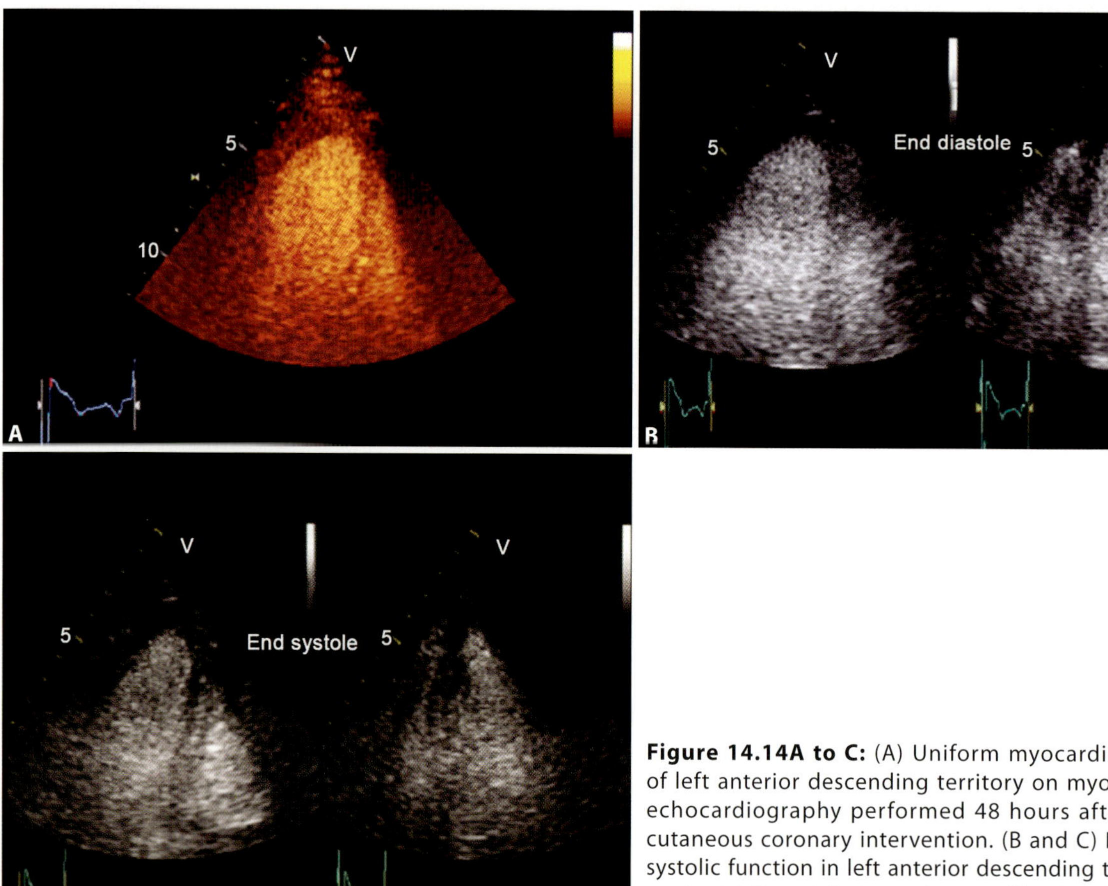


**Figure 14.14A to C:** (A) Uniform myocardial opacification of left anterior descending territory on myocardial contrast echocardiography performed 48 hours after primary percutaneous coronary intervention. (B and C) Late recovery of systolic function in left anterior descending territory seen on contrast left ventricular cavity opacification during follow-up. **(Videos 14.10A to D)**

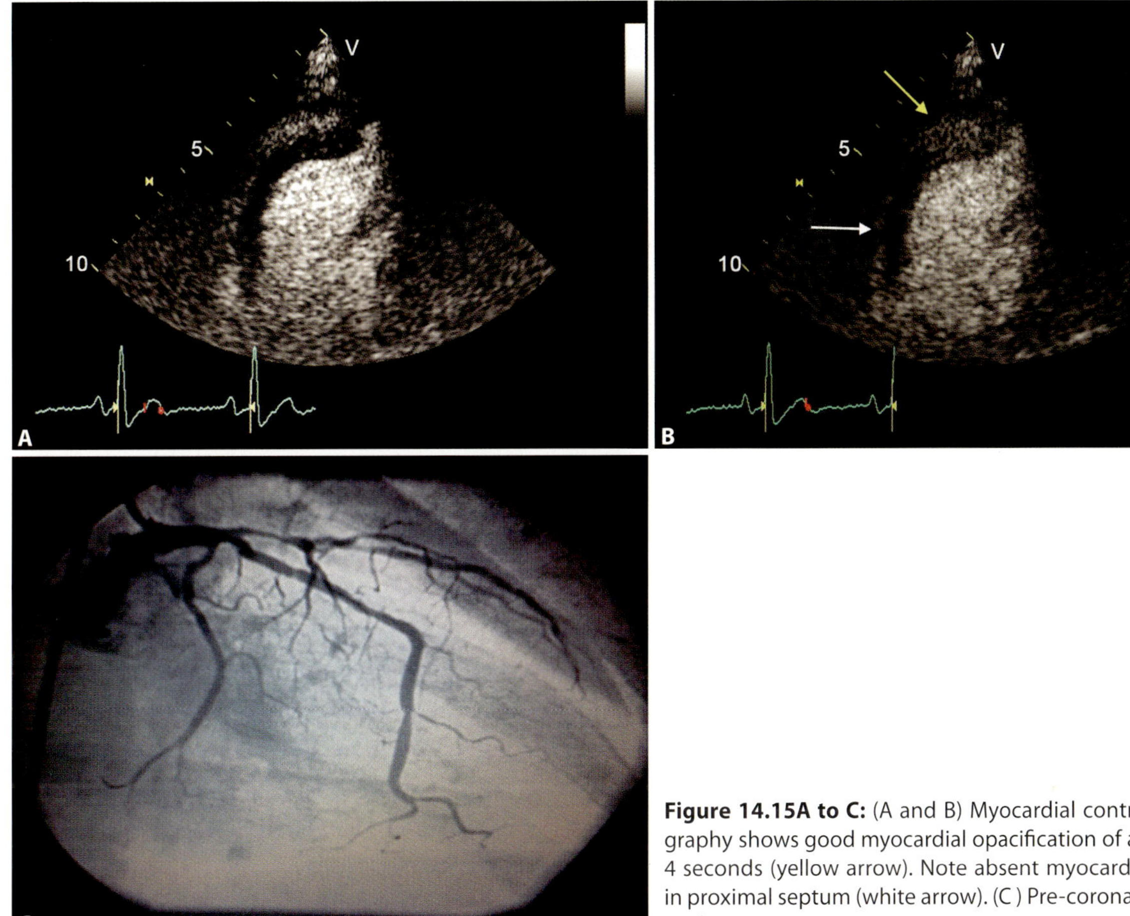


**Figure 14.15A to C:** (A and B) Myocardial contrast echocardiography shows good myocardial opacification of apical septum in 4 seconds (yellow arrow). Note absent myocardial opacification in proximal septum (white arrow). (C) Pre-coronary artery bypass grafting coronary angiogram.

***surprisingly in very stable hemodynamic. The contrast LVO and MCE showed normally contracting mid and apical LV septum with good myocardial opacification limited to distal septum. Only proximal septum showed akinesia with absent perfusion. This suggested normally functioning left internal mammary artery graft with retrograde LAD flow, limiting the infarct caused by acute thrombotic occlusion of the plaque downstream from first septal and old ostial disease. Considering this information along with age and clinical status, conservative approach was taken avoiding unnecessary intervention*** **(Figure 14.15A to C)**.

The MCE with vasodilatory stress is more sensitive than conventional stress echo for RWMA.[31] When MCE is performed with dobutamine or exercise, the regional wall thickening is better appreciated in real-time MCE, because of clear delineation of subendocardial perfusion defects, compared to conventional stress echo with only LVO.[32]

Similar strategy can be used in patients with chest pain, ECG ST/T changes, rise in troponins with or without LV dysfunction where clinically noncoronary cause (Takotsubo or myocarditis) is suspected. A uniform perfusion in akinetic septal-apical territory suggests Takotsubo stress cardiomyopathy.

## *Illustrative Case 9*

***A 60-year-old nonhypertensive, nondiabetic lady presented with acute chest pain and breathlessness within few hours after husband's sudden cardiac death. An ECG in the emergency room showed symmetric, deep T inversions, convex ST segment elevation, and 2D echo showed mid to apical LV cavity dilatation and akinesia. While awaiting emergency coronary angiography for primary PCI, a quick bedside MCE perfusion scan shows good transmural perfusion. This is unlikely in occluded***

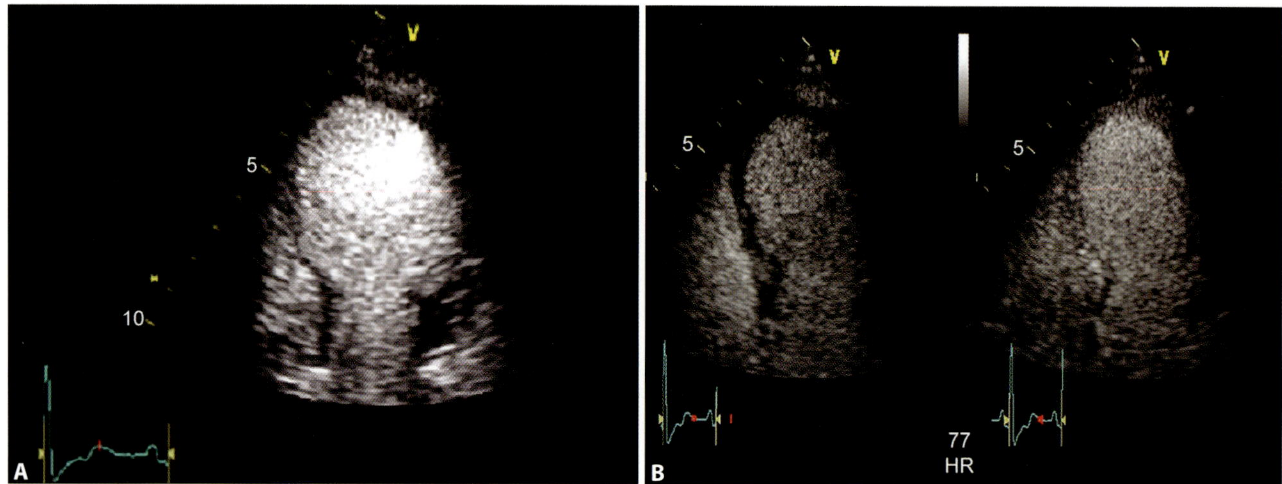


**Figure 14.16A and B:** (A) Takotsubo cardiomyopathy after bereavement. Note typical apical ballooning. (B) Myocardial contrast echocardiography shows delayed but uniform myocardial opacification of left anterior descending territory in 12 seconds. **(Videos 14.11A to D)**

***culprit artery in STEMI and will favor either spontaneous reperfusion or Takotsubo cardiomyopathy. The coronary angiography was normal*** **(Figure 14.16A and B and Videos 14.11A to D)**.

## LIMITATIONS OF CONTRAST

For contrast LVO or MCE, the echo machines are preset at low MI. This makes visualization of valves and atria difficult. No speckle tracking (strain) imaging can be performed on the same set of contrast images due to low frame rate and low MI imaging. Shadowing is very common at basal segments and also due to rib or papillary muscles. Artifactual attenuation in anterior wall due to lung shadowing, or apical segments due to near field destruction, is also a common pitfall.

## VIDEO LEGENDS

**Video 14.1**: An example of normal exercise stress echocardiography. Only systole is shown. The left side images are rest images whereas the right side images are corresponding views obtained immediately after exercise. The upper images show apical 4-chamber view with contrast LVO and the lower images show apical 2-chamber view with contrast LVO.

**Video 14.2:** Abnormal exercise stress echocardiography with stress induced akinesia of postero-lateral wall (LCX territory). A-D: Contrast LVO images are shown (A) Apical 4-chamber view at rest (B) Apical 4-chamber view after exercise (C) Apical long-axis view at rest (D) Apical long-axis view after exercise. Note thinning and bulging of posterolateral wall. (E) Coronary angiogram showing complete occlusion of a large obtuse marginal artery.

**Video 14.3:** A patient with chest pain with abnormal stress echocardiogram (A) Non-contrast harmonic 2D 4-chamber and (B) Apical long-axis view do not show RWMA. (C) Contrast LVO 4-chamber and (D) Apical long-axis views show apical septal akinesia.

**Video 14.4:** LV apical clot on contrast LVO

**Video 14.5:** (A) LV apical clot (B) Minimal residual layer of clot after 2 weeks of anticoagulation.

**Video 14.6:** LV pseudoaneurysm identified with the help of contrast LVO (A) Apical long-axis non-contrast 2D harmonic image does not show the pseudoaneurysm. (B) Apical long-axis contrast LVO and (C) Apical short-axis contrast LVO clearly delineate the pseudoaneurysm and the contained rupture.

**Video 14.7:** (A) Contrast LVO (right panel) clearly shows apical displacement of papillary muscle not visualized on non-contrast 2D harmonic imaging (left panel). (B) Apical displacement of papillary muscle confirmed on cardiac MRI.

**Video 14.8:** Stress cardiomyopathy in a patient of road traffic accident admitted in intensive care unit and on high dose noradrenaline (A) Non-diagnostic bedside 2D echo image on non-contrast 2D harmonic imaging. (B) Bedside contrast LVO clearly shows LV apical ballooning and hypovolemia.

**Video 14.9:** Post CABG patient with hemodynamic instability. (A) Non-diagnostic bedside 2D echo image on harmonic imaging. (B) Bedside contrast LVO clearly shows normally contracting all LV wall segments with hypovolemic LV cavity.

**Video 14.10:** (A) Uniform myocardial opacification of LAD territory on MCE performed 48 hr after primary PCI. (B) Late recovery of systolic function in LAD territory seen on contrast LVO during follow-up. (C) Coronary angiogram prior to PCI. (D) Coronary angiogram immediately after primary PCI.

**Video 14.11:** (A) Takatsubo cardiomyopathy after bereavement. Note typical apical ballooning. (B) MCE shows delayed but uniform myocardial opacification of LAD territory in 12 seconds. (C) and (D) Coronary angiogram confirming absence of significant coronary stenosis.

## REFERENCES


1. Mulvagh SL, Rakowski H, Vannan MA, Abdelmoneim SS, Becher H, Bierig SM, et al. American Society of Echocardiography Consensus Statement on the Clinical Applications of Ultrasonic Contrast Agents in Echocardiography. J Am Soc Echocardiogr. 2008;21(11):1179-201.
2. Patric Coon, James Bednarz, Alan Pearlman, et al. Implementaion of contrast echocardiography in the laboratory. Cardiol Clin. 2004:22(2);199-210.
3. Mulvagh SL, DeMaria AN, Feinstein SB, et al. Contrast echocardiography: Current and future applications. J Am Soc Echocardiogr. 2000;13:331-42.
4. Cohen JL, Cheirif J, Segar DS, Gillam LD, Gottdiener JS, Hausnerova E, et al. Improved left ventricular endocardial border delineation and opacification with Optison (FS069), a new echocardiographic contrast agent: results of a phase III multicenter trial. J Am Coll Cardiol. 1998;32:746-52.
5. Shaw LJ, Gillam L, Feinstein S, et al. Technology assessment in the managed care era: use of an intravenous contrast agent (FS069-Optison) to enhance cardiac diagnostic testing. Am J Manag Care. 1998;4:SP169-76.
6. Linder JR, Dent JM, Moos SP. Enhancement of left ventricular cavity opacification by harmonic imaging after venous injection of Albunex. Am J Cardiol. 1997;79:1657-62.
7. Al-Mansour HA, Mulvagh SL, Foley DA, et al. Is harmonic contrast echocardiography the procedure of choice for optimal endocardial border definition J Am Soc Echocardiogr. 1998;11:527.
8. Porter TR, Xie F, Kricsfeld A, et al. Improved endocardial border resolution during dobutamine stress echocardiography with intravenous sonicated dextrose albumin. J Am Coll Cardiol. 1994;23:1440-3.
9. Leischik R, Kuhlmann C, Bruch C, Jeremias A, Buck T, Erbel R. Reproducibility of stress echocardiography using intravenous injection of ultrasound contrast agent (BY 963). Int J Card Imaging. 1997;13:387-94.
10. Rainbird AJ, Pellikka PA, Mulvagh SL, McCully RB, Oh JK, Klarich KW, et al. Contrast dobutamine stress echocardiographyn 100 consecutive patients: improvement in image quality, wall segment visualization and confidence of interpretation. J Am Coll Cardiol. 1999;33:422A.
11. Hoffmann R, Lethen H, Marwick T, Arnese M, Fioretti P, Pingitore A, et al. Analysis of interinstitutional observer agreement in interpretation of dobutamine stress echocardiograms. J Am Coll Cardiol. 1996;27:330-6.
12. Marwick TH, Nemec JJ, Pashkow FJ, et al. Accuracy and limitations of exercise echocardiography in a routine clinical setting. J Am Coll Cardiol. 1992;19:74-81.
13. Plana JC, Mikati IA, Dokainish H, Lakkis N, Abukhalil J, Davis R, et al. A randomized cross-over study for evaluation of the effect of image optimization with contrast on the diagnostic accuracy of dobutamine echocardiography in coronary artery disease: the OPTIMIZE trial. J Am Coll Cardiol. 2008;1: 145-52.
14. Dolan MS, Riad K, El-Shafei A, Puri S, Tamirisa K, Bierig M, et al. Effect of intravenous contrast for left ventricular opacification and border definition on sensitivity and specificity of dobutamine stress echocardiography compared with coronary angiography in technically difficult patients. Am Heart J. 2001;142:908-15.
15. Cwajg JM, Cwajg E, Nagueh SF, He ZX, Qureshi U, Olmos LI, et al. End-diastolic wall thickness as a predictor of recovery of function in myocardial hibernation: Relation to rest-redistribution Tl-201 tomography and dobutamine stress echocardiography. J Am Coll Cardiol. 2000;35(5): 1152-61.
16. Sabia P, Afrookteh A, Touchstone DA, Keller MW, Esquivel L, Kaul S. Value of regional wall motion abnormality in the emergency room diagnosis of acute myocardial infarction. A prospective study using two-dimensional echocardiography. Circulation. 1991;84(suppl):I85-92.
17. Kontos MC, Arrowood JA, Paulsen WH, et al. Early echocardiography can predict cardiac events in emergency department patients with chest pain. Ann Emerg Med. 1998;31:550-7.
18. Tong KL, Kaul S, Wang XQ, Rinkevich D, Kalvaitis S, Belcik T, et al. Myocardial contrast echocardiography versus thrombolysis in myocardial infarction score in patients presenting to the emergency department with chest pain and a nondiagnostic electrocardiogram. J Am Coll Cardiol. 2005;46: 920-7.
19. Rinkevich D, Kaul S, Wang XQ, Tong KL, Belcik T, Kalvaitis S, et al. Regional left ventricular perfusion and function in patients presenting to the emergency department with chest pain and no ST-segment elevation. Eur Heart J. 2005;26:1606-11.
20. Hundley WG, Kizilbash AM, Afridi I, Franco F, Peshock RM, Grayburn PA. Administration of an intravenous perfluoro-carbon contrast agent improves echocardiographic determination of left ventricular volumes and ejection fraction: comparisonwith cine magnetic resonance imaging. J Am Coll Cardiol. 1998;32:1426-32.
21. Carly Jenkins, Stuart Moir, Jonathan Chan. Left ventricular volume measurement with echocardiography: a comparison of left ventricular opacification, three-dimensional echocardiography, or both with magnetic resonance imaging. Eur Heart J. 2009;30:98-106.
22. Thanigaraj S, Perez JE. Diagnosis of cardiac rupture with the use of contrast-enhanced echocardiography. J Am Soc Echocardiogr. 2000;13:862-5.
23. Nagai T, Atar S, Luo H, et al. The usefulness of second generation ultrasound contrast agent to identify intracardiac thrombus. J Am Coll Cardiol. 1999;33:408A.
24. Thanigaraj S, Schechtman KB, Perez JE. Improved echocardiographic delineation of left ventricular thrombus with the use of intravenous second-generation contrast image enhancement. J Am Soc Echocardiogr. 1999;12:1022-6.

25. Yong Y, Wu D, Fernandes V, Kopelen HA, Shimoni S, Nagueh SF, et al. Diagnostic accuracy and cost-effectiveness of contrast echocardiography on evaluation of cardiac function in technically very difficult patients in the intensive care unit. Am J Cardiol. 2002;89:711-8.
26. Kurt M, Shaikh KA, Peterson L, Kurrelmeyer KM, Shah G, et al. Impact of contrast echocardiography on evaluation of ventricular function and clinical management in a large prospective cohort. J Am Coll Cardiol. 2009;53(9):802-10.
27. Rafter P, Phillips P, Vannan MA. Imaging technologies and techniques. Cardiol Clin. 2004;22;181-97.
28. Porter TR, Xie F. Myocardial perfusion imaging with contrast ultrasound. J Am Coll Cardiol Cardivasc Img. 2010;3:176-87.
29. Dwivedi G, Janardhanan R, Hayat SA, et al. Prognostic value of myocardial viability detected by myocardial contrast echo- cardiography early after acute myocardial infarction. J Am Coll Cardiol. 2007;50:327-34.
30. Galiuto L, Garramone B, Scara A, et al. The extent of micro-vascular damage during myocardial contrast echocardiography is superior to other known indexes of post-infarct reperfusion in predicting left ventricular remodeling. J Am Coll Cardiol. 2008; 51:552-9.
31. Nicola Gaibazzi, Fausto Rigo, Claudio Reverberi, et al. Detection of coronary artery disease by combined assessment of wall motion, myocardial perfusion and coronary flow reserve: A multiparametric contrast stress-echocardiography study. J Am Soc Echocardiogr. 2010;23:1242-50.
32. Dodla S, Xie, F, O'Leary E, et al. Detection of CAD with real time perfusion imaging during exercise and dobutamine stress echocardiography. Circulation. 2008;118S:850.

# Direct Visualization of Coronary Arteries by Echocardiography

*Ty Whitfield, Ayman A Farag, Navin C Nanda*

## INTRODUCTION

Echocardiography has become an essential diagnostic tool for the modern cardiologist. It is excellent at visualizing valvular disease, estimating ejection fraction, and visualizing wall motion abnormalities suggestive of scar or ischemia. However, relatively little has been published regarding direct visualization of coronary arteries and their abnormalities, especially in the patients with coronary narrowing and stenosis. Both two-dimensional (2D) and three-dimensional (3D) transthoracic and transesophageal modalities have been used to directly assess the coronary arteries, and clinical applications have been described in the evaluation of ischemic heart disease, aortic dissection, ischemic stroke, and congenital coronary artery anomalies.

## CORONARY ARTERY STENOSIS

### Two-dimensional Transthoracic Echocardiography

#### *Feasibility*

Direct visualization of coronary arteries with 2D transthoracic echocardiography (TTE) can be very challenging, and published studies tend to have success rates that are higher than are often achieved in day-to-day clinical practice **(Figure 15.1A and B)**.[1-5] The most specific echocardiographic finding for coronary stenosis is high velocity with concomitant flow acceleration and turbulence **(Figure 15.2)**.[1,3,6] A study involving 50 consecutive patients scheduled for coronary angiography was undertaken to evaluate the feasibility of direct 2D TTE evaluation of coronary arteries to diagnose flow-limiting stenosis. Success of visualizing coronary arteries is shown in **Table 15.1**.[3] Significance of stenosis was determined by comparing maximal flow velocities within the stenosis to maximal flow velocity immediately proximal to the stenosis. Doubling of maximal flow velocity was taken as suggestive of significant stenosis. If flow immediately proximal to the stenosis could not be reliably measured, a local velocity of at least 2 m/s was taken as significant. Using this methodology, when vessels were adequately visualized, stenosis could be detected with approximately 62–66% sensitivity and nearly 100% specificity, as shown in **Table 15.2**.[1] Another study of 111 consecutive patients scheduled for cardiac catheterization reported extremely high success rates at visualizing coronary segments. However, this particular study had strict exclusion criteria, including high probability of poor acoustic windows due to obesity or chronic obstructive pulmonary diseases, prior coronary artery bypass grafting, significant valvular disease, or atrial fibrillation. In this highly selected patient population, 2D TTE was extremely successful in imaging coronary arteries. Results are shown in **Table 15.3**.[2]

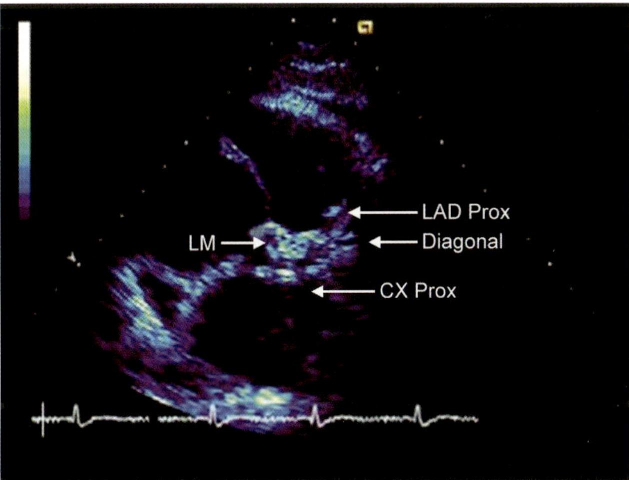


**Figure 15.1A:** Two-dimensional transthoracic echocardiographic assessment of the proximal part of left coronary artery in B-mode, modified parasternal short-axis view.

*Abbreviations:* LM, left main coronary artery; LAD Prox, proximal part of the left anterior descending coronary artery; Cx Prox, proximal part of the left circumflex coronary artery; Diagonal, proximal part of first diagonal artery.

*Source:* Krzanowski M, Bodzon W, Dimitrow PP. Imaging of all three coronary arteries by transthoracic echocardiography. An illustrated guide. Cardiovasc Ultrasound. 2003;1:16, *with permission.*

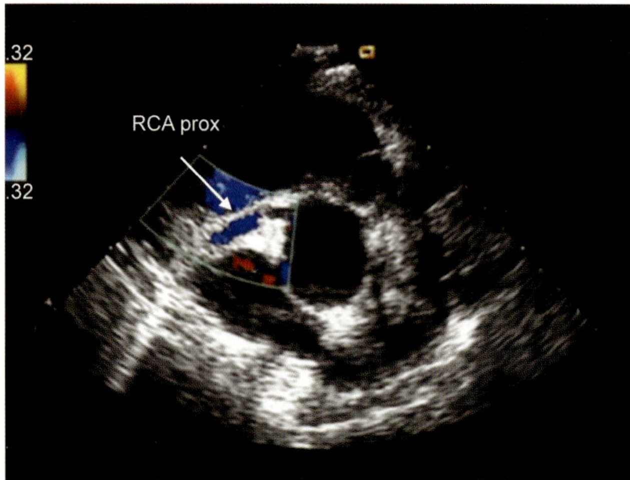


**Figure 15.1B:** Two-dimensional transthoracic echocardiographic assessment of the proximal right coronary artery (RCA Prox) in color Doppler, parasternal short-axis view.
*Source:* Krzanowski M, Bodzon W, et al. Imaging of all three coronary arteries by transthoracic echocardiography. An illustrated guide. Cardiovascular Ultrasound. 2003,1:16. (Figure 29)

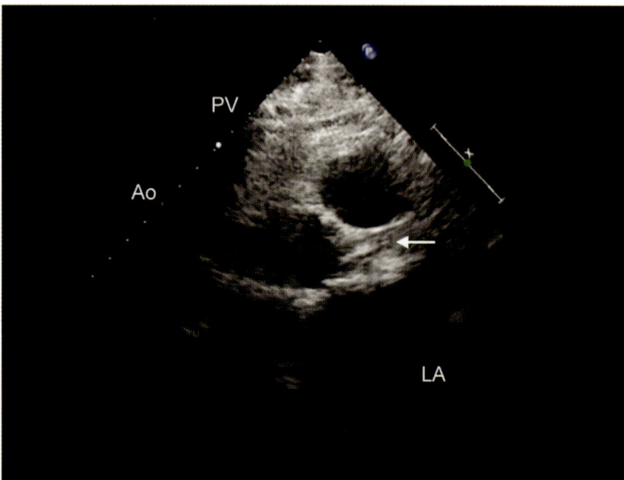


**Figure 15.2:** Left main coronary artery. Two-dimensional transthoracic echocardiography. Parasternal short-axis view at the level of the aorta (Ao) shows a small, left main coronary artery (arrow) with luminal irregularity due to nonobstructive atherosclerotic plaques.
*Abbreviations:* LA, left atrium; PV, pulmonary valve.
*Source:* Nanda NC, Sungur A, Bhagatwala K, et al. Non-standard echocardiographic examination. In: Nanda NC (Ed): Comprehensive Textbook of Echocardiography. New Delhi, India: Jaypee Brothers Medical Publishers (P) Ltd; 2014. pp. 188-223, *with permission*.

**Table 15.1:** Success rate of imaging coronary arteries by transthoracic echocardiography[3]

| *Segment* | *Percentage of patients* |
|---|---|
| LM/Proximal LAD | 55/≥90 |
| Proximal Cx | 88 |
| Middle Cx | 61 |
| Distal Cx | 3 |
| Proximal RCA | 40 |
| Middle RCA | 28 |
| Distal RCA | 54 |

*Abbreviations*: Cx, circumflex coronary artery; LAD, left anterior descending artery; LM, left main coronary artery; RCA, right coronary artery.

**Table 15.2:** When visualization of coronary arteries was obtained by two-dimensional transthoracic echocardiography, stenosis was identified with the below sensitivity and specificity, but the number of subjects in each group was low[1]

| *Vessel* | *Sensitivity (%)* | *Specificity (%)* |
|---|---|---|
| LAD | 64 | 96 |
| Cx | 66 | 100 |
| RCA | 62 | 100 |

*Abbreviations*: Cx, circumflex coronary artery; LAD, left anterior descending artery; RCA, right coronary artery.

**Table 15.3:** Findings of complete visualization of coronary artery segments with antegrade flow or coronary segments found with retrograde flow from a study of 111 consecutive patients scheduled for cardiac catheterization with exclusion criteria as outlined in the text

| *Segment* | *Antegrade flow or retrograde flow (%)* | *Antegrade flow (%)* | *Retrograde flow (%)* |
|---|---|---|---|
| LM | 98 | 98 | 0 |
| pLAD | 96 | 96 | 0 |
| mLAD | 96 | 95 | 1 |
| dLAD | 98 | 91 | 2 |
| pCx | 88 | 88 | 0 |
| mCx | 61 | 61 | 0 |
| dCx | 3 | 3 | 0 |
| pRCA | 40 | 40 | 0 |
| mRCA | 29 | 28 | 1 |
| PDA | 59 | 54 | 5 |

*Abbreviations:* dCx, distal circumflex coronary artery; dLAD distal left anterior descending artery; LM, left main coronary artery; mCx, middle circumflex coronary artery; mLAD, middle left anterior descending artery; mRCA, proximal right coronary artery; pCx, proximal circumflex coronary artery; PDA, posterior descending artery; pLAD, proximal left anterior descending artery; pRCA, proximal right coronary artery.
*Source:* Vegsundvag J, Holt E, Wiseth R, et al. Transthoracic echocardiography for imaging of the different coronary artery segments: a feasibility study. Cardiovasc Ultrasound. 2009;7:58, *with permission.*

**Table 15.4:** Two-dimensional transthoracic (TTE) and two-dimensional transesophageal (TEE) echocardiographic views for examining coronary arteries

| *Stenosis* | *Coronary artery visualization* | |
|---|---|---|
| Coronary artery | TTE optimal view | TEE optimal view |
| LM | High parasternal short-axis, apical five-chamber | Short axis, 0 or 180 degrees, 1–2 cm above aortic valve |
| LAD | High short-axis proximal and directed toward the probe, apical five chamber | Short-axis distal and directed from the probe—near parallel to Doppler beam |
| Cx | High short-axis distal and directed from the probe | Short-axis proximal and directed toward the probe |
| RCA | Parasternal long-axis, parasternal short axis | Short axis, slightly higher than LM ostium and in the aortic long-axis view |

*Abbreviations:* Cx, circumflex coronary artery; LAD, left anterior descending artery; LM, left main coronary artery; RCA, right coronary artery.
*Source:* Wierzbowska-Drabik K, Kasprzak JD. Echocardiographic assessment of coronary arteries: morphology and coronary flow reserve. In: Nanda NC (Ed): Comprehensive Textbook of Echocardiography. New Delhi, India: Jaypee Brothers Medical Publishers (P) Ltd; 2014; pp. 1336-47, *with permission.*

## *Technique*

Typically, the coronary ostia are seen in parasternal short-axis views at the level of the sinuses of Valsalva with additional views of the right coronary ostium seen in parasternal long-axis view. The perpendicular direction of the left main coronary artery (LMCA) in short-axis view in 2D TTE may cause suboptimal detection of flow with underestimation of recorded flow velocity, thus prompting a search for images from additional windows, such as the modified apical 5-chamber view. While the orifice and proximal segment of the LMCA are often visualized, the left anterior descending (LAD) artery is more difficult to visualize, especially the distal segment using standard parasternal approaches. On the other hand, using a nonstandard left parasternal technique in which the transducer is angled from the parasternal long-axis view or a para-apical view to slice a plane that basically "skims" the surface of the heart and transects the right ventricular (RV) but not the left ventricular (LV) cavity often brings into view the mid-segment of LAD. The apical 5-chamber view can also be used in a similar way to visualize the LAD. The circumflex coronary artery (Cx) can be seen with a modified high short-axis view. The right coronary artery (RCA) is extremely difficult to visualize with 2D TTE but can occasionally be seen in parasternal long-axis and short-axis views. Viewing techniques for each coronary artery are shown in **Table 15.4.**[3]

## *Stenosis and Occlusion*

High coronary flow velocity is suggestive of coronary stenosis. Precise cutoff values for coronary flow velocity are not well established at this time. Two sets of proposed cutoff values are provided in **Table 15.5.**[3] Complete coronary occlusion is more challenging to diagnose by echocardiography, as the velocity in the occluded segment would be practically zero. However, detection of diastolic flow reversal by Doppler in the segment distal to occlusion due to retrograde filling by collateral circulation coupled with nonvisualization of the coronary lumen on 2D TTE is useful in making the diagnosis. Sensitivity of this method is limited by the presence of collateral vessels and specificity is limited as collaterals may provide anterograde perfusion. In a study of 110 consecutive patients undergoing coronary angiography for investigation of angina, investigators used 2D TTE prior to angiography to diagnose chronic total coronary occlusion. In this study, investigators searched for flow reversal in epicardial and intramyocardial collaterals. They reported very high sensitivity and specificity for identifying occlusion, although the number of patients with occlusion was relatively low. Results are shown in **Table 15.6.**[6] Experience with this method is limited.

**Table 15.5:** Two sets of proposed cut off values for the echocardiographic diagnosis of coronary stenosis

| *Coronary artery* | *Proposed cut off value* | *Proposed cut-off value* |
|---|---|---|
| LM | >1.23 m/s | >1.40 m/s |
| LAD | >1.10 m/s | >0.9 m/s |
| Cx | >1.40 m/s | >1.10 m/s |
| RCA | >0.53 m/s | – |

*Abbreviations:* Cx, circumflex coronary artery; LAD, left anterior descending artery; LM, left main coronary artery; RCA, right coronary artery.
*Source:* Wierzbowska-Drabik K, Kasprzak JD. Echocardiographic assessment of coronary arteries: morphology and coronary flow reserve. In: Nanda NC (Ed): Comprehensive Textbook of Echocardiography. New Delhi, India: Jaypee Brothers Medical Publishers (P) Ltd; 2014. pp. 1336-47, with permission.

## Three-dimensional Transthoracic Echocardiography

A 3D TTE has been used to evaluate coronary artery disease, especially proximal coronary disease. The 3D imaging has a distinct advantage over 2D echocardiography, which provides only a thin section of cardiac structures such that a significant lesion in a coronary artery can be missed, if the section cuts across a normal portion of the coronary lumen. On the other hand, 3D echocardiography allows cropping in any plane. This enhances visualization for all segments of the coronary artery contained within the 3D dataset and reduces the risk of missing a lesion. Because the full extent of the lumen is visualized, the severity and extent of the stenotic lesion can be more accurately assessed by 3D echocardiography as compared with 2D echocardiography. An oblique 2D cut through a coronary artery may show evidence of narrowing of the lumen when none exists. This, too, can be avoided using 3D echocardiography. The 3D TTE is capable of visualizing blood flow, as in standard 2D TTE/Doppler echocardiography. A potential advantage to this method includes the ability to view coronary arteries in any orientation, including en face. Additionally, in one report by our group, a discrete stenotic lesion was found to be "gel-like" with some mobility consistent with a soft plaque (**Figures 15.3 to 15.5, Video 15.1**). The significance of this finding is unclear at this time; however, it does seem to suggest future plaque instability.[7] The primary limitation, as with 2D TTE, is the ability to acquire appropriate windows. Experience with this technique is extremely limited in published literature, and the role of 3D TTE in the evaluation of coronary artery disease remains to be defined.

**Table 15.6:** Sensitivity and specificity of retrograde flow for diagnosing coronary occlusion. Patients with poor visualization were excluded

| *Occluded vessel* | *Target vessel* | *Sensitivity (%)* | *Specificity (%)* |
|---|---|---|---|
| LAD | dLAD | 78 | 96 |
| LAD | sbLAD | 88 | 75 |
| LAD | dLAD and sbLAD | 89 | 96 |
| Cx | OMB | 80* | 100 |
| RCA | PDA | 79 | 97 |
| RCA | PDA and sbRCA | 89 | 97 |
| RCA | sbRCA | 63 | 35 |

*Abbreviations:* Cx, circumflex coronary artery; dLAD, distal left anterior descending artery; LAD, left anterior descending artery; OMB, obtuse marginal branch; PDA, posterior descending artery; RCA, right coronary artery; sbLAD, side branch LAD; sbRCA, side branch RCA.

*Note OMB was not well visualized in most patients.

*Source:* Boshchenko AA, Vrublevsky AV, Karpov RS. Transthoracic echocardiography in the detection of chronic total coronary artery occlusion. Eur J Echocardiogr. 2009;10:62-8, *with permission.*

## Two-dimensional Transesophageal Echocardiography

2D transesophageal echocardiography (TEE) with color flow and pulsed Doppler produces higher quality images of different coronary segments as compared to 2D TTE, because of the proximity of the cardiac structures to the ultrasound probe located in the esophagus such that a higher frequency transducer can be used. Operator experience is a critical factor in visualizing coronary arteries. With appropriate skill and equipment, images may be obtained of each of the coronary arteries, including LMCA, LAD, Cx, and RCA.[8-10]

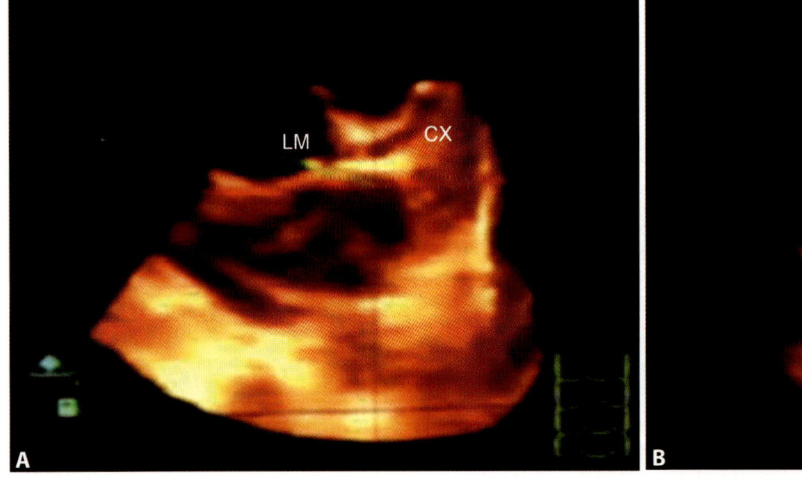


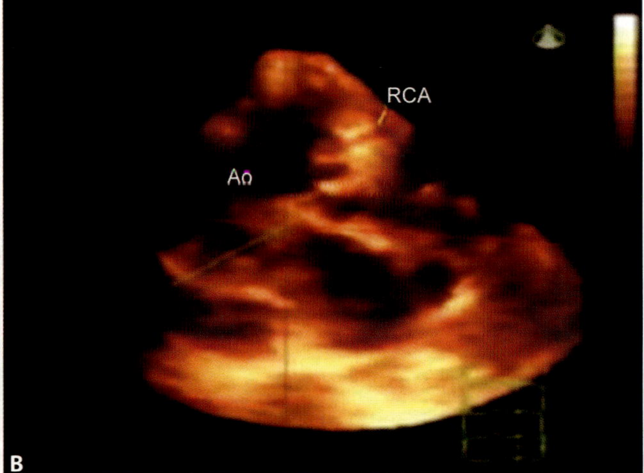


**Figure 15.3A and B:** Live/real time three-dimensional transthoracic echocardiographic assessment of coronary arteries in a 69-year-old female. (A) The pyramidal section has been cropped to show normal left main (LM) and proximal circumflex (Cx) coronary arteries. The left anterior descending coronary artery is located in a different plane. (B) Another section in the same patient demonstrates a normal proximal right coronary artery (RCA).

*Abbreviations:* Ao, aorta; RCA, right coronary artery.

*Source:* Vengala S, Nanda NC, Agrawal G, et al. Live three-dimensional transthoracic echocardiographic assessment of coronary arteries. Echocardiography. 2003;20:751-3, *with permission.*

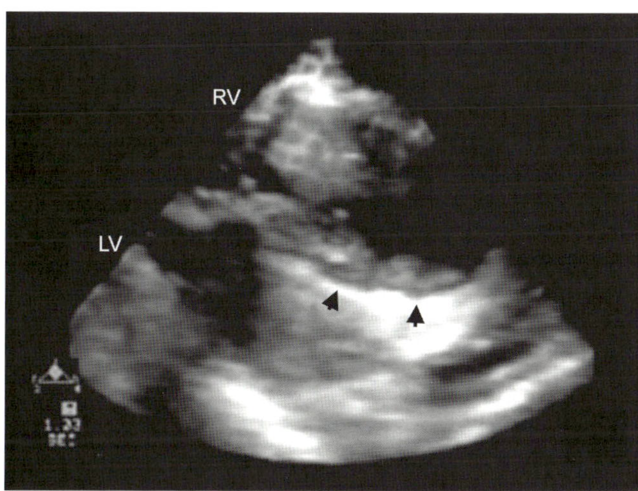


**Figure 15.4:** Live/real time three-dimensional transthoracic echocardiographic assessment of coronary arteries a 26-year-old male. The arrowheads demonstrate the mid-portion of the left anterior descending coronary artery (LAD) located in the anterior interventricular groove.

*Abbreviations:* LV, left ventricle; RV, right ventricle.

*Source:* Vengala S, Nanda NC, Agrawal G, et al. Live three-dimensional transthoracic echocardiographic assessment of coronary arteries. Echocardiography. 2003;20:751-3, *with permission.*

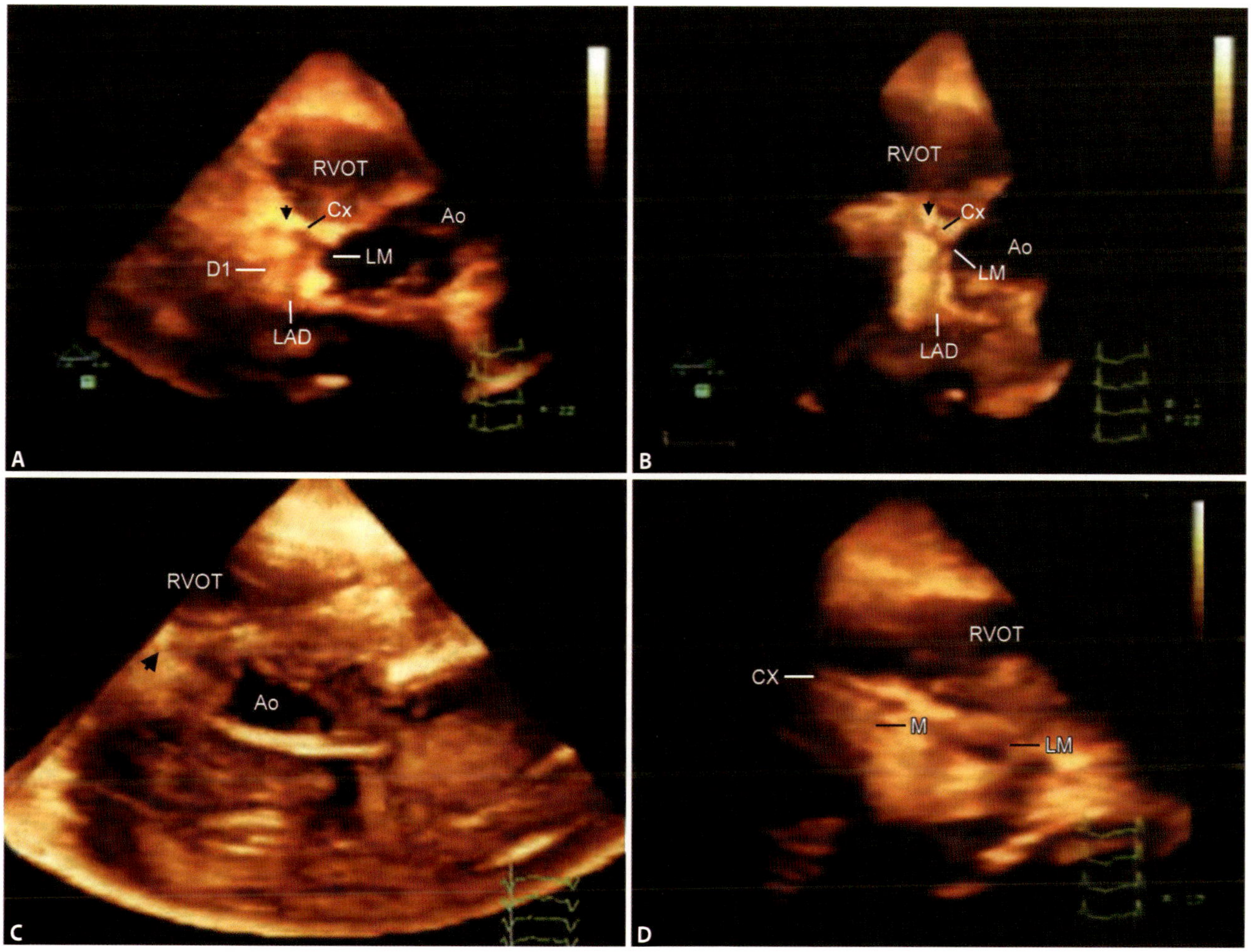

**Figure 15.5A to D**

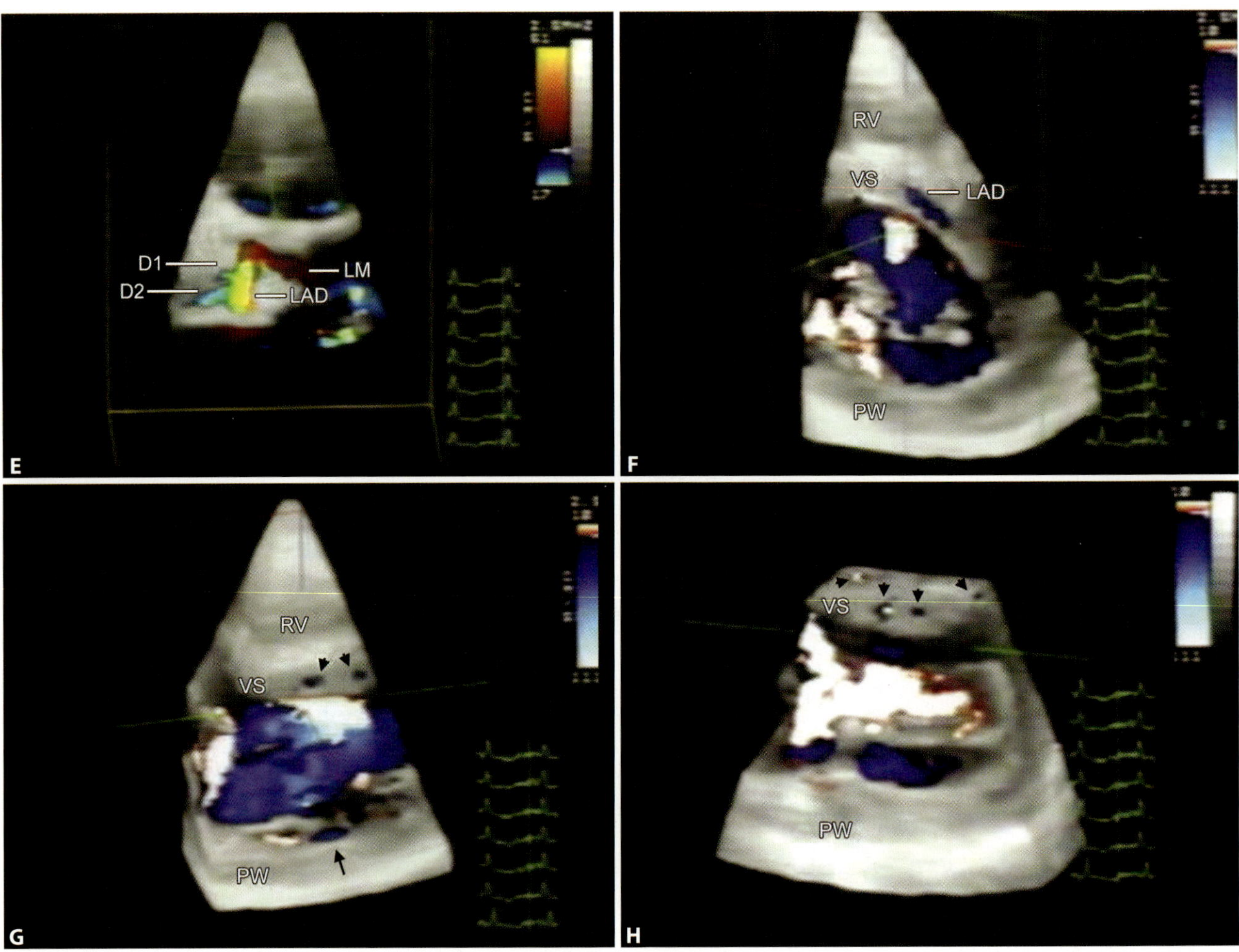


**Figure 15.5E to H**

**Figure 15.5A to H:** Live/real time transthoracic echocardiographic assessment of coronary arteries in a 39-year-old male, status post-orthotopic cardiac transplantation. (A) The arrowhead points to severe stenosis at the origin of the first obtuse marginal branch of Cx. (B) The image in A has been cropped and rotated to provide an en face view of the stenosis (arrowhead). (C) The arrowhead shows almost total stenosis of the proximal RCA. (D) The pyramidal section has been cropped to delineate a longer segment of CX, which shows no significant stenosis. M represents another marginal branch of Cx with a normal lumen. (E) Three-dimensional color Doppler flow imaging shows flow signals in the visualized coronary arteries. Note that the baseline on the color Doppler bar has been shifted to provide an estimate of coronary flow velocities. (F) Three-dimensional color Doppler flow imaging demonstrates a segment of LAD adjacent to ventricular septum (VS). This segment was not visualized by B-mode 3D imaging. (G and H) The arrowheads point to multiple septal perforators imaged in short axis within the VS. Note also the presence of an intramural coronary artery branch (arrow) in the left ventricular posterior wall (PW) in G.

*Abbreviations:* Ao, aorta; Cx, circumflex coronary artery; D1, first diagonal branch of LAD; D2, second diagonal branch of LAD; LAD, left anterior descending artery; LM, left main coronary artery; RV, right ventricle; RVOT, right ventricular outflow tract.

*Source:* Vengala S, Nanda NC, Agrawal G, et al. Live three-dimensional transthoracic echocardiographic assessment of coronary arteries. Echocardiography. 2003;20:751-3, *with permission.*

## *Technique*

Using a basal short-axis view just above the aortic valve leaflets, the LMCA and proximal RCA can be seen. Tilting the probe superiorly and leftward from the basal short axis brings the ostium of the LM into view. Tilting the probe inferiorly with leftward rotation from the basal short axis brings the proximal LMCA into view. Further tilting from the basal short axis reveals the LAD. The Cx can be seen coursing in the atrioventricular groove by using the plane for the LMCA and tilting the probe leftward and superiorly. The RCA ostium can be seen from the basal short-axis view by rightward and inferior tilting of the probe between the 6 o'clock and 7 o'clock position. Due to anatomic variability, one must image to the right or inferiorly from the ostium. The longitudinal scanning plane is helpful for assessing luminal narrowing as it provides a cross-section view of the coronary arteries.[11]

## *Stenosis*

Success rates for visualizing coronary arteries are somewhat variable.[8-11] Approximate reported success rates for each segment are 90% (85–95) for the LMCA, 85% (80–90) for the Cx, 70% (55–80) for LAD, and 65% (50–80) for the RCA **(Figure 15.6A and B)**. Ideally, images clearly reveal the wall and lumen and show the maximum length possible of each segment. Normal arteries appear echolucent with no luminal irregularities. Calcified plaque is seen as "shadowing" on ultrasound. Noncalcified plaque is poorly visualized. Stenosis can be identified on TEE by either apparent luminal narrowing or flow turbulence with increased velocity. The apparent luminal narrowing must be at least a 50% reduction in lumen diameter. In this case, normal lumen must be visualized distal to the stenosed area for comparison **(Figure 15.7A and B)**. For accuracy, multiple measurements are required, both of the stenosis itself and of the coronary width. It is appropriate in this case to use the largest measured diameter as the coronary width, as smaller measurements may include plaque from the vessel wall. Flow turbulence can be identified by either a mosaic flow pattern or aliasing seen on pulsed Doppler **(Figure 15.8A and B)**.

**Table 15.7** enlists results of several studies on the evaluation of proximal coronary artery stenosis by 2D TEE.[6] **Table 15.8** enlists sensitivity and specificity of echocardiographic findings when compared with angiography in identifying coronary artery disease.[8] Proximal coronary artery stenosis includes narrowing of the LMCA, proximal LAD up to the first septal perforator, proximal Cx up to the obtuse marginal, and the proximal third of the RCA.

## *Limitations*

The following limitations exist in directly visualizing coronary artery stenosis by 2D TEE:[9]

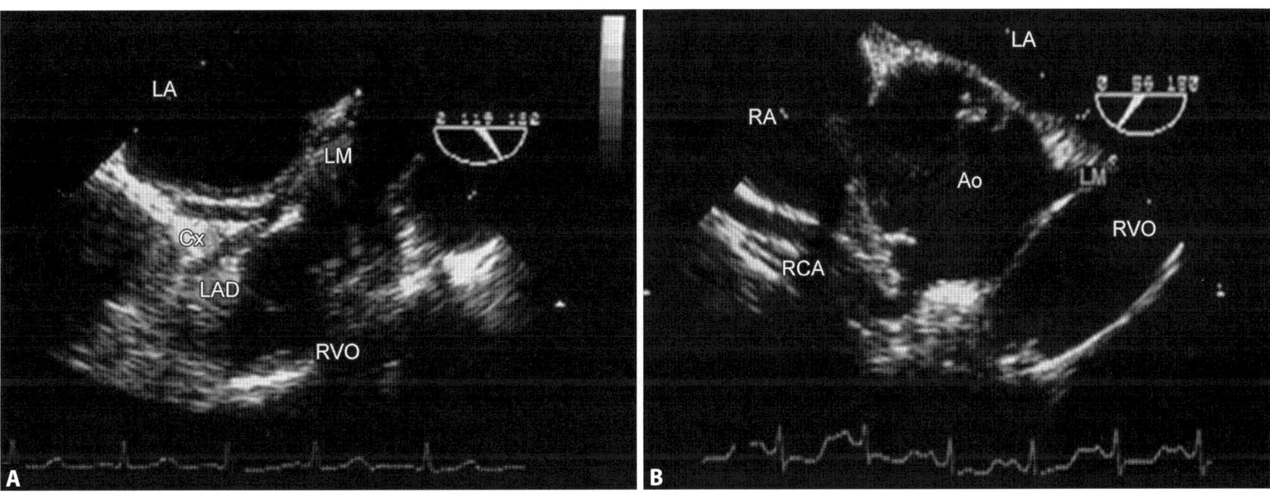


**Figure 15.6A and B:** (A) Transesophageal echocardiographic assessment of normal proximal left-sided coronary arteries. Plane angulation at 119° demonstrate the LMCA and its bifurcation into the LAD and LCx vessels. Note absence of any significant stenosis in the coronary arteries visualized. (B) Transesophageal echocardiographic assessment of normal right coronary artery. Shown at 56° multiplane angle, a long segment of the RCA is visualized without any stenosis in this patient.

*Abbreviations:* Ao, aorta; Cx, circumplex coronary artery; LA, left atrium; LAD, left anterior descending artery; LM, left main coronary artery; RA, right atrium; RCA, right coronary artery; RVO, right ventricular outflow tract.

*Source:* Biederman RWW, Sorrell VL, Nanda NC, et al. Transesophageal echocardiographic assessment of coronary stenosis. A decade of experience. Echocardiography. 2001;18:49-57, *with permission.*

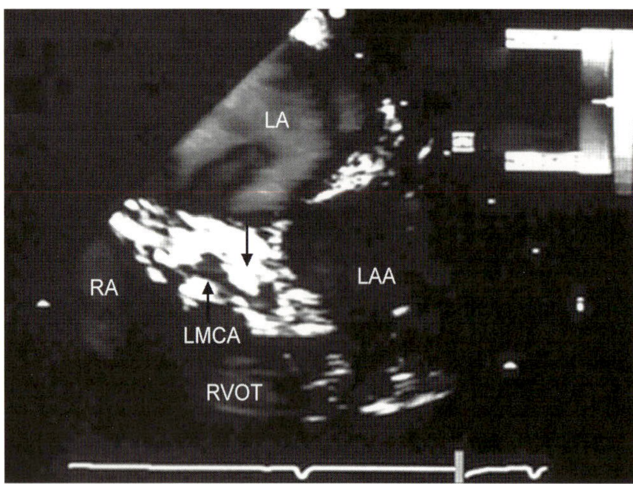


**Figure 15.7A:** Transesophageal echocardiographic assessment of left main stenosis. The bold arrow demonstrates a large atherosclerotic plaque producing 80% stenosis of the LMCA. The small arrow points to absence of significant stenosis proximally.
*Abbreviations:* LAA, left atrial appendage; RVOT, right ventricular outflow tract; LA, left atrium; LMCA, left main coronary artery; RA, right atrium.
*Source:* Nanda NC, Domanski MJ (Eds). Atlas of Transesophageal Echocardiography. Baltimore: Williams & Wilkins, 1998. (Figure 4).

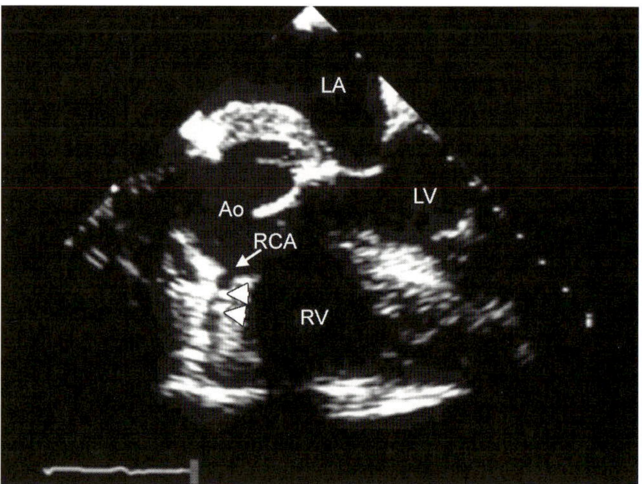


**Figure 15.7B:** Transesophageal echocardiographic assessment of proximal right coronary artery stenosis. The arrowheads point to two discrete areas of severe stenosis in the proximal portion of the RCA.
*Abbreviations:* Ao, aorta; LA, left atrium; LV, left ventricle; RCA, right coronary artery; RV, right ventricle.
*Source:* Nanda NC, Domanski MJ (Eds). Atlas of Transesophageal Echocardiography. Baltimore: Williams & Wilkins, 1998. (Figure 7).

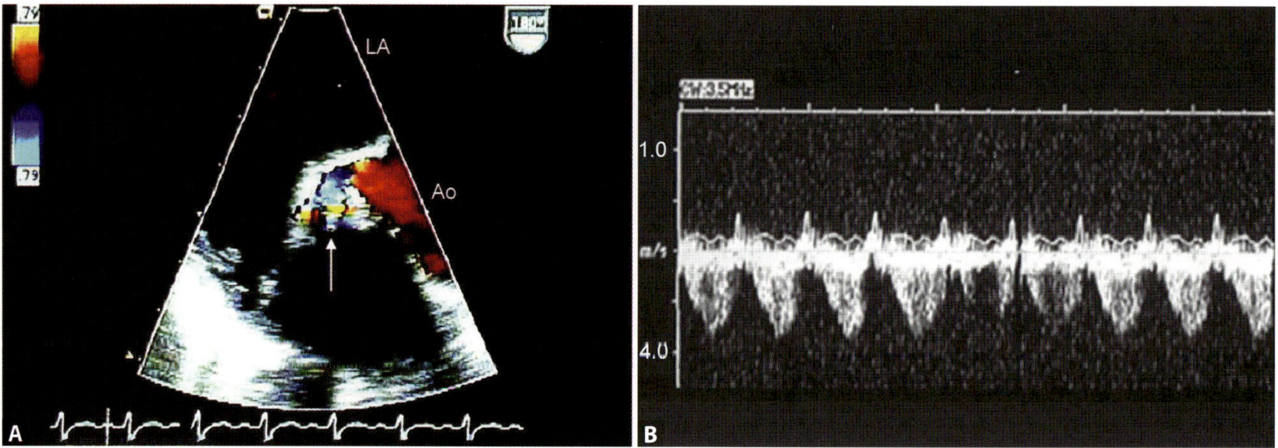


**Figure 15.8A and B:** Transesophageal echocardiographic assessment of proximal left anterior descending coronary artery stenosis. (A) The arrow points to turbulent flow signals at the origin of the LAD coronary artery imaged at 180° multiplane angle. (B) Color Doppler-guided continuous-wave Doppler examination shows a very high peak velocity of 3.8 m/second indicative of severe stenosis.
Coronary angiogram, done subsequently to transesophageal examination, demonstrated a 70% lesion in the proximal LAD in this patient.
*Abbreviations:* Ao, aorta; LA, left atrium.
*Source:* Biederman RWW, Sorrell VL, Nanda NC, et al. Transesophageal echocardiographic assessment of coronary stenosis: A decade of experience. Echocardiography. 2001;18:49-57, (Figure 5).

- Long visualized segments of the arteries are associated with higher sensitivity. However, 2D TEE is not always capable of this, particularly with the RCA.
- Eccentric lesions can pose a challenge. Depending on the scanning plane, the severity of eccentric lesions may appear different in echocardiographic than in angiographic views. Calcified plaques can cause acoustic shadowing, which may also obscure stenotic lesions. False-negative results attributable to eccentric lesions or acoustic shadowing of a calcified plaque are reduced by multiplane echocardiography with its capability of obtaining additional views as compared to biplane imaging.

**Table 15.7:** Assessment of coronary artery stenosis using two-dimensional transesophageal echocardiography by different authors

| *First author (number of patients)* | *LM (%)* | *LAD (%)* | *LCx (%)* | *RCA (%)* | *LM ≥50%* | *Proximal LAD ≥50%* | *Proximal LCx ≥50%* | *Proximal RCA ≥50%* | *Comments* |
|---|---|---|---|---|---|---|---|---|---|
| Zwicky | 100 | – | – | – | – | – | – | – | Awake |
| Yamagishi | 77 | 77 | 54 | 26 | – | – | – | – | Postoperative |
| Pearce | 79 | 62 | 57 | 50 | _ | _ | _ | _ | Intraoperative |
| Yoshida | 90 | – | – | – | 88% (10/12) | – | – | – | Awake |
| Yamagishi | 90 | – | – | – | 94% (16/17) | – | – | – | Awake |
| Schrem | 100 | – | – | – | 100% (4/4) (all ostial) | – | – | – | Awake |
| Reichert | 88 | 52 | 88 | – | 100% (4/4) | 71%(5/7) | 50%(2/4) | – | Postoperative |
| Taams | 95 | 14 | 68 | – | 65% (15/23) | – | 64% (9/14) | – | Awake |
| Samdarshi | 93 | 93 | 93 | 49 | 96% (2k;3/24) | 82%(11/14) | 80%(6/8) | 100%(7/7) | Intraoperative |

*Abbreviations:* LAD, left anterior descending artery; LCx, left circumflex coronary artery; LM, left main coronary artery; RCA, right coronary artery.
*Source:* Samdarshi TE, Nanda NC, Gatewood RP Jr, Ballal RS, Chang LK, Singh HP, et al. Usefulness and limitations of transesophageal echocardiography in the assessment of proximal coronary artery stenosis. J Am Coll Cardiol. 1992;19:572-80, *with permission.*

**Table 15.8:** Two-dimensional transesophageal echocardiography in the assessment of angiography defined proximal coronary artery stenosis irrespective of whether these coronary segments were visualized by echocardiography (total number of stenoses = 75)

| *ANG → TEE↓* | *LM* | | *LAD* | | *Cx* | | *RCA* | |
|---|---|---|---|---|---|---|---|---|
| | + | – | + | – | + | – | + | – |
| + | 23<br>1 | | 11<br>1 | | 6 | 0 | 7 | 0 |
| – | 1<br>78 | | 12<br>79 | | 3<br>94 | | 12<br>36 | |
| Sensitivity, % | 96 | | 48 | | 67 | | 37 | |
| Specificity, % | 99 | | 99 | | 100 | | 100 | |

*Abbreviations:* –, <50% stenosis; +, ≥50% stenosis; ANG, angiography; LAD, left anterior descending artery; LCx, left circumflex coronary artery; LM, left main coronary artery; RCA, right coronary artery.
*Source:* Samdarshi TE, Nanda NC, Gatewood RP Jr, Ballal RS, Chang LK, Singh HP, et al. Usefulness and limitations of transesophageal echocardiography in the assessment of proximal coronary artery stenosis. J Am Coll Cardiol. 1992;19:572-80, *with permission.*

- Cardiac motion can also pose a challenge as the vessel may move in and out of view. This challenge is increased by respiratory motion. Together, these can make measurement of flow velocity during an entire cardiac cycle very challenging.
- Color flow Doppler utilization increases diagnostic sensitivity of 2D TEE. However, color flow may not be appropriately detectable in all visualized segments. Utilizing an echocardiographic contrast agent may circumvent this limitation.

## Contrast Enhancement

Echocardiographic contrast agents consist essentially of microbubbles of a gas, typically a fluorocarbon. When injected intravenously, it is easily detected by ultrasound, because of the strong reflections produced by the gaseous microbubbles. They result in enhancement of both conventional and color Doppler signals permitting an improved assessment of coronary stenotic lesions. One study from our group has highlighted the role of contrast 2D TEE for direct coronary visualization. Before using contrast, patients had 2D TEE revealing variable lengths of LMCA, LAD, and Cx. Intravenous contrast injection enabled visualization of longer segments of the LMCA, LAD, and Cx coronary arteries, and in one patient, significant stenosis was detectable only after administration of contrast. Therefore, contrast echo can improve visualization and may detect coronary stenosis that cannot be directly visualized without contrast **(Figure 15.9)**.[12,13] In another study, some patients with normal findings on 2D TEE were found to have significant coronary disease after administration of an echo contrast agent.[13]

### *Limitations*

- Contrast-enhanced echocardiography shows longer segments of the coronary arteries; however, distal segments are better visualized by intracoronary procedures.
- Contrast enhanced echo has a limited ability to overcome ultrasound masking by calcified plaques.

## Three-dimensional Transesophageal Echocardiography

A 3D TEE reconstruction of coronary arteries has been performed using multiplane 2D TEE. Several studies have demonstrated successful utilization of this modality to identify coronary stenosis **(Figure 15.10 to 15.12)**,[14] although experience is more limited than with traditional 2D imaging. In one particular study, 27 patients had 3D TEE performed followed by coronary angiography. Reconstruction of the entire LMCA was done in all patients. Reconstruction of LAD,

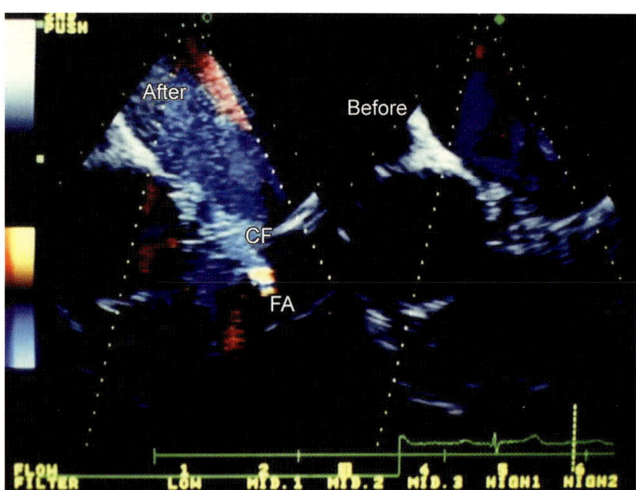


**Figure 15.9:** Transesophageal echocardiographic assessment of proximal coronary arteries after echo contrast enhancement. At baseline (right) virtually no flow signals are noted in the left main coronary artery. After contrast injection (left), prominent flow signals not only completely fill the lumen, but also opacify an additional segment of the proximal left anterior descending coronary vessel that was not visualized at baseline. In addition, flow aliasing (FA) is noted more distally, and its site corresponded to an area of severe stenosis in the left anterior descending artery on the coronary angiogram.
*Abbreviation:* CF, origin of the circumflex vessel.
*Source:* Aggarwal KK, Gatewood RP, Nanda NC, et al. Improved transesophageal echocardiographic assessment of significant proximal narrowing of the left anterior descending and left circumflex coronary arteries using echo contrast enhancement. Am J Cardiol. 1994;73:1131-3, *with permission.*

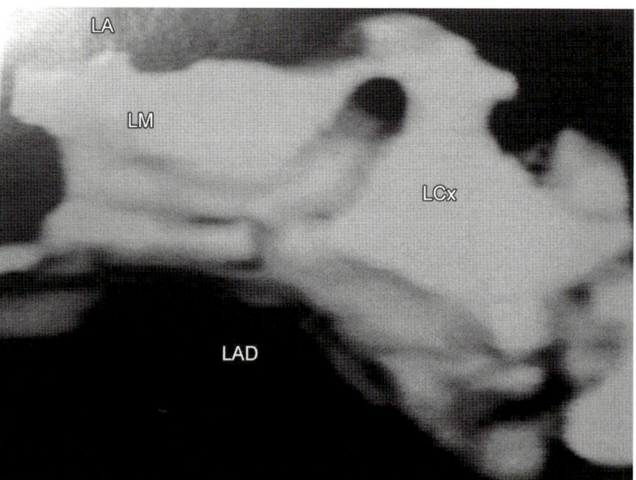


**Figure 15.10:** Transesophageal three-dimensional echocardiographic examination of coronary arteries. The left main (LM) originating from the aortic root as well as the proximal left anterior descending (LAD) and circumflex (LCx) coronary arteries are viewed in long axis in three dimensions. Note short-axis imaging of the more distal portion of the circumflex vessel. There is no evidence of stenosis.
*Abbreviations:* LA, left atrium; LAD, left anterior descending; LCx, left circumflex.
*Source:* Abd El-Rahman SM, Khatri G, Nanda N, et al. Transesophageal three-dimensional echocardiographic assessment of normal and stenosed coronary arteries. Echocardiography. 1996;13:503-10, *with permission.*

Cx, and RCA was also done with a mean visualized length of 0.8 cm (range 0.2–2.5 cm), 0.9 cm (range 0.2–2.8 cm), and 0.9 cm (range 0.2–2.8 cm), respectively. Although the numbers were small in this study, patients with >50% stenosis also had significant stenosis on coronary angiography.[14]

## CORONARY FLOW RESERVE

Coronary flow reserve (CFR) is an important index of coronary artery function. It is a ratio of maximal coronary flow compared to baseline. It can be measured with various modalities, including positron emission tomography, magnetic resonance imaging, as well as echocardiography.[15-17] Normal coronary arteries respond to potent vasodilation with a marked increase in flow, up to 3–5 times their baseline. This response is attenuated in patients with epicardial coronary disease. It is also decreased in patients with hypertension, diabetes mellitus, hypertrophic cardiomyopathy, and syndrome X, that is believed to be due to microvascular disease. In one series, LAD flow velocity was assessed using harmonic color Doppler with contrast enhancement on 2D TTE. Flow velocities at rest and flow velocities after maximal vasodilation with dipyridamole were used to calculate CFR. In an unselected group of consecutive patients undergoing coronary angiography, a peak diastolic CFR of <2.0 had a sensitivity and specificity of 86% and 90%, respectively for the presence of ≥70% LAD stenosis on coronary angiography.[15] Another study compared the wall motion abnormalities and CFR seen on 2D TTE. Coronary flow velocity was measured in the distal LAD before and after dipyridamole infusion. Contrast was used if needed. CFR ≤2 was taken to be suggestive of disease. In this study, CFR compared to wall motion abnormalities had a higher sensitivity (94% vs 72%) but lower specificity (65% vs 95%) for detecting significant LAD stenosis. In patients with both low CFR and wall motion abnormalities, this testing had 94% accuracy in predicting significant LAD stenosis.[17] It should be noted, however, that these studies evaluated CFR in the LAD, not in other vascular beds. A few studies have investigated CFR in all three coronary beds. One such study enrolled 175 patients 6 months after stent implantation. Patients had 2D TTE with visualization of LAD, RCA, and Cx arteries. A value <2.0 was considered significant. Compared to angiography, sensitivity, specificity,

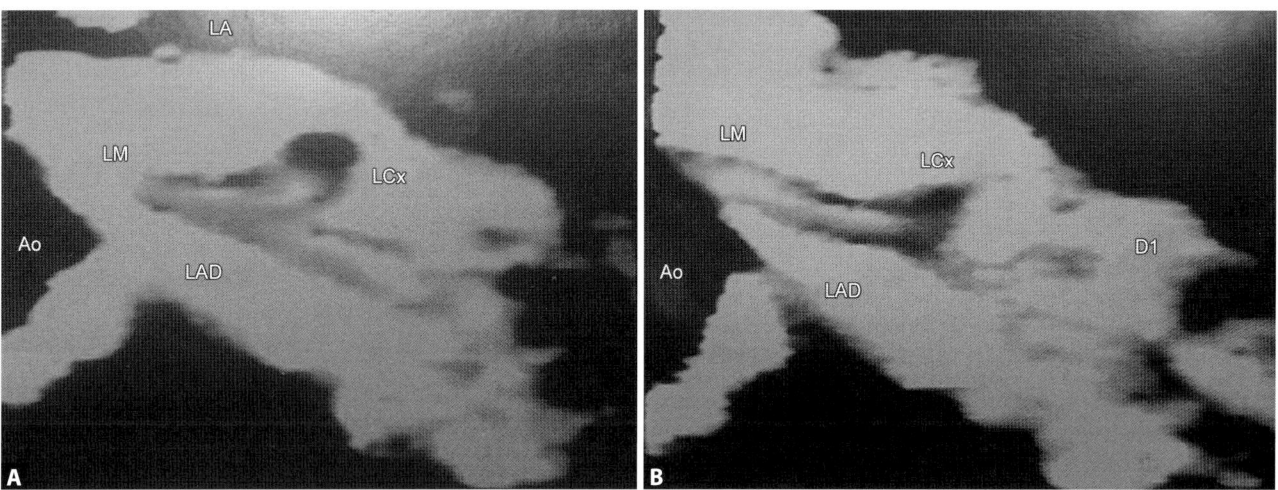


**Figure 15.11A and B:** Transesophageal three-dimensional echocardiographic examination of coronary arteries. Both (A) and (B) represent two different three-dimensional reconstructions of left-sided coronary arteries from the same dataset stored in the computer. Figure B shows delineation of the first diagonal branch (D1), which is not visualized in Figure A.
*Abbreviations:* Ao, aortic root; LA, left artery; LAD, left anterior descending artery; LM, left main coronary artery; LCx, left circumflex coronary artery.
*Source:* Abd El-Rahman SM, Khatri G, Nanda N, et al. Transesophageal three-dimensional echocardiographic assessment of normal and stenosed coronary arteries. Echocardiography. 1996;13:503-10, *with permission*.

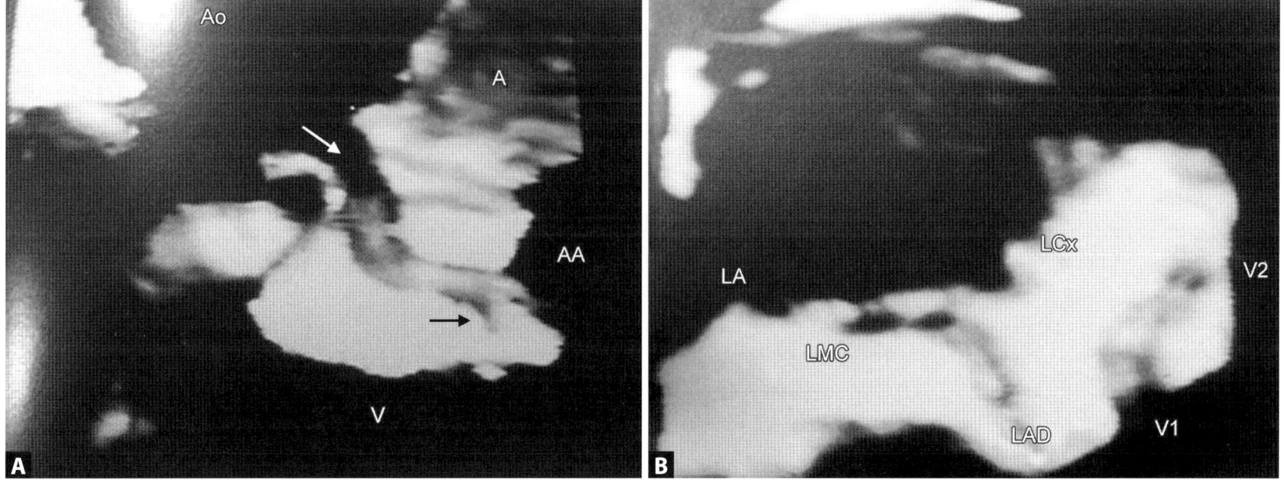


**Figure 15.12A and B:** (A) Transesophageal three-dimensional echocardiographic examination of coronary arteries. The right coronary artery (oblique arrow) is seen arising from the aortic root (Ao) and coursing along the right atrioventricular groove adjacent to the right atrial appendage (AA). The horizontal arrow points to a right ventricular branch. A, right atrium, V, right ventricle. (B) Transesophageal three-dimensional echocardiographic examination of coronary arteries. Both interventricular (V1) and great cardiac (V2) veins are delineated accompanying the left anterior descending (LAD) and circumflex (LCx) coronary arteries.
*Abbreviations:* LA, left artery; LMC, left main coronary artery.
*Source:* Abd El-Rahman SM, Khatri G, Nanda N, et al. Transesophageal three-dimensional echocardiographic assessment of normal and stenosed coronary arteries. Echocardiography. 1996;13:503-10, *with permission*.

and feasibility were 86%, 91%, and 95%, respectively. For RCA, results were 92%, 92%, and 85%, respectively. For Cx, results were 91%, 92%, and 81%, respectively. Overall sensitivity and specificity were 89% and 91%, respectively.[18] The CFR is most often measured with TTE rather than 2D TEE, which is semiinvasive, and not without patient discomfort The clinical role of echocardiographic measurement on CFR is unclear at this time. However, given that it is noninvasive and relatively inexpensive, it may see broader clinical use in the future. At present, it is used mainly in Europe and Japan.

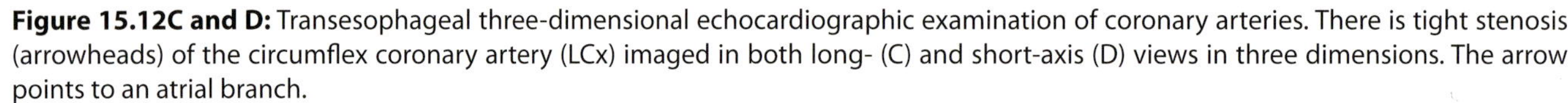

**Figure 15.12C and D:** Transesophageal three-dimensional echocardiographic examination of coronary arteries. There is tight stenosis (arrowheads) of the circumflex coronary artery (LCx) imaged in both long- (C) and short-axis (D) views in three dimensions. The arrow points to an atrial branch.
*Abbreviations:* Ao, aorta; LA, left artery; LMC, left main coronary artery.
*Source:* Abd El-Rahman SM, Khatri G, Nanda N, et al. Transesophageal three-dimensional echocardiographic assessment of normal and stenosed coronary arteries. Echocardiography. 1996;13:503-10, *with permission*.

## ISCHEMIC STROKE

The clinical role of direct visualization of coronary arteries for stenosis by 2D and 3D TEE in patients with stroke referred for TEE for evaluation of a cardiac source of embolization is not entirely clear at this point. Studies have shown that it may guide therapy after ischemic stroke in patients without known coronary disease. Patients, especially elderly, with ischemic stroke due to cerebrovascular disease have a very high prevalence of coronary artery disease, ranging from 28% to 86%. This is no surprise given the underlying pathophysiologic process is the same for atherosclerosis in the coronary system as it is for cerebral arteries. In one particular study from our laboratory, 32 patients with ischemic stroke underwent 2D TEE for evaluation of coronary disease. Successful coronary artery visualization rates were very high **(Table 15.9)**.[19] Of these patients, 17 had changes in their management related to TEE findings, mainly visualization of severe stenosis in the proximal coronary arteries **(Figure 15.13 to 15.15)**. Because of the diagnosis of significant coronary stenosis, 10 patients underwent coronary angiography, which confirmed the 2D TEE diagnosis, and had revascularization.

Although this examination is not a part of routine practice at most centers, it shows great promise and may have a greater role in routine clinical care in the future. In general, it takes only a few additional minutes to quickly evaluate the proximal coronaries for stenosis. Normal unaliased color Doppler flow signals rule out any significant narrowing in the visualized segments of the coronary arteries and obviate the need for additional interrogation by conventional Doppler. When aliasing or flow turbulence is detected, that particular area is then interrogated by pulsed Doppler and, if necessary, continuous wave Doppler to measure the peak

**Table 15.9:** Two-dimensional transesophageal echocardiography (TEE) and coronary angiography correlation

| | *TEE-positive* | *TEE-negative* |
|---|---|---|
| *Left main coronary artery* | | |
| Coronary angiography positive | 4 | 0 |
| Coronary angiography negative | 0 | 27 |
| *Left anterior descending coronary artery* | | |
| Coronary angiography positive | 13 | 0 |
| Coronary angiography negative | 1 | 18 |
| *Left circumflex coronary artery* | | |
| Coronary angiography positive | 2 | 0 |
| Coronary angiography negative | 1 | 27 |
| *Right coronary artery* | | |
| Coronary angiography positive | 2 | 2 |
| Coronary angiography negative | 0 | 19 |

TEE positive, peak diastolic velocity >2 m/s in the narrow segment detected by the 2D TEE.
Coronary angiography positive, stenosis ≥50% of the lumen width.
*Source:* Voros S, Nanda NC, Samal AK, et al. Transesophageal echocardiography in patients with ischemic stroke accurately detects significant coronary artery stenosis and often changes management. Am Heart J. 2001;142:916-22, *with permission*.

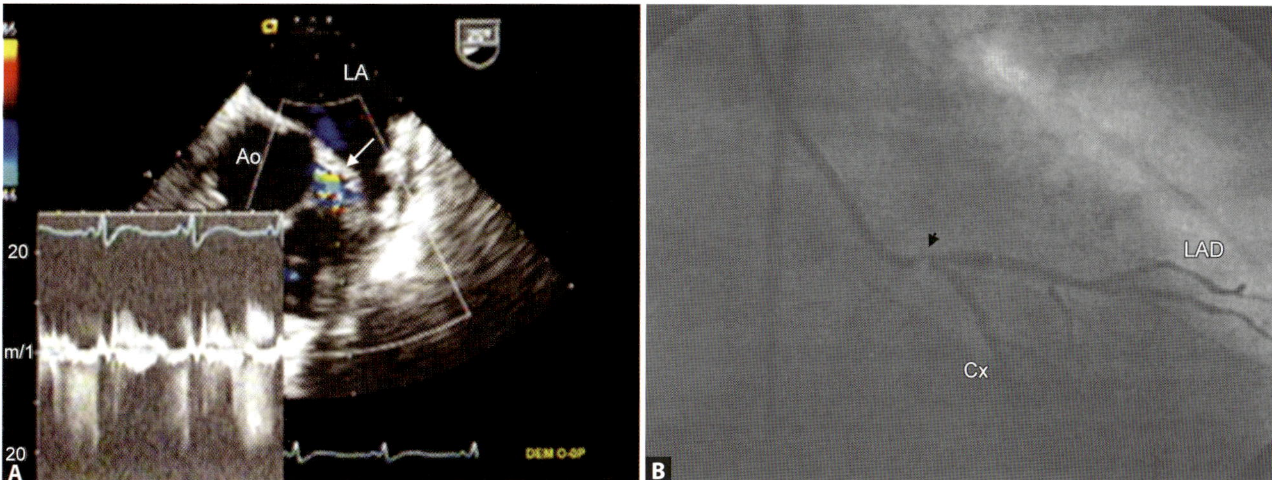


**Figure 15.13A and B:** Transesophageal echocardiographic detection of significant left main coronary artery stenosis. (A) Arrow, Turbulent flow in the left main coronary artery. Inset, Doppler interrogation demonstrates a very high velocity of 2.2 m/s, indicative of severe stenosis. (B) Coronary angiography confirms the presence of severe left main coronary artery stenosis (arrowhead).
*Abbreviations:* Ao, aorta; Cx, left circumflex coronary artery; LA, left atrium; LAD, left anterior descending coronary artery.
*Source:* Voros S, Nanda NC, Samal AK, et al. Transesophageal echocardiography in patients with ischemic stroke accurately detects significant coronary artery stenosis and often changes management. Am Heart J. 2001;142:918-20, *with permission*.

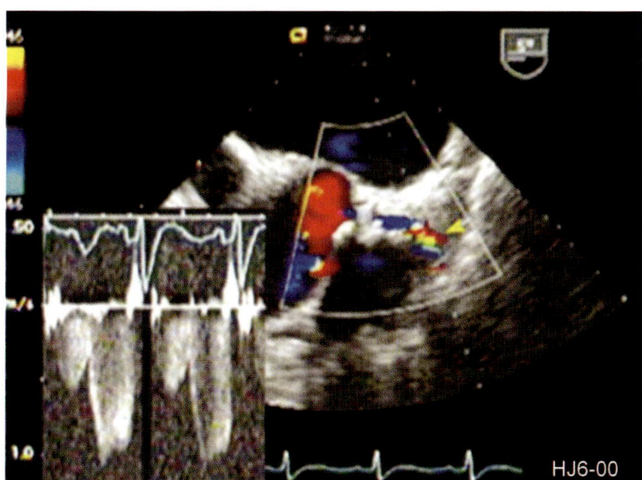


**Figure 15.14:** Transesophageal echocardiographic detection of significant proximal left anterior descending coronary artery stenosis. Arrow, Turbulent flow in the proximal left anterior descending coronary artery. Inset, Doppler interrogation demonstrates a high velocity of 1.2 m/s, indicative of significant stenosis.
*Source:* Voros S, Nanda NC, Samal AK, et al. Transesophageal echocardiography in patients with ischemic stroke accurately detects significant coronary artery stenosis and often changes management. Am Heart J. 2001;142:918-20, *with permission*.

diastolic velocity. If it is high enough, a diagnosis of significant stenosis can be made. Additional demonstration of narrowing on 2D imaging adds to the confidence level of the diagnosis. Reversed diastolic flow may alert one to a completely occluded coronary lumen, especially if this is also associated with no lumen on the B-mode examination. In the presence of severe aortic regurgitation and other high flow states, such as peripheral arteriovenous shunts in patients with chronic kidney disease undergoing dialysis, high diastolic velocities may be found in the coronary arteries, and this should be taken into account when evaluating for stenosis. In these cases, usually the velocities are not very high and the coronary lumen shows no evidence of narrowing on B-mode examination. Coronary veins, which accompany coronary arteries and are located adjacent to them, may also show high velocities, but these are easily differentiated because the velocities are high in both systole and diastole unlike arterial stenosis where the high velocities are predominantly diastolic.[19]

## AORTIC DISSECTION

Aortic dissection is an acute, life-threatening condition requiring prompt diagnosis and treatment. Both 2D and 3D TEE have a high sensitivity not only for the diagnosis of aortic dissection but also for detection of proximal coronary artery involvement **(Figure 15.16 and 15.17, Videos 15.2A and B)**.[11,20,21] Studies show that 10–20% of aortic dissection patients have coronary artery involvement. The dissection flap can obstruct the ostium of LMCA or RCA or the dissection can extend along the walls of the coronary arteries producing narrowing of the lumen. Both can result

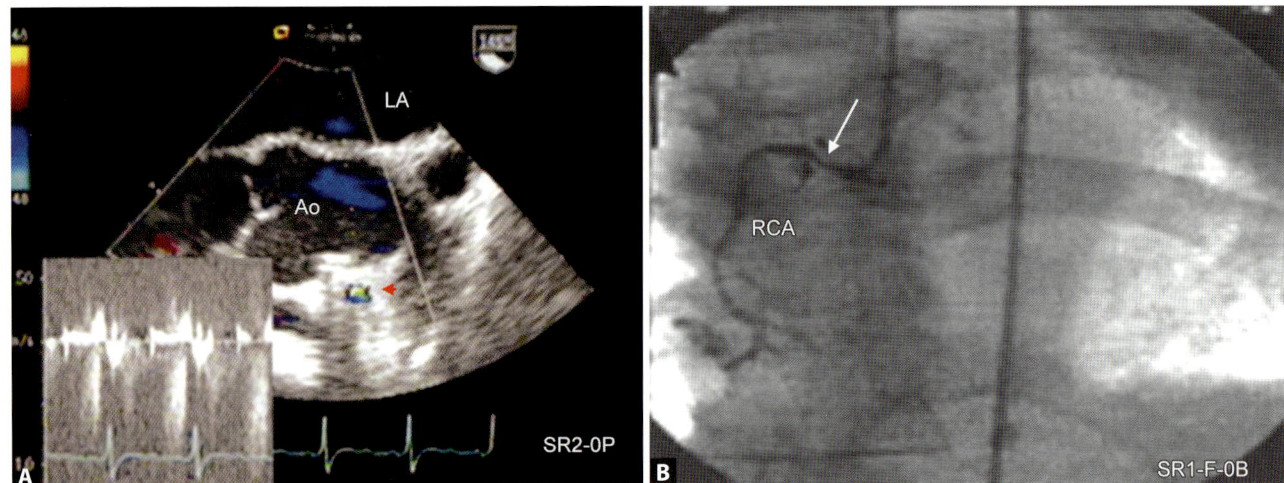


**Figure 15.15A and B:** Transesophageal echocardiographic detection of significant proximal right coronary artery stenosis. (A) Arrow, Turbulent flow in the in the proximal right coronary artery. Inset, Doppler interrogation demonstrates a high velocity of 1.2 m/s, indicative of significant stenosis. (B) Coronary angiography confirms the proximal right coronary artery (RCA) lesion (arrow).
*Abbreviations:* LA, left atrium; AO, aorta.
*Source:* Voros S, Nanda NC, Samal AK, et al. Transesophageal echocardiography in patients with ischemic stroke accurately detects significant coronary artery stenosis and often changes management. Am Heart J. 2001;142:918-20, *with permission*.

in myocardial infarction or ischemia. In some cases, coronary vessel narrowing can be caused by extrinsic compression by a subadventitial hematoma caused by the dissection process. Both 2D and 3D TEE can potentially diagnose and assess not only the stenosis severity but also its mechanism in these patients. The proximity of the TEE probe in the esophagus to the aortic root and aorta facilitates improved visualization of the coronary arteries as compared to 2D TTE. Knowledge of coronary artery involvement in aortic dissection is critical for appropriate surgical planning. In these cases, surgery needs to be performed immediately, because the patient's life is endangered not only by aortic dissection but also by simultaneously occurring reduction in myocardial perfusion from coronary obstruction. Diagnosis of coronary obstruction by echocardiography takes on an even greater importance; because in many patients with aortic dissection, coronary arteriograms are not performed, since the main objective is to save the patient's life, and a delay in taking the patient to surgery after the diagnosis of dissection has been made may result in increased morbidity and even mortality.

In a study involving 34 patients with aortic dissection, 7 patients had coronary involvement at the time of surgery. 2D TEE was able to visualize coronary involvement in 6 of these 7 patients, with 3 having involvement of both LMCA and RCA while 3 had involvement of the RCA only. The patient with a false-negative result on 2D TEE was diagnosed intraoperatively by direct visualization. Of the remaining 27 patients, only 17 (63%) had coronary arteries that could be visualized to show that the dissection did not extend into the proximal coronary arteries. Overall, 2D TEE for detection of coronary artery involvement in aortic dissection is believed to have a sensitivity of 90%, whereas aortography has a sensitivity of only 40%. Overall, both 2D and 3D TEE are very helpful and reliable tests for aortic dissection and can provide essential information regarding coronary involvement prior to operative intervention.[11,20,21]

## CONGENITAL CORONARY ANOMALIES

Congenital coronary anomalies include anomalous origins of coronary arteries as well as fistulous connections of coronary arteries to cardiac chambers or veins. Congenital coronary anomalies are occasionally seen on echocardiography. Typically, they are first appreciated on coronary angiography as an incidental finding, but they can be confirmed echocardiographically. Recognition is important because of associated risk of myocardial ischemia, infarction, syncope, and sudden cardiac death **(Figure 15.18 to 15.25)**.

### Anomalous Origins

Echocardiography has been successfully used to visualize anomalous origins of coronary arteries. Clinical outcomes of adults with anomalous coronary arteries depend greatly on the anatomy of the anomalous vessel. Anomalies that include

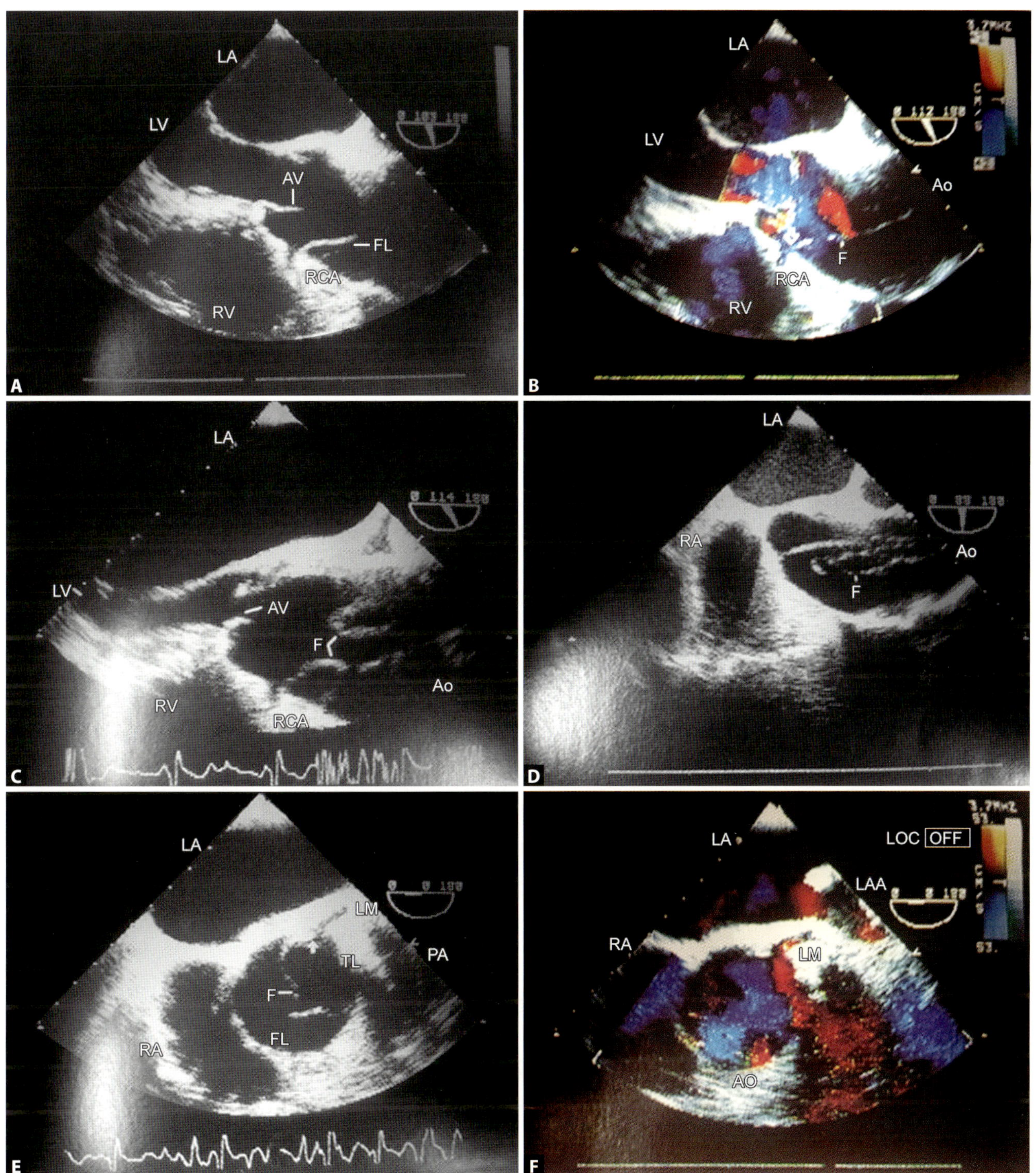


Figure 15.16A to F

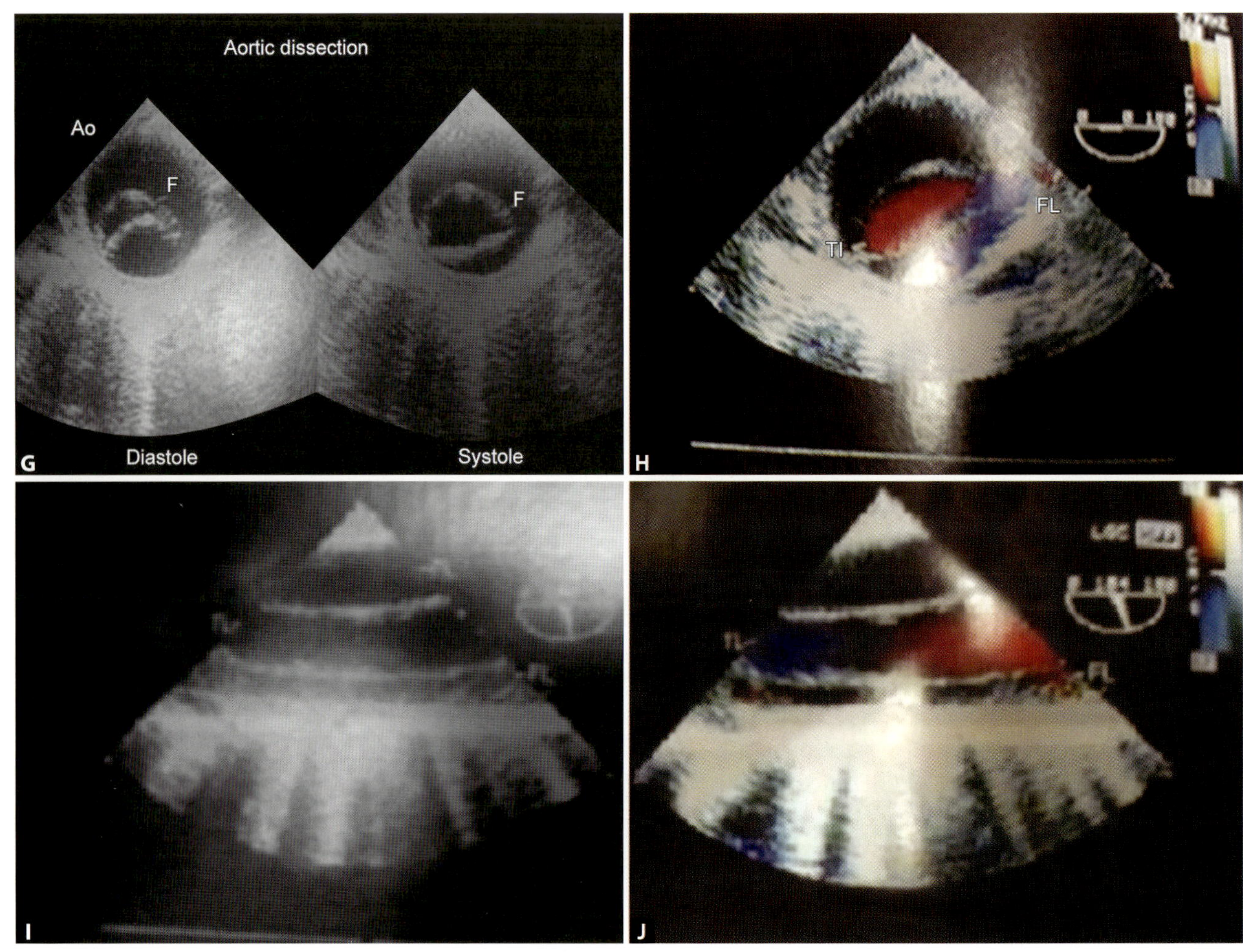


**Figure 15.16G to J**

**Figure 15.16A to J:** Aortic dissection. (A to J) The dissection flap (FL, F) appears to extend up to the origins of the right coronary artery (RCA) and the left main coronary artery (LM). Reduplication of the dissection flap is well seen in Figure D. (G to J) Shows extension of the dissection into the descending thoracic aorta imaged in long-axis and short-axis views. Collapse of the true lumen (TL) in diastole and expansion in systole, as shown in the short-axis view in Figure G, result in a characteristic "help" sign when the descending aorta is viewed in real-time motion.
*Abbreviations:* Ao, aorta, aortic valve; FL, false lumen; LA, left atrium; LAA left atrial appendage; LV, left ventricle; PA, pulmonary artery, RA, right atrium; RV, right ventricle.
*Source:* Nanda NC, Domanski MJ (Eds): Atlas of Transesophageal Echocardiography. Baltimore: Williams & Wilkins; 1998. (Figure 3.41).

a coronary artery origin from the pulmonary artery (PA) or having a proximal course between the PA and the aortic trunk are often associated with worse cardiac outcomes.[22]

The most serious coronary anomalies in adults are origin of the LMCA from the right coronary sinus and origin of the RCA from the left coronary sinus when the anomalous vessel passes between the aorta and the pulmonary trunk. The former is the most common anomaly associated with sudden cardiac death in young adults. These anomalies are often not visible on 2D TTE due to resolution limits but may be visualized on 2D or 3D TEE. Compression of the anomalous vessel between the aorta and PA, especially during exercise has been postulated to be the reason for sudden death in these individuals.

Bland-White-Garland syndrome, also known as anomalous origin of left coronary artery from pulmonary artery (ALCAPA) is a rare congenital malformation. The untreated mortality rate in the first year of life is more than 90%.[23] Those who survive to adulthood are at high risk for sudden death. Given the poor prognosis, early recognition and surgical

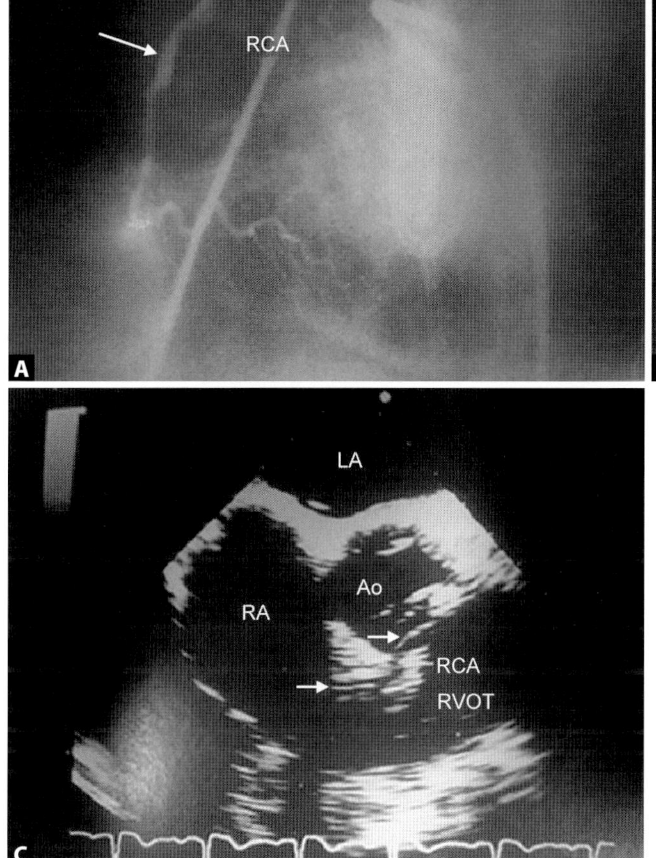


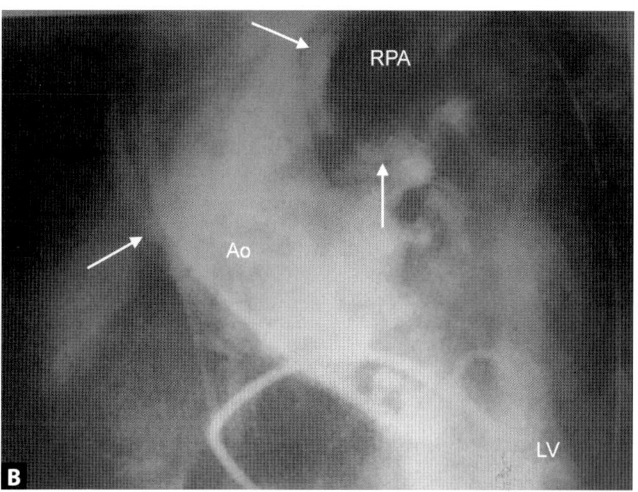


**Figure 15.17A to C:** Proximal right coronary artery dissection extending into the aortic root. (A) Coronary angiogram shows dissection (arrows) of the right coronary artery (RCA). (B) Left ventriculogram shows the contrast dye (arrows) outside the lumen of the ascending aorta (Ao). (C) The aortic short-axis view demonstrates a dissection flap (solid arrow) in the lumen of the RCA as well as in the adjacent portion of the aortic root (open arrow) (Figure 3.37).
*Abbreviations:* LA, left atrium; LV, left ventricle; RA, right atrium; RCA, right coronary artery; RPA, right pulmonary artery; RVOT, right ventricular outflow tract.

correction are of critical importance. In adult patients, this condition is often discovered due to symptoms of palpitations or chest discomfort. In one case series, the following features were found to be common among 6 adult patients with this abnormality:

- An abnormal vessel inserting into the pulmonary trunk was seen in all patients by echocardiography. A continuous shunt was seen on color Doppler mapping with flow from the vessel into the PA prominent during diastole. Branches with retrograde flow into the vessel were visible in several cases.
- Proximal RCA dilatation was seen in all patients with a median RCA: aorta ratio of 0.35 (range 0.29–0.45), whereas normal is approximately 0.20 in adults.[24]
- Numerous septal intramyocardial coronary flow signals were seen in every patient. These were often also seen across the surface of the RV to the root of the PA or within the posterior wall of the LV.
- Patients had varying degrees of LV enlargement with normal contractile function.
- Mitral regurgitation was seen in 4 cases with mitral valve prolapse in three cases.

In the same case series, 2 infants were diagnosed with ALCAPA. Both of them also had endocardial fibroelastosis. Their presenting symptoms tended to be much more dramatic with heart failure in the first half year of life. Electrocardiogram demonstrated ischemic changes. Their RCA: aorta diameter was normal or only mildly dilated. Septal collaterals were not very prominent. They had prominent fibrotic changes of their papillary muscles. They had severe LV dilatation and dysfunction with anterior and lateral wall motion abnormalities. Given the high morbidity and mortality of this condition, echocardiographers must carefully search for and rule out anomalous coronary arteries origins in infants with endocardial fibroelastosis or cardiomyopathy. At this time, cardiac catheterization with aortography is the standard means of diagnosing ALCAPA. However, because infants and young children with this condition often present with acute, severe congestive heart failure, this procedure carries a greater risk of morbidity and mortality. 2D TTE, on the other hand, has very little associated morbidity and mortality.[25] In patients with ALCAPA, 2D TTE is often capable of providing adequate images for diagnosis. However, 3D TTE may be required to clarify subtle anatomic defects. In particular, in a patient with prior surgical repair of ALCAPA, 3D TTE was found to be extremely useful. In this particular patient, the

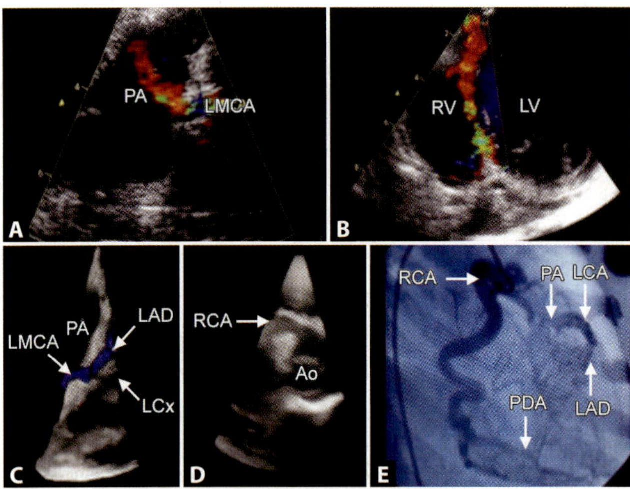


**Figure 15.18A to E:** A 3-year-old boy with older type ALCAPA. (A) Modified parasternal short-axis view identified left main coronary artery from the main pulmonary artery and the red shunt from it to the pulmonary artery. (B) Parasternal short-axis view showed abundant septal collateral signals from right to left coronary artery. (C) Real time three-dimensional echocardiographic imaging showed retrograde flow from left coronary branches and then via main trunk into the pulmonary artery. (D) Real-time three-dimensional echocardiographic imaging showed the dilated right coronary artery arising from the aorta. (E) Aortogram from ascending aorta in frontal projection showed normal origin of a single large right coronary artery. The posterior descending artery gives rise to numerous intercoronary collaterals. These course through the ventricular septum, opacifying in retrograde fashion, the left coronary system, and the main pulmonary artery.
*Abbreviations:* Ao, aorta; LAD, left anterior descending artery; LCA, left coronary artery; LCx, left circumflex artery; LMCA, left main coronary artery; LV, left ventricle; PA, pulmonary artery; PDA, posterior descending artery; RCA, right coronary artery; RV, right ventricle.
*Source:* Yang YL, Nanda NC, Wang XF, et al. Echocardiographic diagnosis of anomalous origin of the left coronary artery from the pulmonary artery. Echocardiography. 2007;24:405-11, *with permission.*

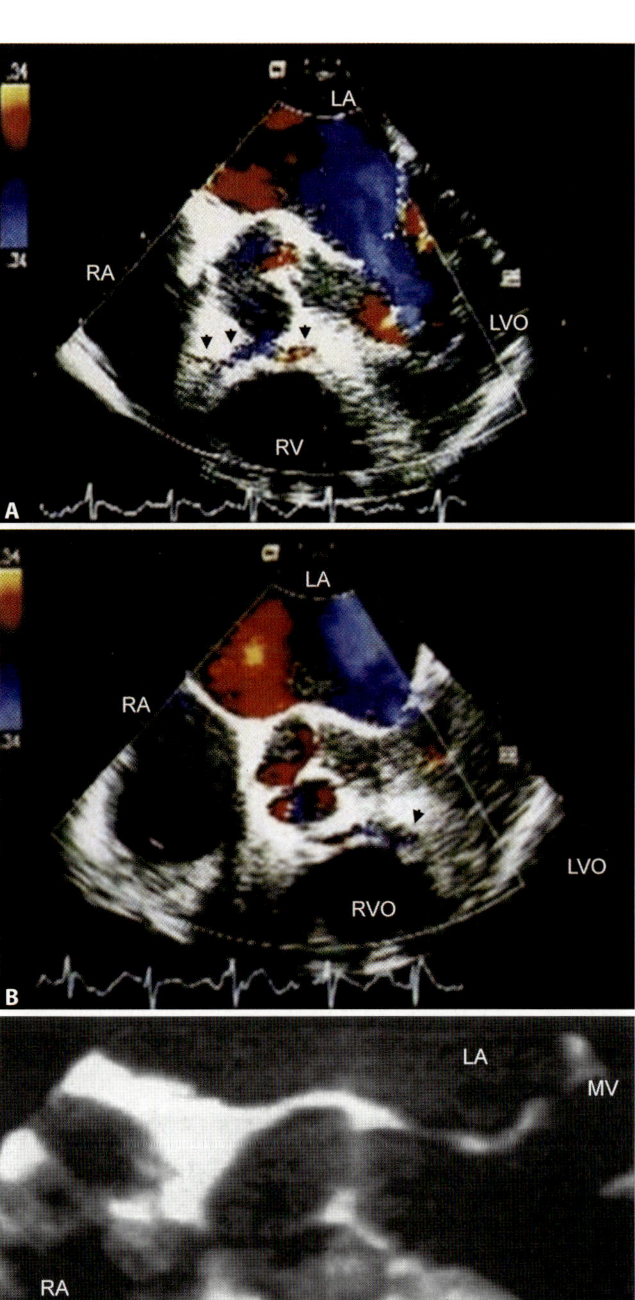


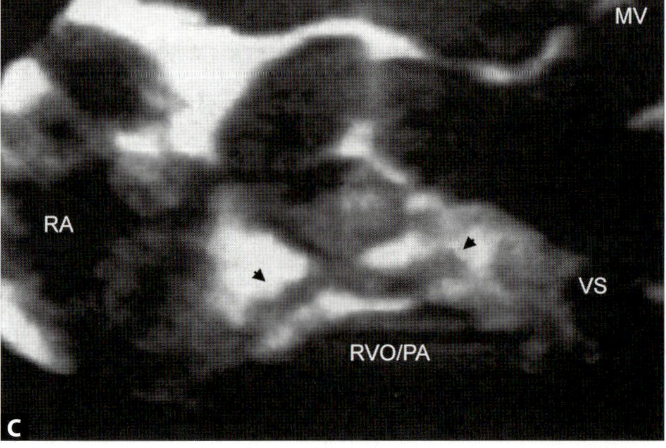


**Figure 15.19A to C**

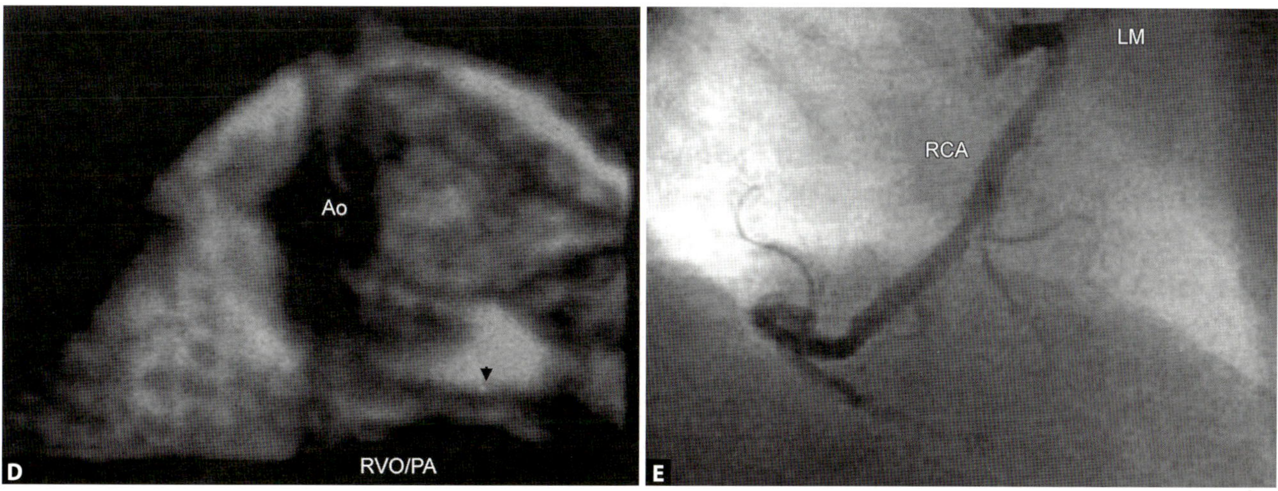


**Figure 15.19D and E**

**Figure 15.19A to E:** Transesophageal two and three-dimensional echocardiography in an adult patient with anomalous coronary artery. (A to D). In this patient, both left main and right coronary arteries (arrowheads) arise from a common ostium in the right sinus with the left main coursing between Ao and RVO/PA. (B) Arrowhead points to intramyocardial course of the LAD coronary artery within the ventricular septum. (E) Coronary angiogram showing the common origin of the left main (LM) and right coronary (RCA) arteries.
*Abbreviations:* LVO, left ventricular outflow tract; MV, mitral valve; RV, right ventricle; Ao, aorta; LA, left atrium; LAD, left anterior descending artery; LM, left main, RA, right atrium; RCA, right coronary artery; PA, pulmonary artery; RVO, right ventricular outflow; VS, ventricular septal.
*Source:* Nanda NC, Bhambore MM, Jindal M, et al. Transesophageal three-dimensional echocardiographic assessment of anomalous coronary arteries. Echocardiography. 2000;17:53-60, *with permission.*

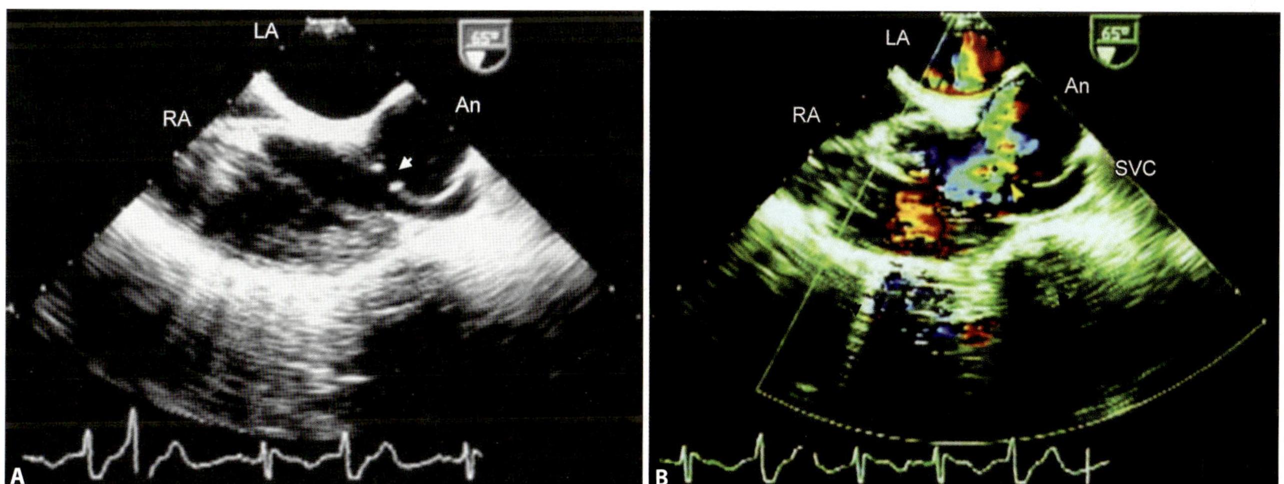


**Figure 15.20A and B:** Transesophageal two-dimensional echocardiographic findings in left main coronary artery fistula. (A) Arrowhead points to the opening of the fistula at the SVC-RA junction. Note localized thickening of the edges of the fistula opening. (B) Color Doppler examination shows turbulent flow signals moving from the AN into RA at the SVC-RA junction (arrowhead).
*Abbreviations:* An, aneurysm; LA, left artery; RA, right artery; SVC, superior vena cava.
*Source:* Nekkanti R, Nanda NC, Angsingkar G, et al. Transesophageal three-dimensional echocardiographic assessment of left main coronary artery fistula. Echocardiography. 2001;18:305-7, *with permission.*

repair included an aortopulmonary window with a tunnel connecting the aorta to the PA and enclosing the orifice of the anomalous coronary artery. On 2D TTE, no abnormalities were seen. However, 3D TTE with color flow Doppler clearly showed a defect in the tunnel which had not been seen on other imaging modalities. For postsurgical changes in patients with ALCAPA, 3D TTE is more capable of demonstrating abnormalities than 2D TTE.[26]

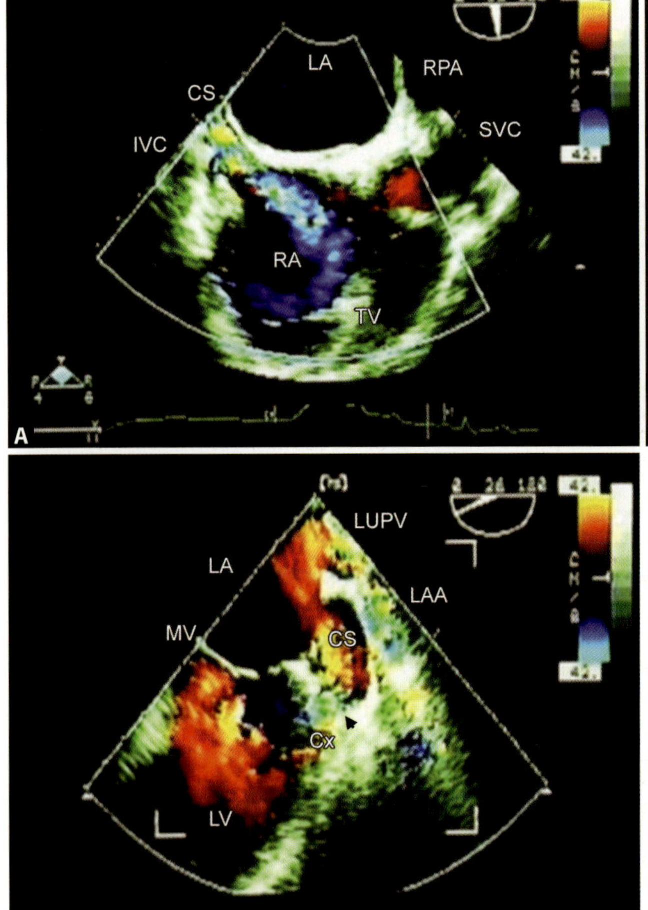


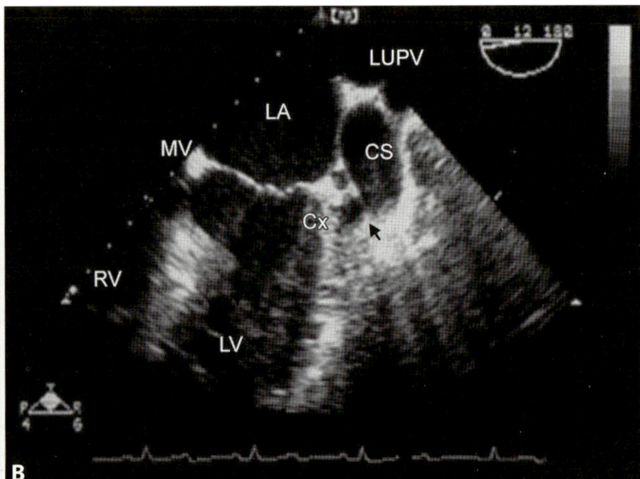


**Figure 15.21A to C:** Left circumflex coronary artery to coronary sinus fistula. Multiplane two-dimensional transesophageal echocardiographic findings. (A) Turbulent flow signals are noted moving into the right atrium (RA) from the coronary sinus (CS), which is dilated. (B and C) Arrowhead points to a possible connection between the left circumflex coronary artery (Cx) and the dilated CS adjacent to the left atrioventricular groove.
*Abbreviations:* IVC, inferior vena cava; LA, left atrium; LAA, left artery appendage; LUPV, left upper pulmonary vein; LV, left ventricle; MV, mitral valve; RA, right artery; RPA, right pulmonary artery; SVC, superior vena cava.
*Source:* Nekkanti R, Mukhtar O, Nanda NC, et al. Transesophageal color Doppler three-dimensional echocardiographic assessment of left circumflex coronary artery fistula. Echocardiography. 2002;19:573-575, *with permission*.

Anomalous origin of the RCA from the pulmonary trunk is another rare congenital abnormality. It is associated with far less morbidity and mortality than ALCAPA. It is often found incidentally at autopsy or during cardiac surgery. However, it is also associated with sudden cardiac death, which appears to be due to "pulmonary steal." Given the associated risks, surgical correction is generally recommended. Visualization of this abnormality with 2D TTE is challenging because artifactual echocardiographic dropouts can masquerade as origin of a coronary artery. However, using color flow Doppler, we have successfully demonstrated in our laboratory continuity of flow between the anomalous channel and pulmonary trunk with dramatic pulsatile beat-to-beat flow seen from the RCA to the pulmonary trunk during diastole.[27]

Cx from the right coronary sinus is a relatively common congenital anomaly and accounts for almost half of all aberrant origins of coronary arteries.[28] It is typically diagnosed by angiography. However, it has successfully been diagnosed with 2D TEE. In this particular instance, the Cx originated from the right coronary sinus, traveled posteriorly behind the aorta, and supplied the Cx system. Visualization was obtained by beginning with a short axis view of the aortic root, and then the transducer was pulled up slightly to visualize the coronary arteries. A coronary artery originating from the left sinus was seen; however, rather than bifurcating into an LAD and Cx, it coursed anteriorly like the LAD. The transducer was then rotated clockwise with rightward angulation to show the RCA. Because the Cx had not been seen bifurcating off of the abnormal LMCA, the echocardiographer searched carefully until he found the origin of the Cx from the right sinus of Valsalva. Color flow easily enabled good visualization of the path of the anomalous Cx. At its origin, it angled sharply posteriorly to lie between the aorta and the left atrium, and

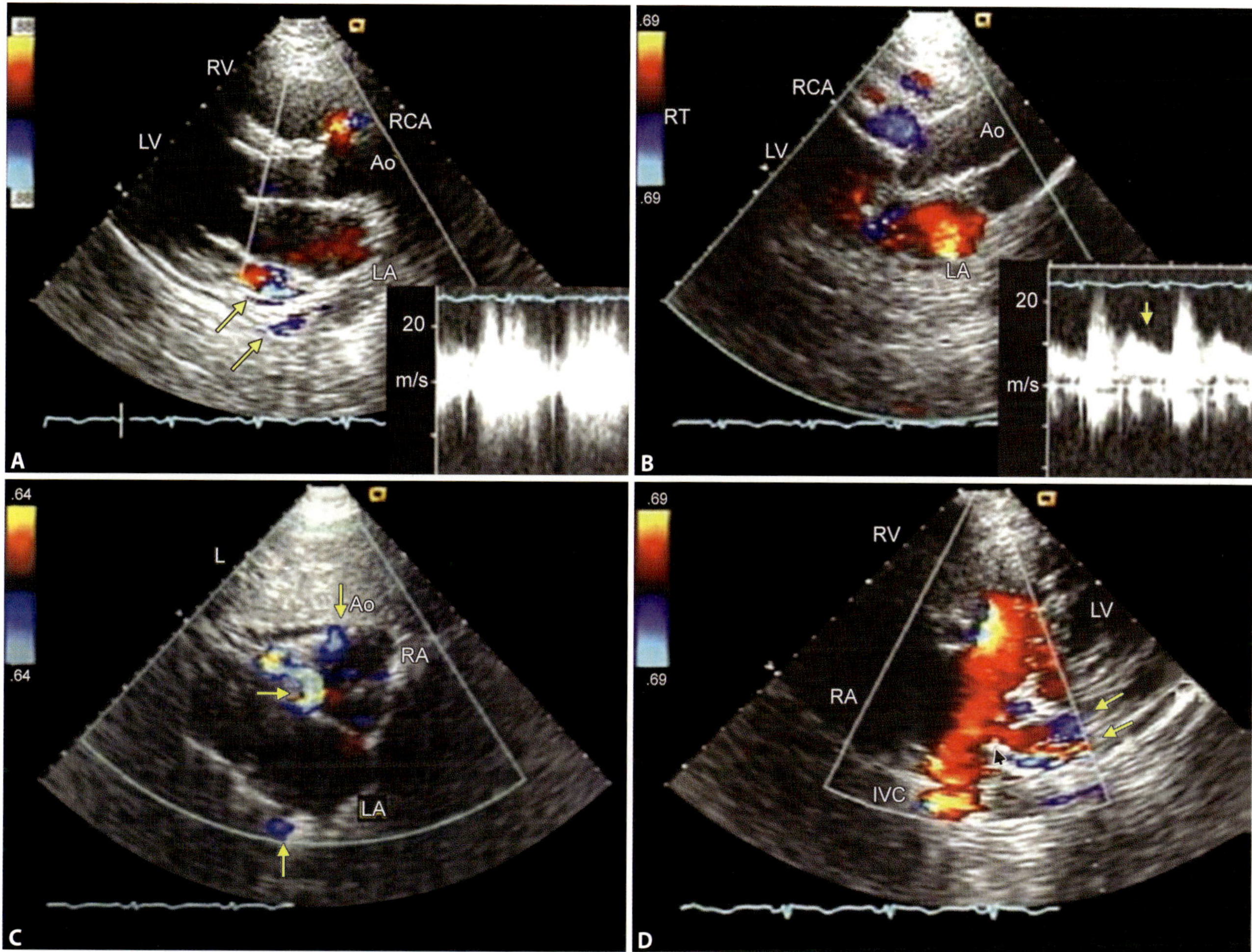


**Figure 15.22A to D:** Transthoracic echocardiogram in a patient with right coronary artery–coronary sinus fistula. (A) Parasternal long-axis view shows flow aliasing/turbulence (arrows) in the region of the left atrial (LA)–left ventricular (LV) posterior wall junction and in the right coronary artery (RCA) consistent with a RCA-coronary sinus fistula in the region of left atrioventricular groove. Continuous wave Doppler interrogation at the LA–LV junction (inset) shows high velocity flow signals throughout the cardiac cycle also consistent with a coronary artery–coronary sinus fistula at this level. (B) Right parasternal examination demonstrates marked enlargement of the RCA, which measures 1.3 cm in width at its origin. Inset shows a high peak diastolic velocity (arrow) of 1.4 m/sec$^2$ obtained by continuous wave Doppler interrogation of the RCA. (C) The arrows point to various segments of the fistula imaged using the subcostal approach. (D) Right ventricular (RV) inflow view shows laminar flow signals (arrowhead) moving from what appears to be the coronary sinus into the right atrium (RA). The arrows point to other adjacent segments of the fistula, some of which demonstrate aliased/turbulent flow signals.

*Abbreviations:* Ao, aorta; IVC, inferior vena cava; L, liver.

*Source:* Mirza S, Nanda NC, Baweja G, et al. Multiple fistulae connecting the right coronary artery to the coronary sinus. Echocardiography. 2004;21:199-202, *with permission.*

then resumed its normal course bordering the posterolateral aspect of the left atrium.[29]

Anomalous separate origin of the Cx coronary artery from a separate ostium in the left coronary sinus can be seen well with 2D TEE and color Doppler. In a 62-year-old gentleman being evaluated prior to replacement of a regurgitant aortic valve with a St. Jude prosthesis, the anomalous origin could be seen by positioning the transducer posterior to the left atrium while obtaining horizontal plane basal short-axis images of the aortic valve. By tilting the transducer up with slight counterclockwise rotation the coronary ostia of the left coronary system could

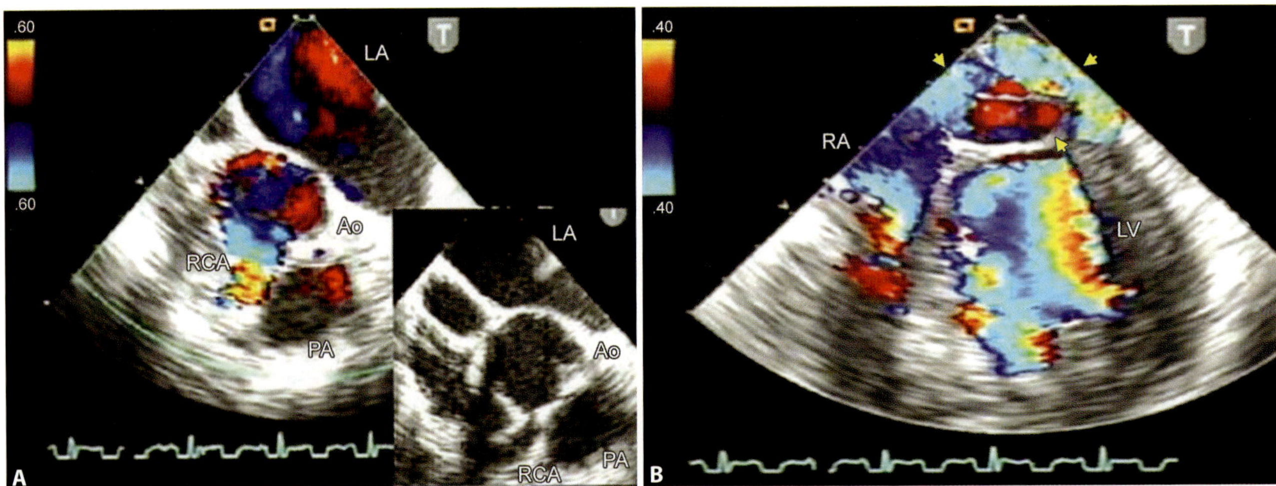


**Figure 15.23A and B:** Transesophageal echocardiogram in the same patient. (A) A dilated RCA. (B) Note laminar flow signals (arrowhead) moving from the coronary sinus into the RA. The arrows point to two other segments of the fistula, one of which shows aliased/turbulent flow signals.

*Abbreviations:* Ao, aorta; LA, left artery; LV, left ventricle; PA, pulmonary artery; RA, right artery; RCA, right coronary artery.

*Source:* Mirza S, Nanda NC, Baweja G, et al. Multiple fistulae connecting the right coronary artery to the coronary sinus. Echocardiography. 2004;21:199-202, *with permission*.

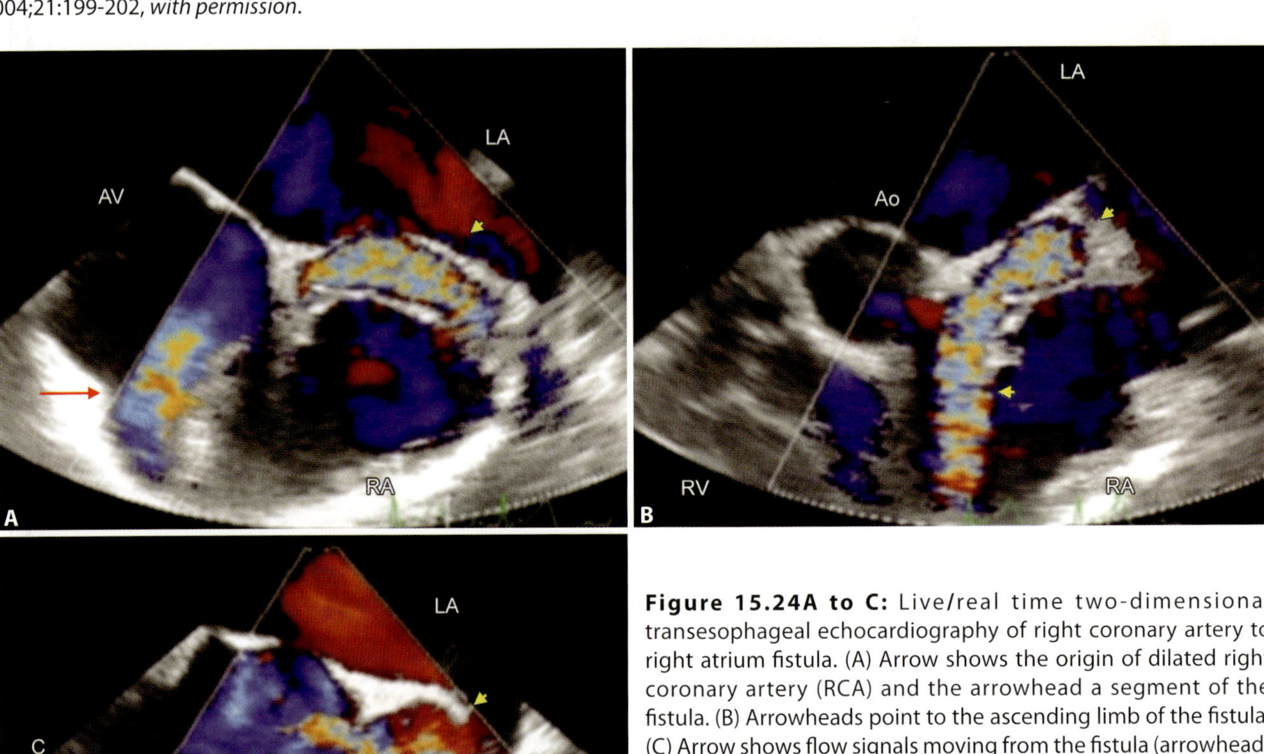


**Figure 15.24A to C:** Live/real time two-dimensional transesophageal echocardiography of right coronary artery to right atrium fistula. (A) Arrow shows the origin of dilated right coronary artery (RCA) and the arrowhead a segment of the fistula. (B) Arrowheads point to the ascending limb of the fistula. (C) Arrow shows flow signals moving from the fistula (arrowhead) into the right atrium (RA). The maximum width of flow signals measured 0.75 cm.

*Abbreviations:* Ao, aorta; AV, aortic valve; C, catheter; LA, left atrium; RV, right ventricle.

*Source:* Mishra J, Puri HP, Hsiung MC, et al. Incremental Value of Live/Real Time Three-Dimensional over Two-Dimensional Transesophageal Echocardiography in the Evaluation of Right Coronary Artery Fistula. Echocardiography. 2011;28:805-8, *with permission*.

be seen above the plane of the aortic valve cusps. In this instance, two adjacent but separate coronary arteries were seen emerging from the left coronary sinus as two pairs of parallel lines. The Cx was positioned posterior to the LAD. Color Doppler revealed parallel flow predominantly during diastole.[30]

The LMCA from the right coronary sinus is another anomalous coronary origin. One particular patient with this anomaly was evaluated with both 2D TEE and angiography. She had been referred due to angina, syncope, and a stress test concerning for ischemia. Coronary angiography was able to visualize the LMCA origin and the initial pathway taken by the artery but could not definitively visualize the more distal path of the artery. In particular, it was unclear after angiogram

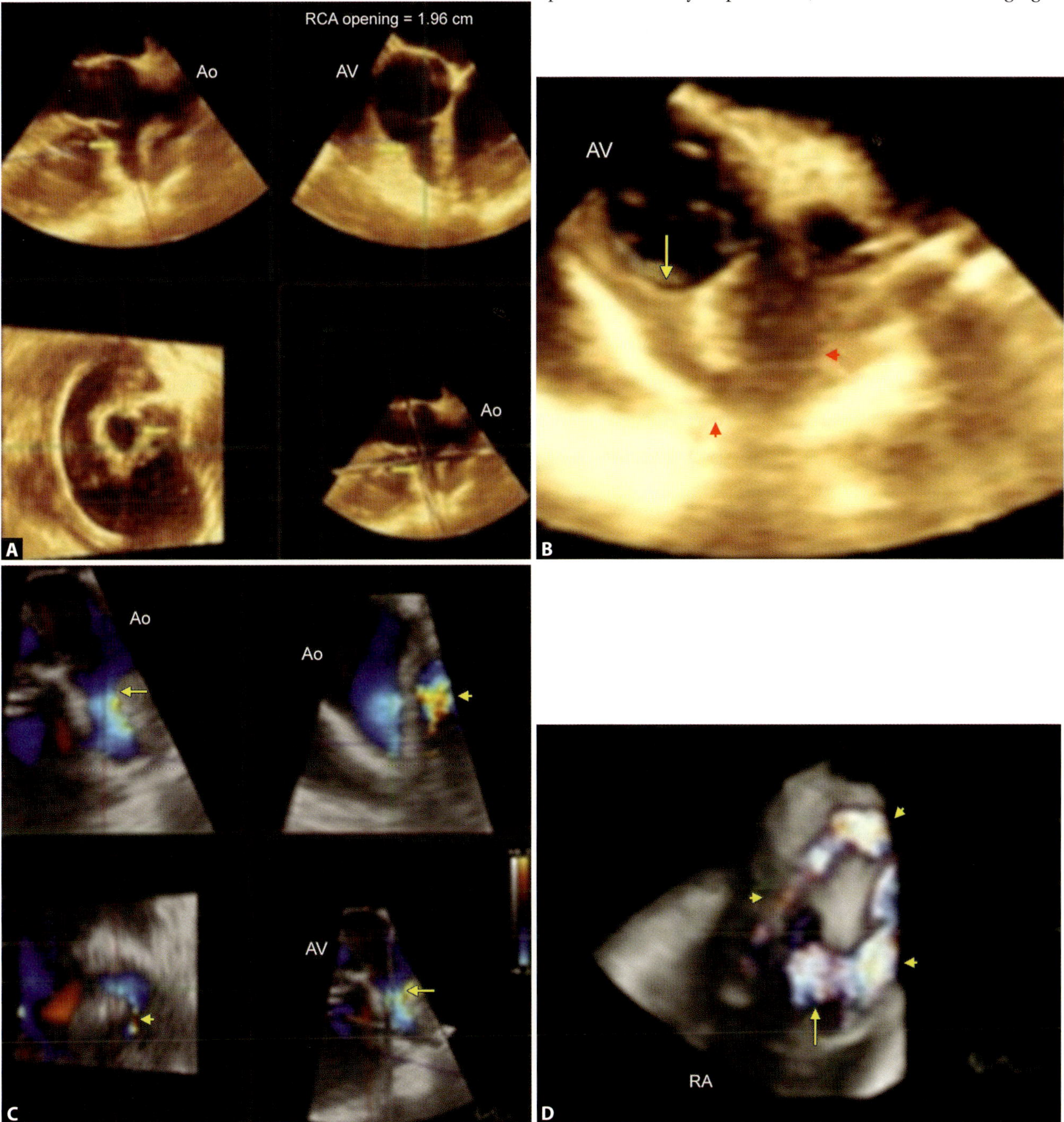


**Figure 15.25A to D**

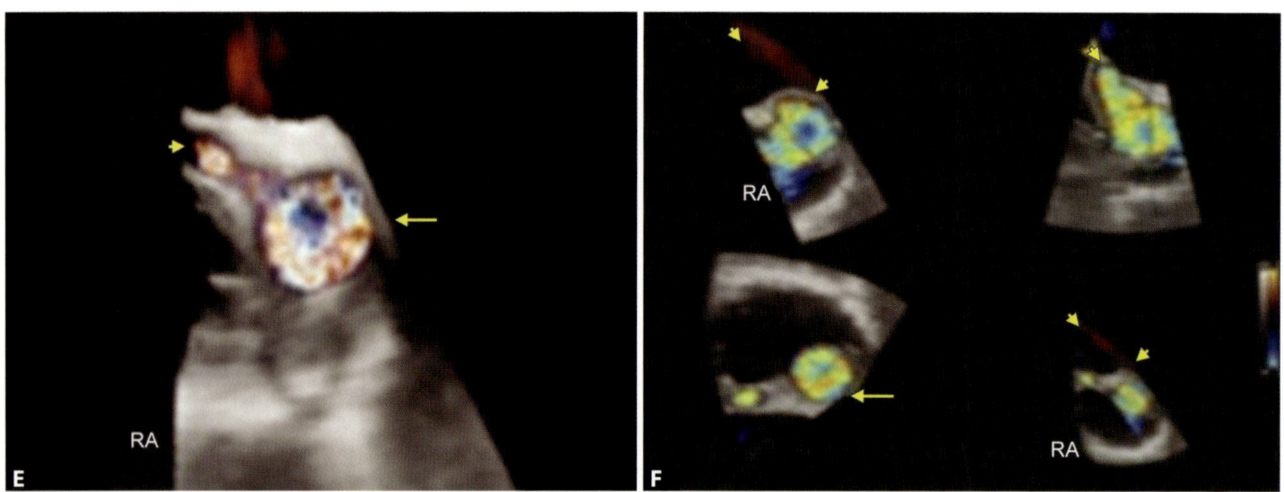


**Figure 15.25E and F**

**Figure 15.25A to F:** Live/real time three-dimensional transesophageal echocardiography of right coronary artery to right atrium fistula. Same patient as Figure 15.24. (A) Qlab study. Top arrows and the bottom right arrow point to the origin of the dilated RCA. The RCA opening viewed en face (arrow in bottom left panel) measured 1.70 cm × 1.55 cm, area 1.96 $cm^2$. (B) Vertical arrowhead shows the continuity of the descending and the ascending (transverse arrowhead) limbs of the fistula. Arrow shows origin of the dilated RCA. (C) Qlab cropping also shows the continuity (lower arrowhead) of the descending and ascending (upper right arrowhead) limbs of the fistula. Arrow in upper left and lower right panels show the origin of dilated RCA. (D) Arrow shows flow signals moving from the fistula (arrowheads) into RA. (E and F) Represent regular (E) and Qlab (F) en face views (arrow) of the opening of fistula into RA. This measured 1.83 cm × 1.43 cm, area 3.94 $cm^2$. Arrowheads show segments of the fistula.
*Abbreviations:* Ao, aorta; AV, aortic valve; RA, right atrium; RCA, right coronary artery.
*Source:* Mishra J, Puri HP, Hsiung MC, et al. Incremental value of live/real time three-dimensional over two-dimensional transesophageal echocardiography in the evaluation of right coronary artery fistula. Echocardiography. 2011;28:805-8, *with permission*.

whether the vessel passed between the aorta and the PA. Multiplane 2D TEE with 3D reconstruction clearly showed a single coronary artery originating from the right sinus, which almost immediately divided into right and left branches with acute angulation. The right branch followed the normal pathway of the RCA, whereas the left branch coursed between the aorta and PA. In another patient undergoing 2D TEE to evaluate for cardiac source of an embolic stroke, 2D TEE was done to evaluate for a cardiac source of the embolism. Angiography had been done in the past and had shown that her LMCA originated from the right sinus of Valsalva; however, it could not be determined with coronary angiography whether the LMCA passed between the aorta and the PA. Multiplane 2D TEE with 3D reconstruction was able to demonstrate a single coronary artery from the right sinus which divided almost immediately with acute angulation into right and left branches. The right branch followed the normal RCA course. However, the left branch was seen coursing between the PA and aorta and then intramyocardially within the ventricular septum.[31]

An RCA originating from the left sinus of Valsalva has also been seen on 2D TEE. In one particular patient with recurrent anginal chest pain and a nuclear stress test concerning for ischemia, the RCA was seen originating from the left sinus of Valsalva on coronary angiography. No significant stenosis was seen. However, it could not be determined whether the RCA passed between the aorta and PA. Using multiplane 2D TEE, a normal LMCA origin as well as another coronary artery originating from the left sinus of Valsalva could be visualized with acute angulation. This anomalous vessel passed within the aortic wall anteriorly between the aorta and PA toward the right sinus before following the normal course of the RCA. Turbulent flow was seen near its origin. The acute angulation was believed to be the cause of the ischemia, and the patient had a single vessel bypass involving the RCA. A similar patient was also referred for angiography due to anginal chest pain and a positive exercise stress test. On angiography, she was found to have an RCA originating from the left sinus. Again, it could not be determined angiographically whether the RCA passed between the aorta and PA. No significant coronary stenosis was seen. 2D TEE with 3D reconstruction showed a normal origin and course of the LMCA. However, a second coronary artery originating from the left sinus very near the origin of the LMCA with acute angulation was seen. It passed within the aortic wall between the aorta and PA toward the right sinus before following the normal path of the RCA.

In the previous 4 cases of anomalous origins of coronary arteries, coronary angiography was unable to delineate the course of the anomalous vessels. Multiplane 2D TEE, on the other hand, clearly showed both the origin and course between the aorta and PA of the anomalous vessels. Three-dimensional reconstruction was able to provide clearer, more vivid images and improve confidence in the diagnosis. In these instances, TEE was found to be superior to coronary angiography for identifying the course of anomalous vessels.[31]

## Fistulous Connections

A coronary arteriovenous fistula is a communication between one of the coronary arteries and a cardiac chamber or vein. Of patients with coronary fistulas, about 55% involve the RCA, 35% the left coronary artery, and 5% both. Communication is usually to the right-sided chambers. Most of these fistulas drain into the right ventricle, right atrium, or coronary sinus. Coronary to PA fistulas are a rare incidental finding.[32] The shunt through the fistula is usually small, and myocardial blood flow may not be compromised, although distal ischemia can occur due to "myocardial steal". Other potential complications include pulmonary hypertension and congestive heart failure if a large left-to-right shunt is present, bacterial endocarditis, and rupture or thrombosis of the fistula or of an associated arterial aneurysm. When coronary fistulas are discovered in childhood, they often present with a loud, superficial, and continuous cardiac murmur. The site of maximal intensity is related to the site of drainage and is usually away from the second left intercostal space, the classic site of a persistent ductus arteriosus. Coronary artery fistulas can be recognized with a high degree of accuracy on echocardiogram when coronary arteries are examined. Findings may include a significantly enlarged feeding coronary artery as well as a continuous turbulent systolic and diastolic flow pattern at the entry site. The 2D TTE is a valuable tool for finding evidence of fistula.[32-36] Common evidence of fistula includes dilation of the coronary arteries proximal to the fistula. If the fistula involves the coronary sinus, it is often dilated as well. Turbulent flow may be seen in any of the involved vessels. However, the fistula itself is usually not localized on 2D TTE. The 2D TEE is capable of providing clearer images and may show the location of the fistula. At this time, angiography is considered the test of choice at most centers for localizing coronary fistulae. However, angiography, too, is occasionally unable to identify the location of the communication. The 3D TEE with color flow Doppler appears to be the most helpful test to accurately define the origin, course, and drainage site of the fistula, and can be very helpful to clarify anatomy if operative intervention is planned.[33-44]

In a series of three patients, one with RCA to coronary sinus fistula and the others with Cx to coronary sinus fistulae, 2D TTE was able to show evidence of the fistula, including dilation of the involved coronary arteries and the coronary sinus. However, it failed to demonstrate the actual fistula. The 2D TEE was then utilized, which was able to show the fistula. Dilation of coronary arteries should raise suspicion for fistula, particularly in patients without a history of percutaneous coronary intervention or Kawasaki's disease. A dilated coronary sinus should also raise suspicion for fistula, especially in the absence of other causes of coronary sinus dilatation, such as left-sided superior vena cava, anomalous pulmonary venous connection to the coronary sinus, or marked right heart enlargement, which can all be excluded with echocardiography. In these patients, a meticulous echocardiographic examination is required, including standard and nonstandard planes, including RV inflow view, examination of the coronary sinus near the left atrial appendage, and following as much as possible of the course of the dilated coronary artery and coronary sinus. The exact site of the fistulous connection may not be visible on coronary angiography. In that case, if intervention is being considered, 2D TEE may help clarify anatomy for assisting in surgical planning. For cases in which other imaging modalities fail to demonstrate the anatomy of the fistula, 3D TEE may be able to clarify the anatomy. In one particular patient, coronary angiography appeared to show a LMCA to right atrium fistula. Using 3D TEE, the fistula was found to be near the junction of the right atrium and the superior vena cava. The 3D TEE was found to be superior to coronary angiography and clearly demonstrated the anatomy of the fistula.[40] In another patient with Cx to coronary sinus fistula, 2D TEE was able to demonstrate evidence of the fistula. However, 3D TEE was able to clearly show the anatomy of the fistula. In yet another patient with small fistulae connecting the RCA to the coronary sinus, no imaging modality was able to visualize the fistulae. Evidence of fistulae was easily seen on 2D and 3D TEE with color flow Doppler, coronary angiography, and cardiac MRI; however, the fistulae themselves were not visualized. Intraoperatively, the coronary sinus was opened, which revealed numerous small fistulae.[42] In another interesting situation, after a stress test suggestive of myocardial ischemia, a patient underwent coronary angiography. The angiogram revealed mild ectasia of the proximal LAD and a small fistula from the proximal segment of the LAD to the PA. The 2D TTE was attempted to clarify the findings on angiography. However, the shunt could not be seen on 2D TTE even with color Doppler. Because each image in 2D TTE represents only a thin slice of the heart, a small area of turbulent flow can easily be missed. In this case, the echocardiographer was aware of the diagnosis but still unable to localize the fistula. However, using 3D TTE, the echocardiographer was able to visualize the anatomy. In this instance, utilizing 3D TTE was a tremendous advantage as it provides a view of a pyramidal section, which can be cropped systematically to find even a small localized area of flow turbulence.[43] Although coronary angiography remains the test of choice for visualizing coronary fistula in most centers, with improvements in echocardiographic equipment and technique, particularly in 3D TEE, this may change in the near future. In our center, we have found 3D TEE to be more accurate at localizing the fistula than angiography, but experience is limited.

## Acquired Coronary Anomalies

Echocardiography has also been able to demonstrate a few acquired coronary anomalies. In a patient with hypertrophic cardiomyopathy with a history of myomectomy, septal perforators to LV fistula were seen on 2D TTE. The septal perforators mimicked aortic regurgitation in some views. Peak diastolic flow velocities in this particular instance were approximately 4 m/s, which is consistent with a coronary-cameral fistula. No preoperative echocardiogram was available; however, it is believed that this anomaly resulted from her septal myomectomy.[45] An 18-year-old male who had emigrated from India was brought to medical attention due to syncope. The syncopal event was preceded by vague substernal chest pain during light exercise. An electrocardiogram showed large Q waves and deeply inverted T waves in leads I and AVL with T wave inversion in leads V5 and V6, suggestive of lateral infarction. The 2D and 3D TTE showed the presence of a huge cystic mass compressing the LV free wall. Color Doppler showed prominent intramyocardial coronary vessels in the compressed LV wall with high velocity flow suggestive of obstruction **(Figure 15.26A to F)**. The cyst was resected and pathology was typical of hydatid disease. In this instance, the echocardiographic finding of intramyocardial coronary flow obstruction prompted early surgical removal.[46] In another patient with a prosthetic aortic valve endocarditis, acute myocardial infarction was diagnosed. The 2D TEE demonstrated a large aortic root abscess that extended into the proximal ventricular septum and tricuspid valve annulus region. Color Doppler demonstrated prominent retrograde diastolic flow signals from the RCA orifice to the aortic root. The peak velocity was abnormally high at 1.4 m/s. The 3D TEE was able to demonstrate a patent but narrowed RCA orifice with complete occlusion immediately downstream from the orifice. Due to the anatomic position and involvement of the proximal RCA by the abscess cavity, the myocardial infarction was attributed to the abscess rather than embolization. The diastolic flow from the RCA to the aortic root was felt to be due to diastolic emptying of the occluded RCA after filling of the proximal portion of the RCA during systole. In this instance, the ability of 3D TEE to clearly demonstrate the anatomy of the abscess cavity and its relationship to the RCA helped explain the unusual diastolic flow pattern seen on 2D TEE with Doppler.[47]

## CONCLUSION

At this time, direct visualization of coronary arteries for stenosis and other abnormalities is not commonly performed using echocardiography in most clinical settings. However, as technology improves, it represents an increasingly useful tool

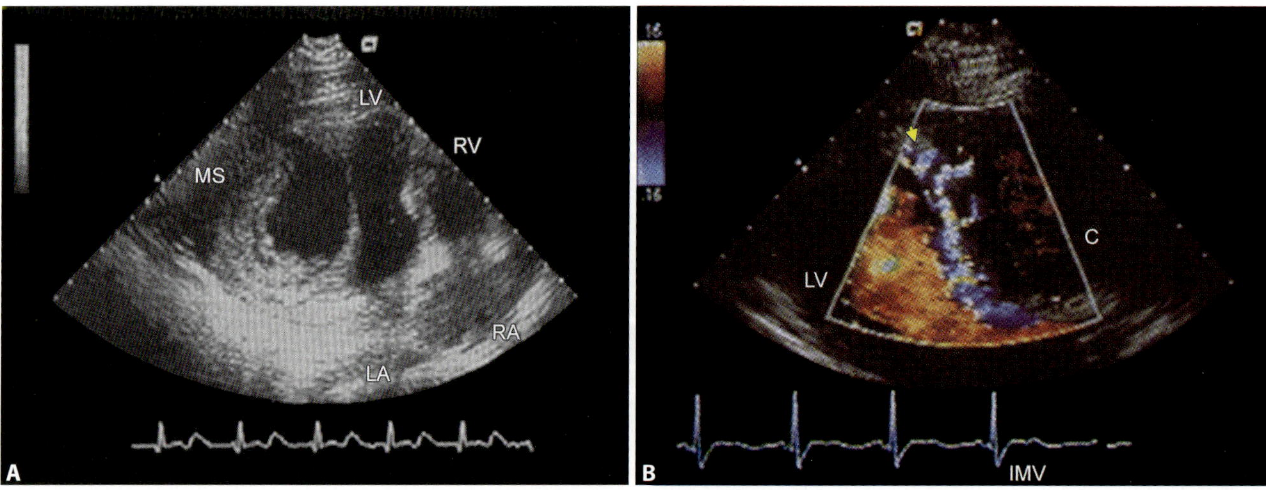


**Figure 15.26A and B**

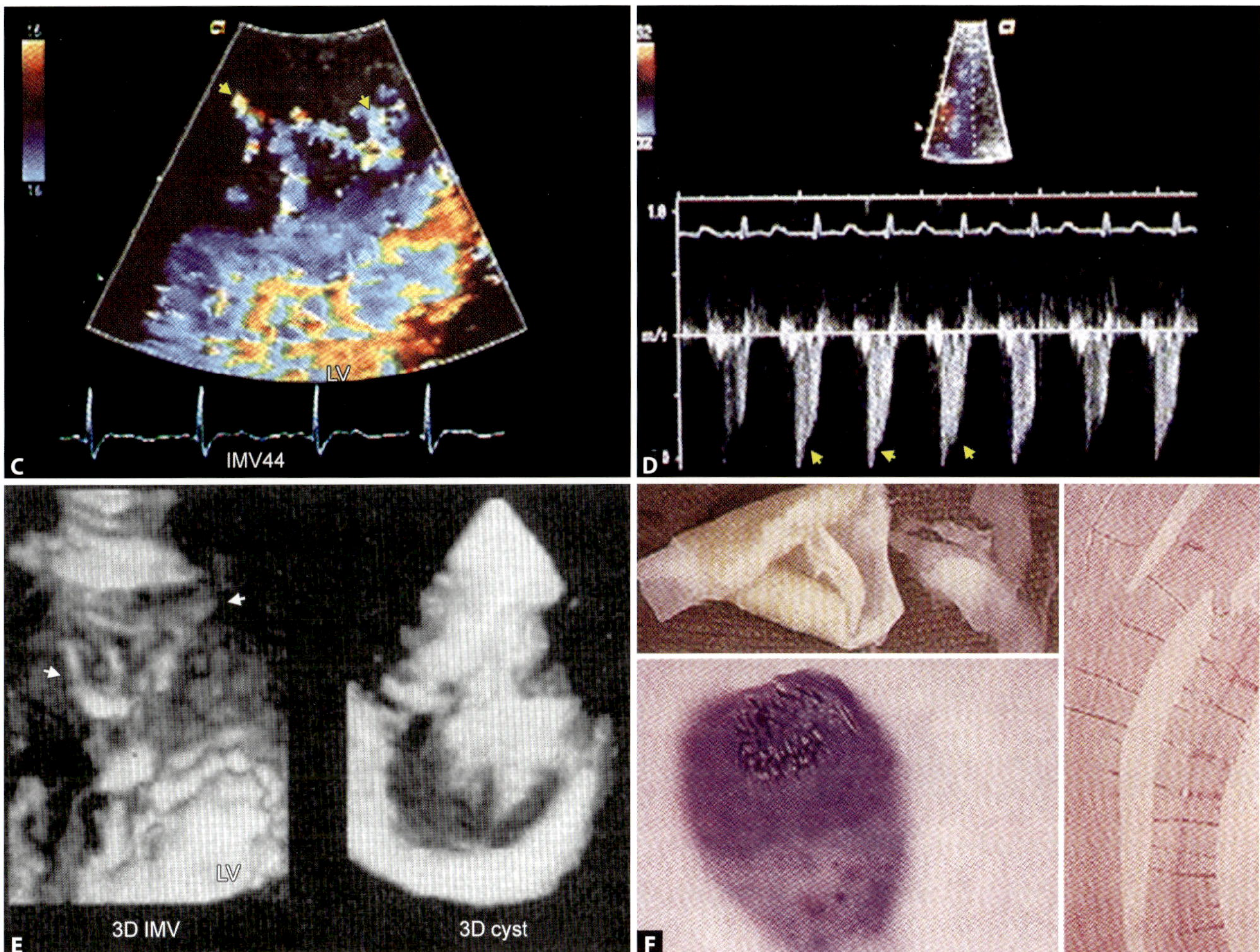


**Figure 15.26C to F**

**Figure 15.26A to F:** (A) Transthoracic echocardiography shows a large pericardial hydatid cyst (MS) compressing the left ventricular (LV) lateral wall. It measures approximately 8 cm in diameter and appears to contain layered solid tissue. (B and C) Arrows point to multiple intramyocardial coronary vessels imaged within the compressed LV free wall. These were visualized using a high resolution color Doppler system. Note that the Nyquist limit is set at a very low velocity of 0.16 m/sec. (D) Arrowheads demonstrate a high velocity of 1.2 m/sec obtained by color Doppler guided pulsed Doppler interrogation of an intramyocardial coronary vessel (normal velocity <0.6 m/sec). (E) Left: Three-dimensional reconstruction demonstrates membrane-like solid tissue in the cyst. Right: Three-dimensional reconstruction of intramyocardial coronary vessels (arrowheads) in the compressed LV wall. (F) Left upper panel: Hydatid cyst wall and surrounding soft tissue. Left lower panel: Close up of hydatid scolex with double rows of hooklets (100X). Right panel: Laminated membrane. C, pericardial cyst.

*Abbreviations:* LA, left atrium; RA, right atrium; RV, right ventricle.

*Source:* Jamil F, Nanda NC, Thakur AC, Malhotra S, Agrawal DI, Reddy VVB, et al. Echocardiographic detection of intramyocardial coronary obstruction produced by pericardial hydatid cyst. Echocardiography. 1997;14:459-60, *with permission*.

for noninvasive evaluation of coronary artery disease. Future advances in transducer technology resulting in superior quality 2D and 3D images may improve visualization rates of stenotic lesions. Utilization of contrast echocardiography appears to be extremely helpful in improving image quality and diagnostic sensitivity. Flow reserve determination helps differentiate normal from abnormal vessels. Further investigation is necessary to clarify the diagnostic role of echocardiography relative to more traditional tools for the detection of coronary artery disease.

## VIDEO LEGENDS

**Video 15.1:** Live/real time transthoracic echocardiographic assessment of coronary arteries. The moving image shows a plaque in the obtuse marginal artery which is somewhat mobile and "wiggling", indicating its soft consistency and probable propensity to rupture. Please refer to Figure 15.5 for detailed description of the findings.

**Video 15.2:** (A) and (B) Live/real time three-dimensional transesophageal echocardiographic assessment of ascending aortic dissection. A mobile dissection flap is seen protruding into the right coronary artery lumen.

## REFERENCES

1. Krzanowski M, Bodzoń W, Brzostek T, et al. The value of TTE for the detection of high-grade coronary artery stenosis: prospective evaluation in 50 consecutive patients scheduled for coronary angiography. J Am Soc Echocardiogr. 2000;13: 1091-9.
2. Vegsundvag J, Holt E, Wiseth R, et al. Transthoracic echocardiography for imaging of the different coronary artery segments: a feasibility study. Cardiovasc Ultrasound. 2009;7:58.
3. Wierzbowska-Drabik K, Kasprzak JD. Echocardiographic assessment of coronary artgeries-morphology and coronary flow reserve. In: Nanda NC (Ed): Comprehensive Textbook of Echocardiography. New Delhi, India: Jaypee Brothers Medical Publishers (P) Ltd; 2014. pp. 1336-47.
4. Krzanowski M, Bodzon W, Dimitrow PP. Imaging of all three coronary arteries by transthoracic echocardiography. An illustrated guide. Cardiovasc Ultrasound. 2003;1:16.
5. Nanda NC, Sungur A, Bhagatwala K, et al. Non-standard echocardiographic examination. In: Nanda NC (Ed): Comprehensive Textbook of Echocardiography. New Delhi, India: Jaypee Brothers Medical Publishers (P) Ltd; 2014. pp. 188-223.
6. Boshchenko AA, Vrublevsky AV, Karpov RS. Transthoracic echocardiography in the detection of chronic total coronary artery occlusion. Eur J Echocardiogr. 2009; 10:62-8.
7. Vengala S, Nanda NC, Agrawal G, et al. Live three-dimensional transthoracic echocardiographic assessment of coronary arteries. Echocardiography. 2003;20: 751-3.
8. Samdarshi TE, Nanda NC, Gatewood RP Jr, Ballal RS, Chang LK, Singh HP, et al. Usefulness and limitations of transesophageal echocardiography in the assessment of proximal coronary artery stenosis. J Am Coll Cardiol. 1992;19:572-80.
9. Ofili EO, Nanda NC. Transesophageal echocardiographic imaging of coronary arteries. In: Maurer G (Ed): Transesophageal Echocardiography. New York: McGraw Hill; 1993. pp.143-57.
10. Biederman RWW, Sorrell VL, Nanda NC, et al. Transesophageal echocardiographic assessment of coronary stenosis. A decade of experience. Echocardiography. 2001;18:49-57.
11. Nanda NC, Domanski MJ (Eds). Atlas of Transesophageal Echocardiography. Baltimore: Williams & Wilkins; 1998.
12. Aggarwal KK, Gatewood RP, Nanda NC, et al. Improved transesophageal echocardiographic assessment of significant proximal narrowing of the left anterior descending and left circumflex coronary arteries using echo contrast enhancement. Am J Cardiol. 1994;73:1131-3.
13. Ofili EO, Aggarwal KK, Nanda NC, et al. Transesophageal echocardiographic assessment of coronary arteries using echo-contrast enhancement. In: Nanda NC, Schlief R (Eds): Advances in Echo Imaging Using Contrast Enhancement. Dordrecht, The Netherlands: Kluwer Academic Publishers; 1993. pp. 301-8.
14. Abd El-Rahman SM, Khatri G, Nanda N, et al. Transesophageal three-dimensional echocardiographic assessment of normal and stenosed coronary arteries. Echocardiography. 1996;13:503-10.
15. Carlo Caiati, Cristiana Montaldo, Norma Zedda, et al. New noninvasive method for coronary flow reserve assessment: contrast-enhanced transthoracic second harmonic echo Doppler. Circulation. 1999;99:771-8.
16. Caiati C, Iliceto S, Nanda NC, et al. Transesophageal echocardiographic assessment of coronary flow reserve and coronary artery stenosis using echo enhancement. In: Nanda NC, Schlief R, Goldberg B (Eds): Advances in Echo Imaging Using Contrast Enhancement, 2nd edition. Dordrecht, The Netherlands: Kluwer Academic Publishers; 1997.pp.309-24.
17. Nohtomi Y, Takeuchi M, Nagasawa K, Arimura K, Miyata K, Kuwata K, et al. Simultaneous assessment of wall motion and coronary flow velocity in the left anterior descending coronary artery during dipyridamole stress echocardiography. J Am Soc Echocardiogr. 2003;16:457-63.
18. Eiichi Hyodo, Kumiko Hirata, Makoto Hirose. Detection of restenosis after percutaneous coronary intervention in three major coronary arteries by transthoracic Doppler Echocardiography. J Am Soc Echocardiogr. 2010;23:553-9.
19. Voros S, Nanda NC, Samal AK, et al. Transesophageal echocardiography in patients with ischemic stroke accurately detects significant coronary artery stenosis and often changes management. Am Heart J. 2001;142:916-22.
20. Joshi D, Bicer EI, Donmez C, Hsiung MC, Nanda NC, Sadat K, et al. Incremental value of live/real time three-dimensional transesophageal echocardiography over the two-dimensional technique in the assessment of aortic aneurysm and dissection. Echocardiography. 2012;29:620-30.
21. Ballal RS, Nanda NC, Gatewood R, et al. Usefulness of transesophageal echocardiography in assessment of aortic dissection. Circulation. 1991;84:1903-14.
22. Dawn B, Talley JD, Prince CR, Hoque A, Morris GT, Xenopoulos NP, et al. Two-dimensional and Doppler transesophageal echocardiographic delineation and flow characterization of anomalous coronary arteries in adults. J Am Soc Echocardiogr. 2003;16:1274-86.
23. Wesselhoeft H, Fawcett JS, Johnson AL. Anomalous origin of the left coronary from the pulmonary trunk. Its clinical spectrum, pathology, and pathophysiology, based on a review of 140 cases with seven further cases. Circulation. 1968;38: 403-25.
24. Koike K1, Musewe NN, Smallhorn JF, et al. Distinguishing between anomalous origin of the left coronary artery from the pulmonary trunk and dilated cardiomyopathy: role of echocardiographic measurement of the right coronary artery diameter. Br Heart J. 1989;61:192-7.

25. Yang YL, Nanda NC, Wang XF, Xie MX, Lu Q, He L, et al. Echocardiographic diagnosis of anomalous origin of the left coronary artery from the pulmonary artery. Echocardiography. 2007;24:405-11.
26. Ilgenli TF, Nanda NC, Sinha A, et al. Live three-dimensional transthoracic echocardiographic assessment of anomalous origin of left coronary artery from the pulmonary artery. Echocardiography. 2007;24:559-62.
27. Shah RM, Nanda NC, Hsiung MC, et al. Identification of anomalous origin of the right coronary artery from pulmonary trunk by Doppler color flow mapping. Am J Cardiol. 1986; 57:366-7.
28. Kimbris D, Iskandrian AS, Segal GL, et al. Anomalous aortic origin of coronary arteries. Circulation. 1978;58:606-15.
29. Samdarshi TE, Hill DL, Nanda NC. Transesophageal color Doppler diagnosis of anomalous origin of left circumflex coronary artery. Am Heart J. 1991;122:571-3.
30. Boogaerts J, Samdarshi TE, Nanda NC, et al. Anomalous separate origin of left circumflex coronary artery from a separate ostium in the left coronary sinus: Identification by transesophageal color Doppler echocardiography. Echocardiography. 1990;7:165-7.
31. Nanda NC, Bhambore MM, Jindal A, et al. Transesophageal three-dimensional echocardiographic assessment of anomalous coronary arteries. Echocardiography. 2000;17: 53-60.
32. Bonow, Robert O, Braunwald E (Eds). Braunwald's Heart Disease a Textbook of Cardiovascular Medicine, Chapter 65. Congenital Heart Disease, 9th edition. Philadelphia, Pa; London: Saunders; 2011.
33. Ashmeik K, Amin J, Pai RG. Echocardiographic characterization of a rare type of coronary artery fistula draining into superior vena cava. J Am Society Echocardiogr. 2000:13:407-11.
34. Barbosa MM, Katina T, Oliveira HG, et al. Doppler echocardiographic features of coronary artery fistula: Report of 8 cases. J Am Soc Echocardiogr. 1999:12:149-54.
35. Sherwood MC, Rockemacher S, Colan SD, et al. Prognostic significance of clinically silent coronary artery fistulas. Am J Cardiol. 1999;83:407-11.
36. Samdarshi TE, Mahan EF, Nanda NC, et al. Transesophageal echocardiographic assessment of congenital coronary artery to coronary sinus fistulas in adults. Am J Cardiol. 1991;68:263-6.
37. Sooudi SK, Ahmed S, Nanda NC, et al. Transthoracic echocardiographic demonstration of septal perforator coronary arteries-left ventricle fistula. Echocardiography. 2003;20:197-8.
38. Sunaga Y, Taniichi Y, Okubo N, Hayashi K, Karakawa M, Sugiura T, et al. Biplane transesophageal echocardiographic study of left coronary artery to right atrium fistula. Am Heart J. 1992;123(4 Pt 1):1058-60.
39. Kuo CT, Chiang CW, Fang BR, Lee CP, Hsu TS, Lee YS, et al. Coronary artery fistula: diagnosis by transesophageal two-dimensional and Doppler echocardiography. Am Heart J. 1992;123:218-20.
40. Nekkanti R, Nanda NC, Angsingkar KG, et al. Transesophageal three-dimensional echocardiographic assessment of left main coronary artery fistula. Echocardiography. 2001;18:305-8.
41. Nekkanti R, Mukhtar O, Nanda NC, et al. Transesophageal color Doppler three-dimensional echocardiographic assessment of left circumflex coronary artery fistula. Echocardiography. 2002;19:573-5.
42. Mirza S, Nanda NC, Baweja G, et al. Multiple fistulae connecting the right coronary artery to the coronary sinus. Echocardiography. 2004;21:199-202.
43. Mehta D, Nanda NC, Vengala S, et al. Live three dimensional transthoracic echocardiographic demonstration of coronary artery to pulmonary artery fistula. Am J Geriatric Cardiol. 2005;14:42-4.
44. Mishra J, Puri HP, Hsiung MC, et al. Incremental value of live/real time three-dimensional over two-dimensional transesophageal echocardiography in the evaluation of right coronary artery fistula. Echocardiography. 2011;28(7):805-8.
45. Sooudi SK, Ahmed S, Nekkanti R, et al. Transthoracic echocardiographic demonstration of septal perforator coronary arteries-left ventricle fistula. Echocardiography. 2003;20:197-8.
46. Jamil F, Nanda NC, Thakur AC, Malhotra S, Agrawal DI, Reddy VVB, et al. Echocardiographic detection of intramyocardial coronary obstruction produced by pericardial hydatid cyst. Echocardiography. 1997;14:459-60.
47. Horton CJ Jr, Nanda NC, Nekkanti R, et al. Prosthetic aortic valve abscess producing total right coronary artery occlusion: diagnosis by transesophageal three-dimensional echocardiography. Echocardiography. 2002;19:395-8.

# Chronic Ischemic Mitral Regurgitation

16
CHAPTER

*Raluca Dulgheru, Patrizio Lancellotti*

## INTRODUCTION

### Secondary Mitral Regurgitation: Definition and Classification

As opposed to primary mitral regurgitation (MR), which is characterized by morphologic abnormalities of the mitral valve (MV), chronic secondary MR (SMR) is exclusively a disease of the left ventricle with direct consequences on MV function. In chronic SMR, the MV is morphologically intact. However, there is marked distortion of the MV and subvalvular apparatus, due to regional or global LV remodeling that leads to valve incompetence during systole.

Chronic SMR may develop in the context of ischemic (chronic ischemic MR) or nonischemic heart disease (chronic nonischemic MR). Irrespective of the scenario, LV remodeling (either local/regional or global) is a prerequisite. Thus, the term "*secondary*" reflects the fact the valve dysfunction is only secondary to an LV disease, while the terms "*ischemic*" and "*nonischemic*" refer to SMR etiology.

This chapter will address the topic of *chronic ischemic MR*, by far the most frequently encountered entity. For further understanding of this chapter some additional term definitions are necessary. Other types of MR that have been described and classified as "*ischemic MR*" are the "*acute ischemic MR*" complicating an acute transmural myocardial infarction (MI) with rupture of the papillary muscle and the "*transient ischemic MR*" complicating a transient myocardial ischemic event (reversible myocardial ischemia involving the LV wall adjacent to the papillary muscles). As opposed to these entities, in *chronic ischemic MR,* there is progressive irreversible damage and remodeling of the left ventricle, months to years, after an MI.

## MECHANISM AND PATHOPHYSIOLOGY

The maintenance of perfect geometrical and functional balance between the MV apparatus and the left ventricle throughout systole is the key to prevent any type of SMR, of either ischemic or nonischemic etiology.

After MI and through a complex remodeling process, the left ventricle can change its "bullet shape" geometry, becoming more spherical. This change in LV geometry may lead to apical and outward displacement of papillary muscles which, in turn, pulls on the MV chordae and leaflets throughout the entire LV systole leading to tethering, restricted systolic leaflet motion and tenting of the leaflets **(Figure 16.1)**. Systolic tethering of the MV leaflets brings the leaflet coaptation line more apically into the LV cavity and can decrease the coaptation surface, thus, leading to valve incompetence **(Figure 16.2, Videos 16.1A and B)**.[1-3]

Classically, it has been hypothesized that in SMR, the relative position of mitral leaflets coaptation line depends on the balance between the forces that work to push the leaflets together and towards the base of the left ventricle (i.e. closing forces) and the forces that pull them apart (pulling them towards the LV apex or sideways).[1]

Little force is needed to seal the normal MV in systole. However, in the presence of tethering, MV leaflet closure is impeded which is further impaired by LV systolic dysfunction. Consequently, a decrease in LV closing forces will favor MR, while preservation of closing forces will work to diminish MR severity.[1,2,4,5] In patients with ischemic MR, "closing forces" typically refer to preservation of LV systolic function[2] and intraventricular/interpapillary muscle synchrony,[6,7] but also to the preservation of the geometry[8] and "sphincteric" function[9] (i.e reduction in annular circumference with systole, which in normal subjects is about 25%[10]) of the MV annulus. Notably, significant SMR does not occur in patients with global LV systolic dysfunction without tethering.[2,11] Otsuji et al. demonstrated that LV dilatation and remodeling was a prerequisite for MR development after MI and that isolated reduction in closing forces without LV dilatation led only to trace MR.[2] Similarly, reduction of mitral annulus "sphincter function" (such as in patients with atrial fibrillation, dilated atria and dilated mitral annuli) did not lead to significant SMR in absence of regional/global LV remodeling.[12] However, both mechanisms promoted SMR in the presence of tethering.

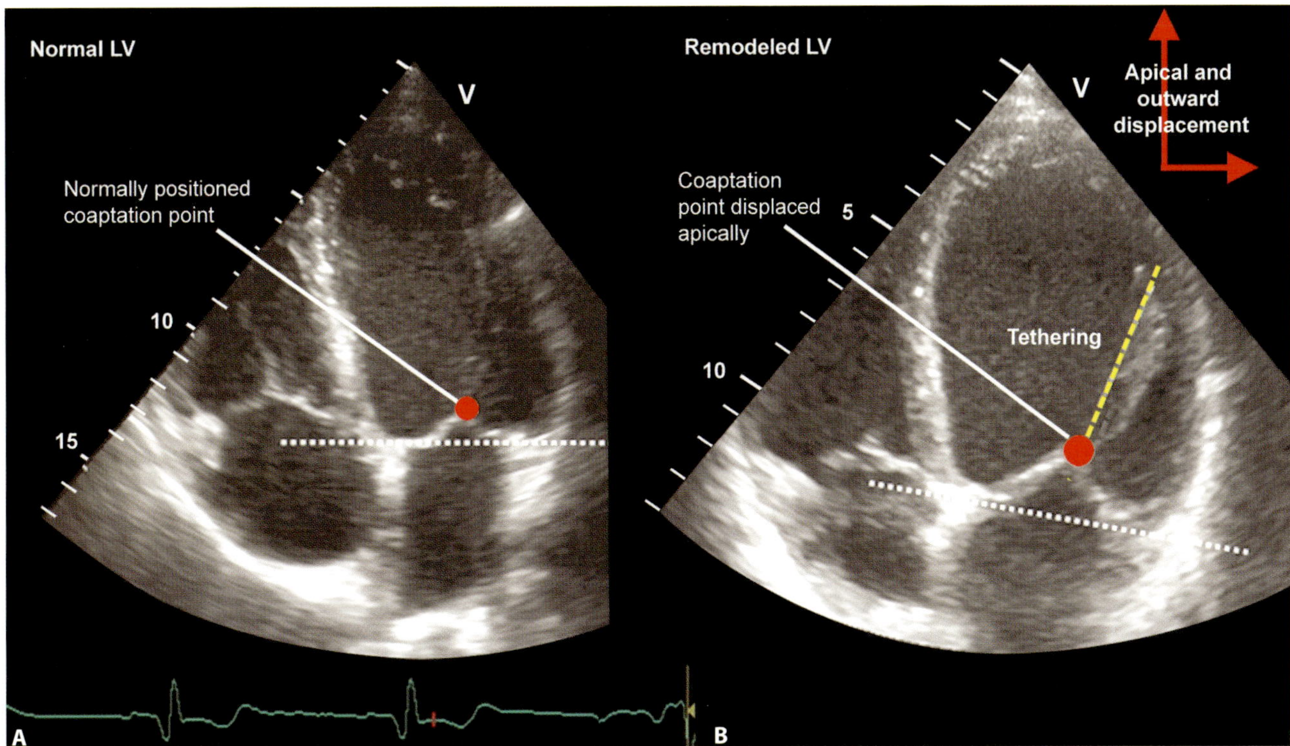


**Figure 16.1A and B:** (A) A patient with normal left ventricular geometry and function and no MR. (B) In contrast, there is systolic apical displacement of mitral leaflets and coaptation point relative to the annular plane (white dashed line) in a patient with ischemic dilated cardiomyopathy and ischemic MR. The red arrows designate the direction of displacement of the papillary muscles and the red dots indicate the coaptation point of the valve leaflets.

*Abbreviations:* LV, left ventricle; MR, mitral regurgitation.

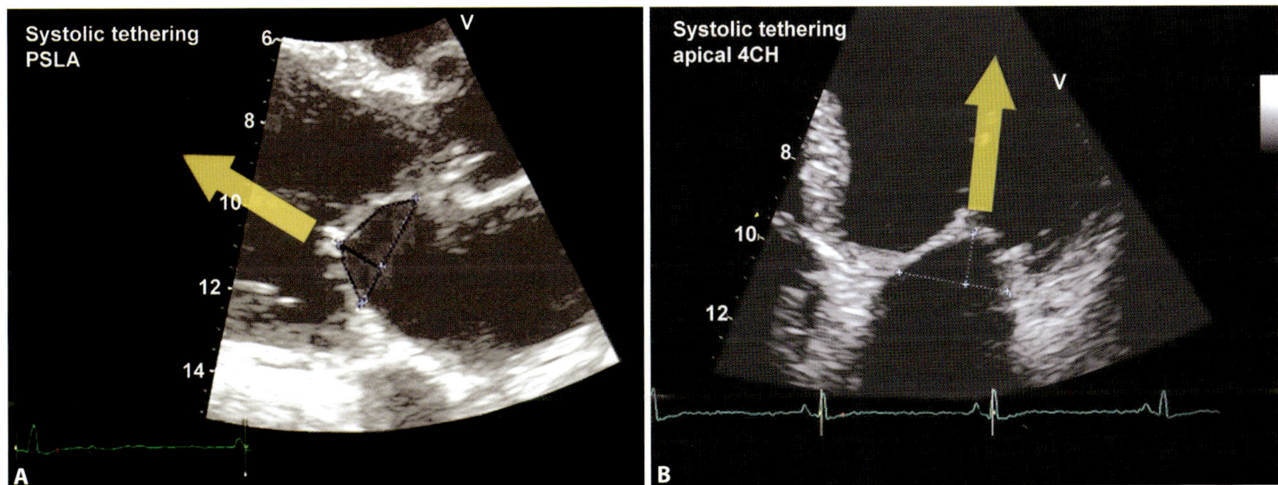


**Figure 16.2A and B:** Systolic tethering of the mitral valve (MV) leaflets which brings the leaflet coaptation line more apically into the left ventricular cavity, seen in the parasternal long-axis view (A) and the apical four-chamber view (B). The yellow arrows indicate that the coaptation line of the MV leaflets is displaced apically; the blue dotted area underneath the MV leaflets represents the tenting created by the leaflet tethering.

*Abbreviations:* 4CH, four-chamber; PSLA, parasternal long-axis.

The MV leaflets enlargement that develops in the presence of chronic leaflet tethering may contribute to the reduction of MR severity in some patients[10,13] and thus, can be categorized as part of the "closing force" mechanisms. In SMR, mitral leaflet area may increase by ≤35% on average but differs in individual patients for a comparable degree of leaflet tethering and LV remodeling.[13] Thus, this adaptative mechanism, aiming to reduce leaflet tethering and improve coaptation, is sometimes overridden and SMR ensues.

Conversely, "tethering forces" refer to all forces that through a complex interplay pull the leaflets apart during systole, preventing effective MV orifice closure. The key "tethering force" in chronic ischemic MR is the local or regional LV remodeling that leads to papillary muscle displacement. Mitral annular dilatation and loss of "saddle-shape" geometry contribute to the development of SMR as an adjunctive mechanism.[8,9] Similarly, the progressive increase in left atrial (LA) pressure may contribute to SMR by pushing the MV leaflets further apically and thus, aggravating valve incompetence.[14]

The pathophysiology of chronic ischemic MR further differs from the pathophysiology of organic MR in the sense that the former imposes a chronic increase in volume overload on an already sick ventricle, less able to cope with this supplementary load and very much in need to maintain its closing forces. A vicious circle is established in the presence of chronic ischemic MR, left ventricle continues to dilate and remodel leading to a progressive increase in MV leaflet tethering and aggravating the MR and so on. Apart from the downstream consequences on the LV, ischemic MR leads to a progressive increase in pulmonary venous pressure, a phenomenon dependent on the degree of LA compliance. In most patients with chronic ischemic MR, left atrium progressively enlarges, and this is why, the increase in pulmonary venous pressure occurs late in the natural history of the disease. Once pulmonary venous pressure has increased, signs and symptoms of pulmonary congestions develop. Moreover, another vicious circle is closed, as the increase in LA pressure will contribute to the worsening of chronic ischemic MR and to further increase in pulmonary venous pressure.

## ECHOCARDIOGRAPHIC DIAGNOSIS

First step to the echocardiographic diagnosis of chronic ischemic MR is to suspect this entity in each patient with regional or global LV remodeling and then to try to identify the mechanisms involved in its genesis. Systolic apical displacement of mitral leaflets and coaptation line is the key change in mitral apparatus geometry **(Figure 16.1 and 16.2)** and the easiest feature that can be identified by echocardiography.[15,16]

Two patterns of leaflet tethering have been classically described—symmetric and asymmetric.[17] If both papillary muscles are displaced apically and outward, both MV leaflets are equally tethered (i.e. symmetric tethering) and a typically central MR jet can be seen **(Videos 16.1A and B)**. Otherwise, when only one of the two papillary muscles is displaced, tethering is predominant on one of the leaflets, usually the posterior leaflet **(Figure 16.3B)**. This leads to asymmetric apposition of the two leaflets over the length of a segment of the coaptation surface and to an eccentric MR jet **(Videos 16.2A and B)**. Commonly, the posteromedial papillary muscle displacement, as in inferior and inferolateral wall MI, will create an asymmetric tethering pattern with severe tethering on the posteromedial scallop of the posterior leaflet (P3), asymmetric apposition of the leaflets at the level of this scallop, and an eccentric, posterior oriented MR jet. Hence, analyzing jet direction by color flow Doppler in patients with chronic ischemic MR can give useful hints about the type of tethering and is therefore an important step in the analysis of MR mechanism **(Figure 16.3)**.

The next step in the complete diagnosis of chronic ischemic MR is the quantification of MR severity. It is mandatory to quantify chronic ischemic MR severity by echocardiography, as a graded relationship between ischemic MR severity and reduced survival has been demonstrated.[18] Quantitative and semiquantitative methods can be used to determine the severity of chronic ischemic MR. However, semiquantitative methods, such as vena contracta width and regurgitant jet area are of little interest due to lower accuracy in eccentric jets and too poor reproducibility, respectively.[19] Quantitative methods, such as the Doppler volumetric method and the proximal isovelocity surface area (PISA) method can grade MR severity more accurately.[20,21] The Doppler volumetric method allows the calculation of regurgitant volume as the difference between mitral and aortic stroke volumes.[20] However, it is rarely performed in the clinical setting because it is time consuming, needs several cumbersome manual measurements, and small errors may lead to significant inaccuracies. The PISA method allows the quantification of both regurgitant volume and effective regurgitant orifice area (EROA)[21] but it too has several limitations that should be acknowledged.[22] First of all, the PISA radius changes during systole, being larger in early and late systole and smaller in midsystole.[23] Performing only one measurement in midsystole will lead to underestimation of EROA and regurgitant volume. Ideally, the PISA radius should be averaged throughout systole, but software capable of performing such a measurement has not been developed yet. Second, the PISA method assumes that the flow convergence area is hemispherical. In practice, flow convergence area is frequently hemielliptic, especially in chronic ischemic MR, and applying the PISA method in this case will lead to underestimation of EROA and

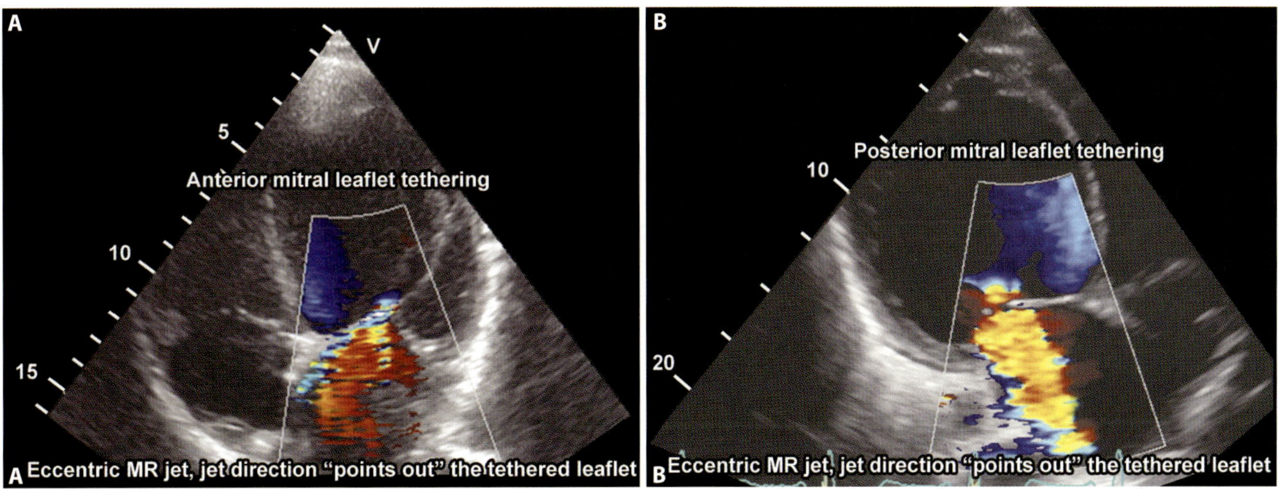


**Figure 16.3A and B:** Depending on which leaflet is predominantly tethered the direction of the regurgitant jet changes, "pointing out" the leaflet that is more severely tethered. (A) Severe tethering of the anterior mitral leaflet with an eccentric jet (asymmetric tethering pattern) towards the interatrial septum. (B) Severe tethering of the posterior leaflet with an eccentric jet towards the posterior atrial wall (asymmetric tethering pattern).
*Abbreviation:* MR, mitral regurgitation.

regurgitant volume.[24,25] Real-time three-dimensional (3D) echocardiography may be a solution to this problem, but large outcome studies are still missing. The problem of multiple jets could also be solved by this particular technique. 3D echocardiography, both transthoracic and transoesophageal, allows measurement of color-Doppler based vena contracta area.[26] A 3D derived vena contracta area of ≥0.41 cm$^2$ seems to indicate severe ischemic MR. However, further validation of this cutoff value is necessary.[27] A more recent and promising technique developed to quantify MR severity, that could be applied to chronic ischemic MR quantification, is 3D derived PISA. It allows computation of a peak 3D EROA from the peak regurgitant jet velocity (as assessed by continuous wave (CW) Doppler) and the direct 3D based measurement (without any geometrical assumption) of the PISA.[28] However, as for the vena contracta area, validation and outcome studies are still needed. Therefore, for everyday clinical practice, for the time being, two-dimensional (2D) echocardiography derived EROA and regurgitant volume using the PISA method or the Doppler volumetric, are the methods recommended to quantify chronic ischemic MR[19] and decision-making is still based on these 2D echocardiography derived cutoff values. Severe ischemic MR is defined as an EROA >20 mm$^2$ or a regurgitant volume >30 mL.[18,19]

Another important step in the echocardiographic evaluation of chronic ischemic MR, with important implications with regard to treatment strategies, is the assessment of MV configuration. With 2D echocardiography, the following parameters can be measured to assess the degree of deformity of the MV apparatus: annular dimensions, tenting area (area of the region enclosed between the annular plane and the mitral leaflets), anterior and posterior leaflets angle **(Figure 16.4A)**, coaptation distance (shortest distance between the mitral annulus plane and the leaflet coaptation point), bending distances and coaptation length.[29] Frequently used in clinical practice and with prognostic implications are tenting area, coaptation distance, posterior leaflet angle, and mitral annulus diameter. An MV tenting area ≥2.5 cm$^2$ or ≥1.6 cm$^2$, a coaptation distance ≥1 cm, a posterior leaflet angle ≥45° and an annulus diameter ≥37 mm predict persistence of MR after restrictive annuloplasty.[30,31] These measurements are usually performed in apical 4-chamber view **(Figure 16.4A)** in mid-systole with the exception of mitral annulus diameter in which the cutoff value was obtained from transesophageal echocardiography in diastole.

3D echocardiography is able to provide all the above-mentioned measurements with better accuracy, because the technique reduces the risk of measurements performed in off-axis planes. However, the major limitation is the dependency on image quality. Mitral annular geometry and dynamics are best assessed by 3D echocardiography.[8] Mitral annular reconstruction is available using commercial software by off-line analysis of the acquired 3D dataset. Annular diameter and area are increased, the annulus is less elliptical and more flattened, and there is a decrease in annular "sphincter" function in patients with SMR as compared to normal subjects.[8] Tenting volume, the volume enclosed between the surface of the mitral leaflets and the annular plane, can be computed from the 3D datasets through off-line analysis with dedicated software. This parameter proved to be closely related to SMR severity and a reliable marker of leaflets tethering severity.[32] With 3D echocardiography, leaflet surface area, leaflet area/closure area and leaflet area/annular area ratios can be assessed. Leaflet surface area has been shown to be higher by at least 35% on average in patients with SMR,[13] while leaflet area/closure area and leaflet area/annular area ratios are lower in patients with significant SMR.[33] Their incremental role compared to 2D echocardiography in predicting outcome after treatment in patients with chronic ischemic MR is still undefined.

Last but not the least, echocardiography helps in the evaluation of LV remodeling in patients with chronic ischemic MR. The following parameters need to be reported: LV volumes, LV ejection fraction, wall motion abnormalities, LV systolic sphericity index (LV short axis-to-long axis diameter ratio measured at end-systole) **(Figure 16.4C)**, the interpapillary muscle distance (the length between the papillary muscles in short axis view at end-systole) **(Figure 16.4B)** and the tethering distance (the distance between the intervalvular fibrosa and the head of the posteromedial papillary muscle at mid-systole). All of these parameters can be measured with 2D echocardiography and the cutoff values with prognostic implications have been reported from 2D echocardiographic studies, but they can also be obtained by 3D echocardiography with the advantage of lower variability of measurement. An LV end-systolic volume ≥145 mL, a systolic sphericity index ≥0.7[34,35] and an interpapillary muscle distance >20 mm measured at end-systole using 2D echocardiography perform well in predicting recurrent MR after undersized annuloplasty for chronic ischemic MR.[36]

## DYNAMIC NATURE

### Role of Stress Echocardiography

Chronic ischemic MR has a dynamic nature.[37] Its severity varies throughout systole, with a decrease of severity in mid-systole that parallels the increase in LV closing forces.[23] Yet, its dynamic nature is best highlighted by the change in SMR severity with different loading conditions. One of the classical examples of preload and afterload dependency of SMR severity was given by Levine et al. who described the vanishing of MR intraoperatively (preload and afterload reduction

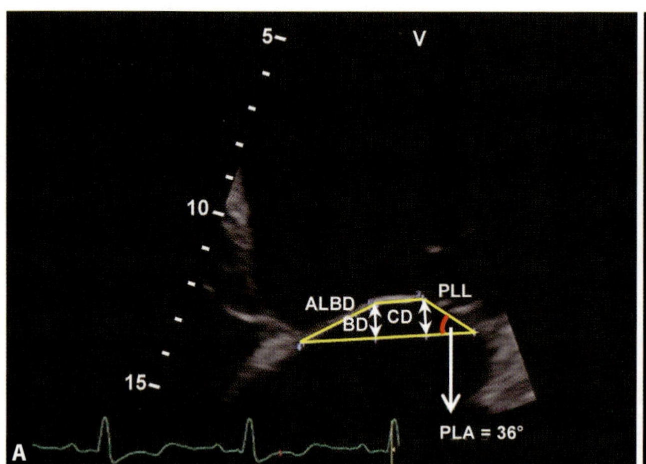


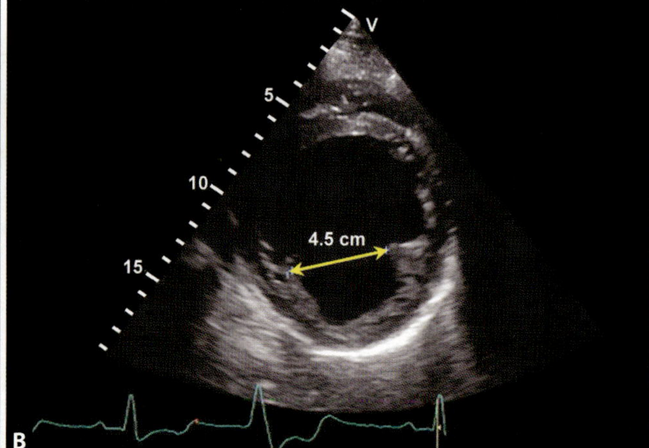


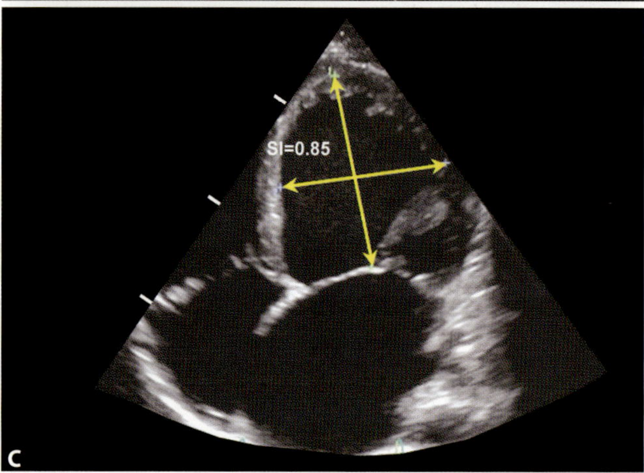


**Figure 16.4A to C:** Echocardiographic evaluation of a patient with dilated cardiomyopathy and secondary mitral regurgitation (MR). (A) Coaptation distance (CD) measures 1.0 cm, the posterior leaflet length (PLL) measures 1.7 cm. Thus, the posterior leaflet angle (PLA) can be calculated applying the formula PLA = $\sin^{-1}$(CD/PLL) = 36°. In this case a CD of 1.0 cm is a predictor of MR persistence after annuloplasty. Moreover, the mitral annulus measures 4.7 cm (>3.7 cm) and is also a predictor of persistence of MR after restrictive annuloplasty. Anterior leaflet bending distance (ALBD) can also be obtained. (B) Interpapillary muscle distance measured at end-systole is 4.5 mm (>2.0 cm). (C) Sphericity index (left ventricular short-axis to long-axis diameter ratio measured at end-systole) is 0.85 (>0.7). Both the interpapillary muscle distance and the sphericity index predict the recurrence of MR after undersized annuloplasty in this patient.

concomitant with increase in contractility due to inotropic agents) in patients with ischemic MR undergoing coronary bypass grafting (CABG).[37] In our experience, exercise stress echocardiography (ESE) is one of the best methods to explore the dynamic behavior of chronic ischemic MR. Exercise alters the loading conditions of the left ventricle by modifying preload, afterload and contractility, and if an exercise test is performed parallel with imaging of the left ventricle and Doppler interrogation of the MV, the mechanisms involved in the dynamic behavior of chronic ischemic MR can be revealed in each individual patient. An ESE is able to provide prognostic information over resting echocardiography, by unmasking patients at high-risk of poor outcome[38,39] and allows matching of MR severity with symptom development.[39] An exercise-induced increase in EROA by ≥13 $mm^2$ proved to be a predictor of mortality and of hospital admission for heart failure in patients with SMR **(Figure 16.5)**.[38]

The most recent guidelines of the European Society of Cardiology (ESC) on the management of valvular heart disease emphasize that "the dynamic component of SMR can be assessed and quantified by exercise echocardiography" and that "in patients capable of exercising, exercise echocardiography should be considered whenever possible" in patients planned for surgical revascularization.[40]

Based on our experience, ESE may be of interest in the following categories of patients: (i) in patients with LV dysfunction who present with exertional dyspnea out of proportion to the severity of resting LV systolic dysfunction or MR, (ii) in patients in whom acute pulmonary edema occurs without any obvious cause, (iii) to unmask patients at high-risk of mortality and heart failure, (iv) before surgical revascularization in patients with moderate ischemic MR, and (v) following surgery, to explain the persistence of pulmonary hypertension and the absence of functional class improvement.

An ESE requires a dedicated tilting table, continuous electrocardiographic monitoring facilities, advanced life support facilities, and medical personnel with adequate expertise in the field. A symptom limited and gradual exercise test (workload increase by 25 watts each 2 minutes) is recommended. In the absence of symptoms, the test should be continued until 85% of the age predicted heart rate is reached. The test should not be performed in patients in New York Heart Association functional class IV, those with uncontrolled blood pressure values at rest (systolic arterial pressure >200 mm Hg or diastolic arterial pressure >110 mm Hg), patients with uncontrolled arrhythmias or those unable or unwilling to perform such a test.

A complete resting echocardiography is performed at rest, prior to exercise. Image acquisition both at rest and during exercise is done with the patient on a tilting table located on the left side of the sonographer. Throughout each step of the test the following imaging sequence is recommended to be recorded: CW Doppler imaging of the tricuspid valve for assessment of peak systolic trans-tricuspid gradient, pulsed-wave Doppler at the level of the mitral leaflet tips for the LV inflow profile, at the level of the mitral annulus and of the LV outflow tract for stroke volume calculation, color Doppler imaging of the MV for PISA radius measurement, CW Doppler imaging of the MR jet and gray scale loops focused on the LV in apical 4-, 2- and 3-chamber view.

During ESE, the following questions should be answered: (i) what happens with the MR: does it increase/decrease or remains unchanged? (ii) does the tethering on MV increase/decrease or remains unchanged? (iii) are there new wall motion abnormalities or is there a recruitment of the hibernating myocardium? (iv) is there a significant and

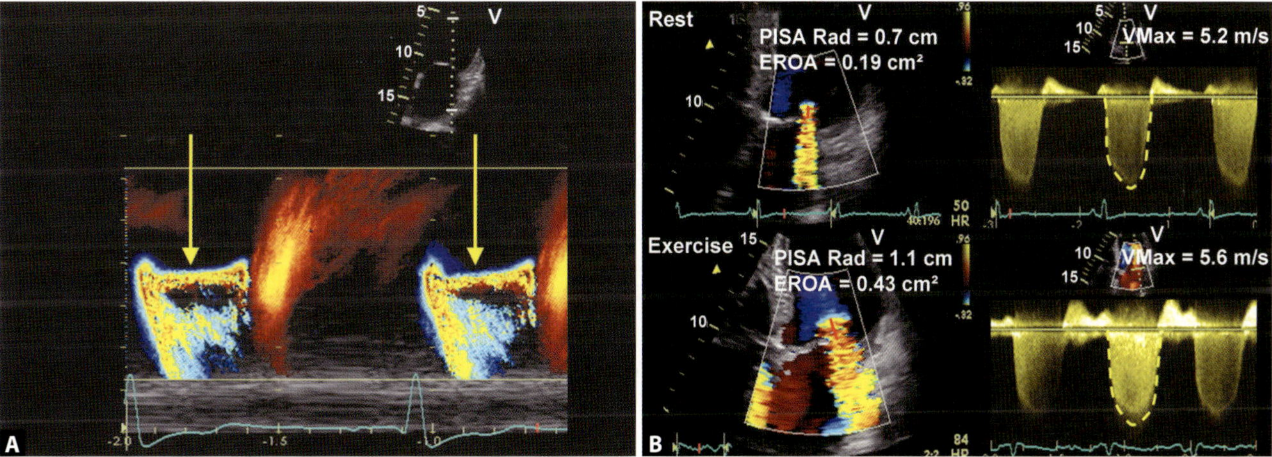


**Figure 16.5A and B:** (A) Dynamic trait of ischemic MR with decrease in MR severity in mid-systole as compared to early and late systole [the arrow indicate that in mid-systole the PISA radius is decreasing as compared to early and late systole] and (B) increase in MR severity during exercise stress echocardiography (more than 13 $mm^2$ exercise-induced increase in EROA) in a patient with ischemic MR.
*Abbreviations:* EROA, effective regurgitant orifice area; MR, mitral regurgitation; PISA Rad, proximal isovelocity surface area radius; Vmax, velocity maximum.

rapid increase in systolic pulmonary artery pressure with exercise? and (v) what is the mechanism of MR behavior during exercise: a decrease in closing forces or an increase in tethering of the MV?

## TIMING AND PATIENT SELECTION FOR SURGICAL CORRECTION

Even though the survival benefit of MV repair compared to myocardial revascularization alone has not been proven in randomized studies, the association of chronic ischemic MR with poor outcome and the fact that myocardial revascularization alone does not correct MR support MV surgery at the time of surgical revascularization in patients with indication for CABG and moderate or severe chronic ischemic MR.[40] Because of a lower mortality rate, MV repair is preferred over MV replacement (6.8% vs. 11.4% when combined with CABG, Fourth European Association for Cardio-Thoracic Surgery adult cardiac surgical database report 2010). According to current guidelines, MV surgical repair is indicated in patients with severe MR and LV ejection fraction >30% undergoing CABG, and it should be considered in moderate MR, especially if there is a high likelihood of reparability or if a significant dynamic component (i.e. increase in EROA with exercise by ≥13 mm²) is documented with ESE.[40] In patients without a clear indication for revascularization, the assessment of myocardial viability and coronary status is mandatory to guide treatment. Symptomatic patients with severe chronic ischemic MR, LV ejection fraction less than 30%, option for revascularization and evidence of myocardial viability should benefit from MV repair. In contrast, symptomatic patients with severe ischemic MR, LV ejection fraction >30%, without possibility of myocardial revascularization, but with low comorbidity, should be operated only if they remain symptomatic despite optimal medical treatment. For others, medical treatment or cardiac transplantation is preferred.[40]

The most common surgical technique to correct chronic ischemic MR is restrictive annuloplasty. Even though chronic ischemic MR is a ventricular and not a valvular disease, and that MV repair using restrictive annuloplasty targets the consequences rather than the cause of the disease, this technique is still largely used and provides good results in terms of MR correction and improvement of symptoms in well-selected patients. However, its major drawbacks are related to the risk of significant residual (*persistent or recurrent*) MR following MV repair with this technique.

*Persistent MR* after MV repair (i.e. MR seen immediately after surgery) can be explained by the reduction of the anteroposterior annular diameter due to the rigid ring that leads to anterior displacement of the posterior annulus and further tethering of the posterior leaflet.[35] Usually, MR jet is eccentric in this case and oriented posteriorly. On the other hand, *recurrent MR* is more related to ongoing LV remodeling happening progressively after surgery, with increasing LV volume and sphericity, further tethering of both leaflets and MR. Usually, in this case, MR jet tends to be more frequently central. Preoperative evaluation of tethering with echocardiography can help to detect patients at risk of persistent or recurrent MR. Asymmetrical tethering pattern with predominant posterior leaflet tethering, is associated with localized LV remodeling and higher risk of *persistent MR*. In contrast, symmetrical pattern, explained by predominant apical tethering of both leaflets, is associated with lack of reverse LV remodeling after revascularization and higher risk of *recurrent MR*.

Several studies attempted to identify the preoperative predictors of MV repair failure. Prediction of *persistent MR* is based on MV geometry assessment, such as MV tenting area ≥2.5 cm² or ≥1.6 cm², coaptation distance ≥1 cm, posterior leaflet angle ≥45° and annulus diameter ≥37 mm.[30,31] An increased posterior leaflet angle was the best predictor of persistent MR and associated with a markedly reduced 3-year event-free survival in one study.[30] *Recurrent MR* is better predicted by LV remodeling parameters such as LV end-systolic volume ≥145 mL, systolic sphericity index ≥0.7[34,35] and an interpapillary muscle distance >20 mm.[36] However, the presence of significant tethering does not preclude annuloplasty if the patients fulfill the ESC criteria for revascularization and valve repair. However, in patients with high-risk of MV repair failure, MV replacement with preservation of the subvalvular apparatus could be contemplated.

Surgical or interventional techniques, addressing the ventricular problem (ventricular plication, polymer injection to reverse myocardial remodeling) or addressing the subvalvular apparatus (secondary chord cutting, repositioning of the papillary muscles) showed promising results but have not yet been accepted by current guidelines.[41-43]

Further studies are needed to conclude on the best therapeutic approach to improve outcomes in patients with significant chronic ischemic MR and at high-risk of residual MR after MV restrictive annuloplasty.

## CONCLUSION

Chronic secondary MR is common after MI and in patients with dilated cardiomyopathy. Prompt recognition of the mechanism and etiology is highly important, as severity grading is different from organic MR. Echocardiography is the key investigation to make the diagnosis, assess severity, and its consequences on the left atrium, left ventricle and pulmonary vascular bed. Based on our experience, an approach to a patient with chronic ischemic MR is summarized in **Flow chart 16.1**.

**Flow chart 16.1:** Management of patients with chronic ischemic mitral regurgitation.

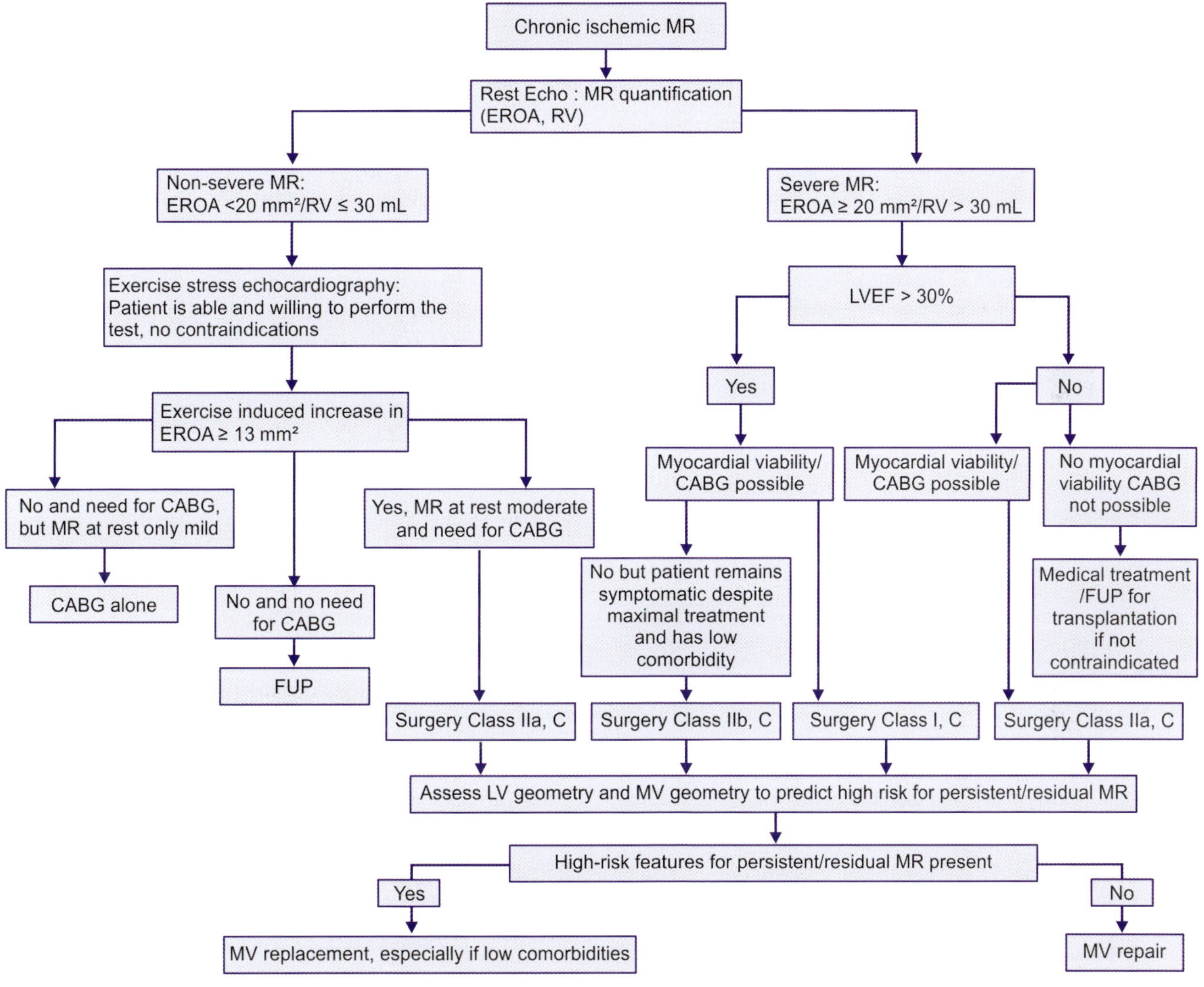


*Abbreviations:* CABG, coronary artery bypass grafting; EROA, effective regurgitant orific area; FUP, follow-up; LV, left ventricular; LVEF, left ventricular ejection fraction; MR, mitral regurgitation; MV, mitral valve; VR, valve replacement; RV, regurgitant volume.

## VIDEO LEGENDS

**Video 16.1:** (A) Severe left ventricular systolic dysfunction resulting in symmetrical tenting of mitral valve leaflets leading to non-coaptation. (B) Central jet of severe mitral regurgitation.

**Video 16.2:** (A) Asymmetric tethering of mitral valve leaflets causing more marked restriction of the posterior mitral leaflet. (B) Eccentric posteriorly directed jet of mitral regurgitation due to malcoaptation of mitral valve leaflets secondary to asymmetric tethering.

## REFERENCES


1. He S, Fontaine A, Schwammenthal E, et al. Integrated mechanism for functional mitral regurgitation. Circulation. 1997;96:1826-34.
2. Otsuji Y, Hanschumacher MD, Liel-Cohen N, et al. Mechanism of ischemic mitral regurgitation with segmental left ventricular dysfunction: three-dimensional echocardiographic studies in models of acute and chronic progressive regurgitation. J Am Coll Cardiol. 2001;37:641-8.

3. Kono T, Sabbah HN, Rosman H, et al. Mechanism of functional mitral regurgitation during acute myocardial ischemia. J Am Coll Cardiol. 1992;19:1101-5.
4. Silbiger JJ. Novel pathogenetic mechanisms and structural adaptations in ischemic mitral regurgitation. J Am Soc Echocardiogr. 2013;26:1107-17.
5. Ciarka A, Van de Veire N. Secondary mitral regurgitation: pathophysiology, diagnosis, and treatment. Heart. 2011;97:1012-23.
6. Ypenburg C, Lancellotti P, Tops LF, et al. Acute effects of initiation and withdrawal of cardiac resynchronization therapy on papillary muscle dyssynchrony and mitral regurgitation. J Am Coll Cardiol. 2007;50:2071-7.
7. Lancellotti P, Melon P, Sakalihasan N, et al. Effect of cardiac resynchronization therapy on functional mitral regurgitation in heart failure. Am J Cardiol. 2004;94:1462-5.
8. Watanabe N, Ogasawara Y, Yamaura Y, et al. Geometric deformity of the mitral annulus in patients with ischemic mitral regurgitation: a real-time three-dimensional echocardiographic study. J Heart Valve Dis. 2005;14:447-52.
9. Daimon M, Gillinov AM, Liddicoat JR, et al. Dynamic change in mitral annular area and motion during percutaneous mitral annuloplasty for ischemic mitral regurgitation: preliminary animal study with real-time 3-dimensional echocardiography. J Am Soc Echocardiogr. 2007;20:381-8.
10. Chaput M, Handschumacher MD, Guerrero J, et al. Mitral leaflet adaptation to ventricular remodeling: prospective changes in a model of ischemic mitral regurgitation. Circulation. 2009; 120 (11 Suppl): S99-103.
11. Otsuji Y, Handschumacher M, Schwammenthal E, et al. Insights from three dimensional echocardiography into the mechanism of functional mitral regurgitation. Circulation. 1997;96:1999-2008.
12. Otsuji Y, Kumanohoso T, Yoshifuku S, et al. Isolated annular dilation does not usually cause important functional mitral regurgitation: comparison between patients with lone atrial fibrillation and those with idiopathic or ischemic cardiomyopathy. J Am Coll Cardiol. 2002;39:1651-6.
13. Chaput M, Handschumacher MD, Tournoux F, et al. Mitral leaflet adaptation to ventricular remodeling: occurrence and adequacy in patients with functional mitral regurgitation. Circulation. 2008;118:845-52.
14. Marechaux S, Pincon C, Poueymidanette M, et al. Elevated left atrial pressure estimated by Doppler echocardiography is a key determinant of mitral valve tenting in functional mitral regurgitation. Heart. 2010;96:289-97.
15. Ogawa S, Hubbard FE, Mardelli TJ, et al. Cross-sectional echocardiographic spectrum of papillary muscle dysfunction. Am Heart J. 1979;97:312-21.
16. Godley R, Wann L, Rogers E, et al. Incomplete mitral leaflet closure in patients with papillary muscle dysfunction. Circulation. 1981;63:565-71.
17. Agricola E, Oppizzi M, Maisano F, et al. Echocardiographic classification of chronic ischemic mitral regurgitation caused by restricted motion according to tethering pattern. Eur J Echocardiogr. 2004;5:326-34.
18. Grigioni F, Enriquez-Sarano M, Zehr KJ, et al. Ischemic mitral regurgitation. Long-term outcome and prognostic implications with quantitative Doppler assessment. Circulation. 2001;103: 1759-64.
19. Lancellotti P, Tribouilloy C, Hagendorff A, et al. Recommendations for the echocardiographic assessment of native valvular regurgitation: an executive summary from the European Association of Cardiovascular Imaging. Eur Heart J Cardiovasc Imaging. 2013;14:611-44.
20. Enriquez-Sarano M, Bailey KR, Seward JB, et al. Quantitative Doppler assessment of valvular regurgitation. Circulation. 1993;87:841-8.
21. Enriquez-Sarano M, Seward JB, Bailey KR, et al. Effective regurgitant origice area: a noninvasive Doppler development of an old hemodynamic concept. J Am Coll Cardiol. 1994;23: 443-51.
22. Enriquez-Sarano M, Miller FA, Hayes SN, et al. Effective mitral regurgitation orifice area: clinical use and pitfalls of the proximal isovelocity surface area method. J Am Coll Cardiol. 1995;25:703-9.
23. Schwammenthal E, Chen C, Benning F, et al. Dynamics of mitral regurgitant flow and orifice area. Physiologic application of the proximal flow convergence method: Clinical data and experimental testing. Circulation. 1994;90:307-22.
24. Song JM, Kim MJ, Kim YJ, et al. Three-dimensional characteristics of functional mitral regurgitation in patients with severe left ventricular dysfunction: a real-time 3-dimensional color Doppler echocardiography study. Heart. 2007;94: 590-6.
25. Yosefy C, Levine RA, Solis J, et al. Proximal flow convergence region as assessed by real-time 3-dimensional echocardiography: challenging the hemispheric assumption. J Am Soc Echocardiogr. 2007;20:389-96.
26. de Agust¡n JA, Marcos-Alberca P, Fernandez-Golfin C, et al. Direct measurement of proximal isovelocity surface area by single-beat three-dimensional color Doppler echocardiography in mitral regurgitation: a validation study. J Am Soc Echocardiogr. 2012;25:815-23.
27. Thavendiranathan P, Phelan D, Thomas J, et al. Quantitative assessment of mitral regurgitation: validation of new methods. J Am Coll Cardiol. 2012;60:1470-83.
28. Grady L, Datta S, Kutter O, et al. Regurgitation quantification using 3D PISA in volume echocardiography. Med Image Comput Comput Assist Interv. 2011;14:512-9.
29. Lancellotti P, Zamorano JL, Vannan MA. Imaging challenges in secondary mitral regurgitation: unsolved issues and perspectives. Circ Cardiovasc Imaging. 2014;7:735-46.
30. Magne J, Pibarot P, Dagenais F, et al. Preoperative posterior leaflet angle accurately predicts outcome after restrictive mitral valve annuloplasty for ischemic mitral regurgitation. Circulation. 2007;115:782-91.
31. Kongsaerepong V, Shiota M, Gillinov AM, et al. Echocardiographic predictors of successful versus unsuccessful mitral valve repair in ischemic mitral regurgitation. Am J Cardiol. 2006;98:504-8.
32. Breithardt OA, Sinha AM, Schwammenthal E, et al. Acute effects of cardiac resynchronization therapy on functional mitral regurgitation in advanced systolic heart failure. J Am Coll Cardiol. 2003;41:765-70.

33. Beaudoin J, Thai WE, Wai B, et al. Assessment of mitral valve adaptation with gated cardiac computed tomography: validation with three-dimensional echocardiography and mechanistic insight to functional mitral regurgitation. Circ Cardiovasc Imaging. 2013;6:784-9.
34. Gelsomino S, Lorusso R, De Cicco G, et al. Five-year echocardiographic results of combined undersized mitral ring annuloplasty and coronary artery bypass grafting for chronic ischaemic mitral regurgitation. Eur Heart J. 2008;94:590-6.
35. Hung J, Papakostas L, Tahta SA, et al. Mechanism of recurrent ischemic mitral regurgitation after annuloplasty: continued LV remodeling as a moving target. Circulation. 2004;110:II85-90.
36. Roshanali F, Mandegar MH, Yousefnia MA, et al. A prospective study of predicting factors in ischemic mitral regurgitation recurrence after ring annuloplasty. Ann Thorac Surg. 2007; 84:745-9.
37. Levine RA, Hung J. Ischemic mitral regurgitation, the dynamic lesion: clues to the cure. J Am Coll Cardiol. 2003;42:1929-32.
38. Lancellotti P, Lebrun F, Pierard LA. Determinants of exercise-induced changes in mitral regurgitation in patients with coronary artery disease and left ventricular dysfunction. J Am Coll Cardiol. 2003;42:1921-8.
39. Pierard LA, Lancellotti P. The role of ischemic mitral regurgitation in the pathogenesis of acute pulmonary edema. N Engl J Med. 2004;351:1627-34.
40. Vahanian A, Baumgartner H, Bax J. Guidelines on the management of valvular heart disease (version 2012): The Joint Task Force on the Management of Valvular Heart Disease of the European Society of Cardiology (ESC) and the European Association for Cardio-Thoracic Surgery (EACTS). Eur Heart J. 2012; 33:2451-96.
41. Fattouch K, Murana G, Castrovinci S, et al. Mitral valve annuloplasty and papillary muscle relocation oriented by 3-dimensional transesophageal echocardiography for severe functional mitral regurgitation. J Thorac Cardiovasc Surg. 2012;143:42.
42. Fattouch K, Castrovinci S, Murana G, et al. Papillary muscle relocation and mitral annuloplasty in ischemic mitral valve regurgitation: Midterm results. J Thorac Cardiovasc Surg. 2014. [Epub ahead of print].
43. Hung J, Chaput M, Guerrero JL, et al. Persistent reduction of ischemic mitral regurgitation by papillary muscle repositioning: structural stabilization of the papillary muscle-ventricular wall complex. Circulation. 2007;116:1259-63.

# Assessment of Myocardial Viability

17
CHAPTER

*Manish Bansal, Ravi R Kasliwal*

## INTRODUCTION

During early 1970s, a few reports emerged that showed that the left ventricular (LV) myocardial dysfunction resulting from previous myocardial infarction (MI) did not necessarily indicate irreversible myocardial necrosis, and that such myocardium could show functional recovery if revascularized in time.[1-3] This was a remarkable discovery as it completely revolutionized the management of patients with chronic ischemic LV systolic dysfunction who were, till then, considered to be unsuitable for any form of myocardial revascularization. From there on, coronary artery bypass graft (CABG) surgery was increasingly offered to these patients and resulted not only in improvement in LV systolic function but also in significant reduction in overall morbidity and mortality.[4-6] However, as CABG itself was associated with a significant risk of operative mortality in these patients, it became imperative to accurately identify the patients who were likely to show LV functional recovery following revascularization and in whom the benefits of CABG outweighed any potential risks. This clinical need led to the concept of myocardial viability assessment and fostered development of several new modalities aimed at predicting recovery of LV contractile function after revascularization.

## WHAT IS MYOCARDIAL VIABILITY?

In the simplest terms, viability can be described as the ability to live. Any myocardial tissue which has the capability to live is therefore viable. However, when used in the context of myocardium, this term is used only for referring to dysfunctional myocardium. The normally contracting myocardium, even though fully alive, is ideally not included in this definition. Thus, viable myocardium is defined as *'dysfunctional myocardium with reduced contractility that has the potential to improve with restoration of adequate coronary blood flow'*. There are two major forms of viable myocardium: stunned myocardium and hibernating myocardium. The knowledge about the pathophysiology of the two and the distinction between them is essential to understand how different diagnostic modalities detect myocardial viability and what their clinical implications are.

When there is acute significant reduction in the blood supply to a myocardial segment, it leads to impairment of contractile function of the affected segment.[7-9] If reperfusion occurs very quickly, i.e. in less than 10 minutes, cardiac function is usually completely and rapidly restored. There is no necrosis and myocardial ultrastructure is maintained. A little prolonged ischemia lasting up to 15–20 minutes also does not cause necrosis, but results in a prolonged, albeit reversible contractile dysfunction, which is known as myocardial stunning **(Flow chart 17.1)**.[10] At cellular level, stunning is characterized by mainly metabolic changes with only minimal alterations in the myocyte structure. Cellular calcium overload, oxygen free radical generation and neutrophil accumulation are the key mechanisms responsible for the development of stunning.[11-13] Although stunning was originally described in animal models,[14] it is a common observation in day-to-day clinical practice also. Some of the commonly encountered clinical settings in which stunning occurs include reperfusion therapy in acute MI, myocardial ischemia during unstable angina and non-ST elevation MI, exercise-induced severe ischemia, etc.[15,16]

In contrast, myocardial hibernation is thought to occur as a result of chronic reduction in myocardial blood supply. The term was first used by Diamond in 1978[17] and was later popularized by Rahimtoola.[18,19] It was believed that hibernation was an adaptive response whereby myocardium downregulated its metabolic activities in order to survive in the face of reduced perfusion. However, more recent studies have shown that this is not necessarily the case.[20] Often the stenosis is not significant enough to produce myocardial ischemia at rest but the myocardial blood flow reserve is severely reduced.[21-23] As a result, repeated episodes of ischemia occur during day-to-day activities which lead to repeated episodes of stunning. And before the myocardium is able to recover from the previous episode of stunning, another episode occurs, resulting in persistent contractile dysfunction **(Flow chart 17.1)**.[24-26] The reduction in resting coronary

**Flow chart 17.1:** Pathogenesis of viable myocardium

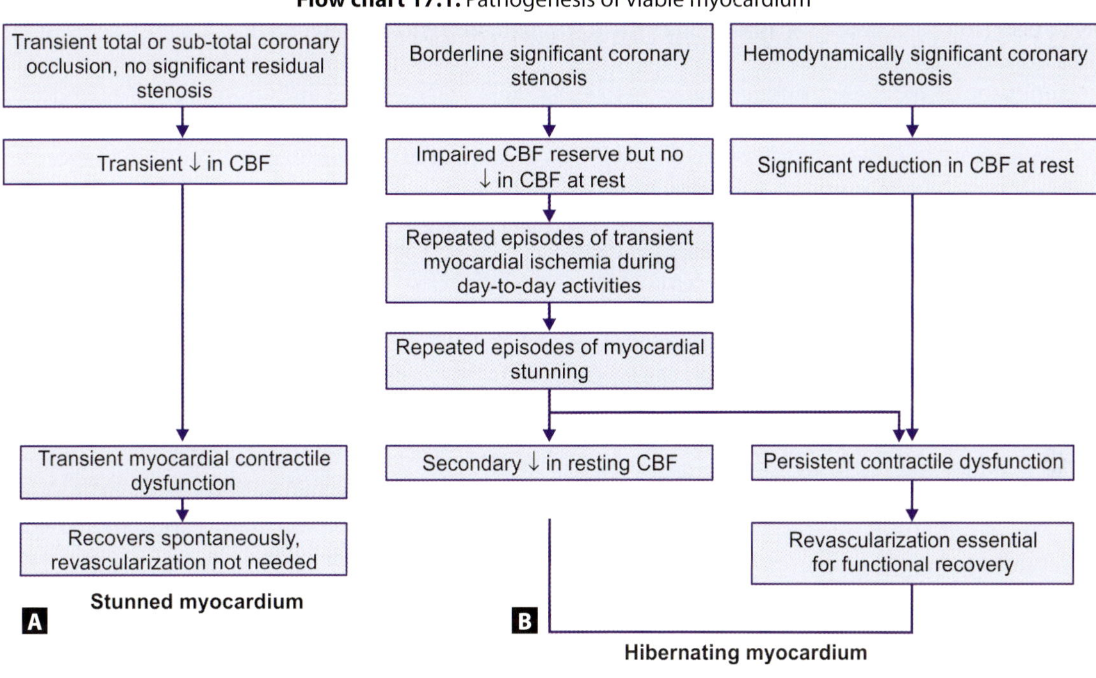


*Abbreviation:* CBF, coronary blood flow.

blood supply may then occur as a secondary event.[21,23,27,28] At ultrastructural level, hibernating myocardium is characterized by several distinct changes: there is a loss of sarcomeres, myofibrils, and contractile proteins; mitochondria are enlarged, nuclei become abnormal, and sarcoplasmic reticulum disappears; glycogen accumulation occurs within the myocytes; and in the interstitium, there may be some degree of collagen deposition.[24,29,30] The extent of these ultrastructural changes determines the likelihood of functional recovery following revascularization.

It is important to note that regardless of the definitions and the underlying mechanisms, both stunning and hibernating myocardium are characterized by 'perfusion-contraction mismatch', i.e. segmental contractile dysfunction which is out of proportion to reduction in the perfusion to that segment. However, while stunning refers to myocardial dysfunction without any residual ischemia, hibernation indicates viable but ischemic myocardium. Accordingly, the stunned myocardium recovers spontaneously, without any need for revascularization, whereas in the case of hibernation, revascularization is essential to salvage the myocardium. If the hibernating myocardium is not revascularized in time, there will be gradual myocyte necrosis and scar formation, resulting in irreversible myocardial damage.

The time course of functional recovery after revascularization is variable. Stunned myocardium with little structural abnormalities recovers mostly within 10 days.[19] However, hibernating myocardium takes longer to recover, depending on the extent of ultrastructural changes.[18,24,29,30] The typical time frame for the recovery of hibernating myocardium is within 6 months, but functional recovery has been reported to occur even up to 2–4 years after revascularization.[31,32]

## ECHOCARDIOGRAPHIC ASSESSMENT OF MYOCARDIAL VIABILITY

Several echocardiographic techniques are currently available for assessment of myocardial viability. These include dobutamine echocardiography, diastolic wall thickness measurement, tissue velocity and strain imaging, and myocardial contrast echocardiography (MCE). Of these, dobutamine echocardiography is the most commonly utilized and the most useful technique for this purpose.

### Dobutamine Echocardiography

Assessment of myocardial viability by dobutamine echocardiography relies on detection of contractile reserve in the dysfunctional myocardium. If a dysfunctional myocardial segment can augment its contractile function when subjected to low-dose dobutamine stimulation, it is likely to be viable and expected to recover after revascularization. In contrast, if there is no improvement in contractility at low-dose dobutamine, the segment is considered to be nonviable.

The technique of performing dobutamine echocardiography is described in detail in Chapter 4. Briefly, incremental doses of dobutamine are administered as intravenous infusion, beginning at 2.5 or 5 µg/kg/minute and increasing every 3 minutes to a maximum dose of 40 µg/kg/minute. Segmental wall-motion analysis is performed at baseline and is repeated at every stage during the dobutamine infusion. At low-dose (i.e. 5–10 µg/kg/min), dobutamine produces only mild inotropic effect with negligible chronotropic effect and hence, there is no increase in myocardial oxygen demand. As a result, the viable segments show improvement in contractility at this dose. However, as the dose increases, there is progressive increase in heart rate with commensurate increase in the myocardial oxygen demand. At peak-dose dobutamine (i.e. 40 µg/kg/min), the increase in myocardial oxygen demand is profound and sufficient enough to precipitate ischemia in segments that have compromised blood supply. Thus, a hibernating myocardial segment, which is viable but ischemic, will show improvement in contractility at low dose but worsening at peak-dose dobutamine **(Figure 17.1, Videos 17.1 and 17.2)**. This biphasic response is the hallmark of myocardial viability and is the most accurate predictor of functional improvement after revascularization.[33] In contrast, a uniphasic response characterized by sustained improvement in contractility at low- and peak-dose dobutamine indicates viable but nonischemic myocardium. In acute setting, this is usually a manifestation of myocardial stunning and indicates high likelihood of spontaneous recovery, without the need for any surgical or percutaneous revascularization. However, in chronic setting, this may just represent viable myocardium with underlying scar and no ischemia. The functional outcome of these segments after revascularization is variable.[33] For this reason, it is important to distinguish between a uniphasic response and a biphasic response. Therefore, even though low-dose response is sufficient to detect myocardial viability, it is advisable to perform a full-dose dobutamine echocardiography in most patients requiring myocardial viability assessment.

Occasionally, there is worsening of contractile function even at low-dose dobutamine. This indicates severe ischemia. Although these segments also tend to improve after revascularization, the response rate is variable.

### *Accuracy*

Numerous studies have evaluated accuracy of dobutamine echocardiography for predicting functional recovery after revascularization. In 1997, Bax et al. performed a pooled analysis of 37 such studies that utilized various imaging modalities for assessment of myocardial viability and reported changes in regional contractile function after revascularization.[34] Dobutamine echocardiography was found to have the highest specificity (81%) among all the modalities included in the analysis. The sensitivity was also excellent (84%), albeit lower than the same for rest-redistribution thallium-201 (Tl-201) perfusion scintigraphy which had the highest sensitivity (90%). In another pooled analysis, Bonow et al. also found dobutamine echocardiography to be the best predictor of functional recovery amongst the modalities studied.[35]

Schinkel et al. performed a larger pooled analysis in 2007.[36] This analysis included a total of 158 studies evaluating the following imaging techniques-dobutamine echocardiography, Tl-201 perfusion scintigraphy, technetium-99m (Tc-99m) perfusion scintigraphy, F-18 fluorodeoxyglucose (FDG) positron emission tomography (PET) and cardiac magnetic resonance imaging (MRI). The analysis showed that the overall accuracy of all the modalities for prediction of regional contractile functional recovery was similar **(Table 17.1)**. However, FDG PET had the highest sensitivity and dobutamine echocardiography had the highest specificity. Nuclear imaging techniques had

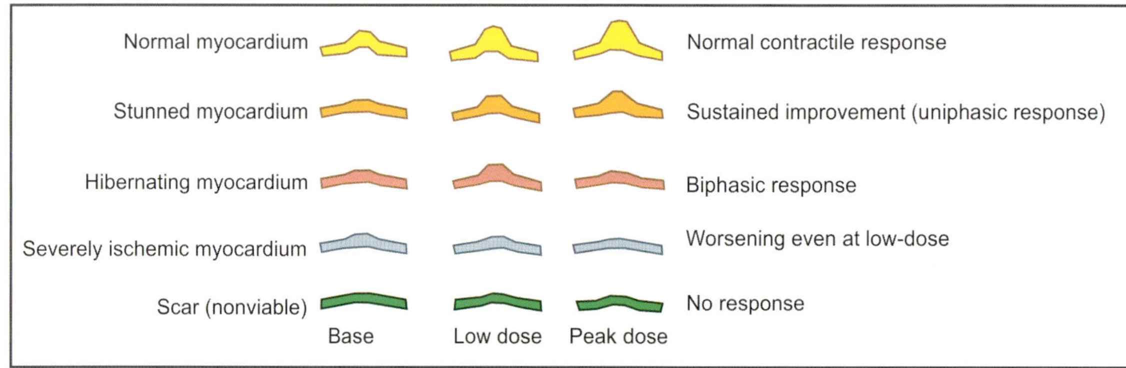


**Figure 17.1:** Interpretation of segment wall-motion response during dobutamine echocardiography for assessment of myocardial viability.

**Table 17.1:** Pooled diagnostic accuracies of commonly used imaging modalities for assessment of myocardial viability[36]

| | *No. of studies/ no. of patients* | *Sensitivity* | *Specificity* | *Positive predictive value* | *Negative predictive value* |
|---|---|---|---|---|---|
| *Recovery of regional contractile function* | | | | | |
| Dobutamine echocardiography | 41/1421 | 80 | 78 | 75 | 83 |
| Thallium-201 perfusion scintigraphy | 40/1119 | 87 | 54 | 67 | 79 |
| Technetium-99m perfusion scintigraphy | 25/721 | 83 | 65 | 74 | 76 |
| F-18 FDG PET | 24/756 | 92 | 63 | 74 | 87 |
| Cardiac magnetic resonance imaging | 13/420 | 84 | 63 | 72 | 78 |
| *Recovery of global left ventricular contractile function* | | | | | |
| Dobutamine echocardiography | 5/195 | 57 | 73 | 63 | 68 |
| Thallium-201 perfusion scintigraphy | 3/95 | 84 | 53 | 76 | 64 |
| Technetium-99m perfusion scintigraphy | 2/98 | 84 | 68 | 74 | 80 |
| F-18 FDG PET | 3/253 | 83 | 64 | 68 | 80 |
| Cardiac magnetic resonance imaging | – | – | – | – | – |

*Abbreviations:* FDG, fluorodeoxyglucose; PET, positron emission tomography.
*Source:* Schinkel AF, Bax JJ, Poldermans D, Elhendy A, Ferrari R, Rahimtoola SH. Hibernating myocardium: Diagnosis and patient outcomes. Curr Probl Cardiol. 2007;32:375-410.

higher sensitivity but lower specificity than dobutamine echocardiography. Positive predictive value (PPV) was highest for dobutamine echocardiography and FDG PET. The FDG PET also had the highest negative predictive value (NPV) whereas Tc-99m scintigraphy had the lowest NPV. Sensitivity, specificity, NPV and PPV of cardiac MRI were intermediate. Similar observations were made for prediction of global LV functional recovery also,[36] although only a few studies had assessed this end-point. In all these studies, an absolute increase of 5% in LV ejection fraction (EF) was used as the cut-off to define global LV functional recovery. Nuclear imaging techniques were found to have a higher sensitivity, whereas dobutamine echocardiography had the lowest sensitivity, in line with the prediction of improvement in regional function. Dobutamine echocardiography appeared to have a higher specificity, but the differences between the techniques were not statistically significant.

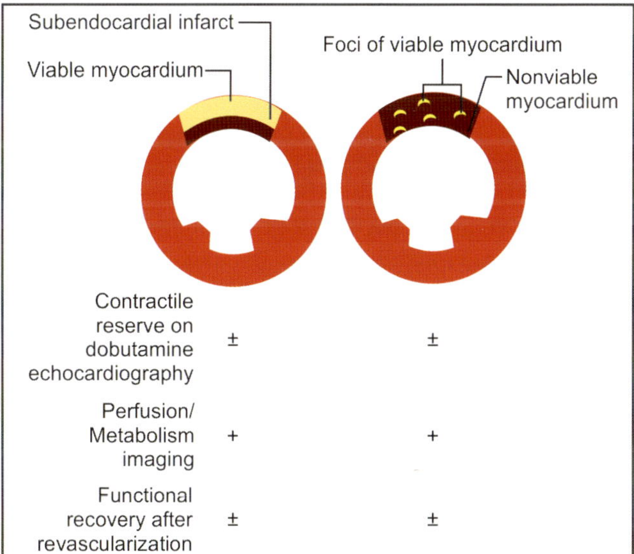


**Figure 17.2:** Potential mechanisms responsible for higher specificity but lower sensitivity of dobutamine echocardiography in comparison to nuclear imaging for prediction of functional recovery.

The greater specificity but lower sensitivity of dobutamine echocardiography, as compared to FDG PET and other nuclear imaging techniques, can be explained by the differences in the targets evaluated by these techniques. Dobutamine echocardiography detects contractile reserve, whereas FDG PET scan and nuclear imaging look for the preserved myocardial metabolism and/or perfusion. Improvement in myocardial contractile function requires presence of a large number of viable cells **(Figure 17.2)**, much more than what is required for detection by nuclear imaging. Thus, if there is a partially infarcted segment, where the viable myocardium constitutes only a fraction of the muscle thickness, it will be unable to demonstrate any improvement in contractile function. On dobutamine echocardiography, such a segment is likely to be regarded as nonviable, but nuclear imaging may find evidence of metabolic activity and identify it as a viable segment. In addition, the location of the infarcted tissue within the myocardium is also important. Normal myocardial contractile function is determined predominantly by the subendocardial segment. Thus, when there is a subendocardial infarction that involves just 20–30% of the wall thickness, the segment may become akinetic even though the remaining myocardium is normal.[37]

Such segments are unlikely to demonstrate any contractile reserve on low-dose dobutamine stimulation and are also unlikely to recover after revascularization **(Figure 17.2)**.

However, several investigators have questioned the rationale of using functional recovery as the end-point for assessing benefit of myocardial viability assessment. It has been argued that though improvement in LVEF following revascularization is associated with improved survival, converse is not true. There are numerous benefits of myocardial revascularization, apart from functional recovery alone.[38] It helps prevent LV remodeling, stabilizes electrical milieu, protects against further episodes of myocardial ischemia and infarction, and results in improvement in LV diastolic function. All these beneficial effects of myocardial revascularization have a favorable impact on clinical outcomes, independent of the improvement in LVEF. These arguments are supported by the studies showing improved survival with CABG despite lack of any measureable improvement in LVEF.[39] Samady et al. studied 135 consecutive patients undergoing CABG and followed them up for 32 ± 23 months. They found that there was no relationship between the change in LVEF and cardiac death rate, symptoms of heart failure, incidence of implantable cardioverter defibrillator discharges, and overall event free survival.[39]

Relatively fewer studies on viability testing have evaluated survival benefit as the end-point.[5, 36] Allman et al. performed a meta-analysis of 24 studies in which long-term survival was evaluated **(Figure 17.3A and B)**.[5] The analysis included 6 studies using Tl-201 perfusion imaging, 11 using FDG PET metabolic imaging and 8 studies using dobutamine echocardiography. A total of 3,088 patients (2,228 men) with mean LVEF 32 ± 8% were included and followed-up for 25 ± 10 months. Nearly one-third (34.9%) of the patients underwent revascularization whereas the remaining 65.1% were treated medically. Myocardial viability was demonstrated in 42.3% patients. The analysis showed that in patients who had evidence of viability, revascularization was associated with 79.6% reduction in annual mortality (16% vs. 3.2%, $p < 0.0001$) compared with medical treatment. There was a direct relationship between severity of LV systolic dysfunction and magnitude of benefit with revascularization. In contrast, the patients without any demonstrable viability had intermediate mortality, which increased slightly with revascularization (7.7% vs. 6.2%, p = NS). Importantly, no statistically significant difference was found among different imaging modalities in their ability to predict mortality benefit with revascularization. Similar findings were noted in the Surgical Treatment of IsChemic Heart Failure (STICH) trial also, as discussed in detail subsequently.[40] Myocardial viability in this study was assessed using dobutamine echocardiography and/or Tl-201 nuclear imaging. There was no interaction between the imaging modality used for viability assessment and the clinical outcomes.

## Diastolic Wall Thickness

The myocardial segments that are transmurally infarcted undergo progressive thinning and fibrosis as time elapses. On echocardiography, these segments will eventually appear echo-dense and thinned out. Such segments are very unlikely

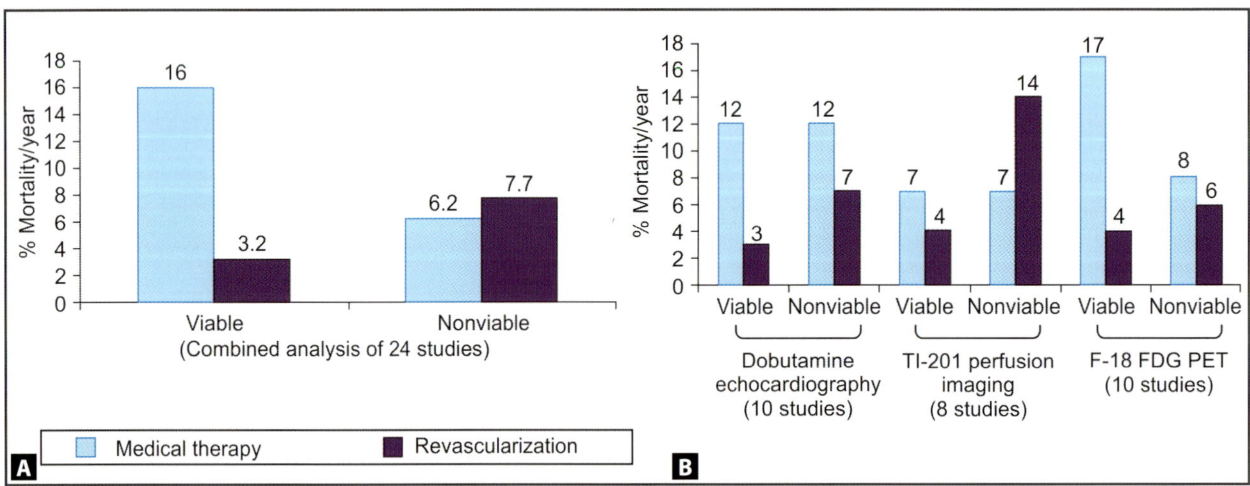


**Figure 17.3A and B:** Annualized mortality rates in patients with viable and nonviable myocardium in relation to treatment (revascularization or medical therapy).[5,36] (A) Pooled analysis combining all imaging modalities. (B) Modality specific outcomes. *Abbreviations:* FDG, fluorodeoxyglucose; PET, positron emission tomography; Tl, thallium.

to recover after revascularization. Thus, segmental wall thinning can be used as a marker of lack of viability. It has been found that reduced diastolic wall thickness <6.0 mm after 4 months of MI has high degree of specificity for scar tissue and indicates lack of viability with a NPV of 93%.[41] However, the PPV of a relatively preserved wall thickness is poor (53%).

## Role of Tissue Velocity and Strain Imaging

One of the major limitations of dobutamine echocardiography is that it is based on visual interpretation of wall motion, which is largely subjective.[42] The subjectivity of this process renders the technique susceptible to intra- and interobserver variability, which remains the 'Achilles' heel' of dobutamine echocardiography. Moreover, visual wall-motion analysis also makes it difficult to detect subtle changes in myocardial contractile function, thereby compromising the sensitivity of the technique.[42,43] Quantitative techniques, such as tissue velocity and strain imaging, impart objectivity to the assessment of myocardial contractility and promise to overcome many of the challenges inherent to visual wall-motion analysis.

Both tissue velocity imaging (TVI) and strain imaging have been used for assessment of myocardial viability. However, TVI is no longer used for this purpose because it only measures myocardial velocity relative to the transducer which is not a true measure of myocardial contractile function. Strain imaging is currently the preferred technique for quantifying myocardial contractile function. As discussed in Chapter 7, strain imaging can be performed using either Doppler-based method or the gray scale-based speckle tracking method. Both have been applied to myocardial viability assessment, and both have their advantages and disadvantages for this purpose.[44,45] The Doppler-based strain imaging allows high frame rates required for peak-dose imaging. However, being a Doppler-based technique, it is dependent on insonation angle. As a result, it does not allow measurement of radial or circumferential strain (RS and CS, respectively) and even for longitudinal strain (LS), the accuracy is seriously compromised if the myocardial motion is not aligned with the Doppler beam, as in case of dilated and distorted ventricles. Speckle tracking echocardiography (STE) on the other hand, is a relatively angle-independent technique and therefore permits comprehensive assessment of LV myocardial deformation. However, STE is heavily dependent on grayscale image quality and seems to have a relatively inferior accuracy in basal LV segments, as discussed subsequently. In addition, STE uses lower frame rates (around 50–70/seconds) as compared to the Doppler-based strain, which may be a limitation at peak-dose dobutamine imaging. However, as peak-dose assessment is generally not required for myocardial viability assessment, the frame rate is usually not an issue.

There are three different ways in which TVI and strain rate imaging have been used for assessment of myocardial viability:[45,46] (i) magnitude and timing of longitudinal deformation at rest, (ii) relative impairment of longitudinal, radial, and circumferential deformation at rest, and (iii) longitudinal deformation as an adjunct to wall-motion analysis during dobutamine echocardiography.

### *Magnitude and Timing of Longitudinal Deformation at Rest*

Numerous studies have shown that the impairment of LS is in proportion to the extent of myocardial injury. Accordingly, the magnitude of LS can be used as a predictor of functional recovery, late LV remodeling and clinical outcomes.

Both segmental and global LS have been used for this purpose.[47-53] Abate et al. performed three-dimensional (3D) STE in 153 patients with acute MI undergoing primary percutaneous coronary intervention (PCI).[47] A cutoff value of –11.1% for segmental 3D LS had 92% sensitivity and 91% specificity for predicting functional improvement at 6 months. Additionally, 3D global LS (GLS) was also found to have incremental value over clinical and conventional echocardiographic variables in predicting global LV function improvement. In yet another study on acute MI patients undergoing primary PCI, Bochenek et al. found that baseline GLS could reliably predict LV remodeling at 3 months with an optimal cutoff value of –12.5%.[53] They also found a graded relationship between segmental LS and the likelihood of functional recovery as confirmed on follow-up echocardiogram at 3 months. Average peak LS was –17.4% ± 7.5% in normal segments, 13.4% ± 6.9% in viable segments and 5.2% ± 6.3% in nonviable segments. In another study on patients undergoing primary PCI, strain imaging was found to have comparable accuracy to late gadolinium enhancement (LGE) on MRI for prediction of global functional recovery and LV remodeling.[54] A GLS cutoff value of –12.9% had 72.2% sensitivity and 69.2% specificity for predicting global functional recovery and 81.8% sensitivity and 80.5% specificity for predicting global LV remodeling. Several other studies have also shown the baseline GLS to be a strong, independent predictor of LV remodeling at follow-up.[51-53]

In addition to predicting LV remodeling and functional recovery, GLS has been shown to be a predictor of clinical outcomes as well. In a study involving 576 patients undergoing primary PCI for acute MI, both GLS and wall-motion score index (WMSI) were found to be independent predictors of the composite end-point of death, hospitalization with reinfarction, congestive heart failure, or stroke at 2 years.[55] Importantly, the predictive accuracy of both GLS and WMSI was superior to that of LVEF and LV end-systolic volume. In yet another study involving 548 patients with acute MI, GLS was found to be the strongest predictor (superior to clinical parameters, LVEF, troponin levels and N-terminal pro-brain natriuretic peptide levels) of in-hospital heart failure.[56]

In addition to the magnitude of LS, other measures of longitudinal deformation have also been evaluated as predictors of functional recovery. The extent of systolic lengthening, postsystolic shortening and early diastolic longitudinal strain rate have all been found to be useful for this purpose.[57-59] Apart from these, a new parameter, longitudinal-global mean strain, has also been promulgated by some investigators.[60] It is the average of LS over the entire cardiac cycle and is thus distinct from GLS which measures the peak systolic LS. In a study on 76 patients with acute MI, longitudinal global mean strain had the best correlation with infarct size and had the best ability to discriminate between different infarct size categories (no infarct, 1–10% transmural infarct, 11–20% transmural infarct and >20% transmural infarct) as measured by LGE on MRI.[60]

### *Relative Impairment of Longitudinal, Radial and Circumferential Deformation at Rest*

Because of the unique architecture of LV myocardium, contraction of muscle fibers in the different myocardial layers results in dissimilar conformational changes in the left ventricle. Thus, while the contraction of subendocardial fibers results predominantly in longitudinal shortening, the contraction of those in the middle and the subepicardial layers brings about circumferential shortening, LV twist, and radial thickening. Since ischemic myocardial injury begins from the subendocardium, LS gets compromised first. The impairment of RS, CS and LV twist occurs late in the process and indicates transmural injury.[45,46]

Several studies have shown that impairment of short-axis dynamics of the left ventricle can be used as a marker of transmural extent of the infarct.[61-64] Chan et al. performed STE and contrast-enhanced MRI in 80 patients with chronic ischemic LV systolic dysfunction. LGE involving >50% of myocardial thickness on MRI was used as a marker of transmural infarct. It was found that only CS and not LS was able to distinguish between subendocardial and transmural infarct segments.[61] Similarly, Rost et al. reported that a cutoff value of –10.5% for segmental CS had 78% sensitivity and 75% specificity for distinguishing between nontransmural and transmural infarcts.[63] In yet another study involving 213 patients with ST-elevation MI, the total number of segments with transmural scar on MRI was inversely related with the peak subepicardial twist.[64]

Since transmurally infarcted segments are less likely to recover despite revascularization, impairment of CS can also be used as a predictor of LV remodeling and functional recovery.[54,65-67] In the aforementioned study on 93 patients undergoing primary PCI, peak systolic CS cutoff of -14.2% had 71.6% sensitivity and 58.1% specificity for predicting segmental functional recovery.[54] The same group also performed layer-specific analysis of CS and correlated it with the extent of LGE on MRI and with the likelihood of functional recovery.[67,68] While the epicardial CS had high accuracy for identifying transmural infarcts, endocardial CS could distinguish between noninfarcted segments and nontransmural infarcts.[68] Furthermore, both endocardial and epicardial CS were significantly higher in segments showing functional recovery as compared with those without functional recovery.[67] These observations were corroborated by the findings from the Valsartan in Acute Myocardial Infarction Trial (VALIANT) echo study.[65] This trial enrolled 603 patients with LV systolic dysfunction, heart failure, or both 5 days after MI. It was found that both longitudinal and circumferential strain rate were independent predictors of clinical outcomes after MI but only circumferential strain rate was predictive of LV reverse remodeling.

### *Strain Imaging as an Adjunct to Wall-motion Analysis during Dobutamine Echocardiography*

Strain imaging has also been used to improve accuracy of wall-motion analysis during dobutamine echocardiography for viability assessment.[69,70] The incremental value of strain imaging for this purpose was first evaluated by Hanekom et al.[70] Fifty-five consecutive patients with ischemic LV dysfunction (mean LVEF 36 ± 8%) who had undergone dobutamine echocardiography for viability assessment and subsequently underwent revascularization were included in the study. Doppler-based strain imaging was performed during the baseline dobutamine echocardiography. Functional recovery of the dysfunctional segments was assessed on a repeat echocardiogram at 9 months after revascularization. It was found that –0.25/s increase in longitudinal strain rate at low-dose dobutamine had 80% sensitivity and 75% specificity for prediction of segmental functional recovery, which was slightly better than that of wall-motion analysis. Combining strain parameters with wall-motion analysis significantly increased the sensitivity of wall-motion analysis alone for prediction of functional recovery, although specificities were comparable.

Bansal et al. studied the clinical utility of STE-based strain imaging in the same patient population as in the above study.[71] Resting and low-dose CS and low-dose LS and longitudinal strain rate were predictive of segmental functional recovery independent of wall-motion analysis. However, STE measurements of strain and strain rate could assess viability mainly in the anterior circulation but not in the posterior circulation. This difference was likely to be due to suboptimal image quality in the basal myocardial segments. In yet another study, Ran et al. evaluated STE strain as an adjunct to adenosine echocardiography. Radionuclide myocardial perfusion/metabolic imaging served as the "gold standard" to define myocardial viability. An increase of LS by 14.6% was found to have a sensitivity of 86.7% and a specificity of 90.2% for identifying myocardial viability on nuclear imaging.[72]

These data indicate that incorporation of strain imaging during echocardiography, both at rest and during pharmacological or vasodilatory stress, has the potential to provide valuable information about infarct size and transmural extent, likelihood of LV reverse remodeling and functional recovery and the risk of adverse clinical events. However, several important challenges exist. The most important of these in the context of coronary artery disease is the unacceptably high variability of segmental strain at present.[44,46] When strain imaging is applied to groups of myocardial segments, it is able to distinguish between less extensive versus more extensive infarcts. However, at the individual segment level, the reproducibility of strain measurements is currently not robust enough to justify routine clinical use. Therefore, at the present moment, the role of strain imaging in the evaluation of coronary artery disease is only adjunctive to conventional echocardiography.

### Role of MCE for Myocardial Viability Assessment

The main application of echocardiographic contrast is for improving endocardial border delineation in patients with suboptimal acoustic window. Although not currently approved, the addition of contrast imaging to echocardiography also permits assessment of myocardial perfusion, which is not otherwise feasible with conventional echocardiography.

MCE requires specific protocols for administration of contrast agents, image acquisition and for image interpretation. These issues are discussed in greater details in Chapter 6. Using quantitative techniques, peak myocardial contrast density as well as rate of contrast filling (an index of myocardial blood flow) can be measured which provide an estimate of myocardial viability. Unlike the normally perfused regions that show rapid and dense appearance of contrast, viable but ischemic areas show delayed appearance of contrast. Shimoni et al. compared quantitative MCE with dobutamine echocardiography and Tl-201 imaging in 20 patients undergoing CABG.[73] Segmental functional recovery was assessed on a repeat echocardiogram at 3–4 months after CABG. MCE had 90% sensitivity for prediction of segmental functional recovery, which was similar to that of Tl-201 scintigraphy (92%) or of any contractile reserve on dobutamine echocardiography (80%). However, the specificity of MCE (63%) was higher than that for Tl-201 imaging (45%) or dobutamine echocardiography (54%). When quantitative techniques are not available, mere appearance of contrast in a dysfunctional myocardial segment can itself be used as a crude marker of intact capillary circulation, and thus, the presence of viability. This can be of great help in rapid assessment of adequacy of reperfusion in patients undergoing primary PCI or thrombolysis for acute ST-elevation MI. Absence of myocardial contrast opacification in the infarct territory indicates no reflow at microvasculature level and is a strong predictor of LV remodeling and adverse clinical outcomes. Conversely, good contrast filling in the infarcted segments suggests largely salvaged myocardium with favorable clinical outcomes.[74,75]

## CLINICAL UTILITY OF MYOCARDIAL VIABILITY ASSESSMENT: THE CURRENT UNDERSTANDING

As discussed earlier, a large number of studies over the past 30 years have demonstrated value of myocardial viability assessment in predicting functional recovery and improvement in survival with revascularization. A common message from these studies, individually as well as in pooled analyses, is that the patients with myocardial viability, when treated medically have the worst outcome and those subjected to revascularization have the best outcomes. In comparison, the patients without myocardial viability have intermediate mortality risk and CABG in these patients may indeed result in harm rather than any benefit. However, all these studies were singe-center, small size, nonrandomized and retrospective in nature. There were significant differences between the patients treated medically and those treated surgically and often the decision to subject the patients to CABG was itself influenced by the results of myocardial viability testing. Because of these limitations, there has always been a concern about the true value of myocardial viability in predicting clinical outcomes.[40,76-78] These concerns have only grown with time as there have been significant advancements in medical therapy, PCI and surgical revascularization techniques resulting in ever improving outcomes of the patients with ischemic severe LV systolic dysfunction.

However, much as it is vital to assess the true value of myocardial viability assessment in the contemporary clinical practice, it has now become virtually impossible to perform a randomized study to address this issue. Given the available evidence supporting prognostic significance of myocardial viability and the prevailing wisdom on this topic, it would be ethically unacceptable to randomize a patient with significant LV systolic dysfunction and evidence of myocardial viability to medical therapy. Similarly, it will also be hard to randomize a patient without evidence of myocardial viability to CABG. These challenges were well illustrated by the recent studies performed to evaluate the clinical value of viability testing.[40,79,80]

Nonetheless, there have been a few recent, large trials that have attempted to assess the role of myocardial viability assessment in guiding clinical decisions in patients with severe LV systolic dysfunction.[40,79,81] Although all these trials had several limitations, they have provided valuable insights into this complex clinical issue.

## Surgical Treatment of Ischemic Heart Failure Trial[40,82]

The STICH was the largest randomized trial comparing medical therapy with CABG in patients with ischemic heart disease and moderate to severe LV systolic dysfunction.[82] This also remains the largest trial so far to assess the prognostic significance of myocardial viability in such patients.[40]

A total of 1,212 patients with LVEF ≤35% (median LVEF 28%) and coronary artery disease amenable to CABG were randomly assigned to medical therapy alone (602 patients) or medical therapy plus CABG (610 patients).[82] The patients in both the groups were treated effectively with high use of guideline directed medical therapy in all patients and the use of at least 2 grafts in 88% patients and at least one arterial graft in >90% patients undergoing CABG. All-cause mortality was the primary outcome of the study. After a median follow-up of 56 months, no difference was found between the two groups in the primary end-point (41% in the medical-therapy group vs. 36% In the CABG group; $p = 0.12$). The cardiovascular mortality showed a trend towards reduction in the CABG group (28% vs. 33%, $p = 0.05$), whereas the composite of death from any cause or hospitalization for cardiovascular causes decreased significantly in the CABG group (58% vs. 68%, $P < 0.001$). Thus, prima facie this trial did not show any mortality benefit of CABG over optimized medical therapy in patients with significant LV systolic dysfunction. However, it is noteworthy that 9% of the patients randomized to CABG arm did not undergo the procedure, whereas 17% of the patients randomized to medical therapy arm underwent CABG. When data were analyzed according to the actual treatment received, there was significant reduction in all-cause mortality in the CABG group (32.7% vs. 43.8%, hazard ratio 0.70, $p = <0.001$).[82]

In the STICH trial, all randomized patients were also eligible for viability testing. Tl-201 perfusion imaging and/or dobutamine echocardiography were allowed for this purpose. However, the decision to perform viability testing and the choice of the imaging modality were left at the discretion of the treating physician. On Tl-201 imaging, viability was defined as the presence of relative tracer activity in at least 11 of the 17 segments, whereas on dobutamine echocardiography viability was diagnosed if ≥5 dysfunctional segments (in a 16 segment model) demonstrated contractile reserve with dobutamine.

Of 1,212 patients, 618 underwent viability testing, of which 601 studies were interpretable.[40] Tl-201 imaging was performed in 417 patients and dobutamine echocardiography in 280 patients (150 patients underwent both the procedures). Of the 601 patients with interpretable studies, 487 (81%) were found to have viability whereas the remaining 19% were not. The patients with viability had significantly higher LVEF (28% vs. 23%, $p = <0.001$) and lower LV end-diastolic and end-systolic volumes. Nearly half of the patients in both the groups underwent revascularization. In the overall group, the patients who had viability had significantly lower all-cause mortality, but this difference was no longer significant when adjusted for the differences in the baseline parameters. Additionally, there was no difference in clinical outcomes between the two treatment groups, neither in patients with viability nor in those without viability. The choice of imaging modality used for viability testing also had no impact on clinical outcomes.

However, there were several important limitations to the STICH trial, in particular the viability substudy, that merit consideration: (i) very small proportion of the patients who were eligible for the study were actually randomized (on average, only 2 patients per site per year), raising concerns about significant enrolment bias, (ii) viability testing was not mandatory and was at the treating clinicians' discretion, (iii) patients were not randomized according to viability status, (iv) significant differences were observed between those who underwent viability testing and those who did not, (v) the definitions of viability used in the trial were also controversial; specifically, even the normal myocardium was included in the viability definition on nuclear imaging, whereas on dobutamine echo, no distinction was made between biphasic response and uniphasic response, (vi) multiple Tl-201 perfusion imaging protocols were used at the 217 participating sites, and (vii) viability was defined in a dichotomous manner. Furthermore, the changes in LVEF and volumes during follow-up were also not reported. Thus, the STICH trial ended up raising more questions about viability testing than what it actually answered.

### Positron Emission Tomography and Recovery Following Revascularization-2 Study[79]

The Positron Emission Tomography and Recovery following Revascularization-2 (PARR-2) study was a randomized study performed to examine the utility of FDG PET-guided revascularization in patients with severe LV systolic dysfunction.[79] A total of 430 patients were randomized to FDG PET-assisted management and 212 to standard care. In the FDG PET arm, recommendations were provided about the need to perform revascularization based on FDG PET results, but the actual decision was left at the treating clinicians' discretion. Viability testing was permitted in the standard care arm also but not using FDG PET imaging. Primary end-point was the composite of cardiac death, MI, and hospital readmission for heart disease at 1 year. No difference was found in the primary outcome between the two arms (30% in the PET arm vs. 36% in the standard care arm, p = NS).[79] However, it was noted that a significant number of patients (25%) in the FDG PET arm were not managed according to the PET results. Those who had relatively less extensive viability were more likely to be managed medically despite a recommendation to revascularize. When such patients were excluded and only those in whom there was adherence to the PET recommendations were included, a significant reduction in adverse outcomes was observed with revascularization.[79] Additional analysis from this study showed that there was a graded relationship between the extent of hibernating myocardium on FDG PET imaging and the benefit with revascularization.[83] Clear benefit with revascularization was observed when more than 7% of the LV myocardium showed evidence of hibernation. Finally, this study also demonstrated the value of expertise in interpreting FDG PET results and in incorporating these findings in the patients' management. Among the 111 patients who were treated at a large integrated facility with experienced PET readers, cardiologists and surgeons, there was substantial reduction in the composite end-point with PET-directed management compared with standard care (19% versus 41%, p = 0.005).[84] This benefit was observed despite the fact that these patients were older and had lower LVEF than those at the other centers. No such benefit was observed at the other centers.

### Other Studies

A large prospective observational study evaluating role of PET imaging for viability assessment was recently published.[81] The study included 648 patients (mean age 65 years, 77% male) who had ischemic LV systolic dysfunction (mean LVEF 31%) and were undergoing PET perfusion and metabolic imaging (using rubidium-82 and F-18 FDG, respectively) with automated analysis. Hibernation was defined as flow-metabolism mismatch. Early revascularization (i.e. within 92 days of PET imaging) was performed in 199 patients (33%). The patients were followed up for 2.8 years. It was found that the patients who had >10% hibernating myocardium had significant survival advantage with early revascularization.

The Heart Failure Revascularization Trial (HEART) was a multicentric trial conducted in the UK with a plan to enroll 800 patients with LVEF <35% and evidence of substantial viability on any standard imaging test.[80] However, the trial was prematurely discontinued because of very poor enrolment rate. The Imaging Modalities to Assist with Guiding therapy and the Evaluation of patients with Heart Failure (IMAGE HF) Study is a collaborative Canadian/Finnish funded study that is currently recruiting patients.[85] It aims to study patients with ischemic heart disease and heart failure who are undergoing evaluation by PET imaging, cardiac computed tomography or cardiac MRI and compare these advanced imaging modalities with conventional single photon emission compute tomographic nuclear imaging. The end-point is a composite of cardiac death, MI, resuscitated cardiac arrest, and cardiac rehospitalization.

## HOW MUCH VIABILITY IS ENOUGH?

While the overall value of viability testing itself remains debatable, another pertinent question is that how much viability should be there to accrue benefit from revascularization. The answer to this question has also been difficult to come by with widely different thresholds used for defining viability in different studies. A meta-analysis was performed including 29 studies reporting survival in relation to viability results.[86] It was found that the optimal threshold for the extent of viability for predicting survival benefit was 25.8% for perfusion-metabolism mismatch on FDG PET imaging, 35.9% for contractile reserve or ischemic response on dobutamine echocardiography, and 38.7% for perfusion imaging with Tl-201 or Tc-99m. However, these thresholds appear to be much higher than what have been reported by more recent studies. For FDG PET imaging, several studies have shown that the presence of 7–10% hibernating myocardium indicates high likelihood of improvement in survival with early revascularization.[81,83] Similarly, for Tl-201 imaging, evidence of viability in approximately 15% or more of myocardial mass is required to afford significant improvement in LVEF and overall prognosis following revascularization.[87] The higher threshold suggested by the aforementioned meta-analysis for Tl-201 imaging is due to the fact that in many studies even normal myocardium was also included in the definition of viable myocardium.

The threshold for viability on dobutamine echocardiography also seemed to be inappropriately high in the above meta-analysis. It was likely to be due to inclusion of ischemic response in the definition of viability. Afridi et al. showed significant improvement in survival if there was viability (determined by biphasic response or worsening on dobutamine echocardiography) in >4 myocardial segments (i.e. >25% of LV myocardium).[6] Bax et al. also showed improvement in event free survival with >4 segments showing viability.[88] However, they included sustained improvement also as an indicator of viability. Roxy senior et al. showed survival benefit in presence of viability in >5 segments but they included even the normal segments in assessment of viability.[4] These findings suggest that the presence of contractile reserve in at least 3–4 dysfunctional myocardial segments is required to afford survival benefit with revascularization.

## WHEN TO LOOK FOR MYOCARDIAL VIABILITY IN ROUTINE CLINICAL PRACTICE?

It is evident from the earlier discussion that the true value of myocardial viability assessment in routine clinical practice is highly controversial. While a large number of single-center studies have demonstrated clear benefit of revascularization in patients with evidence of viable myocardium, these studies were limited by retrospective and nonrandomized nature, wide heterogeneity in the patient populations studied, modalities used for viability testing, definitions of viability adopted and in the treatment protocols. The large STICH trial showed no impact of myocardial viability on clinical outcomes, but this study itself had major limitations.[40] The study by Ling et al.[81] and the PARR-2 study[79] showed benefit of viability assessment, but they used only FDG PET imaging and no other modality for viability assessment. These differences among trials and the conflicting results make it rather difficult to decide in what patient subgroups viability testing should be performed.

However, on the basis of the insights gained from all the small and large trials conducted so far, two distinct scenarios can be identified in which viability assessment seem to have a definite role. First is the group of patients who are expected to have high operative morality, either because of the severity of LV systolic dysfunction itself or because of various comorbidities, in particular renal dysfunction. In such patients, lack of significant viability would argue against revascularization and would favor optimized medical therapy. Second is the group of patients in whom a decision needs to be taken about the mode of revascularization. The absence of significant myocardial viability in the left anterior descending artery territory would favor less invasive percutaneous approaches instead of CABG.

The imaging modality used for viability assessment seems to have little influence over clinical outcomes. Therefore, the choice of the imaging modality in a particular patient should be based mainly on the availability of local expertise. Dobutamine echocardiography has lower sensitivity than other modalities but is more specific for predicting functional recovery following revascularization.

## CONCLUSION

Although the results of the STICH trial have cast doubts on the clinical utility of myocardial viability assessment, a large body of evidence exists to support the prognostic significance of the presence and the extent of myocardial viability. Therefore, until more data emerge, assessment of myocardial viability will continue to remain an integral component of evaluation of the patients with ischemic severe LV systolic dysfunction. Dobutamine echocardiography is a commonly employed technique for this purpose. It has the highest specificity among all the modalities used for viability assessment, though its sensitivity is lower. The incorporation of newer modalities, such as strain imaging and MCE promises to further enhance the accuracy of echocardiography for assessment of myocardial viability. However, the role of these techniques is only adjunctive at the present moment.

## VIDEO LEGENDS

**Video 17.1:** Apical four-chamber view at different stages during dobutamine echocardiography. Mid and apical lateral segments are hypokinetic at rest (upper left), improve at low-dose (upper right) but worsen at peak-dose (lower left). This is a typical biphasic response and suggests viability with ischemia (hibernation). In comparison, interventricular septum is akinetic (except for a small segment in the mid part) with no response to dobutamine infusion, which is suggestive of nonviable myocardium.

**Video 17.2:** Apical two-chamber view at different stages during dobutamine echocardiography in the same patient as in Video 17.1. Typical biphasic response is seen in mid and apical anterior wall.

## REFERENCES

1. Saltiel J, Lesperance J, Bourassa MG, Castonguay Y, Campeau L, Grondin P. Reversibily of left ventricular dysfunction following aorto-coronary by-pass grafts. Am J Roentgenol Radium Ther Nucl Med. 1970;110:739-46.
2. Chatterjee K, Swan HJ, Parmley WW, Sustaita H, Marcus HS, Matloff J. Influence of direct myocardial revascularization on left ventricular asynergy and function in patients with coronary heart disease. With and without previous myocardial infarction. Circulation. 1973;47:276-86.
3. Chatterjee K, Swan HJ, Parmley WW, Sustaita H, Marcus H, Matloff J. Depression of left ventricular function due to acute myocardial ischemia and its reversal after aortocoronary saphenous-vein bypass. N Engl J Med. 1972;286:1117-22.

4. Senior R, Kaul S, Lahiri A. Myocardial viability on echocardiography predicts long-term survival after revascularization in patients with ischemic congestive heart failure. J Am Coll Cardiol. 1999;33:1848-54.
5. Allman KC, Shaw LJ, Hachamovitch R, et al. Myocardial viability testing and impact of revascularization on prognosis in patients with coronary artery disease and left ventricular dysfunction: A meta-analysis. J Am Coll Cardiol. 2002;39:1151-8.
6. Afridi I, Grayburn PA, Panza JA, Oh JK, Zoghbi WA, Marwick TH. Myocardial viability during dobutamine echocardiography predicts survival in patients with coronary artery disease and severe left ventricular systolic dysfunction. J Am Coll Cardiol. 1998;32:921-6.
7. Gallagher KP, Kumada T, Koziol JA, McKown MD, Kemper WS, Ross J. Significance of regional wall thickening abnormalities relative to transmural myocardial perfusion in anesthetized dogs. Circulation. 1980;62:1266-74.
8. Gallagher KP, Matsuzaki M, Koziol JA, et al. Regional myocardial perfusion and wall thickening during ischemia in conscious dogs. Am J Physiol. 1984;247:H727-38.
9. Vatner SF. Correlation between acute reductions in myocardial blood flow and function in conscious dogs. Circ Res. 1980;47:201-7.
10. Heyndrickx GR, Millard RW, McRitchie RJ, et al. Regional myocardial functional and electrophysiological alterations after brief coronary artery occlusion in conscious dogs. J Clin Invest. 1975;56:978-85.
11. Kusuoka H, Marban E. Cellular mechanisms of myocardial stunning. Annu Rev Physiol. 1992;54:243-56.
12. Bolli R. Myocardial 'stunning' in man. Circulation. 1992;86:1671-91.
13. Engler R, Covell JW. Granulocytes cause reperfusion ventricular dysfunction after 15-minute ischemia in the dog. Circ Res. 1987;61:20-8.
14. Bolli R. Oxygen-derived free radicals and postischemic myocardial dysfunction ("stunned myocardium"). J Am Coll Cardiol. 1988;12:239-49.
15. Camici P, Araujo LI, Spinks T, et al. Increased uptake of 18f-fluorodeoxyglucose in postischemic myocardium of patients with exercise-induced angina. Circulation. 1986;74:81-8.
16. Renkin J, Wijns W, Ladha Z, et al. Reversal of segmental hypokinesis by coronary angioplasty in patients with unstable angina, persistent t wave inversion, and left anterior descending coronary artery stenosis. Additional evidence for myocardial stunning in humans. Circulation. 1990;82:913-21.
17. Diamond GA, Forrester JS, deLuz PL,et al. Post-extrasystolic potentiation of ischemic myocardium by atrial stimulation. Am Heart J. 1978;95:204-9.
18. Rahimtoola SH. A perspective on the three large multicenter randomized clinical trials of coronary bypass surgery for chronic stable angina. Circulation. 1985;72:V123-35.
19. Rahimtoola SH. The hibernating myocardium. Am Heart J. 1989;117:211-21.
20. Nowak B, Schaefer WM, Koch KC, et al. Assessment of myocardial viability in dysfunctional myocardium by resting myocardial blood flow determined with oxygen 15 water pet. J Nucl Cardiol. 2003;10:34-45.
21. Camici PG, Rimoldi OE. Myocardial blood flow in patients with hibernating myocardium. Cardiovasc Res. 2003;57:302-11.
22. Camici PG, Dutka DP. Repetitive stunning, hibernation, and heart failure: Contribution of pet to establishing a link. Am J Physiol Heart Circ Physiol. 2001;280:H929-36.
23. Camici PG, Prasad SK, Rimoldi OE. Stunning, hibernation, and assessment of myocardial viability. Circulation. 2008;117:103-14.
24. Vanoverschelde JLJ, Wijns W, Borgers M, et al. Chronic myocardial hibernation in humans: From bedside to bench. Circulation. 1997;95:1961-71.
25. Vanoverschelde JL, Wijns W, Depre C, et al. Mechanisms of chronic regional postischemic dysfunction in humans. New insights from the study of noninfarcted collateral-dependent myocardium. Circulation. 1993;87:1513-23.
26. Sun KT, Czernin J, Krivokapich J, et al. Effects of dobutamine stimulation on myocardial blood flow, glucose metabolism, and wall motion in normal and dysfunctional myocardium. Circulation. 1996;94:3146-54.
27. Canty JM Jr, Suzuki G. Myocardial perfusion and contraction in acute ischemia and chronic ischemic heart disease. J Mol Cell Cardiol. 2012;52:822-31.
28. Canty JM Jr, Fallavollita JA. Hibernating myocardium. J Nucl Cardiol. 2005;12:104-19.
29. Haas F, Jennen L, Heinzmann U, et al. Ischemically compromised myocardium displays different time-courses of functional recovery: Correlation with morphological alterations? Eur J Cardiothorac Surg. 2001;20:290-8.
30. Vanoverschelde JL, Pasquet A, Gerber B, Melin JA. Pathophysiology of myocardial hibernation. Implications for the use of dobutamine echocardiography to identify myocardial viability. Heart. 1999;82(Suppl 3):III1-7.
31. Kasliwal RR, Paul B, Mustaqueem A, et al. Low-dose dobutamine echocardiography predicts recovery of left ventricular systolic function following revascularization even in presence of low contractile reserve. Indian Heart J. 2006;58:120-5.
32. Rizzello V, Poldermans D, Biagini E, et al. Prognosis of patients with ischaemic cardiomyopathy after coronary revascularisation: Relation to viability and improvement in left ventricular ejection fraction. Heart. 2009;95:1273-7.
33. Afridi I, Kleiman NS, Raizner AE, et al. Dobutamine echocardiography in myocardial hibernation. Optimal dose and accuracy in predicting recovery of ventricular function after coronary angioplasty. Circulation. 1995;91:663-70.
34. Bax JJ, Wijns W, Cornel JH, Visser FC, Boersma E, Fioretti PM. Accuracy of currently available techniques for prediction of functional recovery after revascularization in patients with left ventricular dysfunction due to chronic coronary artery disease: Comparison of pooled data. J Am Coll Cardiol. 1997;30:1451-60.
35. Bonow RO. Identification of viable myocardium. Circulation. 1996;94:2674-80.
36. Schinkel AF, Bax JJ, Poldermans D, Elhendy A, Ferrari R, Rahimtoola SH. Hibernating myocardium: Diagnosis and patient outcomes. Curr Probl Cardiol. 2007;32:375-410.
37. Lieberman AN, Weiss JL, Jugdutt BI, et al. Two-dimensional echocardiography and infarct size: relationship of regional wall

motion and thickening to the extent of myocardial infarction in the dog. Circulation. 1981;63:739-46.
38. Braunwald E. Myocardial reperfusion, limitation of infarct size, reduction of left ventricular dysfunction, and improved survival. Should the paradigm be expanded? Circulation. 1989;79:441-4.
39. Samady H, Elefteriades JA, Abbott BG, Mattera JA, McPherson CA, Wackers FJ. Failure to improve left ventricular function after coronary revascularization for ischemic cardiomyopathy is not associated with worse outcome. Circulation. 1999; 100:1298-304.
40. Bonow RO, Maurer G, Lee KL, et al. Myocardial viability and survival in ischemic left ventricular dysfunction. N Engl J Med. 2011;364:1617-25.
41. Cwajg JM, Cwajg E, Nagueh SF, et al. End-diastolic wall thickness as a predictor of recovery of function in myocardial hibernation: Relation to rest-redistribution t1-201 tomography and dobutamine stress echocardiography. J Am Coll Cardiol. 2000;35:1152-61.
42. Picano E, Lattanzi F, Orlandini A, et al. Stress echocardiography and the human factor: the importance of being expert. J Am Coll Cardiol. 1991;17:666-9.
43. Hoffmann R, Lethen H, Marwick T, et al. Analysis of interinstitutional observer agreement in interpretation of dobutamine stress echocardiograms. J Am Coll Cardiol. 1996; 27:330-6.
44. Mor-Avi V, Lang RM, Badano LP, et al. Current and evolving echocardiographic techniques for the quantitative evaluation of cardiac mechanics: ASE/eae consensus statement on methodology and indications endorsed by the Japanese Society of Echocardiography. J Am Soc Echocardiogr. 2011;24:277-313.
45. Geyer H, Caracciolo G, Abe H, et al. Assessment of myocardial mechanics using speckle tracking echocardiography: fundamentals and clinical applications. J Am Soc Echocardiogr. 2010;23:351-69.
46. Bansal M, Sengupta PP. Longitudinal and circumferential strain in patients with regional LV dysfunction. Curr Cardiol Rep. 2013;15:339.
47. Abate E, Hoogslag GE, Antoni ML, et al. Value of three-dimensional speckle-tracking longitudinal strain for predicting improvement of left ventricular function after acute myocardial infarction. Am J Cardiol. 2012;110:961-7.
48. Mollema SA, Delgado V, Bertini M, et al. Viability assessment with global left ventricular longitudinal strain predicts recovery of left ventricular function after acute myocardial infarction. Circ Cardiovasc Imaging. 2010;3:15-23.
49. Ingul CB, Malm S, Refsdal E, Hegbom K, Amundsen BH, Stoylen A. Recovery of function after acute myocardial infarction evaluated by tissue Doppler strain and strain rate. J Am Soc Echocardiogr. 2010;23:432-8.
50. Antoni ML, Mollema SA, Atary JZ, et al. Time course of global left ventricular strain after acute myocardial infarction. Eur Heart J. 2010;31:2006-13.
51. Zaliaduonyte-Peksiene D, Vaskelyte JJ, Mizariene V, et al. Does longitudinal strain predict left ventricular remodeling after myocardial infarction? Echocardiography. 2012;29:419-27.
52. D'Andrea A, Cocchia R, Caso P, et al. Global longitudinal speckle-tracking strain is predictive of left ventricular remodeling after coronary angioplasty in patients with recent non-ST elevation myocardial infarction. Int J Cardiol. 2011;153:185-91.
53. Bochenek T, Wita K, Tabor Z, et al. Value of speckle-tracking echocardiography for prediction of left ventricular remodeling in patients with ST-elevation myocardial infarction treated by primary percutaneous intervention. J Am Soc Echocardiogr. 2011;24:1342-8.
54. Altiok E, Tiemann S, Becker M, et al. Myocardial deformation imaging by two-dimensional speckle-tracking echocardiography for prediction of global and segmental functional changes after acute myocardial infarction: a comparison with late gadolinium enhancement cardiac magnetic resonance. J Am Soc Echocardiogr. 2014;27: 249-57.
55. Munk K, Andersen NH, Terkelsen CJ, et al. Global left ventricular longitudinal systolic strain for early risk assessment in patients with acute myocardial infarction treated with primary percutaneous intervention. J Am Soc Echocardiogr. 2012;25:644-51.
56. Ersboll M, Valeur N, Mogensen UM, et al. Relationship between left ventricular longitudinal deformation and clinical heart failure during admission for acute myocardial infarction: a two-dimensional speckle-tracking study. J Am Soc Echocardiogr. 2012;25:1280-9.
57. Vartdal T, Pettersen E, Helle-Valle T, et al. Identification of viable myocardium in acute anterior infarction using duration of systolic lengthening by tissue Doppler strain: a preliminary study. J Am Soc Echocardiogr. 2012;25:718-25.
58. Fujimoto H, Honma H, Ohno T, et al. Longitudinal Doppler strain measurement for assessment of damaged and/or hibernating myocardium by dobutamine stress echocardiography in patients with old myocardial infarction. J Cardiol. 2010;55:309-16.
59. Park SM, Hong SJ, Park JS, et al. Relationship between strain rate imaging and coronary flow reserve in assessing myocardial viability after acute myocardial infarction. Echocardiography. 2010;27:977-84.
60. Grenne B, Eek C, Sjoli B, et al. Mean strain throughout the heart cycle by longitudinal two-dimensional speckle-tracking echocardiography enables early prediction of infarct size. J Am Soc Echocardiogr. 2011;24:1118-25.
61. Chan J, Hanekom L, Wong C, Leano R, Cho GY, Marwick TH. Differentiation of subendocardial and transmural infarction using two-dimensional strain rate imaging to assess short-axis and long-axis myocardial function. J Am Coll Cardiol. 2006;48:2026-33.
62. Kansal MM, Panse PM, Abe H, et al. Relationship of contrast-enhanced magnetic resonance imaging-derived intramural scar distribution and speckle tracking echocardiography-derived left ventricular two-dimensional strains. Eur Heart J Cardiovasc Imaging. 2012;13:152-8.
63. Rost C, Rost MC, Breithardt OA, et al. Relation of functional echocardiographic parameters to infarct scar transmurality by magnetic resonance imaging. J Am Soc Echocardiogr. 2014;27:767-74.
64. Abate E, Hoogslag GE, Leong DP, et al. Association between multilayer left ventricular rotational mechanics and the

development of left ventricular remodeling after acute myocardial infarction. J Am Soc Echocardiogr. 2014;27:239-48.
65. Hung CL, Verma A, Uno H, et al. Longitudinal and circumferential strain rate, left ventricular remodeling, and prognosis after myocardial infarction. J Am Coll Cardiol. 2010;56:1812-22.
66. Iwahashi N, Gohbara M, Kataoka S, et al. Global longitudinal strain by 3d speckle tracking after ST-elevation myocardial infarction is useful for predicting left ventricular remodeling: Comparison with Tc99m-sestamibi. J Am Coll Cardiol. 2015;65:A1228.
67. Altiok E, Becker M, Zwicker C, et al. Layer-specific analysis of myocardial deformation with 2D speckle-tracking echocardiography for prediction of functional recovery in acute myocardial infarction. J Am Coll Cardiol. 2012;59:E1142.
68. Altiok E, Neizel M, Tiemann S, et al. Layer-specific analysis of myocardial deformation for assessment of infarct transmurality: comparison of strain-encoded cardiovascular magnetic resonance with 2D speckle tracking echocardiography. Eur Heart J Cardiovasc Imaging. 2013;14:570-8.
69. Voigt JU, Arnold MF, Karlsson M, et al. Assessment of regional longitudinal myocardial strain rate derived from Doppler myocardial imaging indexes in normal and infarcted myocardium. J Am Soc Echocardiogr. 2000;13:588-98.
70. Hanekom L, Jenkins C, Jeffries L, et al. Incremental value of strain rate analysis as an adjunct to wall-motion scoring for assessment of myocardial viability by dobutamine echocardiography: a follow-up study after revascularization. Circulation. 2005;112:3892-900.
71. Bansal M, Jeffriess L, Leano R, et al. Assessment of myocardial viability at dobutamine echocardiography by deformation analysis using tissue velocity and speckle-tracking. JACC Cardiovasc Imaging. 2010;3:121-31.
72. Ran H, Zhang PY, Fang LL, Ma XW, Wu WF, Feng WF. Clinic value of two-dimensional speckle tracking combined with adenosine stress echocardiography for assessment of myocardial viability. Echocardiography. 2012;29:688-94.
73. Shimoni S, Frangogiannis NG, Aggeli CJ, et al. Identification of hibernating myocardium with quantitative intravenous myocardial contrast echocardiography: Comparison with dobutamine echocardiography and thallium-201 scintigraphy. Circulation. 2003;107:538-44.
74. Galiuto L, Garramone B, Scara A, et al. The extent of microvascular damage during myocardial contrast echocardiography is superior to other known indexes of post-infarct reperfusion in predicting left ventricular remodeling: Results of the multicenter amici study. J Am Coll Cardiol. 2008;51:552-9.
75. Dwivedi G, Janardhanan R, Hayat SA, et al. Prognostic value of myocardial viability detected by myocardial contrast echocardiography early after acute myocardial infarction. J Am Coll Cardiol. 2007;50:327-34.
76. Chareonthaitawee P, Gersh BJ, Panza JA. Is viability imaging still relevant in 2012? JACC Cardiovasc Imaging. 2012;5:550-8.
77. Allman KC. Noninvasive assessment myocardial viability: Current status and future directions. J Nucl Cardiol. 2013;20:618-37.
78. Lim SP, Mc Ardle BA, Beanlands RS, et al. Myocardial viability: It is still alive. Semin Nucl Med. 2014;44:358-74.
79. Beanlands RS, Nichol G, Huszti E, et al. F-18-fluorodeoxyglucose positron emission tomography imaging-assisted management of patients with severe left ventricular dysfunction and suspected coronary disease: A randomized, controlled trial (PARR-2). J Am Coll Cardiol. 2007;50:2002-12.
80. Cleland JG, Calvert M, Freemantle N, et al. The heart failure revascularisation trial (heart). Eur J Heart Fail. 2011;13:227-33.
81. Ling LF, Marwick TH, Flores DR, et al. Identification of therapeutic benefit from revascularization in patients with left ventricular systolic dysfunction: Inducible ischemia versus hibernating myocardium. Circulation: Cardiovascular Imaging. 2013;6:363-72.
82. Velazquez EJ, Lee KL, Deja MA, et al. Coronary-artery bypass surgery in patients with left ventricular dysfunction. N Engl J Med. 2011;364:1607-16.
83. D'Egidio G, Nichol G, Williams KA, et al. Increasing benefit from revascularization is associated with increasing amounts of myocardial hibernation: A substudy of the PARR-2 trial. JACC Cardiovasc Imaging. 2009;2:1060-8.
84. Abraham A, Nichol G, Williams KA, et al. 18F-FDG PET imaging of myocardial viability in an experienced center with access to 18F-FDG and integration with clinical management teams: The ottawa-five substudy of the PARR 2 trial. J Nucl Med. 2010;51:567-74.
85. O'Meara E, Mielniczuk LM, Wells GA, et al. Alternative imaging modalities in ischemic heart failure (AIMI-HF) image HF project I-a: Study protocol for a randomized controlled trial. Trials. 2013;14:218.
86. Inaba Y, Chen JA, Bergmann SR. Quantity of viable myocardium required to improve survival with revascularization in patients with ischemic cardiomyopathy: A meta-analysis. J Nucl Cardiol. 2010;17:646-54.
87. Ragosta M, Beller GA, Watson DD, et al. Quantitative planar rest-redistribution 201Tl imaging in detection of myocardial viability and prediction of improvement in left ventricular function after coronary bypass surgery in patients with severely depressed left ventricular function. Circulation. 1993;87:1630-41.
88. Bax JJ, Poldermans D, Elhendy A, et al. Improvement of left ventricular ejection fraction, heart failure symptoms and prognosis after revascularization in patients with chronic coronary artery disease and viable myocardium detected by dobutamine stress echocardiography. J Am Coll Cardiol. 1999;34:163-9.

# Role in Patients Undergoing Cardiac Resynchronization Therapy



*Qing Zhang, Yu-Jia Liang, Cheuk-Man Yu*

## INTRODUCTION

Cardiac resynchronization therapy (CRT) is an established therapeutic option for patients with advanced heart failure. It is a pacing modality characterized by biventricular pacing with the left ventricular (LV) lead implanted through the coronary sinus to the LV free wall region. It harmonizes the ventricular activation pattern and restore a more coordinated contraction to improve LV function of the heart as a pump.[1]

CRT is one of the most rapidly evolving fields in heart failure management over the last decade.[2] It is recommended in patients with reduced LV ejection fraction (EF) (<35%) and prolonged QRS complex (≥120 ms for New York Heart Association (NYHA) class III/IV and ≥130 ms for NYHA class II) and left bundle branch block QRS morphology.[3] Evidences from multicenter clinical trials have shown that CRT improves hemodynamic status, heart failure symptoms, exercise capacity, quality of life, and cardiac function in heart failure patients.[4-11] More importantly, CRT induces LV reverse remodeling with reduction in LV volume and LV mass.[7,8,12,13] In fact, LV reverse remodeling has been shown to predict a better long-term prognosis after CRT in terms of reduced mortality and heart failure hospitalization.[11,14] However, it remains to be a major problem that about one-third of patients did not respond to CRT clinically, and more than 40% patients did not have LV reverse remodeling response.[15,16] Ischemic etiology of heart failure has been identified as a predictor of nonresponse to CRT.[17] Studies have reported that patients with ischemic etiologies of heart failure often have a worse response to CRT, in particular with regard to LV reverse remodeling.[18]

Echocardiography has a prominent role in the era of CRT by virtue of its noninvasive nature with high feasibility and reproducibility. More importantly, it permits serial assessment after device implantation. The clinical applications include patient selection before device implantation, guidance of LV lead placement during device implantation, optimization of the device settings, as well as assessments of acute hemodynamic changes and responses to CRT after device implantation.

## ECHOCARDIOGRAPHY BEFORE CARDIAC RESYNCHRONIZATION THERAPY IMPLANTATION

The echocardiographic evaluation before CRT implantation has the following roles: confirming the presence of LV systolic dysfunction, assessing the severity of systolic dyssynchrony, evaluating the severity of prepacing functional mitral regurgitation (MR), and assessing myocardial viability in patients with ischemic etiology of heart failure.

### Assessment of Left Ventricular Systolic Function

Based on the current inclusion criteria, echocardiography is the very first step to confirm and assess the severity of LV systolic dysfunction, in particular identify patients with reduced EF. Echocardiography has been considered as the most useful diagnostic test in the evaluation of heart failure patients according to the American College of Cardiology/ American Heart Association guideline.[19] The LVEF could be calculated from the apical 4- and 2-chamber views by two-dimensional (2D) echocardiography, using biplane Simpson's method. For patients who have suboptimal 2D echocardiographic images (≥2 segments unseen), contrast echo should be applied to optimize LV endocardial borders and facilitate the measurement of ventricular volume.[20] M-mode estimation of LVEF is not recommended in these patients as dyssynchrony septal motion will substantially increase the error of such method. On the other hand, three-dimensional (3D) echocardiography may assure a more accurate determination of LV volume and function.[21-23] As LVEF is one of the single most important predictor of poor prognosis in heart failure, an accurate measure of EF will ensure more suitable candidates to receive CRT and render a higher cost-effectiveness of the therapy.

### Assessment of Mechanical Dyssynchrony

In patients with heart failure and reduced EF, LV conduction delay occurred in about one-quarter of the patients and manifested as prolonged QRS duration. The electrical conduction delay typically resulting in a "U-shaped" depolarization which starts from the septal wall, propagate to the apex, and lately the lateral wall of the LV. This results in uncoordinated contraction and reduction of LV systolic function. There are three different levels of dyssynchrony which are closely linked and may coexist, and can be assessed by echocardiography, namely atrioventricular dyssynchrony, interventricular dyssynchrony and intraventricular dyssynchrony.[24] Resynchronization of the heart and correction of different aspects of dyssynchrony LV is the cornerstone and pathophysiological basis for CRT.[25,26]

A number of echocardiographic tools have been described for the assessments of systolic dyssynchrony in heart failure, including conventional M-mode **(Figure 18.1)** and Doppler echocardiography **(Figure 18.2A and B)**, tissue Doppler imaging (TDI) **(Figure 18.3)** and its derived measures, such as tissue synchronization imaging, and more advanced technology, such as the assessment of myocardial deformation patterns by speckle tracking imaging **(Figure 18.4)** or endocardial motion by 3D echocardiography. **Table 18.1** summarizes the commonly used parameters of dyssynchrony assessment and their suggested cutoff values.

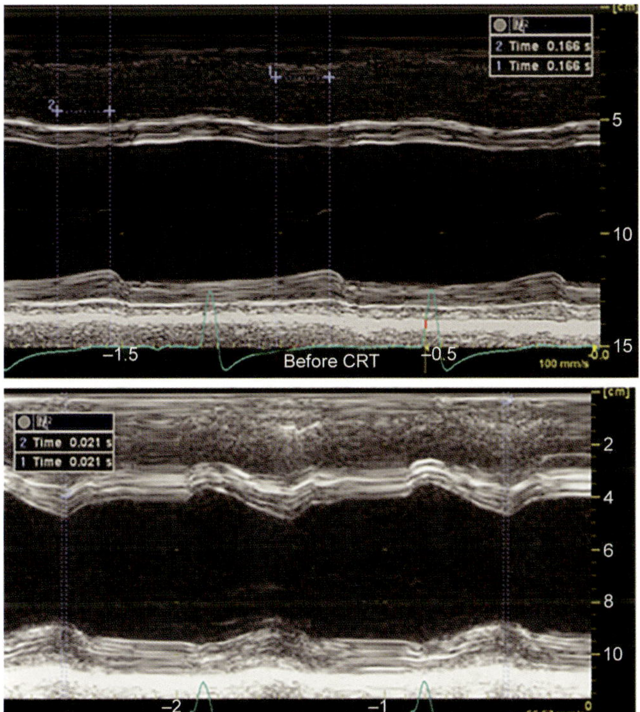


**Figure 18.1:** Left ventricular septal to posterior wall motion delay (SPWMD) by M-mode. With improvement of systolic function and systolic dyssynchrony after cardiac resynchronization therapy (CRT), the SPWMD was substantially improved.

Echocardiographic assessment of mechanical dyssynchrony is potentially helpful in selection of patients for CRT. A comprehensive echocardiographic assessment of systolic dyssynchrony by experienced experts, with integration of mechanical dyssynchrony parameters, myocardial viability and prepacing functional MR can help identify patients with a higher probability to respond to CRT.[27-29]

Moreover, echocardiographic assessment of dyssynchrony helps identification of the site of latest mechanical contraction, which may provide useful information for optimal LV lead placement. In addition, preimplant assessment of systolic dyssynchrony may provide insight on how likely a patient may respond favorably to CRT, in particular in comparison with the postimplant level of dyssynchrony. Finally, a high level of prepacing systolic dyssynchrony predicts a good response after CRT with improvement of mortality and heart failure hospitalization when compared with those with lower level of mechanical dyssynchrony. Useful techniques will include TDI for septal to lateral wall delay >65 ms, TDI with standard deviation of time to systolic velocity of 12 LV segments (Ts-SD or Yu Index) >33 ms, and 2D speckle tracking with septal to posterior wall delay >130 ms.[30-32]

## Assessment of Mitral Regurgitation

MR is frequently observed in patients with ischemic heart disease. It was reported that MR occur in 8–74% of patients after myocardial infarction by color Doppler echocardiography.[33-42] The prevalence of MR depends on the timing of examination after myocardial infarction and heterogeneity of the study population. Risk factors for developing MR after myocardial infarction include advancing age, female gender, history

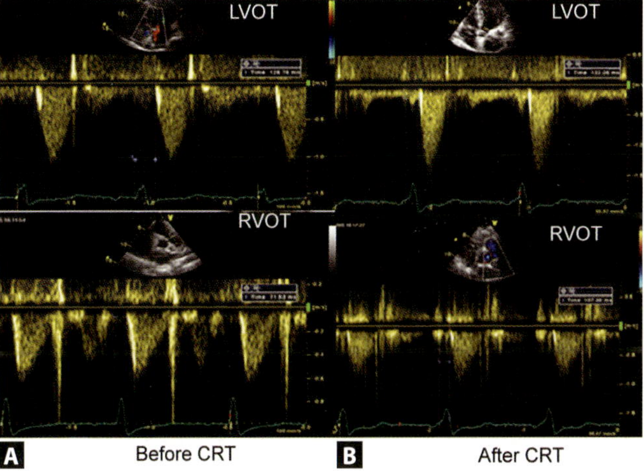


**Figure 18.2A and B:** Interventricular conduction delay (IVCD) by Doppler echocardiography at left (LVOT) and right ventricular outflow tract (RVOT). The IVCD was (A) 50 ms before cardiac resynchronization therapy (CRT), which was reduced to (B) 25 ms after the therapy.

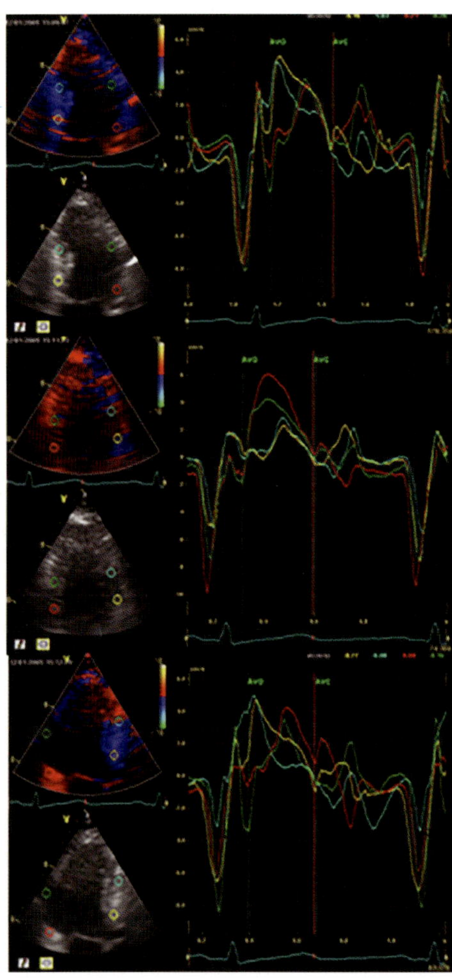

**Figure 18.3:** Tissue Doppler imaging at apical 4-chamber, apical 2-chamber, and apical long-axis views showing delay in systolic contraction at the lateral, inferior and posterior walls, respectively. The standard deviation of 6-basal and 6-mid left ventricular segments in ejection phase (Ts-SD or Yu index) was 43 ms, which falls well above the normal cutoff value of <33 ms indicating significant systolic dyssynchrony.

of inferior or a combined anterior and inferior myocardial infarction, multiple vessel coronary artery disease, congestive heart failure, recurrent ischemia as well as a large infarct size.

Pathogenesis of MR in heart failure is mainly due to LV remodeling, which results in systolic retraction of the papillary muscles toward the apex, inhibits complete leaflet coaptation, particularly when there is a simultaneous decrease in systolic closing force.[43-46] In addition, wall motion abnormalities in the inferior/posterior regions can result in papillary muscle dysfunction with occurrence of MR.[47,48] Recently, it has been shown that LV systolic dyssynchrony is another independent factor that contributes to the development of MR.[49] Besides, a prolonged atrioventricular interval delays the onset of LV contraction and causes delay in mitral valve closure with the occurrence of diastolic MR.[50-53]

For patients who had myocardial infarction, the presence of MR is associated with an increased risk of heart failure and mortality.[33,54,55] Prepacing severity of MR has also been suggested to be a determinant of CRT response. In a prospective study of 143 patients followed for 6 months, independent predictors for lack of CRT response included severe functional MR at baseline, ischemic heart disease, and LV end-diastolic diameter ≥75 mm.[17] Furthermore, those patients who had significant pretreatment MR, which was successfully improved after CRT, have been shown to have the greatest propensity of LV reverse remodeling at follow-up, while being the least for those patients with who did not have improvement of MR.[56] Therefore, assessment of severity of pretreatment MR by echocardiography has a potential role in patient selection and evaluation of prognosis in CRT. In addition, as reduction of MR is a favorable response of CRT, assessment of preimplant MR may facilitate evaluation of treatment efficacy after CRT.

## Assessment of Myocardial Viability

Response to CRT is directly related to the extent of myocardial viability. Extensive scar tissue in the LV posterolateral wall is associated with poor response to CRT.[57,58] Many imaging techniques have been employed for the assessment of myocardial viability, in particular cardiac magnetic resonance imaging (cMRI), radionuclear imaging, and echocardiography. With respect to echocardiography, myocardial viability is commonly assessed using measures of LV wall thickness or myocardial contractile reserve. Assessment of myocardial perfusion using contrast echocardiography, 3D echocardiography, strain and strain rate imaging in order to define myocardial viability is more challenging and is still subject under investigation.

Measuring the LV wall thickness is a simple technique used to predict viability. It has been demonstrated that severely thinned walls most likely represent scar tissue, segments with LV end-diastolic wall thicknesses of less than 6 mm have a low likelihood of recovery of LV function.[59] Dobutamine stress echocardiography has also been shown to predict recovery of LV function in patients with stable coronary artery disease. A biphasic response was found to predict recovery of LV functional following revascularization, after given dobutamine infusion from 5 to 40 μg/kg/minute. On the other hand, worsening of LV systolic function after dobutamine infusion was associated with low rate of recovery after revascularization.[60]

With respect to contrast echocardiography, myocardial contrast defect is the most powerful echocardiographic predictor of future LV adverse remodeling following

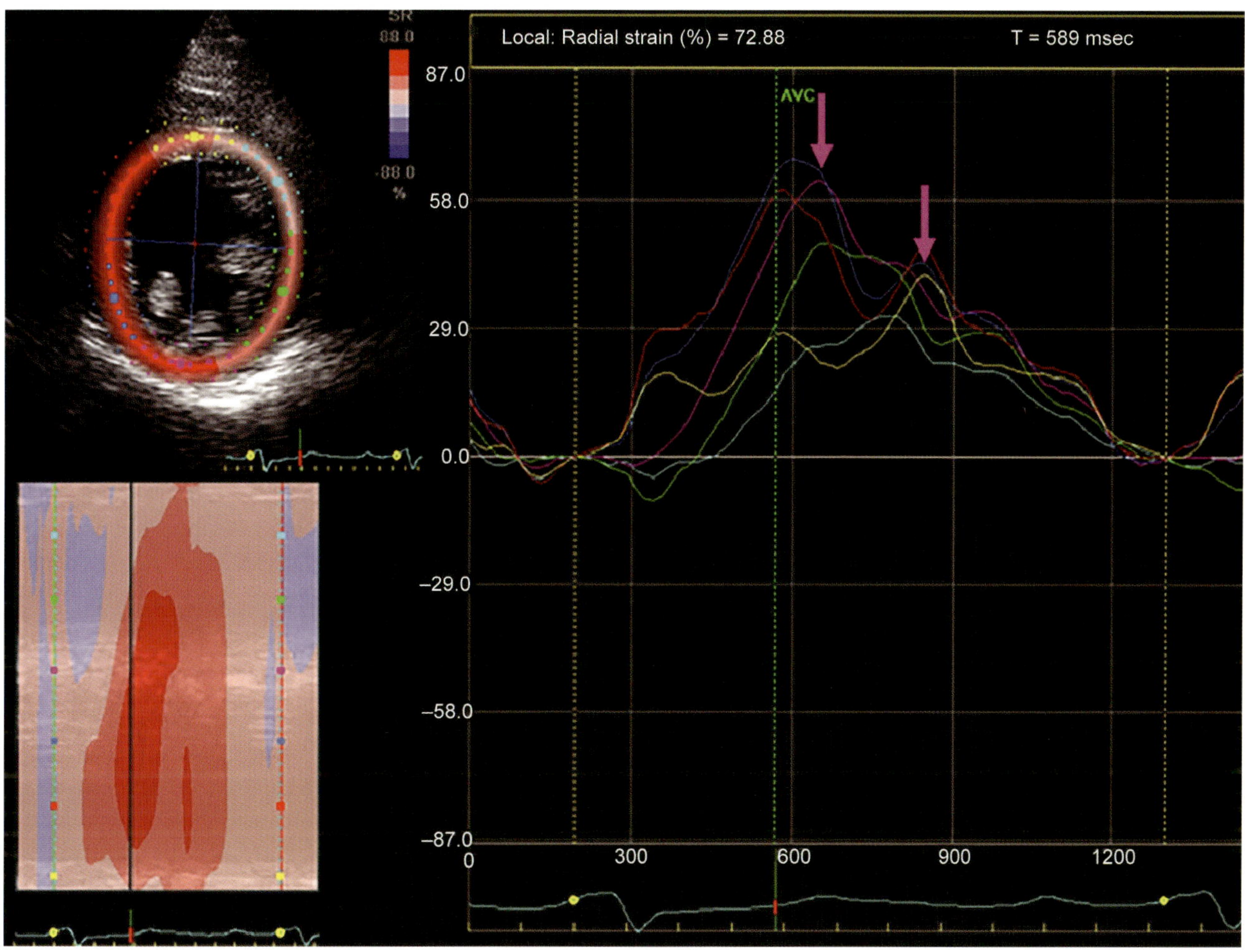


**Figure 18.4:** Two-dimensional speckle tracking assessment of radial strain at mid left ventricular level. There was significant delay among these 6 segments with a maximal difference of 170 ms. *Abbreviation:* AVC, aortic valve closure.

myocardial infarction when compared to wall-motion abnormalities and LVEF.[61]

The 3D echocardiography increased the accuracy of assessing LV morphology, volumes and mass when compared to 2D imaging. Furthermore, contrast-enhanced 3D echocardiography has a sensitivity of 78% and specificity of 99% for detecting myocardial scar tissue when validated against cMRI with late gadolinium enhancement.[62]

Systolic myocardial strain can be used to further assess myocardial viability. Strain imaging correlates with the degree of microvascular integrity which predicts myocardial viability.[63] Study by Mollema et al. has found that global LV systolic strain assessed by automated function imaging derived from 2D speckle tracking has a predictive value for improvement of LV systolic function following myocardial infarction.[64] A baseline global LV systolic longitudinal strain value of –13.7% had a sensitivity of 86% and a specificity of 74% to predict improvement of LVEF at 1 year after myocardial infarction. Strain imaging during dobutamine stress echocardiography can add incremental value over wall-motion analysis for prediction of myocardial viability.[65] An increase in strain rate by more than –0.23 (1/s) with low-dose dobutamine (10 μg/kg/minute) had a sensitivity of 83% and a specificity of 84% to predict viability when validated against FDG PET.[66] In the same study, longitudinal strain and strain rate imaging at rest and low-dose dobutamine were found to be predictors of functional recovery after revascularization.[65]

Myocardial contractile reserve has been suggested to be a predictor of LV reverse remodeling after CRT. In a prospective study of 31 patients who had been followed up for 6 months, a cutoff value of >7.5% increase in dobutamine-induced LVEF before CRT implantation exhibited a sensitivity of 76% and a specificity of 86% to predict a ≥15% reduction in LV end-systolic volume after 6 months of therapy.[67] The improvement

**Table 18.1:** Commonly used parameters of dyssynchrony and their cutoff values

| | | *Dyssynchrony indices* | *Echo techniques* | *Views* | *Cutoff values* |
|---|---|---|---|---|---|
| Intraventricular dyssynchrony | Short-axis | Septal-to-posterior wall mechanical delay (SPWMD) | M-mode | Parasternal mid-LV views | ≥130 ms |
| | | Septal-to-posterior delay | 2D speckle tracking<br>Time-to-peak systolic radial strain (6 segments) | Short-axis mid-LV view | ≥130 ms |
| | | 3D dyssynchrony indices | 3D echo | Apical | |
| | Long-axis | Septal to lateral delay in ejection phase | Tissue Doppler imaging<br>Time to peak systolic velocity (4 segments) | Apical 4-chamber view | ≥65 ms |
| | | Standard deviation of the 6-basal, 6-mid LV segments in ejection phase (Ts-SD or Yu index) | Tissue Doppler imaging<br>Time-to-peak systolic velocity (12 segments) | Apical 4-, 2-chamber, and long-axis views | ≥33 ms |
| | | Maximal delay of the 6-basal, 6-mid LV segments in ejection phase | Tissue Doppler imaging<br>Time-to-peak systolic velocity (12 segments) | Apical 4-, 2-chamber, and long-axis views | ≥100 ms |
| Interventricular dyssynchrony | | Interventricular mechanical delay (IVMD) | Doppler echo<br>QRS to the onset of aortic flow minus QRS to the onset of pulmonary flow | LV and RV outflow tract views | ≥40 ms |

*Abbreviations:* LV, left ventricular; RV, right ventricular; 2D, two-dimensional; 3D, three-dimensional.

of LV short-axis function also contributes to the improvement in global LV function and geometry after CRT. In a 2D speckle study of 39 patients who had been followed up for 3 months after CRT, responders of LV reverse remodeling had higher baseline circumferential strain than nonresponders, who also had improvement in circumferential and radial strain after CRT. The increase in circumferential strain correlated with increase in LVEF and decrease in mid-cavity width. A baseline mean circumferential strain of ≥6.5% predicted a gain in LVEF ≥5%, with a sensitivity of 73% and a specificity of 71%.[68] This study also illustrated the concept of having a critical mass of viable myocardial in order to have effective CRT response. In particular, if both long- and short-axis myocardial function is too much impaired, the LV has probably gone beyond the point of no return, and CRT will not be effective.

## ECHOCARDIOGRAPHY DURING CARDIAC RESYNCHRONIZATION THERAPY IMPLANTATION

The optimal placement of the LV lead represents one of the most challenging issues of CRT implantation. Suboptimal LV lead location has been shown to contribute to the lack of response to CRT. In a study that assessed reasons for lack of CRT response, suboptimal LV lead position was implicated in 21% of patients.[69] There is increasing evidence that selection of specific LV sites for pacing may improve responses to CRT. Two randomized studies showed that patients who had LV lead placed at the LV free wall with most significant mechanical delay according to 2D speckle tracking strain assessment will have a lower mortality and heart failure hospitalization when compared to the conventional approach without echocardiographic guidance.[70,71] Such approach also resulted in a greater extent of LV reverse remodeling.

The general consensus is that in patients with ischemic etiology, placing the LV lead in the posterolateral wall with a transmural scar tissue will substantially reduce the response to CRT.[57] However, cMRI with delay gadolinium enhancement might not be performed in the majority of centers who implant CRT due to cost and resource implication. Nowadays, 2D speckle assessment may also provide similar information of lack of myocardial viability. A study found that a radial strain <16.5% corresponding to >50% transmurality of the scar tissue by cMRI.[32] Patients received CRT who had a radial strain below this cutoff value (i.e. a better radial strain) had significantly lower all-cause mortality and heart failure hospitalization than those above the cutoff valve as it signifies a higher scar burden.[32] The same study also found that assessment of LV systolic dyssynchrony, the placement of LV lead over the most delayed mechanical position, and the assessment of scar burden by strain echocardiography carry incremental prognostic value in CRT population.[32]

In addition, in the operative setting, when coronary sinus cannulation has failed by fluoroscopy alone or when structural anomalies are suspected, echocardiography may provide information that facilitates coronary sinus cannulation. In this setting, transesophageal echocardiography and intracardiac echocardiography have been proven to be useful.[72-74]

## ECHOCARDIOGRAPHY AFTER CARDIAC RESYNCHRONIZATION THERAPY IMPLANTATION

### Optimization of Device Programming after Cardiac Resynchronization Therapy

#### *Optimization of Atrioventricular Interval*

Improvement of atrioventricular dyssynchrony is one of the mechanisms of benefit from CRT. This is particularly helpful in patients with first-degree atrioventricular block where diastolic filling time will further be jeopardized.[24] About half of heart failure patients who have prolonged QRS duration also have accompanied first-degree atrioventricular block. Optimization of atrioventricular interval (AV interval) is an attempt to ensure atrioventricular synchrony and close to 100% ventricular pacing in individual patients. It allows a longest LV filling time and maximal cardiac output but abolishes the "wasted" presystolic time after completion of atrial contraction thus reduces diastolic MR.[75,76] Usually, AV interval optimization is performed shortly after the device implantation, i.e. at the predischarge period. However, reoptimization of AV interval at intermediate (e.g. 3 months) and long-term (e.g. 12–18 months) follow-up may be necessary to further improve cardiac performance.[77] The two commonly employed methods of AV interval optimization by Doppler echocardiography are based on the principles of optimal LV diastolic filling or maximal cardiac output. The former principle can be achieved by the methods described by Ritter or Ishikawa.[75,76] For either method, it aims at enforcing mitral valve closure to occur right after atrial filling is completed in order to reverse the aforementioned deleterious effect of prolonged AV interval. When a discernible A wave is obtained from the transmitral inflow at apical 4-chamber view by pulse Doppler echocardiography, Ritter's method[76] is preferred **(Figure 18.5A and B)**. It is based only on the programmed "long" and "short" AV intervals and their corresponding Q-A intervals (from the onset of QRS complex to the completion of A wave). The optimal AV interval is calculated by the following equation:

$$\text{Optimal AV interval} = \text{Short AV interval} + [(\text{Long AV interval} + \text{Q-A}_{long}) - (\text{Short AV interval} + \text{Q-A}_{short})],$$

where $\text{Q-A}_{long}$ represents for the Q-A interval at the programmed "long" AV interval and $\text{Q-A}_{short}$ for that at the "short" AV interval:

In the situation where the A wave was too small or too noisy that its completion were not discernable, the AV interval can be optimized based on reiterative cardiac output method. Cardiac output is calculated by pulse Doppler echocardiography at the LV outflow tract by the continuity equation. Starting from 30 ms, AV interval is programmed at incremental steps of 20 ms until the ventricular sensing occurs. The AV interval with the largest cardiac output is regarded as the optimal one. One can then reverse the AV interval at steps of –10 ms at the range close to the peak cardiac output to verify the optimal AV interval.

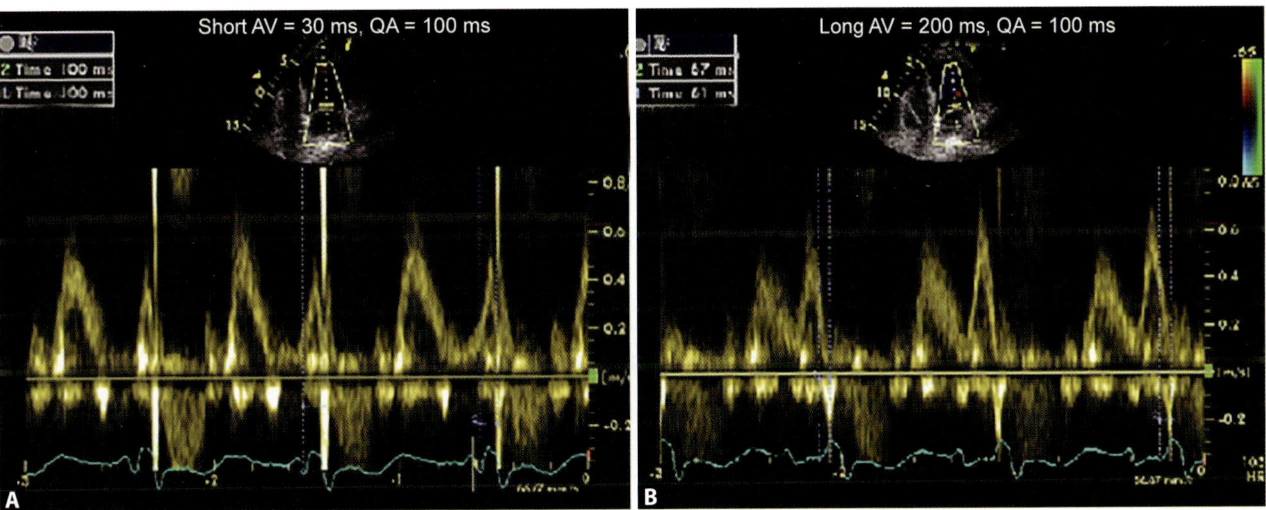


**Figure 18.5A and B:** Atrioventricular (AV) optimization by Ritter's method. Note that during the short AV interval, there is partial truncation of A wave (A), while reverse of E and A wave is seen during a long AV interval (B). The calculated optimal AV interval is 160 ms in this patient.

### *Optimization of Interventricular Interval*

Optimization of interventricular interval (V–V interval) after CRT may further improve intraventricular dyssynchrony, although it has no effect on interventricular dyssynchrony. However, this may further enhance systolic function and reduces MR. Currently, the reiterative cardiac output method is the most commonly used. As a number of V–V interval settings with LV or RV preexcitation need to be programmed where cardiac output are measured, it is quite time consuming. It is recommended to optimize the AV interval before the V–V interval so that the AV dyssynchrony in the LV will remain unchanged when different V–V intervals are tested. In general, it is believed that the need for V–V interval optimization is much less when than the need for AV interval optimization.

## Assessment of Beneficial Effects of Cardiac Resynchronization Therapy

### *Assessment of Acute Hemodynamic Changes*

The CRT immediately improves ventricular contraction patterns and thus results in hemodynamic changes. The acute hemodynamic benefits after CRT implantation can be monitored by echocardiography. Studies in the acute setting have confirmed that CRT immediately improves LV systolic function, which is evident by a reduction in LV end-systolic volume and a more rapid rise of LV pressure (+dP/$dt_{max}$, between 15% and 35%).[78-80] It is well demonstrated by various imaging techniques that the acute hemodynamic benefit is associated with both the magnitude of prepacing mechanical dyssynchrony as well as the extent of mechanical resynchronization during CRT.[81,82] Patients are likely to benefit from CRT in the long-term if there is a reduction in LV systolic dyssynchrony together with improved hemodynamic status and contractile function soon after CRT. In a recent analysis from MADIT-CRT (Multicenter Automatic Defibrillator Implantation Trial with Cardiac Resynchronization Therapy), each 20 ms decrease in LV mechanical dyssynchrony by peak transverse strain was associated with a 7% reduction in all-cause mortality or new heart failure-related events.[83]

### *Assessment of Responses to Cardiac Resynchronization Therapy*

One of the objective criteria to confirm a favorable response to CRT is the occurrence of LV reverse remodeling, which is signified by a decrease of LV volume and increase in LVEF during serial echocardiographic assessment, usually after CRT for 3–6 months.[7,84] LV end-systolic volume (LVESV) measured by biplane Simpson's method is commonly employed and is regarded as the best prognostic predictor in heart failure patients.[85] The average reduction of LV end-systolic volume at 3 months after CRT is about 22%, while the reduction of LV end-diastolic volume is about 15%[7] **(Figure 18.6A and B)**. The average gain in LVEF is about 8% based on biplane Simpson's method. Reduction of LV end-systolic and end-diastolic diameters was constantly observed in large, multicenter trials, and it continue to occur for at least 18 months after CRT.[8] While using a vigorous definition of reduction in LVESV ≥15% as volumetric response, responders occurred in up to 60% of the patients who received CRT in previous studies.[84,86-88] Furthermore, patients who exhibited LV reverse remodeling response at 3–6 months after CRT showed a highly favorable long-term prognosis with significantly lower all-cause mortality, cardiovascular mortality, and heart failure hospitalization.[89]

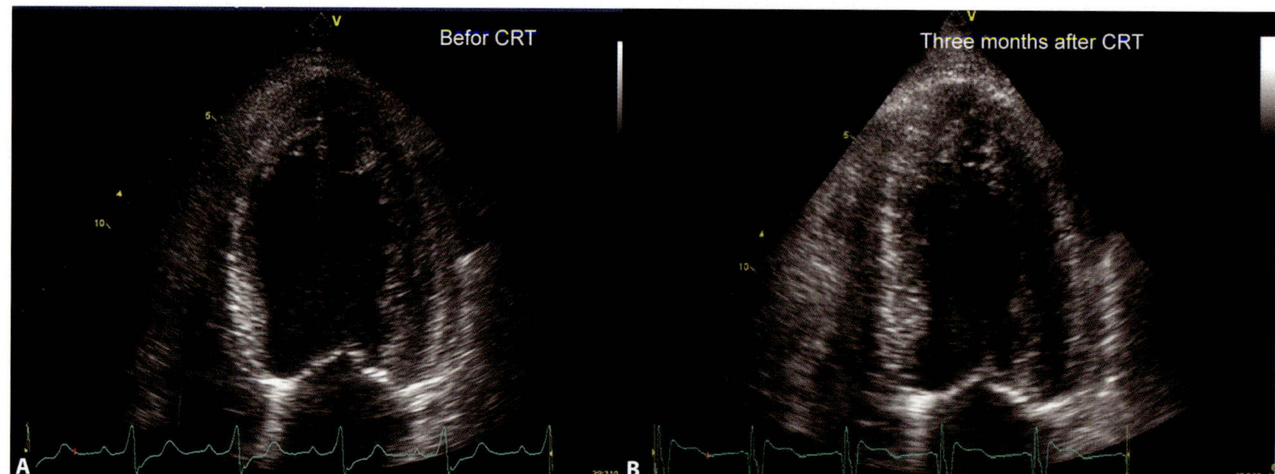


**Figure 18.6A and B:** Left ventricular (LV) reverse remodeling after cardiac resynchronization therapy (CRT). When compared with (A) pretreatment echocardiography, there was (B) significant reduction of LV end-systolic volume after CRT for 3 months and the LV is less enlarged and more slender in shape.

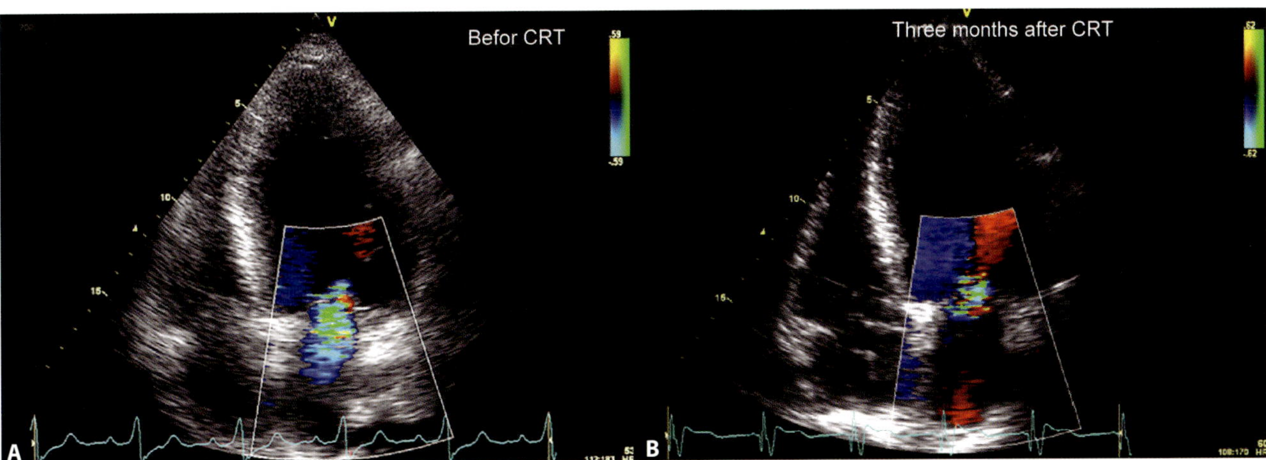


**Figure 18.7A and B:** Improvement of mitral regurgitation (MR) after cardiac resynchronization therapy (CRT). There was significant reduction in the MR jet area at apical 4-chamber view when compared between (A) pretreatment echocardiography and (B) 3 months after CRT.

## Assessment of MR Reduction after CRT

A significant reduction in MR has been reported after CRT **(Figure 18.7A and B)**. An effective CRT can reduce functional MR immediately by about 30% and continue to decrease by an additional 10–20% up to 6 months after device therapy.[7,90,91] MR was reduced significantly in responders of CRT and to a greater extent than the nonresponders.[7,92] Of note, a lesser degree of reduction in MR was reported for CRT in ischemic than nonischemic patients.[10]

The immediate reduction in the degree of systolic MR after CRT is associated with an acute hemodynamic improvement[90] which is related to increase in ventricular closing force as well as both global resynchronization of the left ventricle and regional resynchronization of the papillary muscle contractions. In a previous study, patients were examined by echocardiography during brief reprogramming of a CRT device.[90] The changes in MR severity were compared to the changes in LV systolic function (LV peak positive rate of pressure rise, LV $+dP/dt_{max}$). A inverse linear relationship between severity of MR and LV $+dP/dt_{max}$ was observed. It was concluded that an improved transmitral pressure gradient (the closing force on the mitral leaflet) reduces severity of MR by earlier and more effective mitral leaflet closure.[90] In another study, deformation sequence of the papillary muscles was studied by strain rate imaging.[91] A direct relationship between the interpapillary muscle activation time delay and the improvement in the degree of MR by CRT was reported. Thus, the immediate reduction in MR severity can be attributed to the improvement of coordination of ventricular contraction, including resynchronized papillary muscle activation, which results in improved systolic function and reduced mitral leaflet tethering forces.[91] In addition, reduction of diastolic MR by optimizing of the atrioventricular interval also contributes to the acute improvement of MR after CRT. The long-term improvement of MR is probably attributed to LV reverse remodeling in addition to the aforementioned factors.[93] Systolic dyssynchrony is another factor contributing to the pathogenesis of MR in heart failure patients, especially global systolic dyssynchrony of the left ventricle.[49] Improvement of LV global dyssynchrony was found to be a potential mechanism of reduction in MR after CRT.[56]

In conclusion, echocardiography has an indispensable role in patients receiving CRT. Before device implantation, echocardiography helps select suitable heart failure candidates for the therapy. It also helps identify the best location of LV lead placement. After implantation, echocardiography has a unique role of device optimization as well as evaluating treatment response. In addition, echocardiography is also useful to predict acute therapy response and long-term clinical outcome. With technological advancement, quantitative analyses of multiple imaging modalities provide a complementary role in the assessment of CRT candidates by a "one-stop" service.

## REFERENCES

1. Cazeau S, Ritter P, Bakdach S, Lazarus A, Limousin M, Henao L, et al. Four-chamber pacing in dilated cardiomyopathy. Pacing Clin Electrophysiol. 1994;17:1974-9.
2. Yu CM HD, Auricchio A (Eds). Cardiac Resynchronization Therapy, Second edition. Hoboken, NJ: Wiley-Blackwell; 2008.
3. McMurray JJ, Adamopoulos S, Anker SD, Auricchio A, Böhm M, Dickstein K, et al. ESC guidelines for the diagnosis and treatment of acute and chronic heart failure 2012. Eur J Heart Fail. 2012;14:803-69.

4. Cazeau S, Leclercq C, Lavergne T, Walker S, Varma C, Linde C, et al. Effects of multisite biventricular pacing in patients with heart failure and intraventricular conduction delay. New Eng J Med. 2001;344:873-80.
5. Abraham WT, Fisher WG, Smith AL, Delurgio DB, Leon AR, Loh E, et al. Cardiac resynchronization in chronic heart failure. New Eng J Med. 2002;346:1845-53.
6. Gras D, Leclercq C, Tang AS, Bucknall C, Luttikhuis HO, Kirstein-Pedersen A. Cardiac resynchronization therapy in advanced heart failure the multicenter inSync clinical study. New Eng J Med. 2002;4:311-20.
7. Yu C-M, Chau E, Sanderson JE, Fan K, Tang M-O, Fung W-H, et al. Tissue Doppler echocardiographic evidence of reverse remodeling and improved synchronicity by simultaneously delaying regional contraction after biventricular pacing therapy in heart failure. Circulation. 2002;105:438-45.
8. Sutton MGSJ, Plappert T, Abraham WT, Smith AL, DeLurgio DB, Leon AR, et al. Effect of cardiac resynchronization therapy on left ventricular size and function in chronic heart failure. Circulation. 2003;107:1985-90.
9. Bradley DJ, Bradley EA, Baughman KL, Berger RD, Calkins H, Goodman SN, et al. Cardiac resynchronization and death from progressive heart failure: A meta-analysis of randomized controlled trials. JAMA. 2003;289:730-40.
10. Bristow MR, Saxon LA, Boehmer J, Krueger S, Kass DA, De Marco T, et al. Cardiac-resynchronization therapy with or without an implantable defibrillator in advanced chronic heart failure. New Eng J Med. 2004;350:2140-50.
11. Cleland JG, Daubert J-C, Erdmann E, Freemantle N, Gras D, Kappenberger L, et al. The effect of cardiac resynchronization on morbidity and mortality in heart failure. New Eng J Med. 2005;352:1539-49.
12. Saxon LA, De Marco T, Schafer J, Chatterjee K, Kumar UN, Foster E. Effects of long-term biventricular stimulation for resynchronization on echocardiographic measures of remodeling. Circulation. 2002;105:1304-10.
13. Zhang Q, Fung JW-H, Auricchio A, Chan JY-S, Kum LC, Wu LW, et al. Differential change in left ventricular mass and regional wall thickness after cardiac resynchronization therapy for heart failure. New Eng J Med. 2006;27:1423-30.
14. Yu C-M, Bleeker GB, Fung JW-H, Schalij MJ, Zhang Q, van der Wall EE, et al. Left ventricular reverse remodeling but not clinical improvement predicts long-term survival after cardiac resynchronization therapy. Circulation. 2005;112: 1580-6.
15. Birnie DH, Tang AS. The problem of non-response to cardiac resynchronization therapy. Curr Opin Cardiol. 2006;21:20-6.
16. Tang AS, Ellenbogen KA. A futuristic perspective on clinical studies of cardiac resynchronization therapy for heart failure patients. Curr Opin Cardiol. 2006;21:78-82.
17. Díaz-Infante E, Mont L, Leal J, García-Bolao I, Fernández-Lozano I, Hernández-Madrid A, et al. Predictors of lack of response to resynchronization therapy. Am J Cardiol. 2005;95: 1436-40.
18. Woo GW, Petersen-Stejskal S, Johnson JW, Conti JB, Aranda Jr JA, Curtis AB. Ventricular reverse remodeling and 6-month outcomes in patients receiving cardiac resynchronization therapy: Analysis of the miracle study. J Interv Card Electrophysiol. 2005;12:107-13.
19. Hunt SA, Abraham WT, Chin MH, Feldman AM, Francis GS, Ganiats TG, et al. ACC/AHA 2005 guideline update for the diagnosis and management of chronic heart failure in the adult a report of the American College of Cardiology/American Heart Association Task Force on practice guidelines (writing committee to update the 2001 guidelines for the evaluation and management of heart failure): Developed in collaboration with the American College of Chest Physicians and the International Society for Heart and Lung Transplantation: Endorsed by the Heart Rhythm Society. Circulation. 2005;112:e154-e235.
20. Wei K, Mulvagh SL, Carson L, Davidoff R, Gabriel R, Grimm RA, et al. The safety of definity and optison for ultrasound image enhancement: a retrospective analysis of 78,383 administered contrast doses. J Am Soc Echocardiogr. 2008;21:1202-6.
21. Ilercil A, O'Grady MJ, Roman MJ, Paranicas M, Lee ET, Welty TK, et al. Reference values for echocardiographic measurements in urban and rural populations of differing ethnicity: The strong heart study. J Am Soc Echocardiogr. 2001;14:601-11.
22. Palmieri V, Dahlöf B, DeQuattro V, Sharpe N, Bella JN, de Simone G, et al. Reliability of echocardiographic assessment of left ventricular structure and function: The preserve study. J Am Coll Cardiol. 1999;34:1625-32.
23. Chuang ML, Hibberd MG, Salton CJ, Beaudin RA, Riley MF, Parker RA, et al. Importance of imaging method over imaging modality in noninvasive determination of left ventricular volumes and ejection fraction: assessment by two-and three-dimensional echocardiography and magnetic resonance imaging. J Am Coll Cardiol. 2000;35:477-84.
24. Auricchio A, Abraham WT. Cardiac resynchronization therapy: Current state of the art cost versus benefit. Circulation. 2004;109:300-7.
25. Bleeker GB, Mollema SA, Holman ER, Van De Veire N, Ypenburg C, Boersma E, et al. Left ventricular resynchronization is mandatory for response to cardiac resynchronization therapy analysis in patients with echocardiographic evidence of left ventricular dyssynchrony at baseline. Circulation. 2007;116:1440-8.
26. Smiseth OA, Russell K, Skulstad H. The role of echocardiography in quantification of left ventricular dyssynchrony: state of the art and future directions. Eur Heart J Cardiovasc Imaging. 2012;13:61-8.
27. Lafitte S, Reant P, Zaroui A, Donal E, Mignot A, Bougted H, et al. Validation of an echocardiographic multiparametric strategy to increase responders patients after cardiac resynchronization: A multicentre study. Eur Heart J. 2009;30:2880-7.
28. Breithardt OA, Claus P, Sutherland GR. Do we understand who benefits from resynchronisation therapy? Eur Heart J. 2004; 25:535-6.
29. Stockburger M, Fateh-Moghadam S, Nitardy A, Celebi O, Krebs A, Habedank D, et al. Baseline Doppler parameters are useful predictors of chronic left ventricular reduction in size by cardiac resynchronization therapy. Europace. 2008;10:69-74.
30. Zhang Q, Van Bommel R, Fung JW, Chan JY, Bleeker GB, Ypenburg C, et al. Tissue Doppler velocity is superior to strain imaging in predicting long-term cardiovascular events after cardiac resynchronisation therapy. Heart. 2009;95:1085-90.

31. Gorcsan J, Oyenuga O, Habib PJ, Tanaka H, Adelstein EC, Hara H, et al. Relationship of echocardiographic dyssynchrony to long-term survival after cardiac resynchronization therapy. Circulation. 2010;122:1910-8.
32. Delgado V, van Bommel RJ, Bertini M, Borleffs CJW, Marsan NA, Ng AC, et al. Relative merits of left ventricular dyssynchrony, left ventricular lead position, and myocardial scar to predict long-term survival of ischemic heart failure patients undergoing cardiac resynchronization therapy. Circulation. 2011;123:70-8.
33. Bursi F, Enriquez-Sarano M, Nkomo VT, Jacobsen SJ, Weston SA, Meverden RA, et al. Heart failure and death after myocardial infarction in the community the emerging role of mitral regurgitation. Circulation. 2005;111:295-301.
34. Bhatnagar S, Al Yusuf A. Significance of a mitral regurgitation systolic murmur complicating a first acute myocardial infarction in the coronary care unit? Assessment by colour Doppler flow imaging. Eur Heart J. 1991;12:1311-5.
35. Barzilai B, Gesslr C, Pérez JE, et al. Significance of Doppler-detected mitral regurgitation in acute myocardial infarction. Am J Cardiol. 1988;61:220-3.
36. Vicente VT, Valdés CM, García AA, Soria AF, Fernández PJ, Pérez LF, et al. Mitral valve insufficiency in acute myocardial infarction. Assessment with pulsed and coded Doppler color. Arch Inst Cardiol Mex. 1991;61:117-21.
37. Van Dantzig JM, Delemarre BJ, Koster RW, et al. Pathogenesis of mitral regurgitation in acute myocardial infarction: importance of changes in left ventricular shape and regional function. Am Heart J. 1996;131:865-71.
38. Ma HH, Honma H, Munakata K, et al. Mitral insufficiency as a complication of acute myocardial infarction and left ventricular remodeling. Jpn Circ J. 1997;61:912-20.
39. Feinberg MS, Schwammenthal E, Shlizerman L, Porter A, Hod H, Freimark D, et al. Prognostic significance of mild mitral regurgitation by color Doppler echocardiography in acute myocardial infarction. Am J Cardiol. 2000;86:903-7.
40. Nešković AN, Marinković J, Bojić M, et al. Early predictors of mitral regurgitation after acute myocardial infarction-the mitral valve. Am J Cardiol. 1999;3:329-32.
41. Golia G, Anselmi M, Rossi A, Cicoira MA, Tinto M, Marino P, et al. Relationship between mitral regurgitation and myocardial viability after acute myocardial infarction: their impact on prognosis. Intern J Cardiol. 2001;78:81-90.
42. Alam M, Thorstrand C, Rosenhamer G. Mitral regurgitation following first-time acute myocardial infarction—early and late findings by Doppler echocardiography. Clin Cardiol. 1993;16:30-4.
43. Yiu SF, Enriquez-Sarano M, Tribouilloy C, et al. Determinants of the degree of functional mitral regurgitation in patients with systolic left ventricular dysfunction a quantitative clinical study. Circulation. 2000;102:1400-6.
44. Otsuji Y, Handschumacher MD, Schwammenthal E, Jiang L, Song J-K, Guerrero JL, et al. Insights from three-dimensional echocardiography into the mechanism of functional mitral regurgitation direct in vivo demonstration of altered leaflet tethering geometry. Circulation. 1997;96:1999-2008.
45. Otsuji Y, Handschumacher MD, Liel-Cohen N, Tanabe H, Jiang L, Schwammenthal E, et al. Mechanism of ischemic mitral regurgitation with segmental left ventricular dysfunction: Three-dimensional echocardiographic studies in models of acute and chronic progressive regurgitation. J Am Coll Cardiol. 2001;37:641-8.
46. He S, Fontaine AA, Schwammenthal E, et al. Integrated mechanism for functional mitral regurgitation leaflet restriction versus coapting force: In vitro studies. Circulation. 1997;96:1826-34.
47. Gorman JH, Gorman RC, Plappert T, Jackson BM, Hiramatsu Y, John-Sutton MGS, et al. Infarct size and location determine development of mitral regurgitation in the sheep model. J Thorac Cardiovasc Surg. 1998;115:615-22.
48. Kumanohoso T, Otsuji Y, Yoshifuku S, Matsukida K, Koriyama C, Kisanuki A, et al. Mechanism of higher incidence of ischemic mitral regurgitation in patients with inferior myocardial infarction: Quantitative analysis of left ventricular and mitral valve geometry in 103 patients with prior myocardial infarction. J Thorac Cardiovasc Surg. 2003;125:135-43.
49. Liang Y-J, Zhang Q, Fang F, Lee AP-W, Liu M, Yan BP-Y, et al. Incremental value of global systolic dyssynchrony in determining the occurrence of functional mitral regurgitation in patients with left ventricular systolic dysfunction. Eur Heart J. 2013; 34:767-74.
50. Ishikawa T, Sumita S, Kimura K, Kuji N, Nakayama R, Nagura T, et al. Critical PQ interval for the appearance of diastolic mitral regurgitation and optimal PQ interval in patients implanted with DDD pacemakers. Pacing Clin Electrophysiol. 1994;17:1989-94.
51. Ishikawa T, Kimura K, Nihei T, Usui T, Kashiwagi M, Ishii M. Relationship between diastolic mitral regurgitation and PQ intervals or cardiac function in patients implanted with DDD pacemakers. Pacing Clin Electrophysiol. 1991;14:1797-802.
52. Panidis IP, Ross J, Munley B, et al. Diastolic mitral regurgitation in patients with atrioventricular conduction abnormalities: A common finding by Doppler echocardiography. J Am Coll Cardiol. 1986;7:768-74.
53. Ishikawa T, Kimura K, Miyazaki N, Tochikubo O, Usui T, KAshiwagi M, et al. Diastolic mitral regurgitation in patients with first-degree atrioventricular block. Pacing Clin Electrophysiol. 1992;15:1927-31.
54. Grigioni F, Enriquez-Sarano M, Zehr KJ, et al. Ischemic mitral regurgitation long-term outcome and prognostic implications with quantitative Doppler assessment. Circulation. 2001;103: 1759-64.
55. Grigioni F, Detaint D, Avierinos JF, Scott C, Tajik J, Enriquez-Sarano M. Contribution of ischemic mitral regurgitation to congestive heart failure after myocardial infarction. J Am Coll Cardiol. 2005;45:260-7.
56. Liang YJ, Zhang Q, Fung JWH, Chan JYS, Yip GWK, Lam YY, et al. Impact of reduction in early- and late-systolic functional mitral regurgitation on reverse remodelling after cardiac resynchronization therapy. Eur Heart J. 2010;31: 2359-68.
57. Bleeker GB, Kaandorp TA, Lamb HJ, Boersma E, Steendijk P, de Roos A, et al. Effect of posterolateral scar tissue on clinical and echocardiographic improvement after cardiac resynchronization therapy. Circulation. 2006;113:969-76.
58. Hummel JP, Lindner JR, Belcik JT, Ferguson JD, Mangrum JM, Bergin JD, et al. Extent of myocardial viability predicts response

to biventricular pacing in ischemic cardiomyopathy. Heart Rhythm. 2005;2:1211-7.
59. Schinkel AF, Bax JJ, Boersma E, Elhendy A, Vourvouri EC, Roelandt JR, et al. Assessment of residual myocardial viability in regions with chronic electrocardiographic q-wave infarction. Am Heart J. 2002;144:865-9.
60. Cornel JH, Bax JJ, Elhendy A, Maat AP, Kimman G-JP, Geleijnse ML, et al. Biphasic response to dobutamine predicts improvement of global left ventricular function after surgical revascularization in patients with stable coronary artery disease: implications of time course of recovery on diagnostic accuracy. J Am Coll Cardiol. 1998;31:1002-10.
61. Agati L, Funaro S, Madonna M, Montano M, Berardi E, Picardi MN, et al. Tissue viability by contrast echocardiography. Eur J Echocardiogr. 2006;7:S22.
62. Montant P, Chenot F, Goffinet C, Poncelet A, Vancraeynest D, Pasquet A, et al. Detection and quantification of myocardial scars by contrast-enhanced 3D echocardiography. Circ Cardiovasc Imaging. 2010;3:415-23.
63. Park SM, Hong SJ, Park JS, Lim SY, Ahn CM, Lim DS, et al. Relationship between strain rate imaging and coronary flow reserve in assessing myocardial viability after acute myocardial infarction. Echocardiography. 2010;27:977-84.
64. Mollema SA, Delgado V, Bertini M, Antoni ML, Boersma E, Holman ER, et al. Viability assessment with global left ventricular longitudinal strain predicts recovery of left ventricular function after acute myocardial infarction. Circ Cardiovasc Imaging. 2010;3:15-23.
65. Bansal M, Jeffriess L, Leano R, et al. Assessment of myocardial viability at dobutamine echocardiography by deformation analysis using tissue velocity and speckle-tracking. JACC Cardiovasc Imaging. 2010;3:121-31.
66. Hoffmann R, Altiok E, Nowak B, Heussen N, Kühl H, Kaiser H-J, et al. Strain rate measurement by Doppler echocardiography allows improved assessment of myocardial viability inpatients with depressed left ventricular function. J Am Col Cardiol. 2002;39:443-9.
67. Ypenburg C, Sieders A, Bleeker GB, Holman ER, van der Wall EE, Schalij MJ, et al. Myocardial contractile reserve predicts improvement in left ventricular function after cardiac resynchronization therapy. Am Heart J. 2007;154:1160-5.
68. Zhang Q, Fung JW, Yip GW, Chan JY, Lee AP, Lam Y, et al. Improvement of left ventricular myocardial short-axis, but not long-axis function or torsion after cardiac resynchronisation therapy: An assessment by two-dimensional speckle tracking. Heart. 2008;94:1464-71.
69. Mullens W, Grimm RA, Verga T, Dresing T, Starling RC, Wilkoff BL, et al. Insights from a cardiac resynchronization optimization clinic as part of a heart failure disease management program. J Am Coll Cardiol. 2009;53:765-73.
70. Khan FZ, Virdee MS, Palmer CR, Pugh PJ, O'Halloran D, Elsik M, et al. Targeted left ventricular lead placement to guide cardiac resynchronization therapy: the target study. A randomized, controlled trial. J Am Coll Cardiol. 2012;59:1509-18.
71. Saba S, Marek J, Schwartzman D, Jain S, Adelstein E, White P, et al. Echocardiography-guided left ventricular lead placement for cardiac resynchronization therapy results of the speckle tracking assisted resynchronization therapy for electrode region trial. Circ Heart Fail. 2013;6:427-34.
72. Bashir JG, Frank G, Tyers O, et al. Combined use of transesophageal echo and fluoroscopy for the placement of left ventricular pacing leads via the coronary sinus. Pacing Clin Electrophysiol. 2003;26:1951-4.
73. Cohen TJ, Juang G. Utility of intracardiac echocardiography to facilitate transvenous coronary sinus lead placement for biventricular cardioverter-defibrillator implantation. J Invasive Cardiol. 2003;15:685-6.
74. Shalaby AA. Utilization of intracardiac echocardiography to access the coronary sinus for left ventricular lead placement. Pacing Clin Electrophysiol. 2005;28:493-7.
75. Ishikawa T, Sumita S, Kimura K, Kikuchi M, Kosuge M, Kuji N, et al. Prediction of optimal atrioventricular delay in patients with implanted DDD pacemakers. Pacing Clin Electrophysiol. 1999;22:1365-71.
76. Ritter P, Padeletti L, Gillio-Meina L, et al. Determination of the optimal atrioventricular delay in DDD pacing. Comparison between echo and peak endocardial acceleration measurements. Europace. 1999;1:126-30.
77. Zhang Q, Fung JW-H, Chan Y-S, Chan HC-K, et al. The role of repeating optimization of atrioventricular interval during interim and long-term follow-up after cardiac resynchronization therapy. Intern J Cardiol. 2008;124: 211-7.
78. Auricchio A, Stellbrink C, Block M, Sack S, Vogt J, Bakker P, et al. Effect of pacing chamber and atrioventricular delay on acute systolic function of paced patients with congestive heart failure. Circulation. 1999;99:2993-3001.
79. Kass DA, Chen C-H, Curry C, Talbot M, Berger R, Fetics B, et al. Improved left ventricular mechanics from acute VDD pacing in patients with dilated cardiomyopathy and ventricular conduction delay. Circulation. 1999;99: 1567-73.
80. Nelson GS, Curry CW, Wyman BT, Kramer A, Declerck J, Talbot M, et al. Predictors of systolic augmentation from left ventricular preexcitation in patients with dilated cardiomyopathy and intraventricular conduction delay. Circulation. 2000;101:2703-9.
81. Breithardt OA, Stellbrink C, Kramer AP, Sinha AM, Franke A, Salo R, et al. Echocardiographic quantification of left ventricular asynchrony predicts an acute hemodynamic benefit of cardiac resynchronization therapy. J Am Coll Cardiol. 2002;40: 536-45.
82. Verbeek XA, Auricchio A, Yu Y, Ding J, Pochet T, Vernooy K, et al. Tailoring cardiac resynchronization therapy using interventricular asynchrony. Validation of a simple model. Am J Physiol Heart Circ Physiol. 2006;290:H968-77.
83. Pouleur A-C, Knappe D, Shah AM, Uno H, Bourgoun M, Foster E, et al. Relationship between improvement in left ventricular dyssynchrony and contractile function and clinical outcome with cardiac resynchronization therapy: The MADIT-CRT trial. Eur Heart J. 2011;32:1720-9.
84. Notabartolo D, Merlino JD, Smith AL, DeLurgio DB, Vera FV, Easley KA, et al. Usefulness of the peak velocity difference by tissue Doppler imaging technique as an effective predictor of

response to cardiac resynchronization therapy. Am J Cardiol. 2004;94:817-20.
85. White HD, Norris R, Brown MA, Brandt P, Whitlock R, Wild C. Left ventricular end-systolic volume as the major determinant of survival after recovery from myocardial infarction. Circulation. 1987;76:44-51.
86. Stellbrink C, Breithardt O-A, Franke A, Sack S, Bakker P, Auricchio A, et al. Impact of cardiac resynchronization therapy using hemodynamically optimized pacing on left ventricular remodeling in patients with congestive heart failure and ventricular conduction disturbances1. J Am Coll Cardiol. 2001; 38:1957-65.
87. Pitzalis MV, Iacoviello M, Romito R, Massari F, Rizzon B, Luzzi G, et al. Cardiac resynchronization therapy tailored by echocardiographic evaluation of ventricular asynchrony. J Am Coll Cardiol. 2002;40:1615-22.
88. Yu C-M, Gorcsan J, Bleeker GB, Zhang Q, Schalij MJ, Suffoletto MS, et al. Usefulness of tissue Doppler velocity and strain dyssynchrony for predicting left ventricular reverse remodeling response after cardiac resynchronization therapy. Am J Cardiol. 2007;100:1263-70.
89. Chung ES, Leon AR, Tavazzi L, Sun J-P, Nihoyannopoulos P, Merlino J, et al. Results of the predictors of response to CRT (prospect) trial. Circulation. 2008;117:2608-16.
90. Breithardt OA, Sinha AM, Schwammenthal E, Bidaoui N, Markus KU, Franke A, et al. Acute effects of cardiac resynchronization therapy on functional mitral regurgitation in advanced systolic heart failure. J Am Coll Cardiol. 2003;41:765-70.
91. Kanzaki H, Bazaz R, Schwartzman D, Dohi K, Sade LE, Gorcsan J. A mechanism for immediate reduction in mitral regurgitation after cardiac resynchronization therapy: Insights from mechanical activation strain mapping. J Am Coll Cardiol. 2004;44:1619-25.
92. Yu C-M, Fung W-H, Lin H, Zhang Q, Sanderson JE, Lau C-P. Predictors of left ventricular reverse remodeling after cardiac resynchronization therapy for heart failure secondary to idiopathic dilated or ischemic cardiomyopathy. J Am Coll Cardiol. 2003;91:684-8.
93. Nof E, Glikson M, Bar-Lev D, Gurevitz O, Luria D, Eldar M, et al. Mechanism of diastolic mitral regurgitation in candidates for cardiac resynchronization therapy. J Am Coll Cardiol. 2006; 97:1611-4.

# Role of Echocardiography in the Evaluation and Follow-up of Patients Receiving Ventricular Assist Devices

19
CHAPTER

*M Sonia Jain, Sunil Mankad*

## INTRODUCTION

For appropriate patients with refractory, end-stage heart failure, cardiac transplantation is considered the first-line therapy to improve long-term survival and decrease morbidity. However, limited donor organ availability of <2500 hearts per year in North America poses a logistical challenge. For carefully selected patients, durable mechanical circulatory support with a surgically implanted left ventricular assist device (LVAD) or biventricular assist device (BiVAD) has emerged as a reasonable alternative. Initially, assist devices were indicated as a 'bridge to transplantation' (BTT) to support patients with end-stage heart failure, as they awaited transplantation. North American and European guidelines endorse this as a Class I B recommendation. For a significant proportion of patients, LVAD may be implanted as a 'bridge to decision'. Such patients may suffer severe but potentially reversible, end-organ damage that may preclude their transplant candidacy, but who might recover cardiac function after a period of mechanical circulatory support. Occasionally, LVADs may be implanted as a 'bridge to recovery', to support the heart as it recovers from an acute, overwhelming injury, such as myocarditis. In successful cases, the LVAD can be explanted after sufficient myocardial recovery, thereby avoiding cardiac transplantation altogether. In 2003, there was a landmark approval by the US Food and Drug Administration (FDA) of the pulsatile-flow Thoratec HeartMate (HM) XVE for destination therapy (DT).[1] In 2010, the FDA approved the continuous flow LVAD (CF-LVAD) Thoratec HM-II for DT.[2] The LVAD as DT is increasingly implanted in patients with severe, symptomatic end-stage heart failure, on optimal medical and device therapy and deemed ineligible for transplantation, but with a life-expectancy of greater than one year. A HM-II device is shown in **Figure 19.1**. The LVADs improve heart failure symptoms, reduce morbidity, lower heart failure hospitalizations and improve mortality.

## A BRIEF OVERVIEW OF VENTRICULAR ASSIST DEVICES

The LVAD technology is a fascinating and rapidly evolving field.[3] The LVADs are classified as pulsatile flow or continuous flow devices. The first generation devices provide pulsatile flow utilizing pulsatile volume displacement pumps. They were bulkier, heavier, more challenging to implant, prone to complications, and less durable in the long-term. Examples include the HM-I, the Thoratec paracorporeal ventricular assist device, and the Novacor. These devices are rather obsolete in contemporary clinical practice, having been superseded by the newer generation continuous-flow devices. The FDA approved the continuous-flow HM-II (Thoratec, Pleasanton, CA) as BTT in 2008 and DT in 2010, and the HVAD (HeartWare International, Inc., Framingham, MA) as BTT therapy in 2012,[4] resulting in a remarkable technological dominance in clinical practice.[2,5] Since 2010, >95% of all implanted LVADs and 100% of DT devices are CF-LVADs. It is estimated that >2000 continuous-flow devices are implanted per year in the US, with DT accounting for 40% of overall implants.[6] Among CF-LVADs, the actuarial survival is 80% at the end of 1 year, and 70% at the end of 2 years.[6] Compared to pulsatile-flow devices, continuous-low devices have a dramatically improved durability, thereby decreasing reoperation rates, and a lower overall adverse event burden.[2,3,6,7] However, major adverse events, such as infection, bleeding, device malfunction, stroke or death remain a challenge.

The HM-II and HVAD have 3 serial intracorporeal components—an "LVAD pump" (consisting of a mechanical rotating impeller and motor), that is situated in an abdominal pocket and connected proximally to a titanium inflow cannula (IC) that is inserted into the LV apex, and distally to an outflow cannula (OC), which is a vascular graft anastomosed to the ascending aorta. This mechanical impeller is connected by a

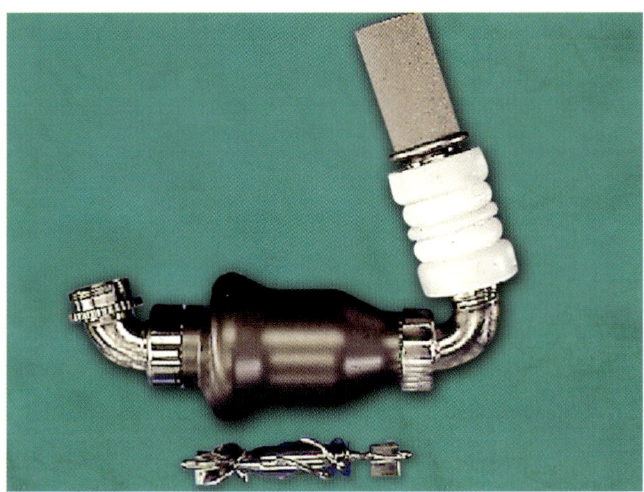

**Figure 19.1:** HeartMate II left ventricular assist device. It utilizes a high-speed rotary pump and can be utilized in small adults and children in addition to larger adults due to its significantly smaller size.

percutaneous driveline to an external battery and controller that are worn on a belt and shoulder backpack. Modifiable variables, such as pump flow, pump speed (in revolutions per minute or rpm), and power consumption are used to regulate pump function. Operating pump speeds for the HM-II are between 6,000 and 15,000 rpm with a maximum pump flow of 10 L/minute.

Echocardiography, both transthoracic (TTE) and transesophageal (TEE), plays an important role in 4 key phases, as endorsed by current guidelines.[8,9]

1. Preoperative TTE for the assessment of patients undergoing LVAD candidacy evaluation.
2. Perioperative management (TEE).
3. Postoperative assessment (TTE and TEE), and
4. Long-term periodic surveillance (serial TTE) for monitoring native myocardial and LVAD function, and troubleshooting alerts.

The TTE, TEE, and occasionally epicardial echocardiography can be utilized. A comprehensive understanding of the unique imaging characteristics and pitfalls is essential for the echocardiographer participating in the care of these complex patients.

## Role of Preoperative Echocardiography in Determining Candidacy

TTE is the most commonly used imaging modality for assessment of potential LVAD candidates. In acutely decompensated or technically challenging cases, TEE may be preferable. Echocardiography should be performed in all patients undergoing evaluation for candidacy of LVAD therapy for an assessment of ventricular structure and function, hemodynamics, cardiac valves and identifying specific findings that may affect the decision-making. A comprehensive echocardiography with an emphasis on obtaining requisite data as part of a "preimplantation" study should be completed. A detailed preimplantation TTE protocol is recommended in the 2015 American Society of Echocardiography (ASE) guidelines.[8]

There are several "red-flag findings" that might pose relative or absolute contraindications to LVAD implantation. In addition to performing a comprehensive study, attention must be focused on ruling out these out. These include the following:

- Morphological features of the left ventricle (small cavity, presence of extensive trabeculations, LV aneurysm, presence of intracardiac masses or thrombus, left atrial [LA] appendage thrombus).
- Acquired or congenital heart defects (atrial septal defect, ventricular septal defect, patent ductus arteriosus, or dictation of aorta).
- Significant valvular heart disease (prosthetic cardiac valves, greater than moderate valvular stenosis, greater than moderate mitral, tricuspid or pulmonary insufficiency, greater than mild aortic insufficiency).
- Aortic pathology (ascending aortic dilatation, aneurysm, dissection or atheroma, coarctation of aorta).
- Agitated saline contrast injection should be performed at rest and with Valsalva, to rule out the presence of patent foramen ovale (PFO) and significant intrapulmonary shunts. An example in which a PFO was not completely closed at the time of LVAD implantation is shown in **Figure 19.2A and B (Videos 19.1A and B)**.

### *Left Ventricular Function*

A detailed assessment of regional and global LV systolic and diastolic function should be performed.[8] The biplane method of disks (modified Simpson's rule) with appropriate use of microbubble contrast opacification is recommended for two-dimensional (2D) determination of LV ejection fraction (LVEF). When anatomically feasibility and expertise permits, three-dimensional (3D) volumetric quantification of LVEF is recommended. The LV end-diastolic dimension (LVEDD) should be accurately measured as it has prognostic significance. In one study, a relatively small LV cavity size (LVEDD <63 mm) was predictive of worse 30-day postoperative outcomes including prolonged inotropic support and death, but actuarial survival after 18 months was comparable to patients with larger ventricles.[10]

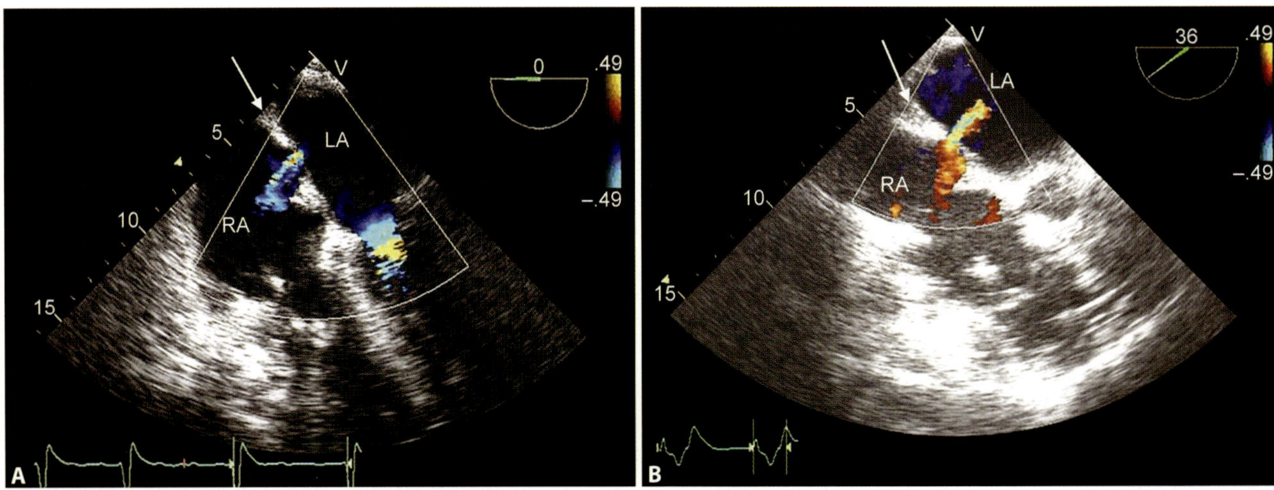


**Figure 19.2A and B:** The perioperative transesophageal echocardiographic images in a patient undergoing LVAD. (A) A left-to-right intra-atrial shunt by color Doppler through a patent foramen ovale pre-LVAD implantation. Closure of the shunt was initially unsuccessful at the time of LVAD implantation. (B) Post-LVAD imaging and now the shunt has reversed and was right-to-left as shown by color Doppler due to lowering of left atrial pressure with appropriate LVAD function. This led to significant hypoxia postoperatively and the shunt was subsequently closed percutaneously. The arrows point out the atrial septum.
*Abbreviations:* LA, left atrium; LVAD, left ventricular assist device; RA, right atrium.

### *Right Ventricular Function*

A thorough evaluation of right ventricular (RV) function is imperative, as it provides important prognostic information for surgical planning and perioperative outcomes. RV dysfunction detrimentally impacts survival, particularly early mortality. Such patients would benefit from pre-emptive BiVAD, rather than LVAD alone, implantation. Postoperative RV failure after LVAD implantation is associated with worse perioperative outcomes and long-term survival.[6] Postoperative complications include prolonged intravenous inotropic support, need for RV mechanical circulatory support with extracorporeal membrane oxygenation or RV assist device (RVAD) placement, and prohibitive perioperative mortality rate of 19–43%. Therefore, identifying preoperative variables that might predict postoperative RV failure is prognostically crucial and might influence candidacy or pre-empt the elective placement of a BiVAD. RV failure is due to complex pathophysiologic mechanisms, and predicting it preoperatively can be challenging. Risk scores incorporating clinical variables with echocardiographic and invasive hemodynamic parameters have been developed.[11] Multiple studies have shown that preoperative RV systolic dysfunction predicts postoperative RV failure.[11] Other potential predictors include RV absolute peak longitudinal strain of <9.6%,[12] an RV: LV end-diastolic diameter ratio of >0.75,[13] a short duration of tricuspid regurgitation (TR),[10] and RV tissue Doppler and strain imaging.[14] A detailed assessment of RV function and hemodynamics, incorporating quantitative parameters when possible, is recommended.[8,15]

### *Intracardiac Masses*

Intracardiac thrombi and masses increase the risk of thromboembolic stroke during device implantation, and they should be meticulously sought for. Microbubble contrast should be utilized, if necessary. Infectious endocarditis and active bacteremia are absolute contraindications to LVAD placement. Any suspicion of it should prompt an extensive evaluation, including multimodality imaging with TEE, computed tomography or magnetic resonance imaging, as indicated.[16]

### *Valvular Heart Disease*

An assessment for specific valvular issues is essential as it may have significant implications for surgical planning.[16] It is important to remember the pitfall that flow dependent Doppler derived hemodynamic data, such as gradients, velocities, regurgitant volume calculations, color flow Doppler profiles may be unreliable in the presence of a severely depressed cardiac index. Greater than moderate mitral stenosis will limit the transmitral LVAD inflow and therefore needs to be corrected with a bioprosthetic valve replacement.[16] Aortic stenosis (AS) is typically well-tolerated, because the OC bypasses the aortic valve, except in the event of severe pump failure when there will be insufficient de novo cardiac output through the native aortic valve. Patients with severe AS may be considered for valve replacement. A competent aortic valve is necessary for efficient LVAD function. An incompetent aortic valve creates a "wasteful" circulatory loop by redirecting a portion of the blood exiting the OC

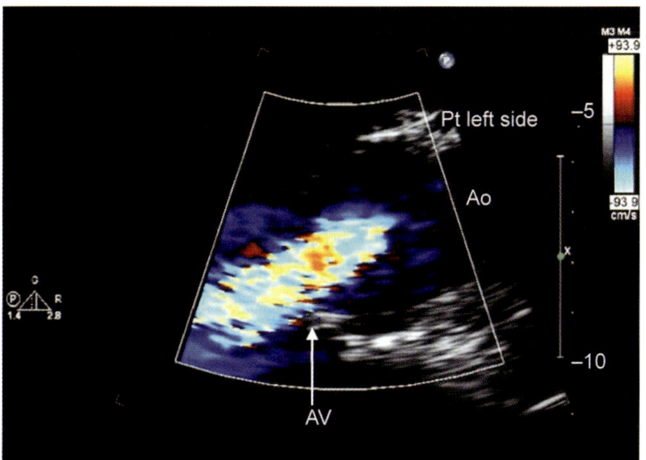


**Figure 19.3:** A zoomed-in parasternal long-axis image demonstrating moderately severe aortic regurgitation by color Doppler. This required placement of a "Park's stitch" (suture closure of the aortic valve) at the time of LVAD implantation.
*Abbreviations:* Ao, aorta; AV, aortic valve; LVAD, left ventricular assist device; Pt, patient.

back into the left ventricle, therefore increasing pump flow and decreasing effective stroke volume. An assessment of the degree of aortic regurgitation (AR), direction of the jet (central or eccentric), the integrity of the aortic valve cusps, and the presence of aortic root dilatation should be completed. The AR severity can be easily underestimated. If there is greater than mild AR, the heart failure team needs to be alerted so that TEE imaging and surgical correction of the incompetent valve can be undertaken before LVAD implantation.[16] Most cases can be corrected by a simple, central coaptation "Park stich" for central AR.[17] If the structural integrity of the aortic valve is compromised, strategies include patch closure, bioprosthetic valve replacement or possibly, transcatheter aortic valve replacement.[18] An example of moderately severe AR is shown which required surgical treatment at the time of LVAD implantation in **Figure 19.3 (Video 19.2)**. Moderate or greater tricuspid or pulmonary regurgitation may portend RV dysfunction, and may prompt tricuspid valve repair at the time of implant.[16] Significant mitral regurgitation (MR) is common in heart failure patients and often improves after LVAD due to improved ventricular hemodynamics. Prosthetic heart valves should be assessed by TTE and TEE, as indicated.[8] Even a normally functioning mechanical valve is at high risk of post-LVAD thrombosis due to low flow, and may warrant replacement with a bioprosthesis prior to LVAD implantation.

### *Thoracic Aorta*

The TEE is superior to TTE for the evaluation of aortic root enlargement that might predispose to AR, ascending aortic aneurysmal dilatation, and atheromatous disease.

### *Congenital Heart Disease*

Patients with congenital heart disease (CHD) and heart failure who are being considered for LVAD should undergo a thorough study by a team with expertise in CHD echocardiography. A meticulous search for interatrial and interventricular communications should be performed as they can lead to major postoperative complications when the left ventricle is decompressed, such as significant right-to-left shunting with systemic hypoxemia and paradoxical embolus, and if found, are often closed prior to LVAD implantation. An interatrial communication [PFO or atrial septal defects] should be probed for color flow imaging, and intravenous agitated saline injection with Valsalva release to simulate increased right atrial (RA) pressure. Similarly, a color Doppler evaluation of the interventricular septum (IVS) in multiple views may reveal a ventricular septal defect (congenital, postoperative or ischemic).

## Perioperative Transesophageal Echocardiography

### *Preimplantation*

A comprehensive perioperative TEE with imaging prior to, during, and post-LVAD implantation, should be performed by a cardiologist or anesthesiologist with advanced echocardiographic training.[8,19] The TEE is helpful to confirm the TTE findings, or may serve as the primary imaging modality in patients who are undergoing emergent device placement. Again, a detailed exam with emphasis on "checklist" parameters is recommended. Interatrial shunts, aortic pathology, intracardiac thrombus, infective endocarditis, native and prosthetic valves are better assessed by TEE rather than TTE. The use of anesthetic agents may interfere with the reliability of Doppler-derived hemodynamics, particularly with quantification of valve disease. On the preimplant images, the presence and degree of AR, interatrial shunt, mitral stenosis, TR, RV dysfunction, intracardiac thrombus, and ascending aorta pathology are specifically sought for, as these impact surgical planning and procedure. An AR is dependent on systemic blood pressure, and transitory inotrope use to augment systemic blood pressure may "unmask" its severity. The PFO detection should be emphasized. Following LVAD implantation, the left ventricle is "unloaded", resulting in a fall in LA pressures, thereby resulting in a right-to-left shunt, with two major attendant risks: paradoxical embolus with the potential for acute device thrombosis or delayed device malfunction and severe hypoxemia due to the shunting. The PFO identification will allow the surgeon to repair it prior to implantation and prevent these potentially disastrous consequences. Due to the significantly elevated LA pressures preimplant, PFO detection may be elusive. The PFO detection requires a focused interrogation of the interatrial septum with 2D and color Doppler with injection of intravenous agitated saline contrast with and without a ventilator aided breath hold and release to simulate the Valsalva maneuver. A visible increase in motion of the interatrial septum toward the left suggests an increase in RA pressure. The sensitivity of detection is increased by saline injection into a femoral vein. The rapid appearance of 3 or more bubbles within the left atrium (within 3 beats) after opacification of the right atrium is consistent with a diagnosis of an interatrial shunt. If the bubbles appear after a delay of 3–8 beats, it is indicative of an intrapulmonary shunt. However, the timing of bubble appearance depends on the size of the shunt and does not reliably distinguish between an interatrial and intrapulmonary shunt.[19,20]

## Postimplantation

Assesses for (i) specific surgical complications, (ii) native cardiac function, and (iii) immediate functioning of the implanted LVAD.

1. *Intracardiac air*: The surgical technique involves marked manipulation of the heart and coring of the LV apex to insert the IC. Hence, there is considerable air bubble entrapment, which appear as white refractors. A careful inspection of the cardiac chambers, LV apex, inflow and outflow cannulas, anastomotic sites, aortic root, and the ascending and descending aorta should be undertaken to ensure adequate deairing, prior to pump activation, in order to minimize the risk of air embolization. Air preferentially embolizes the anteriorly located right coronary artery, causing acute RV dysfunction or severe TR. This might necessitate reinstitution of the cardiopulmonary pump and further deairing.
2. *The left ventricular assist device function*: As soon as the pump is activated, the images should be annotated with the device name and pump speed (updated as indicated). An important clue to the optimal functioning of the new LVAD is the position of the IVS and relative sizes of the left and right ventricles. As the new implant starts to function, it invariably "unloads" the left heart and decreases the LA and LV pressures. This is visibly manifested as a slight leftward shift of the intra-atrial and interventricular septa. Rightward shift of the septum showed raise the suspicion of suboptimal pump function, or an issue with the IC. Alternatively, an extreme leftward septal shift suggests excessive LV unloading or very high pump speed, or markedly elevated right-sided pressures. The appearance of spontaneous echo contrast in the left chambers suggests device malfunction.
3. *Right ventricular dysfunction and severe tricuspid regurgitation*: Acute RV dysfunction may appear as a dilated, hypocontractile right ventricle with severe TR, and a consequent decrease in preload and suboptimal LVAD function. Careful examination for RV dysfunction and significant TR is essential, as it might influence the decision to place an RVAD.
4. *Interatrial shunt*: Up to 20% of patients with no detectable PFO on the preimplant TEE might have evidence of it postimplant due to the hemodynamic changes described above. Sudden hypoxemia on instituting the LVAD is a clue to a PFO. Imaging with agitated saline administration must routinely be repeated postimplant. If a PFO is found, it should be surgically closed.[16]
5. *Inflow cannula*: The tip of the IC is positioned at or near the LV apex and should optimally be aligned with the mitral inflow and demonstrate laminar flow with color flow Doppler. Sometimes, a slight angulation towards the septum may be seen. This is best visualized in the 2D orthogonal planes (midesophageal 4-chamber and 2-chamber views), and real-time 3D echocardiographic imaging can be complementary. Pulsed-wave (PW) and continuous-wave (CW) Doppler profile and velocities should be examined. A normal Doppler profile is low velocity, laminar, continuous with systolic predominance, and a diastolic nadir. The normal PW Doppler inflow filling velocity is 1–2 m/s for HM-II. HVAD inflow velocities cannot be measured due to artifact. The IC can be obstructed due to thrombus or anatomic malpositioning (abutment against the ventricular septum or muscle trabeculae) or a "suction" effect from an excessively decompressed left ventricle (high pump speeds) or an under filled left ventricle that causes a portion of the myocardium to impinge on the IC orifice. In these scenarios, there will be turbulent color flow with aliasing at the IC orifice and elevated peak velocities >2 m/s.
6. *Outflow cannula*: An OC is placed as an end-to-side anastomosis in the right anterolateral ascending aorta and best seen in the long axis view of the ascending aorta. The proximal portion cannot be visualized. Both PW and CW Doppler interrogation should be performed with the PW sample volume placed 1 cm proximal to the anastomosis. The typical peak velocity is 1–2 m/s.
7. *Aortic regurgitation*: An AR that was previously underappreciated can become more apparent post-implant due to favorable hemodynamics. Once the pump is activated, the AR duration depends on the aortic valve opening and pump speed; it can be intermittent, phasic or continuous. An M-mode interrogation in the long axis at a slow sweep speed of 25 m/s is recommended. AR duration, vena contracta width, the AR jet height, CW spectral Doppler imaging should be assessed. Because the LVAD flow is continuous and AR can extend into systole, diastolic flow reversal in the descending aorta is unreliable.

Due to significant lability of LV diastolic filling pressures, the pressure half-time method is not recommended in LVAD patients.

## Postoperative Troubleshooting

The differential diagnosis of postoperative instability includes hypovolemia, acute RV dysfunction, pulmonary embolus, tamponade, and LVAD malfunction. Bedside echocardiography can assist with rapid troubleshooting. With hypovolemia, the right and left ventricles will be underfilled and small in size. The features of acute RV dysfunction are described above. Diagnosing cardiac tamponade or constriction in the post-LVAD patient is challenging as the echocardiographic features of interventricular dependence will be absent. The tamponade may be isolated to a particular chamber (such as right atrium, left atrium or right ventricle) due to localized hematomas. Isolated chamber compression or unexplained pockets of echogenicity may be the only clue. A computed tomographic imaging is helpful in pulmonary embolus and confirming hematomas. The septal position, relative ventricular chamber sizes, appearance of spontaneous contrast in the left atrium, inflow and outflow cannula, and aortic valve opening can cumulatively provide clues to the etiology of LVAD malfunction.

## Left Ventricular Assist Device Surveillance Echocardiography

The first surveillance TTE study is recommended within two weeks of implant or prior to hospital discharge, followed by periodic imaging at specified intervals. The two primary goal of surveillance echocardiography are to assess (i) LVAD function and (ii) native cardiac function. The study should comprise a comprehensive baseline examination with additional LVAD-specific imaging such as inflow and outflow cannula location, color flow, PW and CW Doppler analysis at the baseline pump speed.[8,9,21] Based on the indication, additional imaging at other speeds for an 'LVAD speed change or optimization' protocol maybe needed. The LVAD type and pump speed in rpm should be annotated on the screen and included in the report. In CF- LVADs, cuff blood pressure measurement may not be possible due to a very narrow pulse pressure and impalpable pulse. Postoperatively, several patients will have invasively measured blood pressure available. In stable outpatients, a noninvasive handheld Doppler derived device to interrogate peripheral pulse accurately measures blood pressure.[22]

## Left Ventricular Size and Systolic Function

The LVADs result in a direct unloading of the left ventricle. In stable patients with normally functioning HM-II CF-LVADs, a significant decrease in LV size, LV mass, mitral valve deceleration time, and an average increase in LVEF of 15% can be expected at 3 months.[23] Linear 2D measurement of LVEDD and end-systolic diameter (LVESD), based on electrocardiographic timing, in the parasternal long axis view, is recommended. An LVEDD has been shown to be reasonably reproducible and serial measurements should be reported to reflect temporal changes in LV size (at similar pump speeds). A small left ventricle may indicate excessive LV unloading or diminished stroke volume. Quantification of LV volumes can be underestimated, even with the use of microbubble contrast, due to challenges posed by IC artifact and apical dropout. Where possible, the biplane method of disks is preferred for calculation of LVEF. If the cardiac apex cannot be adequately visualized due to the IC, the Quinones method, which assumes an akinetic apex, can be used. If the apical views are suboptimal, the fractional area change method (LV end-diastolic area – LV end-systolic area/LV end-diastolic area) measured in the parasternal short-axis view, at the mid-papillary muscle level, can be helpful.[21] The mitral valve deceleration time has been shown to increase in LVAD patients reflecting improved LV diastolic filling pressures.[23] Standard diastolic function parameters have not been validated in patients with CF-LVAD support.

### *Right Ventricle*

RV dimensions and function are assessed as per the guidelines of the ASE.[15] Suggested parameters specific to this patient population include RV fractional area change (RVFAC) and tricuspid annular plane systolic excursion (TAPSE). Studies evaluating improvement of RVFAC following LVAD placement have shown discrepant results.[23,24] A recent study suggests that TAPSE may not distinguish patients with RV dysfunction.[25]

### *Aortic Valve*

Aortic valve opening is thought to depend on the interplay between preload, afterload, native cardiac contractility, and the efficiency of LV unloading by the LVAD. If the aortic valve fails to open at relatively low pump speeds, it suggests poor myocardial function. The frequency and duration of aortic valve opening is best assessed by M-mode acquisition over 5–6 cardiac cycles at a slow sweep speed of 25–50 mm/s. The aortic valve can open with every cardiac cycle, intermittently or not at all. A persistently closed aortic valve predisposes to stasis and thrombus formation in the aortic root and development of new onset or de novo AR. New onset AR can occur in a substantial proportion, up to 33% of patients.[26-29] Comprehensive imaging incorporating multiple parameters for quantification of AR with emphasis on aortic root dimension, and valve morphology should be performed.[30,31]

In the parasternal long-axis view, the measurement of vena contracta and relative jet width is recommended. A ratio of regurgitant jet width/LV outflow tract width >45% suggests more than moderate AR. A recent paper by Cowger et al. provided a comprehensive review of AR in LVAD patients.[32]

### Mitral Valve

Typically, the severity of MR is markedly reduced in LVAD supported patients, due to favorable LV hemodynamics and decrease in LV size. An increase in MR severity deserves attention to LV decompression parameters and IC anatomical interference with the subvalvular apparatus.

### Tricuspid Valve

As with MR, TR typically decreases in stable patients maintained on LVAD support. An increase in TR may portend RV dysfunction or unfavorable hemodynamics and should be assessed in a standard method.[30]

## Interventricular Septal Position

Understanding the relevance of the interventricular septal position in LVAD patients is vital. It should be reported as neutral, leftward shifted or rightward shifted. A leftward shift is seen in RV dysfunction, decreased LV preload, excessive LV unloading (high pump speeds). A rightward shift suggests elevated LV diastolic pressures from inadequate decompression (low pump speeds), pump malfunction, or severe AR. These are discussed below.

### Inflow Cannula

The alignment and Doppler interrogation of the IC is performed in the apical four-chamber and two-chamber views. Color flow, PW and CW Doppler are used to assess the LVAD Doppler profile and maximal systolic and diastolic velocities, as described above. An example of a normally functioning IC is shown in **Figure 19.4A and B (Videos 19.3A and B)**. Velocities less than 2 m/s are generally considered normal **(Figure 19.4C)**.

### Outflow Cannula

The high left parasternal long-axis view (for the end-to-side anastomosis in the mid ascending aorta), and the right parasternal view with the patient in the right lateral decubitus position (for the long axis of the OC) are suggested. Color flow, PW and CW Doppler interrogation is required, with the PW sample volume placed at least 1 cm proximal to the anastomosis. Shown in **Figure 19.5A and B (Videos 19.4A and B)** is a normally functioning OC. An in vitro study demonstrated that pump flow can be noninvasively calculated as the product of the PW Doppler velocity time integral and cross sectional area of the OC, and correlated well with measured flow.[33]

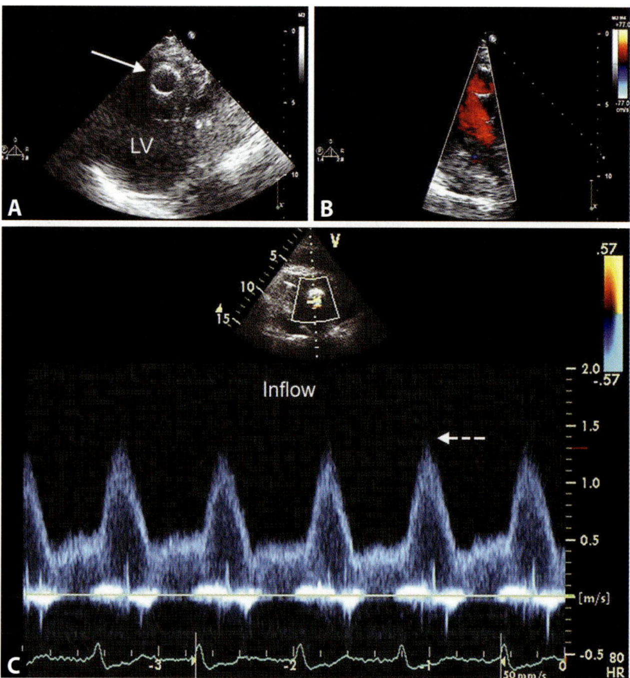


**Figure 19.4A to C:** (A) An apical image of the left ventricle. The inflow cannula of the LVAD can be seen with no evidence of thrombus (arrow). (B) Nice laminar, nonturbulent color Doppler flow. (C) Normal pulsed Doppler velocities of the inflow cannula (1.5 m/s, dashed arrow).

*Abbreviations:* LV, left ventricle; LVAD, left ventricular assist device.

## Troubleshooting Left Ventricular Assist Device Malfunction

When LVAD malfunction is suspected, an expedient evaluation for the etiology should be pursued due to the potential for significant morbidity and mortality, and even surgery for urgent pump replacement.[8,34]

### Low Pump Flow with Increased Power

In this setting, the primary issues are pump failure (due to pump or OC obstruction) or an abnormal increase in afterload. A rightward IVS, spontaneous echo contrast in the left atrium and left ventricle, aortic valve opening with each cycle, and low flow velocities (<20 cm/s) with regurgitant flow in the inflow and outflow cannulas are echocardiographic clues.

1. *Outflow cannula obstruction*: The TEE is preferable for evaluation of the OC. The peak velocity will be >2 m/s

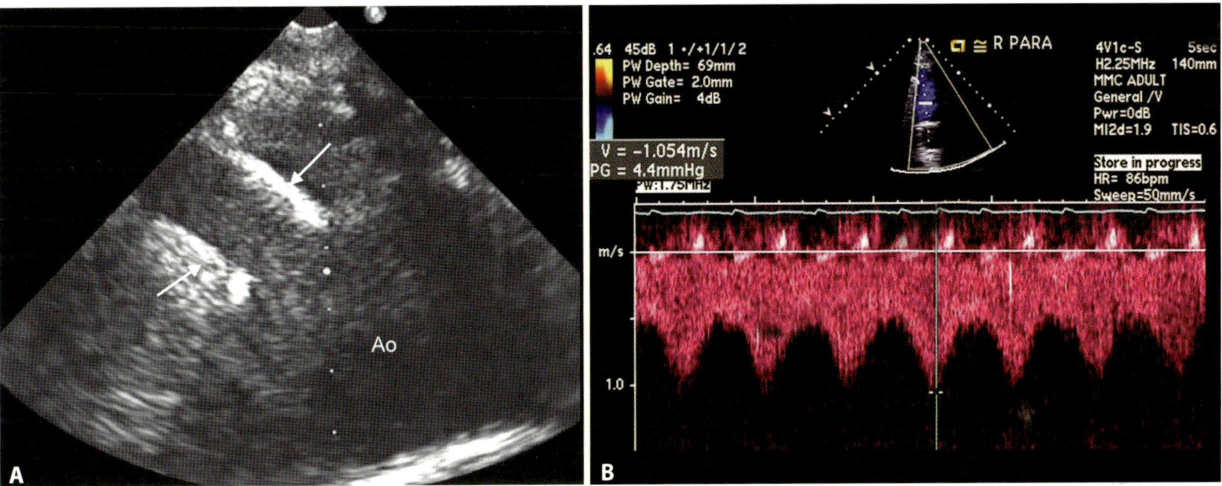


**Figure 19.5A and B:** (A) A right parasternal view demonstrating the LVAD outflow cannula (arrows) entering the aorta (Ao). (B) Pulsed-Doppler velocities are shown and are again noted to be normal (<2 m/s).
*Abbreviations:* Ao, aorta; LAVD, left ventricular assist device.

in the event of obstruction. With kinking of the OC, the Doppler signal cannot be obtained in any view.

2. *Intracardiac thrombus:* Typical locations are the LA appendage, a pocket of the LV apex close to the IC, the IVS and inferior wall and the aortic root or anastomosis site. An example of an LV thrombus obstructing the IC is shown in **Figure 19.6 (Video 19.5)**.
3. *Pump obstruction*: The significant acoustic shadowing from the impeller precludes adequate visualization. Pump thrombosis is typically a diagnosis based on incorporation of clinical variables, and ruling out thrombus in other locations.
4. *Increased afterload states*: This could be due to increased systemic vascular resistance from poorly controlled hypertension, or significant compensatory systemic vasoconstriction (hypovolemia, acute blood loss). The LV unloading is compromised with a rightward shift of the IVS, increased LV size, worsening MR, decreased aortic valve opening with each cycle, and increased peak OC velocity (>2.0 m/s).

### Low Pump Flow with Normal Power

The differential includes etiologies that impede LV filling, such as RV dysfunction, severe TR, hypovolemia or IC obstruction. This should be assessed as previously described.

### High Pump Flow with Low Cardiac Output

When the LVAD output exceeds the estimated forward cardiac output, significant AR should be suspected.

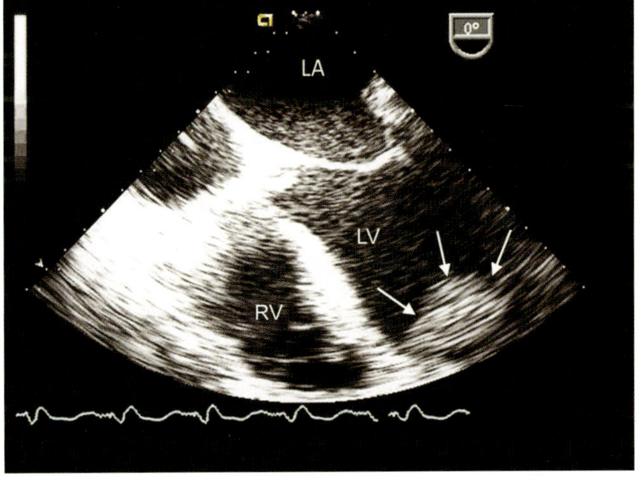


**Figure 19.6:** A transesophageal echocardiographic 4-chamber view demonstrating a left ventricular apical thrombus (arrows). The thrombus was partially obstructing the LVAD inflow cannula which was also at the apex, and this led to abnormal LVAD function. This required surgical intervention with restoration of normal LVAD function after removal of the clot.
*Abbreviations:* LA, left atrium; LV, left ventricle; LAVD, left ventricular assist device; RV, right ventricle.

## SUMMARY

Echocardiography is an indispensable imaging modality in the care of LVAD patients at different stages: the evaluation of patients for LVAD candidacy, perioperative guidance, postoperative troubleshooting, and post-LVAD long-term surveillance. It should be performed and interpreted by sonographers and echocardiographers with appropriate training and experience, and complemented by multimodality imaging, where necessary. A meticulous "checklist" approach and focused communication with the heart failure team is recommended to avoid missing pertinent data that might impact patient management. Familiarity with the fundamentals of LVAD technology and echocardiographic findings is encouraged, because of the rapid increase in implanted mechanical circulatory support.

## VIDEO LEGENDS

**Video 19.1:** Perioperative transesophageal echocardiographic images in a patient undergoing LVAD (same as in Figure 19.2). (A) A left to right intra-atrial shunt by color Doppler through a patent foramen ovale pre-LVAD implantation. Closure of the shunt was initially unsuccessful at the time of LVAD implantation. (B) Post-LVAD imaging and now the shunt has reversed and was right to left as shown by color Doppler due to lowering of left atrial pressure with appropriate LVAD function. This led to significant hypoxia postoperatively and the shunt was subsequently closed percutaneously.

**Video 19.2:** A zoomed in parasternal long-axis color Doppler image demonstrating moderately-severe aortic regurgitation. This required placement of a "Park's stitch" (suture closure of the aortic valve) at the time of LVAD implantation.

**Video 19.3:** (A) The inflow cannula of the LVAD can be seen with no evidence of thrombus. (B) Nice laminar, nonturbulent color Doppler flow.

**Video 19.4:** (A) Right parasternal view demonstrating the LVAD outflow cannula entering the aorta. (B) Color Doppler image showing normal flow through the outflow cannula.

**Video 19.5:** A transesophageal echocardiographic 4-chamber view demonstrating an LV apical thrombus (same patient as in Figure 19.6). The thrombus was partially obstructing the LVAD inflow cannula which was also at the apex and this led to abnormal LVAD function. This required surgical intervention with restoration of normal LVAD function after removal of the clot.

## REFERENCES


1. Rose EA, Gelijns AC, Moskowitz AJ, et al. Long-term use of a left ventricular assist device for end-stage heart failure. New Eng J Med. 2001;345:1435-43.
2. Slaughter MS, Rogers JG, Milano CA, et al. Advanced heart failure treated with continuous-flow left ventricular assist device. New Eng J Med. 2009;361:2241-51.
3. Stewart GC, Givertz MM. Mechanical circulatory support for advanced heart failure: patients and technology in evolution. Circulation. 2012;125:1304-15.
4. Aaronson KD, Slaughter MS, Miller LW, et al. Use of an intrapericardial, continuous-flow, centrifugal pump in patients awaiting heart transplantation. Circulation. 2012;125:3191-200.
5. Miller LW, Pagani FD, Russell SD, et al. Use of a continuous-flow device in patients awaiting heart transplantation. New Eng J Med. 2007;357:885-96.
6. Kirklin JK, Naftel DC, Pagani FD, et al. Sixth INTERMACS annual report: a 10,000-patient database. J Heart Lung Transplant. 2014;33:555-64.
7. Park SJ, Milano CA, Tatooles AJ, et al. Outcomes in advanced heart failure patients with left ventricular assist devices for destination therapy. Circulation. Circ Heart Fail. 2012;5:241-8.
8. Stainback RF, Estep JD, Agler DA, et al. Echocardiography in the Management of Patients with Left Ventricular Assist Devices: Recommendations from the American Society of Echocardiography. J Am Soc Echocardiogr. 2015;28:853-909.
9. Ammar KA, Umland MM, Kramer C, et al. The ABCs of left ventricular assist device echocardiography: a systematic approach. Eur Heart J Cardiovasc Imaging. 2012;13:885-99.
10. Topilsky Y, Oh JK, Shah DK, et al. Echocardiographic predictors of adverse outcomes after continuous left ventricular assist device implantation. JACC Cardiovasc Imaging. 2011;4:211-22.
11. Matthews JC, Koelling TM, Pagani FD, et al. The right ventricular failure risk score a pre-operative tool for assessing the risk of right ventricular failure in left ventricular assist device candidates. J Am Coll Cardiol. 2008;51:2163-72.
12. Grant AD, Smedira NG, Starling RC, et al. Independent and incremental role of quantitative right ventricular evaluation for the prediction of right ventricular failure after left ventricular assist device implantation. J Am Coll Cardiol. 2012;60:521-8.
13. Vivo RP, Cordero-Reyes AM, Qamar U, et al. Increased right-to-left ventricle diameter ratio is a strong predictor of right ventricular failure after left ventricular assist device. J Heart Lung Transplant. 2013;32:792-9.
14. Kato TS, Jiang J, Schulze PC, et al. Serial echocardiography using tissue Doppler and speckle tracking imaging to monitor right ventricular failure before and after left ventricular assist device surgery. JACC Heart Fail. 2013;1:216-22.
15. Rudski LG, Lai WW, Afilalo J, et al. Guidelines for the echocardiographic assessment of the right heart in adults: a report from the American Society of Echocardiography endorsed by the European Association of Echocardiography, a registered branch of the European Society of Cardiology, and the Canadian Society of Echocardiography. J Am Soc Echocardiogr. 2010;23:685-713.
16. Feldman D, Pamboukian SV, Teuteberg JJ, et al. The 2013 International Society for Heart and Lung Transplantation Guidelines for mechanical circulatory support: executive summary. J Heart Lung Transplant. 2013;32:157-87.
17. Park SJ, Liao KK, Segurola R, et al. Management of aortic insufficiency in patients with left ventricular assist devices: a simple coaptation stitch method (Park's stitch). J Thoracic Cardiovasc Surg. 2004;127:264-6.
18. Seiffert M, Diemert P, Koschyk D, et al. Transapical implantation of a second-generation transcatheter heart valve in patients with noncalcified aortic regurgitation. JACC Cardiovasc Interv. 2013;6:590-7.
19. Hahn RT, Abraham T, Adams MS, et al. Guidelines for performing a comprehensive transesophageal echocardiographic examination: recommendations from the American Society of Echocardiography and the Society of Cardiovascular Anesthesiologists. J Am Soc Echocardiogr. 2013;26:921-64.

20. Woods TD, Patel A. A critical review of patent foramen ovale detection using saline contrast echocardiography: when bubbles lie. J Am Soc Echocardiogr. 2006;19:215-22.
21. Estep JD, Chang SM, Bhimaraj A, et al. Imaging for ventricular function and myocardial recovery on nonpulsatile ventricular assist devices. Circulation. 2012;125:2265-77.
22. Bennett MK, Roberts CA, Dordunoo D, et al. Ideal methodology to assess systemic blood pressure in patients with continuous-flow left ventricular assist devices. J Heart Lung Transplant. 2010;29:593-4.
23. Topilsky Y, Oh JK, Atchison FW, et al. Echocardiographic findings in stable outpatients with properly functioning HeartMate II left ventricular assist devices. J Am Soc Echocardiogr. 2011;24:157-69.
24. Lam KM, Ennis S, O'Driscoll G, et al. Observations from non-invasive measures of right heart hemodynamics in left ventricular assist device patients. J Am Soc Echocardiogr. 2009;22:1055-62.
25. Raina A, Seetha Rammohan HR, Gertz ZM, et al. Postoperative right ventricular failure after left ventricular assist device placement is predicted by preoperative echocardiographic structural, hemodynamic, and functional parameters. J Cardiac Fail. 2013;19:16-24.
26. Pak SW, Uriel N, Takayama H, et al. Prevalence of de novo aortic insufficiency during long-term support with left ventricular assist devices. J Heart Lung Transplant. 2010;29:1172-6.
27. Cowger J, Pagani FD, Haft JW, et al. The development of aortic insufficiency in left ventricular assist device-supported patients. Circ Heart Fail. 2010;3:668-74.
28. Aggarwal A, Raghuvir R, Eryazici P, et al. The development of aortic insufficiency in continuous-flow left ventricular assist device-supported patients. Ann Thoracic Surg. 2013;95: 493-8.
29. Jorde UP, Uriel N, Nahumi N, et al. Prevalence, significance, and management of aortic insufficiency in continuous flow left ventricular assist device recipients. Circ Heart Fail. 2014;7:310-9.
30. Zoghbi WA, Enriquez-Sarano M, Foster E, et al. Recommendations for evaluation of the severity of native valvular regurgitation with two-dimensional and Doppler echocardiography. J Am Soc Echocardiogr. 2003;16:777-802.
31. Lancellotti P, Tribouilloy C, Hagendorff A, et al. European Association of Echocardiography recommendations for the assessment of valvular regurgitation. Part 1: aortic and pulmonary regurgitation (native valve disease). Eur J Echocardiogr. 2010;11:223-244.
32. Cowger J, Rao V, Massey T, et al. Comprehensive review and suggested strategies for the detection and management of aortic insufficiency in patients with a continuous-flow left ventricular assist device. J Heart Lung Transplant. 2015; 34:149-57.
33. Schwarz KQ, Parikh SS, Chen X, et al. Non-invasive flow measurement of a rotary pump ventricular assist device using quantitative contrast echocardiography. J Am Soc Echocardiogr. 2010;23:324-9.
34. Catena E, Milazzo F, Montorsi E, et al. Left ventricular support by axial flow pump: the echocardiographic approach to device malfunction. J Am Soc Echocardiogr. 2005;18:1422.

# Transesophageal Echocardiography for Heart Transplantation and Mechanical Circulatory Support

20

CHAPTER

*Alina Nicoara, Madhav Swaminathan*

## HEART FAILURE, SURGERY AND THE ROLE OF ECHOCARDIOGRAPHY

Heart failure is a global phenomenon that often has the word 'epidemic' associated with it to indicate the relentless nature of its spread. The burden of heart failure is expected to increase as a result of an aging population combined with the improved survival from other cardiovascular diseases that lead to left ventricular (LV) dysfunction (e.g. myocardial infarction). Increasingly, these patients who survive a serious cardiac injury, but have persistent ventricular dysfunction precluding normal end-organ function experience a poor quality of life and high rates of morbidity and mortality. In 2010, heart failure noted in 1 out of 9 death certificates in the US.[1] At the age of 40, the lifetime risk of developing heart failure is 20%, and the 1-year heart failure mortality rate is 20%. The estimated annual cost of heart failure is about $32 billion, indicating the magnitude of its burden on the global economy.[1]

Most heart failure patients are managed medically. A proportion of those with end-stage heart failure that continue to decompensate despite optimal medical therapy will require surgical management. While orthotopic heart transplantation (OHT) remains the cornerstone of surgical therapy for heart failure, not all patients will qualify for this option and may become candidates instead for various forms of mechanical circulatory support (MCS). Continuing advances in donor and recipient selection, organ procurement, and immunosuppressant therapy have led to an increase in short- and long-term survival among OHT recipients. However, the chronic shortage of suitable organ donors remains the rate-limiting step in providing OHT as an option for all qualified patients. With parallel and rapid advances in the development of devices, MCS has therefore emerged as a valuable and viable option in the management of heart failure patients.

Echocardiography remains a valuable imaging tool in the donor organ selection process and preoperative screening, perioperative management, and post-transplant follow-up of recipients. In the operating room, transesophageal echocardiography (TEE) provides valuable structural and functional information on the newly transplanted heart. In patients undergoing MCS implantation, TEE not only provides information that would impact device operation, but also assists with device orientation and functional effects.

## HEART TRANSPLANTATION

In the field of heart transplantation, the role of TEE can be grouped according to the timing of its use. It can be useful as a diagnostic and monitoring instrument in the following time periods:

- Cardiac donor screening.
- Intraoperative monitoring prior to transplantation.
- Intraoperative assessment of early allograft functions immediately following transplantation.
- Hemodynamic management during the early post-operative period in surgical intensive care.

### Donor Screening

The chronic shortage of suitable donor hearts has led to liberalized acceptance criteria to include higher-risk (marginal) donor hearts.[2] Older donors are increasingly considered suitable despite the potential for transmitting atherosclerotic, hypertensive, and valvular heart diseases. This approach has proved to be valuable when matching marginal donors with higher-risk recipients that have a greater risk of short-term mortality or those with significant comorbidities.

While transthoracic echocardiography (TTE) remains the mainstay of donor heart evaluations, TEE has been shown to be useful in providing consistent high-quality imaging when TTE has proved inadequate, such as in ventilated organ donors.

The goals of the initial echocardiographic assessment are to (a) rule out structural defects, (b) assess global ventricular function, and (c) exclude significant wall-motion abnormalities (WMA). Therefore, the initial evaluation should be performed only after adequate hemodynamic optimization with minimal inotropic support.

### Structural Lesions

The prognostic significance of LV hypertrophy, defined as a wall thickness greater than 11 mm in the absence of underfilling of the ventricle (pseudohypertrophy) is unclear. While there is some evidence that LV hypertrophy can adversely impact post-OHT outcome, others have refuted this claim.[2-4] While most structural abnormalities will preclude eligibility for transplantation, mild lesions, such as mitral valve prolapse in the absence of significant regurgitation, a functionally normal bicuspid aortic valve, or a small secundum-type atrial septal defect or patent foramen ovale are exceptions.

### Global Function

While the minimum acceptable LV ejection fraction (EF) for qualifying as a suitable donor is not defined, an EF greater than 45% without significant inotropic support is desirable.[5] When the EF is assessed as below 45%, the donor is usually classified in the marginal list. One relevant etiology of global LV dysfunction in heart donors is brain death. Following brain death, up to 42% of patients can present with LV dysfunction. However, one study found that there was significant improvement over time in ventricular function in over half of the brain dead patients eventually leading to transplantation.[6]

### Regional Function

The assessment of segmental WMAs assumes significance due to the risk of accelerated graft vasculopathy in the transplanted heart. Given the high incidence of coronary artery disease (CAD) within 5 years of transplantation, donors with significant CAD should be excluded. Segmental WMAs in donor hearts may be due to CAD, myocardial contusion, or ventricular dysfunction following traumatic brain injury. While myocardial contusion may be indistinguishable from an infarction, ventricular dysfunction after spontaneous intracranial hemorrhage often spares the LV apex owing to the pattern of sympathetic LV innervation.[7] Transplantation of hearts with segmental WMAs can be associated with significant early graft failure.[8]

## Intraoperative Monitoring Prior to Transplantation

The role of TEE during the immediate pretransplant period is directed more towards monitoring than diagnosis as the surgical decision has already been made on extensive preoperative diagnostic imaging. The emphasis during this time is on hemodynamic management and identification of embolic risk.

### Hemodynamic Management

While most patients present with idiopathic or ischemic cardiomyopathy, the occasional recipient will present with hypertrophic cardiomyopathy or severe noncompaction.[9,10] A common feature of those with ischemic or idiopathic cardiomyopathy is global cardiac dilatation, hence the term, *dilated cardiomyopathy*. Hemodynamic parameters in these patients are delicately poised and critically dependent on adequate preload and optimized afterload to enable maximal stroke volumes. The induction of general anesthesia can upset this delicate balance. Hence, TEE can be extremely valuable in assisting with hemodynamic management in the anesthetized state. Patients with hypertrophic hearts often display restrictive physiology and depend on adequate afterload, heart rate, and sinus rhythm. The anesthetized state combined with the effects of positive pressure ventilation and dynamic valvular lesions lead to poor correlation between measured filling pressures and intracardiac volume. Intraoperative hemodynamic management in these patients is therefore greatly enhanced by the presence of TEE which can be used as an adjunct to invasive pressure monitors. It may also be extremely useful when placement of the pulmonary artery (PA) catheter is challenging owing to large dilated ventricles, incompetent tricuspid valves, and the low cardiac output state. Additionally, the presence of right ventricular (RV) hypertrophy in the recipient is suggestive of long-standing pulmonary hypertension which should alert the intraoperative team to the risk of acute RV dysfunction in the transplanted heart.

A subset of patients will present for transplantation with pre-existing MCS devices in situ. In these patients, TEE can be useful in distinguishing whether hemodynamic compromise is a result of inadequate preload, afterload or malpositioned MCS cannulae.[11]

### Identification of Embolic Risk

Embolic risk in the recipient may be increased by the presence of thrombi in the LV apex or left atrial appendage **(Figure 20.1)**. The presence of sluggish blood flow in the dilated LV, characterized by spontaneous echo contrast or "smoke", is accompanied by a high incidence of apical thrombus formation **(Figure 20.2)**. While TEE is not the ideal imaging modality to determine the presence of an apical thrombus, it should be ruled out as far as possible and extreme caution exercised in handling of the LV prior to cardiopulmonary bypass (CPB). The frequent presence of atrial fibrillation in these patients should prompt the search for possible thrombi in the left atrial appendage.

Another potential source of embolism includes detachment of atheromatous plaque from the ascending aorta during aortic cannulation **(Figure 20.3)**. The ascending

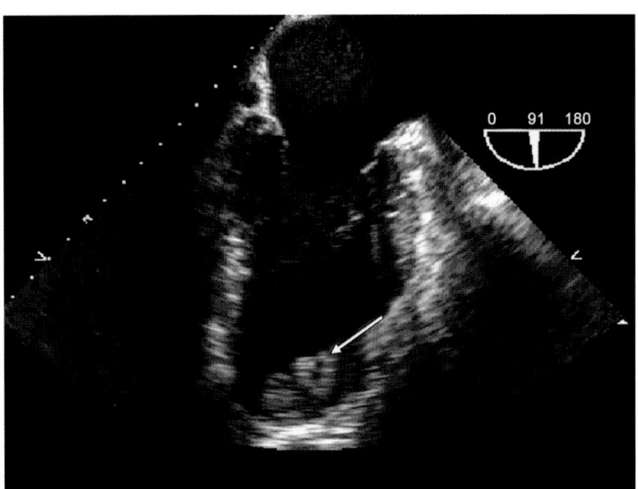


**Figure 20.1:** Mid-esophageal 2-chamber view demonstrating a thrombus in the apical region (arrow) adjacent to the anterior wall of the left ventricle.

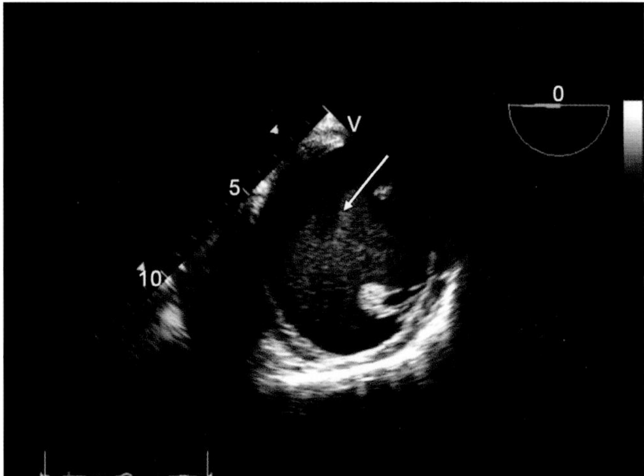


**Figure 20.3:** A large atheromatous plaque (arrow) can be seen adherent to the aortic intima in this upper esophageal ascending aorta short-axis view.

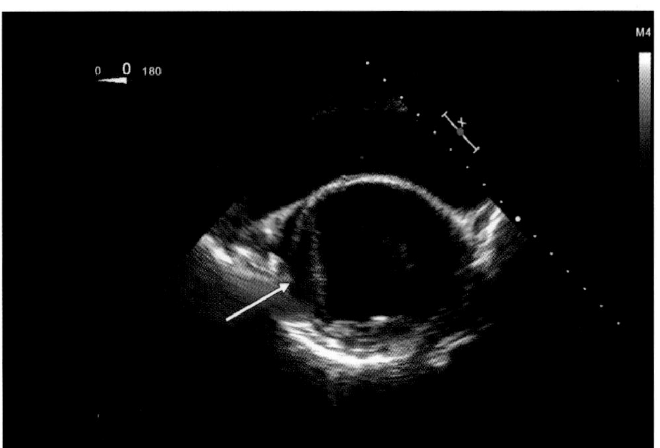


**Figure 20.2:** Transgastric mid-short-axis view of the left ventricle demonstrating a dilated chamber with spontaneous contrast due to sluggish flow (arrow).

aorta should be examined for atherosclerotic plaque before aortic cannulation using epiaortic ultrasound if required.[12] Air entrainment during explantation of a pre-existing MCS device may also lead to systemic embolization of air bubbles, and TEE can be particularly sensitive in detection of intracardiac air.

## Intraoperative Post-transplantation Monitoring

The immediate post-transplant period probably represents the most important period where TEE imaging provides valuable diagnostic information with prognostic implications. The imaging approach with TEE begins in the period just before discontinuation of CPB, proceeds with a structural and functional assessment of the allograft taking into account the atria, ventricles and anastomotic sites. An imaging approach with TEE is suggested in **Table 20.1**. However, the proper imaging approach is critically dependent on an understanding of the surgical technique.

### *Surgical Technique*

The biatrial technique of Lower and Shumway was the primary method for nearly 30 years.[13] This has been then largely supplanted by the bicaval anastomotic technique as the method of choice in adults.[14] The bicaval anastomotic technique is associated with preserved atrial geometry and function, improved cardiac output, and less disruption in the geometry of the atrioventricular valves. This results in reduced valvular regurgitation, fewer conduction abnormalities, less thrombus formation in the left atrium, and decreased perioperative mortality.[15] In the standard technique of Lower and Shumway, most of the native atrial walls and the interatrial septum are left in situ, leaving the inferior and superior vena cavae, and pulmonary veins undisturbed. In the donor heart, a left atrial cuff is created by incising through the pulmonary vein orifices, whereas the right atrial cuff is created by incising through the inferior vena caval orifice and extending the incision towards the base of the right atrial appendage. With the bicaval anastomotic technique, most of the native atrial tissue is excised, thereby creating inferior and superior vena caval cuffs for end-to-end anastomoses with the donor vena cavae. Anastomoses of the aorta and PA remain the same in both techniques.

**Table 20.1:** Imaging approach using transesophageal echocardiography to assess a newly transplanted heart

| *Assessment goal* | *Useful imaging views* |
|---|---|
| Intracardiac air | ME4C, MELAX, bicaval, ME AVLAX |
| LV structure and function | TG mid-SAX, ME4C, MELAX |
| RV structure and function | ME4C, RV inflow outflow |
| LV diastolic function | Mitral annular and transmitral flow velocities |
| Atrioventricular valves | Most ME views with CFD/spectral Doppler |
| Pulmonary venous anastomoses | Modified ME4C focused on LAA and LUPV, Bicaval to view RUPV |
| Pulmonary arterial anastomosis | Ascending aorta SAX, UE aortic arch SAX |

*Abbreviations:* AVLAX, aortic valve long-axis; CFD, color flow Doppler; LAA, left atrial appendage; LAX, long-axis; LUPV, left upper pulmonary vein; LV, left ventricular; ME, mid-esophageal; ME4C, mid-esophageal 4-chamber; RUPV, right upper pulmonary vein; RV, right ventricular; SAX, short-axis; TG, transgastric; UE, upper-esophageal.

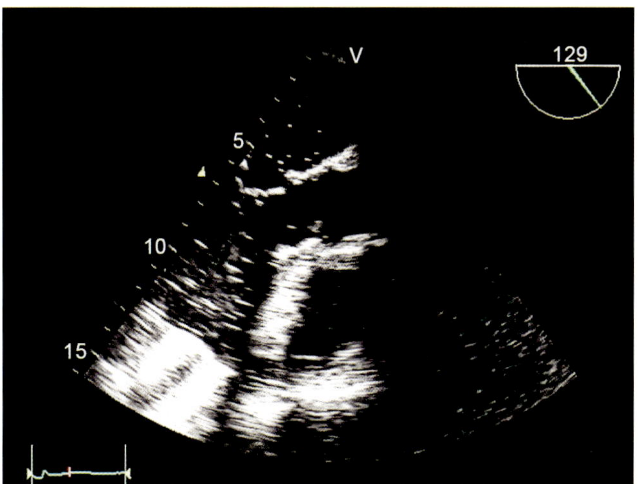


**Figure 20.4:** Mid-esophageal long-axis view in a patient with a left ventricular assist device. The inflow cannula can be seen as an echo bright structure at the left ventricular apex while multiple air bubbles can be seen as bright 'dots' throughout the left ventricle and left atrium.

## *Before Discontinuation of Cardiopulmonary Bypass*

Prior to weaning from CPB, TEE can be useful in monitoring the extent of intracardiac air and assist with de-airing strategies. The resumption of ventilation will result in a sudden increase in entrained air in the left ventricle with the most common sites of retention being the right and left upper pulmonary veins, the LV apex close to the interventricular septum, the left atrium adjacent to the interatrial septum, and the coronary sinus. With its ostium at a more superior location, the right coronary artery is a common site of air embolism, frequently resulting in RV dysfunction and accompanying ST-segment changes in the inferior ECG leads. This is a common finding in any open chamber surgical procedure and transplantation is no exception **(Figure 20.4)**.

**Box 20.1:** Factors determining allograft function

| | |
|---|---|
| 1. | Baseline function before brain death |
| 2. | Cardiac damage before and during harvesting |
| 3. | Extent of donor inotropic support |
| 4. | Ischemic time |
| 5. | Myocardial protection during ischemic time |
| 6. | Reperfusion injury |
| 7. | Cardiac denervation |
| 8. | Donor–recipient heart size mismatch |
| 9. | Pulmonary hypertension in recipient |

## *Functional Assessment*

### *Left Ventricle*

*Systolic function:* There are several factors that determine allograft function **(Box 20.1)**. Normally, the function of the allograft is expected to be normal or at the very least similar to the last assessment of the donor heart. However, ischemic injury or acute rejection can lead to impaired function. Intraoperative echocardiographic assessment of LV systolic function early after discontinuation of CPB can predict requirements for inotropic and mechanical support, especially when ischemic times are prolonged.[16] The early occurrence of segmental WMAs is concerning and could reflect transient ischemia from air emboli in the right coronary artery, or coronary atherosclerosis that could be a cause of postoperative morbidity.

*Diastolic function:* Diastolic dysfunction in a transplanted heart portends a poor outcome.[17] Transient ischemia or reperfusion injury often lead to a decrease in diastolic function in the early postoperative period. Another less frequent cause of diastolic dysfunction could be an allograft size-mismatch with a larger organ in a restricted pericardial space, limiting diastolic distensibility. The assessment of diastolic function using Doppler techniques can be limited by several factors, including native atrial activity leading to asynchronous contractions, and altered pulmonary venous flow patterns. Furthermore, higher heart rates may preclude an accurate assessment of transmitral flow velocities. Tissue Doppler assessment of myocardial velocities may yield more reliable information on diastolic function. While a comprehensive discussion on assessment of diastolic dysfunction is beyond the scope of this chapter, there are important caveats to the use of tissue Doppler techniques in a newly transplanted heart. While a transmitral early flow velocity (E) to early lateral mitral annular tissue velocity (e') ratio of greater than 15 is associated with high LV filling pressures in native hearts,[18] an

E/e' value of greater than 22 was able to identify patients with a PA wedge pressure greater than 12 with 95% specificity in one study.[19] Therefore, 'normal' E/e' ratios should be interpreted with caution in transplant recipients. Another study found that the ratio or transmitral E to propagation velocity was the most accurate indicator of wedge pressure.[20] A high e' value, however, reliably excludes severe rejection.[21]

*Right Ventricle*

Patients with end-stage heart failure usually have high PA pressure that places the thin-walled RV in the allograft at risk during ischemia and reperfusion. Therefore, acute RV failure is one of the most common and feared complications after transplantation.[22] Intraoperative TEE can be useful in ruling out PA stenosis as a potential cause of acute RV failure. Additionally, TEE can be helpful in optimizing hemodynamics by avoiding volume overload of the RV while monitoring its response to inotropes and pulmonary vasodilator therapy. Continued RV failure with maximized pharmacologic therapy with a normally functioning LV should then prompt consideration of a MCS device for the right heart.

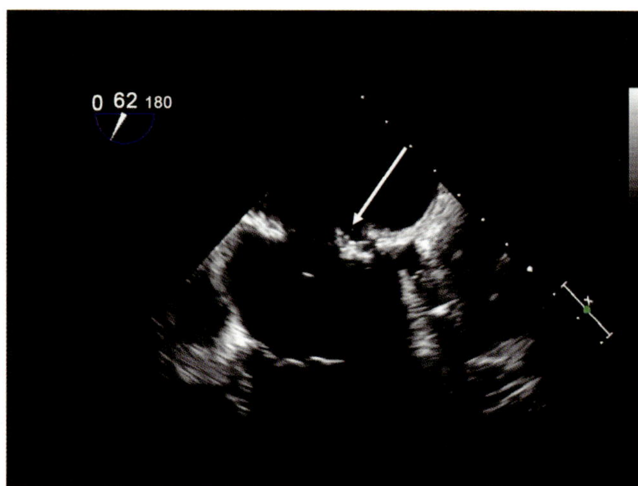


**Figure 20.5:** Mid-esophageal mitral commissural view in a patient post-heart transplant. Portions of the native atrial cuff can be seen (arrow) in the left atrium.

## *Structural Assessment*

*Imaging planes:* A comprehensive structural assessment of the allograft is complicated by factors unique to the transplantation process. Imaging planes can be challenging owing to a more medially rotated heart since the allograft is frequently smaller in size compared to the native dilated heart. Therefore, standard imaging planes may only be obtained at more rotated scan planes.[23]

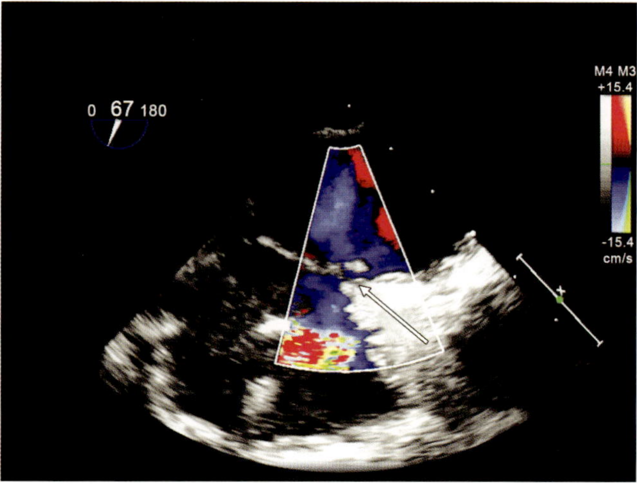


**Figure 20.6:** Left-to-right shunt flow (arrow) in a patient with a patent foramen ovale. Note the reduced color flow scale to enable visualization of low velocity flows.

*Atria:* Both atria can appear large due to portions of the native atria that are left in situ. Invagination of the left atrial cuff can mimic a left atrial appendage thrombus **(Figure 20.5)**.[24] Thrombi can also occur along suture lines within the left atrial component and are associated with spontaneous echo contrast within the left atrium. The risk is reduced with the bicaval anastomotic technique. More extensive tissue within the left atrium can lead to acquired cor triatriatum.[25] This is characterized by an enlarged left atrial remnant, reduced LV volume, turbulent flow by color-flow Doppler, and mitral valve leaflet fluttering. As the right-sided pressures rise from transient RV dysfunction and elevated right atrial pressure, a previously unsuspected patent foramen ovale can become an obvious source of right-to-left shunting. This should be assessed either using color-flow Doppler **(Figure 20.6)** or agitated saline to determine cross-atrial flow. Once identified, a left-to-right atrial shunt should be surgically addressed since it can lead to progressive volume overloading of the RV and worsening tricuspid regurgitation (TR).

*Pulmonary vessels:* Donor-recipient allograft size mismatch can rarely lead to torsion or kinking along the PA anastomosis which in turn can lead to acute RV failure.[26] The anastomotic site at the level of the main PA should be assessed using color flow Doppler and a gradient obtained by continuous wave Doppler. The upper esophageal aortic arch short-axis view can be helpful in this assessment as the Doppler beam aligns well with flow through the main PA **(Figure 20.7)**. The integrity of flow across the pulmonary veins should also be assessed using color-flow and pulsed-wave Doppler.

*Valvular function:* The most common valve lesion following heart transplantation is TR which occurs in up to 84% recipients.[27] The presence of TR can be confirmed

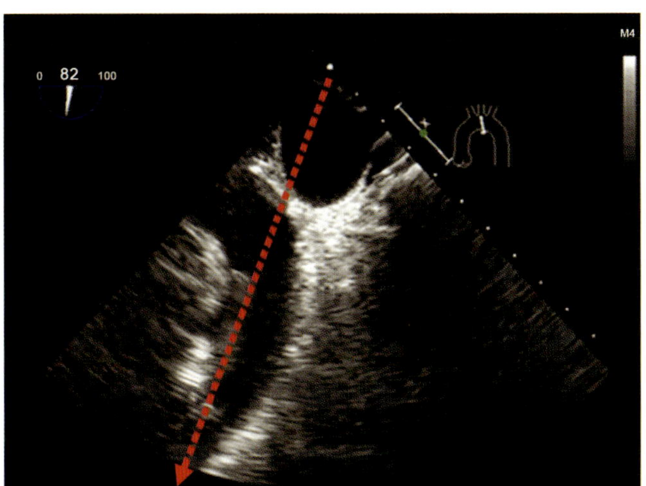

**Figure 20.7:** The upper esophageal aortic arch short-axis view demonstrating the optimal view that permits alignment of the Doppler beam (red dotted arrow) with transpulmonic flow.

qualitatively using color flow Doppler. The TR can be best quantified by the ratio of jet area to right atrial area.[28] The presence of systolic flow reversal in the hepatic veins may also be seen **(Figure 20.8A and B)**. However, its absence may not exclude severe TR. While some degree of TR is almost always expected, moderate TR or worse can signal worsening RV function and need for escalating pharmacological support or adding an MCS device for the right heart. Mitral regurgitation (MR) is also common but not as frequently seen as TR. Mild-to-moderate MR can be seen as an eccentric jet but can be difficult to quantify due to the presence of native atrial tissue in the scan plane. Regurgitation of the tricuspid and mitral valves is attributed to distortion of annular geometry. The distortion is more significant with the standard technique, which results in disturbed atrial geometry and function, while in the bicaval technique, the distortion is attributed to donor heart and recipient pericardial cavity size mismatch.[27,29] Consequently, the incidence and severity of TR and MR have decreased after the bicaval technique was introduced.

The progression of TR in these patients seems to mimic that in other pathological settings. The incidence and severity of TR appears to increase with time, and when refractory to medical management, may require valve repair or replacement. Damage to the tricuspid valve or its support apparatus during follow-up, heart biopsy may also result in worsening of TR. These patients usually have worse right heart function, persistent congestive heart failure and higher mortality than patients without hemodynamically significant TR.[27,29]

### Hemodynamic Management in Surgical Intensive Care

Management of the hemodynamically unstable patient can be challenging for the heart transplant recipient. Most patients will be admitted after surgery with some amount of inotropic support. While in a majority of cases, the support will be gradually tapered off without significant impact, hemodynamics may deteriorate in a smaller proportion of patients due to progressive right heart dysfunction, acute rejection leading to LV failure, or cardiac tamponade. Bedside TEE can be invaluable under these circumstances, and TTE windows should be challenging.

## MECHANICAL CIRCULATORY SUPPORT

MCS devices include intra-aortic balloon pumps and ventricular assist devices that may be inserted for supporting the failing left and/or right ventricle. The following text will describe the value of intraoperative TEE during surgery for heart failure that includes placement of MCS devices, specifically, ventricular assist devices.

### Current Mechanical Circulatory Support Technology

Rapid advances in the last few years have seen devices that have a spectrum of mechanisms of action, individualized support capabilities and variable placement options. While there is no single universal classification system based on consensus, MCS devices can be categorized in several ways. They can be grouped by device mechanism of action (centrifugal or axial), method of implantation (surgical or percutaneous), intended duration of support (temporary or long-term), location of placement (extracorporeal or intracorporeal), and chamber supported (left, right, or biventricular). Patients that are candidates for MCS therapy will usually present in one of the categories described by the Interagency Registry for Mechanically Assisted Circulatory Support (INTERMACS) **(Table 20.2)**.[30] For purposes of intraoperative TEE, the MCS devices will be considered according to the ventricle they support and the essential elements of imaging when MCS devices are placed, irrespective of indication.

### Left Ventricular Assist Devices

Imaging with TEE can be crucial prior to MCS placement for hemodynamic management, detection of interatrial shunts and determination of aortic and tricuspid valve pathology. It also plays an important role during separation from CPB and assessment of device function in the postoperative period.

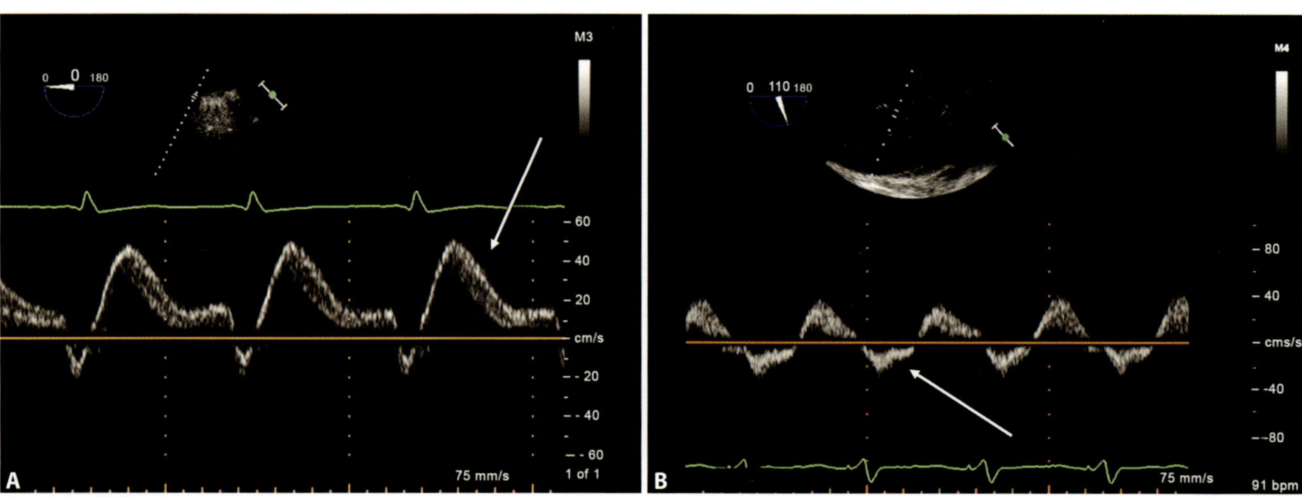


**Figure 20.8A and B:** Hepatic vein flow with transesophageal echocardiography using pulsed-wave Doppler. A normal flow pattern is shown in the left panel while systolic flow reversal is seen in the patient on the right panel. Arrows on both panels indicate systolic flow. Forward flow is towards the transducer and is directed upwards (A), while reverse flow is directed away from the transducer and is directed below the baseline (B).

**Table 20.2:** Interagency Registry for Mechanically Assisted Circulatory Support (INTERMACS) profiles for patient selection for device placement

| *Level* | *Definition* | *Description* | *Urgency of intervention* |
|---|---|---|---|
| 1. | Critical cardiogenic shock | Life-threatening hypotension despite high inotropic support and worsening end-organ perfusion (crash and burn) | Immediate, within hours |
| 2. | Progressive decline | Declining function despite optimal inotropic support; worsening renal function (sliding on inotropes) | Early, within days |
| 3. | Stable but inotrope dependent | Stable hemodynamics on continuous intravenous inotropes or temporary circulatory assist; repeated inability to wean support | Elective, within weeks/months |
| 4. | Resting home symptoms | Stabilized on medical management but in NYHA class IV with fluctuating diuretic use | Elective, within weeks/months |
| 5. | Exertion intolerant | Stable at reset and with ADL, but home-bound and unable to exert | Variable, depends on maintenance of organ function |
| 6. | Exertion limited | Stable at rest, with ADL and minimal external activities but rapid deterioration with further exertion | Variable, depends on maintenance of organ function |
| 7. | Advanced NYHA Class III | Unspecified at this time (reserved for future use) | Device support not indicated |

*Abbreviations:* ADL, activities of daily living; NYHA, New York Heart Association.

## *Pre-left Ventricular Assist Device Placement Assessment*

*Imaging approach:* The patient presenting for left ventricular assist device (LVAD) placement by definition has a failing heart and is hemodynamically fragile following induction of general anesthesia. Imaging with TEE can help with monitoring of left and right heart function to optimize inotropic management prior to institution of cardiopulmonary bypass. Some patients may present with malfunctioning LVADs that require device replacement. In these patients, imaging would be focused on device function and optimization of preload and afterload. There are a few structural lesions that are important to exclude or define prior to device placement as they could adversely impact LVAD function and reduce its benefit to the failing heart. These include the search for any intracardiac shunt especially a patent foramen ovale, determination of aortic valve insufficiency, mitral valve stenosis, TR, and left heart thrombus.

*Patent foramen ovale:* This is the most common intracardiac shunt and is important to diagnose and repair for reducing the risk of paradoxical embolism or hypoxemia following LVAD placement. After placement, an LVAD will significantly reduce LV diastolic and left atrial pressures while right-sided filling pressures can remain abnormally high. A right-to-left shunt and hypoxemia can result from an unrepaired patent foramen ovale (PFO).

Normally, the foramen ovale is best seen in a midesophageal bicaval view in which it appears as a thin slice of tissue bound by thicker ridges of tissue, one of which appears as a "flap". Evaluation of the patency of a foramen ovale can be performed using two-dimensional (2D) assessment for flap movement, color-flow Doppler assessment with optimal low velocity flow detection settings **(Figure 20.6)** and an agitated saline (a bubble study) along with a Valsalva maneuver to provoke right-to-left shunting. In a patient receiving positive pressure ventilation, agitated saline should be injected following a Valsalva maneuver that decreases right atrial volume. The Valsalva should then be released thereby transiently generating pressures higher in the right compared to left atrium. Microbubbles can then be visualized as they enter the right atrium. The bubble study is positive (PFO present), if bubbles appear in the left atrium within five cardiac cycles **(Figure 20.9A to C)**. The search for a PFO by examining passage of agitated saline contrast can be complicated by high left atrial pressures preoperatively. Color flow Doppler in these situations can be useful in identifying left-to-right shunt through a PFO, if present. Small PFOs also need to be surgically repaired due to significant risk of shunting in patients with LVADs.

*Aortic pathology:* A comprehensive examination of the ascending aorta is essential as the LVAD outflow cannula is typically placed in this region (except for the Jarvik 2000, which may be attached to the descending aorta). The ascending aorta is best seen in the midesophageal ascending aortic short- and long-axis views. Pathology in the ascending aorta may include aneurysmal dilatation that must be repaired during CPB prior to LVAD placement,[31] and protruding or mobile atheroma **(Figure 20.3)** that increases the risk of stroke and may require modification of surgical approach. An epiaortic ultrasound scan of the ascending aorta may be useful in patients at high risk of atherosclerosis at the site of cannulation as digital palpation may not be as sensitive in atheroma detection.[12]

*Aortic regurgitation:* Significant aortic regurgitation (AR) results in chronic volume overload of the LV with consequent ventricular dilation and dysfunction. Echocardiographic estimation of severity of AR can be confounded by several factors. The size of the regurgitant jet can be affected by an elevated LV end-diastolic pressure that reduces the transvalvular gradient. Similarly, the pressure half time (PHT) of the AR jet can be affected by a lower afterload typically seen after induction of anesthesia (shorter PHT), or a higher afterload as a result of vasopressor administration (prolonged PHT). In patients with an LVAD, the degree of AR can be increased in two ways: (i) pressure in the ascending aorta is increased as a result of blood returning from the LVAD directly just above the aortic valve and (ii) LV end-diastolic pressure is now lower as a result of the LVAD-induced decompression of the LV. These two factors can combine to increase the net regurgitant volume. When this volume exceeds 1–2 L/minute, patients may remain in clinical heart failure despite the LVAD, since this volume is not delivered systemically but remains within a shunt formed by the LV, LVAD, and the ascending aorta. The midesophageal aortic valve short- and long-axis views are the most ideal imaging planes to assess AR. Concomitant aortic valve repair or replacement may be necessary even for patients with mild AR.[32] The advantage of an aortic valve replacement may be counterbalanced by a higher procedural mortality associated with this additional procedure. Other considerations include presence of concomitant aortic valve calcification, characteristics of the regurgitant jet, and planned duration of LVAD support. The presence of calcification can

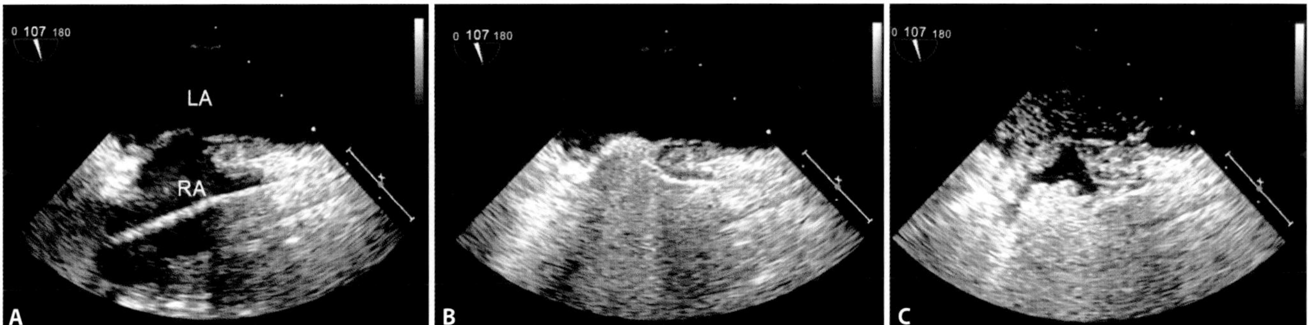


**Figure 20.9A to C:** (A) Saline contrast study showing a bicaval view with left and right atria labeled (LA and RA). (B) Agitated saline is injected into a vein and can be seen opacifying the RA. (C) Bubbles can be seen to cross over into the LA (see text for details).

render an AR jet more eccentric which may worsen after LVAD placement. For short-term LVADs, mild AR may be well tolerated until device explantation, while patients with long-term or destination LVADs, AR may progress and may mitigate any benefit of the device.[33]

Surgical options for the aortic valve include replacement or repair. Replacement is the most durable option and a biologic prosthesis is preferred over a mechanical one. The potential for thrombus formation is higher with a mechanical valve due to leaflet immobility during most LVAD cycles and subsequent risk of embolization with intermittent opening.[34] Aortic valve repair may be partial or complete, with complete ligation reserved for patients with no expected possibility of recovery of native heart function. Expectedly, long-term survival of patients receiving complete aortic valve closure is inferior compared with aortic valve replacement.[34] Echocardiographic examination of the repaired or replaced aortic valve in LVADs should follow the same guidelines as for prosthetic aortic valves in other settings.[35] Another emerging option for addressing a pathological aortic valve is transcatheter aortic valve replacement, which may be suitable in select patients.[36,37]

*Mitral valve stenosis:* While mitral valve stenosis is uncommon in this group of patients, rheumatic disease is more common globally and the presence of a significant mitral gradient must be excluded. Any prosthesis that restricts flow into the LV should be examined in detail, since it could impair LV filling and lead to persistently elevated pulmonary venous pressures and consequent heart failure. Intraoperative TEE should evaluate for the presence of any flow restriction across the mitral valve, whether as a result of native stenosis or pathological obstruction of a prosthetic valve.

*Tricuspid regurgitation:* The presence of severe TR, which may be preset in up to 50% of LVAD candidates, usually warrants concomitant tricuspid valve repair, as elimination of TR improves forward flow and LVAD filling.[38] The presence of TR can be assessed using the mid-esophageal 4-chamber and the mid-esophageal RV inflow–outflow views. The presence of systolic flow reversal in the hepatic veins can also be useful in confirming the presence of severe TR. Surgical correction of significant TR can improve survival following LVAD placement compared with uncorrected TR, which may progress over time.[39]

*Left heart thrombus:* Patients with heart failure are at risk for thrombus formation in the LV apex **(Figure 20.1)** and left atrial appendage. A thorough scan with TEE for intracardiac thrombi can be useful in alerting the surgical team to the potential for embolic phenomenon during cardiac manipulation and ventriculotomy.[40]

*Right ventricular dysfunction:* The filling of an LVAD is dependent on the same factors that impact LV filling and include an RV that is optimally functional. The RV may be assessed using 2D views including the mid-esophageal 4-chamber and RV inflow–outflow views. A useful metric to evaluate systolic RV performance is the RV fractional area change (RVFAC). A normal RVFAC is greater than 40%, and most LVAD candidates have an RVFAC of 20–30%. Studies suggest that an RVFAC less than 20% predicts a high risk for RV failure following LVAD placement.[41] Acute RV failure remains a significant complication that limits the success of MCS support for left heart failure.[42]

## *Separation from Cardiopulmonary Bypass*

The TEE examination can be useful during separation from CPB primarily to assist in the de-airing process. Following any open chamber procedure, ambient air **(Figure 20.4)** can be retained and visualized in the LV apex, the left atrial appendage, the right coronary sinus of Valsalva, and the PA. The assessment of intracardiac air has been described previously in context of heart transplantation. In patients undergoing LVAD placement, an additional source of air retention is when the LVAD pump function is initiated prior to discontinuation of CPB. Since LVADs are capable of generating negative pressure, they can entrap extracardiac ambient air. Hence, separation from CPB is a complex process with requirement for gradual reduction in venous reservoir filling and increase in native heart venous return. This ensures a gradual preload delivery to the left ventricle and LVAD. The LVAD is then started with low pump speeds. It is at this time when air entrainment is seen on TEE. The consequences of intracardiac air are most serious when RV function is compromised from air emboli induced impairment of right coronary artery flow. Acute RV failure in this setting can be disastrous for LV filling. Therefore, a careful titration of inotropes and pulmonary vasodilators is required to ensure continued optimization of RV function. Other maneuvers, such as de-airing needles and vents can help reduce the embolic burden of intracardiac air.

## *Post-left Ventricular Assist Device Placement Assessment*

Immediately after separation from CPB, there should be search for any intracardiac shunt, assessment of aortic valve and RV function, and position of LVAD cannulae.

*Patent foramen ovale:* While a PFO should be excluded prior to CPB, the complex interplay of pressure differences between the left- and right-sided chambers may preclude an accurate assessment. The reduction in left-sided pressures following LVAD placement may result in unmasking of a previously unrecognized PFO. This could be seen more commonly in a setting when an LVAD is placed emergently for post-cardiotomy shock and an assessment for PFO has not been performed pre-CPB. Any significant right-to-left shunt may require reinstitution of CPB and repair of the PFO.

*Aortic valve:* While significant AR should have been excluded pre-CPB, an increased transvalvular diastolic gradient associated with reduction of the LV end-diastolic pressure and increased flow into the ascending aorta through the outflow graft may worsen pre-existing AR. An additional feature of the echocardiographic examination of the aortic valve is the determination of frequency of aortic valve opening. The combination of a decompressed left ventricle with inadequate native ejectile force and an elevated aortic pressure can lead to complete immobility of the aortic valve leaflets. However, intermittent opening of the aortic valve is desirable to avoid thrombus formation on the aortic valve and risk of subsequent systemic embolization.[43]

*Right ventricular function:* With normalization of left heart output after LVAD placement, the amount of blood flow to the right ventricle is increased. A judicious combination of inotropes and pulmonary vasodilators can help optimize RV function. However, as mentioned earlier, several factors can lead to reduced RV function and even acute RV failure with reduced LVAD flow and output. A properly functioning LVAD may decrease RV afterload by reducing pulmonary venous and left atrial pressures. On the other hand, an excessive LVAD pump speeds can result in loss of ventricular interdependence and adversely affect RV performance leading to acute RV failure.[44] When it occurs, the most common short-term solution is a temporary reduction in LVAD flow which can increase LV diastolic dimensions thereby restoring the position of the interventricular septum and improving RV function.

*Inflow cannula:* The inflow cannula is normally positioned in a way that directs it anteroseptally and toward the mitral valve opening but away from the interventricular septum and lateral wall **(Figure 20.10)**. Proper inflow cannula position can be assessed in the mid-esophageal 4-chamber and mid-esophageal long-axis views. Color flow Doppler can help identify turbulent flow into the LVAD inflow cannula or even abnormal regurgitant flow in rare circumstances. Continuous wave Doppler can be useful if high flows or obstruction are suspected. Laminar flows with peak velocities less than 2.5 m/s should be seen in properly functioning devices **(Figure 20.11)**. Malposition of the inflow cannula can be surgically corrected as soon as it is recognized after termination of CPB and prior to chest closure.[11] The inflow cannula position should be examined after chest closure to ensure that it remains correctly positioned.

*Outflow cannula:* The mid-esophageal ascending aorta short- and long-axis views are ideal for assessing the outflow graft **(Figure 20.12A and B)**. Pulsed- or continuous-wave Doppler can be used to examine flows across the graft. The peak velocity of graft flow should be 1.0–2.0 m/s for a continuous flow device. Unusual complications of outflow graft placement include internal obstruction due to thrombus or vegetation, and external obstruction due to kinking or compression of the graft.[45-47] Persistent air in the ascending aorta near the outflow cannula may indicate graft perforation.[31]

*Left ventricle:* The final step in a comprehensive post-CPB assessment is an examination of proper LV emptying. A gradual increase in pump flows will reduce LV diastolic dimensions, and this may be monitored with TEE. The interventricular septum should remain in a neutral position.

**Figure 20.10:** Mid-esophageal 2-chamber view in a patient with a left ventricular assist device in situ. The inflow cannula can be seen (arrow) positioned appropriately at the apex pointing towards the mitral valve.

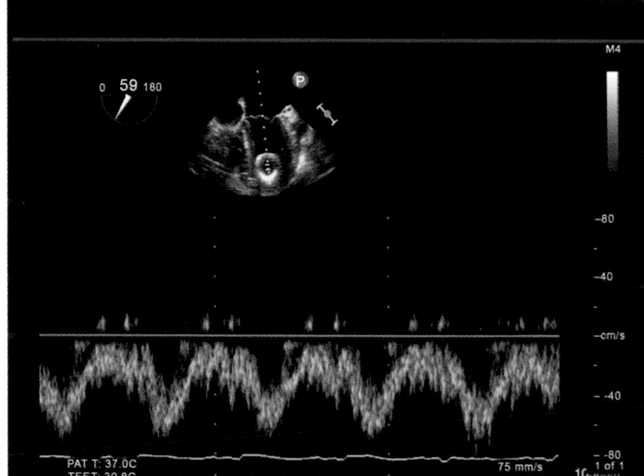


**Figure 20.11:** Pulsed-wave Doppler profile of flow through the inflow cannula of a left ventricular assist device showing laminar, low velocity flow directed away from the probe, into the device and below the spectral baseline.

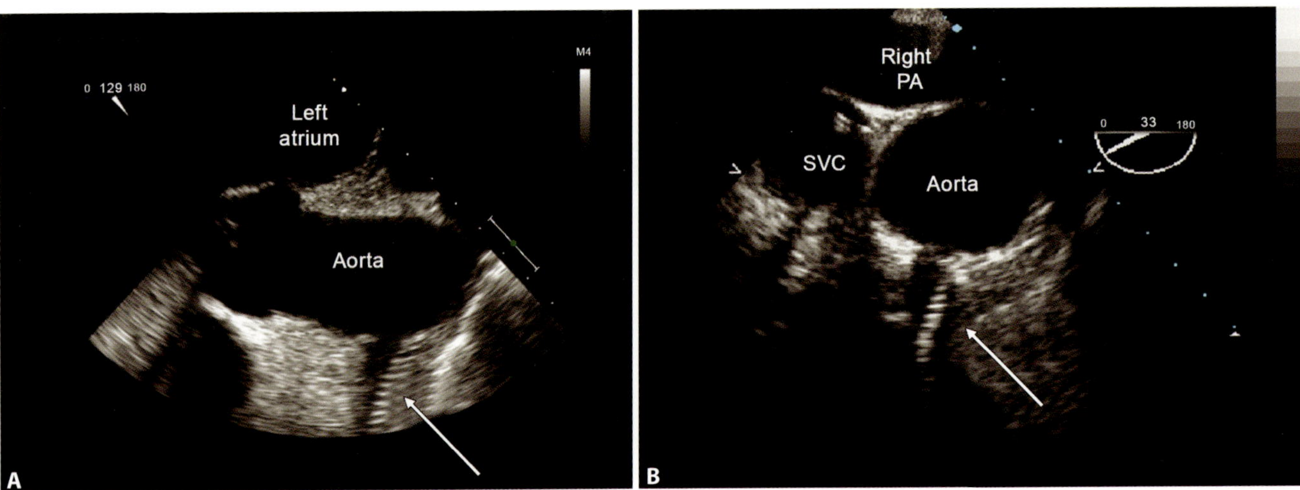


**Figure 20.12A and B:** Position of the outflow graft (arrows) from the left ventricular assist device seen in the ascending aorta long- and short-axis views (Figure A and B, respectively). Other structures, including the right pulmonary artery (PA) and superior vena cava (SVC) can also be seen.

Any deviation of the septum towards the right ventricle should indicate inadequate LV emptying, which may be corrected by increasing increased pump speed is warranted. However, excessive septal displacement towards the left ventricle suggests excessive LV unloading and may worsen RV function as previously discussed.

## Right Ventricular Assist Devices

The use of MCS for right ventricle has increased in recent years as more options become available for the failing right heart. Assist devices to support the right ventricle (right ventricular assist devices or RVADs) may be indicated when RV failure occurs in isolation or following LVAD placement as described above. The relatively lower frequency of RV failure compared to LV failure has resulted in fewer durable RVAD options. Common indications for RVAD support include RV failure following LVAD placement, unsuccessful separation from CPB during other cardiac surgeries, notably heart transplantation or following large RV infarction.[48,49] Following cardiac surgery, acute RV failure is more frequently due to poor RV protection during CPB or right coronary artery embolism.[50-52] The essential imaging principles from a TEE perspective remain analogous to those for LVAD assessment.

The RVAD inflow cannula is usually placed via the right atrial appendage. Infrequently, it can also be placed in the RV outflow tract. This inflow cannula may be easily visualized in the mid-esophageal bicaval view **(Figure 20.13)**. The RVAD outflow cannula is most commonly anastomosed to the main PA. Other surgical options for this cannula include attachment to the right PA or cannulas placed directly across the RV through the pulmonic valve into the main PA. The outflow graft attached to the main PA can be visualized in the upper esophageal ascending aortic short-axis view or in the mid-esophageal RV inflow-outflow view. As with the LVAD outflow cannula, color flow Doppler should reveal laminar flow with unidirectional low-blood flow velocity on spectral Doppler examination.[31,48]

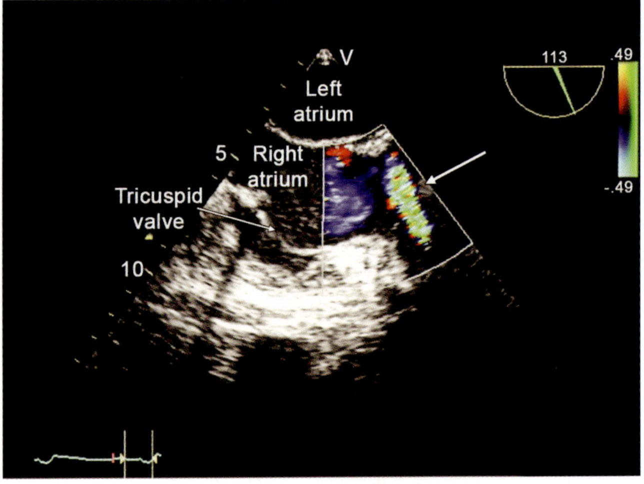


**Figure 20.13:** Modified bicaval view in a patient with a right ventricular assist device with color flow Doppler demonstrating flow through the inflow cannula (arrows) positioned in the right atrial appendage.

## Biventricular Assist Devices

Mechanical support for both ventricles may be indicated for biventricular failure following cardiac surgery, persistent ventricular dysrhythmias, and restrictive cardiomyopathies. Devices that can be used for biventricular MCS include the Syncardia Total Artificial Heart (Syncardia Inc, Tucson, AZ, USA), Thoratec® PVAD (Thoratec Corporation, Pleasanton, CA, USA), a paracorporeal ventricular assist device which can be configured to replace both the right and the left ventricles, and the Thoratec Centrimag, which can be placed in the right ventricle for up to 30 days, and the Abiocor (Abiomed Inc, Danvers, MA, USA) artificial heart. Removal of both ventricles and placement of implantable LVADs such as the HeartWare® HVAD ventricular assist device (HeartWare Inc., Framingham, MA, USA) is another option.

TEE can be crucial during placement of these devices since both pumps need to have balanced flows in order to avoid malfunctioning of either side. Furthermore, invasive hemodynamic monitoring catheters may not be useful or even possible to place with a functioning RVAD. Excessive RVAD flows with inadequate LVAD flows can lead to pulmonary edema while the reverse will lead to signs of acute RV failure. Inadequate flows from the RVAD to the LVAD will result in inadequate systemic output and reduced end-organ perfusion. After termination of CPB, TEE can be used to examine the relative dimensions of the right and left ventricles, loading conditions for both ventricles and opening of the aortic and pulmonic valves.

In total artificial heart devices, such as the Syncardia, examination of the vena cavae and pulmonary veins is important to evaluate device filling. Additionally, electrocardiographic gating may be rendered useless in the absence of ventricular rhythm. Additionally acoustic shadowing can complicate several views and transgastric views are not possible.

## SUMMARY

The global epidemic of heart failure will result in more patients requiring both medical and surgical management. The availability of MCS devices that are smaller, implantable, durable, and more affordable will also likely result in their more frequent surgical placement, especially in areas of the world where donors are in short supply, or the infrastructure is inadequate or culture unsupportive of heart transplantation. TEE has an established role as a monitoring modality for the patient with advanced heart failure and remains invaluable in transplantation or MCS device placement. In addition to aiding placement and ensuring proper functioning of MCS devices, TEE is also valuable in the early detection and troubleshooting of patient or device-related complications. Postoperatively, TEE can also assist in heart transplant recipients with rapid diagnosis of hemodynamic instability and in MCS recipients, with device function, and importantly, for decision making regarding appropriateness or timing of device explantation.[53,54]

The importance of TEE in the perioperative management of the critically ill heart failure patient undergoing transplantation or MCS placement now includes its use in monitoring, patient selection, outcome prediction, and long-term management. Perioperative imaging with TEE can help improve outcomes in this increasingly complex heart failure patient population.

## REFERENCES

1. Go AS, Mozaffarian D, Roger VL, Benjamin EJ, Berry JD, Blaha MJ, et al. Heart disease and stroke statistics--2014 update: A report from the American Heart Association. Circulation. 2014;129:e28-e292
2. Goland S, Czer LS, Kass RM, Siegel RJ, Mirocha J, De Robertis MA, et al. Use of cardiac allografts with mild and moderate left ventricular hypertrophy can be safely used in heart transplantation to expand the donor pool. J Am Coll Cardiol. 2008;51:1214-20.
3. Aziz S, Soine LA, Lewis SL, Kruse AP, Levy WC, Wehe KM, et al. Donor left ventricular hypertrophy increases risk for early graft failure. Transpl Int. 1997;10:446-50.
4. Kuppahally SS, Valantine HA, Weisshaar D, Parekh H, Hung YY, Haddad F, et al. Outcome in cardiac recipients of donor hearts with increased left ventricular wall thickness. Am J Transplant. 2007;7:2388-95.
5. Lima B, Rajagopal K, Petersen RP, Shah AS, Soule B, Felker GM, et al. Marginal cardiac allografts do not have increased primary graft dysfunction in alternate list transplantation. Circulation. 2006;114:I27-32.
6. Borbely XI, Krishnamoorthy V, Modi S, Rowhani-Rahbar A, Gibbons E, Souter MJ, et al. Temporal changes in left ventricular systolic function and use of echocardiography in adult heart donors. Neurocritical Care. 2015;23:66-71.
7. Vedrinne JM, Vedrinne C, Coronel B, Mercatello A, Estanove S, Moskovtchenko JF. Transesophageal echocardiographic assessment of left ventricular function in brain-dead patients: Are marginally acceptable hearts suitable for transplantation? J Cardiothorac Vasc Anesth. 1996;10:708-12.
8. Young JB, Hauptman PJ, Naftel DC, Ewald G, Aaronson K, Dec GW, et al. Determinants of early graft failure following cardiac transplantation, a 10-year, multi-institutional, multivariable analysis. J Heart Lung Transplant. 2001;20:212.
9. Biagini E, Spirito P, Leone O, Picchio FM, Coccolo F, Ragni L, et al. Heart transplantation in hypertrophic cardiomyopathy. Am J Cardiol. 2008;101:387-92.
10. Al-Kindi SG, El-Amm C, Ginwalla M, Hoit BD, Park SJ, Oliveira GH. Heart transplant outcomes in patients with left ventricular non-compaction cardiomyopathy. J Heart Lung Transplant. 2015;34:761-5.
11. Nicoara A, Mackensen GB, Podgoreanu MV, Milano CA, Mathew JP, Swaminathan M. Malpositioned left ventricular assist device cannula: Diagnosis and management with transesophageal echocardiography guidance. Anesth Analg. 2007;105:1574-6.

12. Glas KE, Swaminathan M, Reeves ST, Shanewise JS, Rubenson D, Smith PK, et al. Guidelines for the performance of a comprehensive intraoperative epiaortic ultrasonographic examination: Recommendations of the American Society of Echocardiography and the Society of Cardiovascular Anesthesiologists; endorsed by the Society of Thoracic Surgeons. J Am Soc Echocardiogr. 2007;20:1227-35.
13. Shumway NE, Lower RR, Stofer RC. Transplantation of the heart. Advances in Surgery. 1966;2:265-84.
14. Blanche C, Czer LS, Valenza M, Trento A. Alternative technique for orthotopic heart transplantation. Ann Thorac Surg. 1994; 57:765-7.
15. Schnoor M, Schafer T, Luhmann D, et al. Bicaval versus standard technique in orthotopic heart transplantation: a systematic review and meta-analysis. J Thorac Cardiovasc Surg. 2007;134:1322-31.
16. Kaye DM, Bergin P, Buckland M, et al. Value of postoperative assessment of cardiac allograft function by transesophageal echocardiography. J Heart Lung Transplant. 1994;13:165-72.
17. Tallaj JA, Kirklin JK, Brown RN, Rayburn BK, Bourge RC, Benza RL, et al. Post-heart transplant diastolic dysfunction is a risk factor for mortality. J Am Coll Cardiol. 2007;50: 1064-9.
18. Nagueh SF, Appleton CP, Gillebert TC, Marino PN, Oh JK, Smiseth OA, et al. Recommendations for the evaluation of left ventricular diastolic function by echocardiography. J Am Soc Echocardiogr. 2009;22:107-33.
19. Broch K, Al-Ani A, Gude E, et al. Echocardiographic evaluation of left ventricular filling pressure in heart transplant recipients. Scand Cardiovasc J. 2014;48:349-56.
20. Lopez B, Sanchez V, Delgado JF, Casares SF, Mora L, Garcia J, et al. Accuracy of noninvasive estimation of pulmonary wedge pressure by echocardiographic indices in heart transplant recipients. Transplant Proc. 2012;44:2639-41.
21. Stengel SM, Allemann Y, Zimmerli M, Lipp E, Kucher N, Mohacsi P, et al. Doppler tissue imaging for assessing left ventricular diastolic dysfunction in heart transplant rejection. Heart. 2001;86:432-7.
22. Hosenpud JD, Bennett LE, Keck BM, et al. The Registry of the International Society for Heart and Lung Transplantation: Seventeenth official report-2000. J Heart Lung Transplant. 2000;19:909-31.
23. Martinelli SM, Rogers JG, Milano CA. Transesophageal echocardiography for heart failure surgery. In: JP M, Ayoub CM, Swaminathan M (Eds): Clinical Manual and Review of Transesophageal Echocardiography. New York, NY: McGraw Hill; 2010. pp. 387-405.
24. Winstead KB, Arora H, Kumar PA. An unusual finding after cardiac transplantation. J Cardiothorac Vasc Anesth. 2013;27: 404-5.
25. Law Y, Belassario A, West L, Coles J, Taylor G, Benson L. Supramitral valve obstruction from hypertrophied native atrial tissue as a complication of orthotopic heart transplantation. J Heart Lung Transplant. 1997;16:922-5.
26. Wolfsohn AL, Walley VM, Masters RG, Davies RA, Boone SA, Keon WJ. The surgical anastomoses after orthotopic heart transplantation: Clinical complications and morphologic observations. J Heart Lung Transplant. 1994;13:455-65.
27. Wong RC, Abrahams Z, Hanna M, Pangrace J, Gonzalez-Stawinski G, Starling R, et al. Tricuspid regurgitation after cardiac transplantation: An old problem revisited. J Heart Lung Transplant. 2008;27:247-52.
28. Zoghbi WA, Enriquez-Sarano M, Foster E, Grayburn PA, Kraft CD, Levine RA, et al. Recommendations for evaluation of the severity of native valvular regurgitation with two-dimensional and doppler echocardiography. J Am Soc Echocardiogr. 2003;16:777-802.
29. Berger Y, Har Zahav Y, Kassif Y, Kogan A, Kuperstein R, Freimark D, et al. Tricuspid valve regurgitation after orthotopic heart transplantation: prevalence and etiology. J Transplant. 2012;2012:120702.
30. Kirklin JK, Naftel DC, Stevenson LW, Kormos RL, Pagani FD, Miller MA, et al. Intermacs database for durable devices for circulatory support: First annual report. J Heart Lung Transplant. 2008;27:1065-72.
31. Chumnanvej S, Wood MJ, MacGillivray TE, et al. Perioperative echocardiographic examination for ventricular assist device implantation. Anesth Analg. 2007;105:583-601.
32. Atkins BZ, Hashmi ZA, Ganapathi AM, Harrison JK, Hughes GC, Rogers JG, et al. Surgical correction of aortic valve insufficiency after left ventricular assist device implantation. J Thorac Cardiovasc Surg. 2013;146:1247-52.
33. Rajagopal K, Daneshmand MA, Patel CB, Ganapathi AM, Schechter MA, Rogers JG, et al. Natural history and clinical effect of aortic valve regurgitation after left ventricular assist device implantation. J Thorac Cardiovasc Surg. 2013;145:1373-9.
34. Robertson JO, Naftel DC, Myers SL, Prasad S, Mertz GD, Itoh A, et al. Concomitant aortic valve procedures in patients undergoing implantation of continuous-flow left ventricular assist devices: An intermacs database analysis. J Heart Lung Transplant. 2015;34:797-805.
35. Zoghbi WA, Chambers JB, Dumesnil JG, Foster E, Gottdiener JS, Grayburn PA, et al. Recommendations for evaluation of prosthetic valves with echocardiography and Doppler ultrasound: A report from the American Society of Echocardiography's guidelines and Standards Committee and the Task Force on Prosthetic Valves, developed in conjunction with the American College of Cardiology Cardiovascular Imaging Committee, Cardiac Imaging Committee of the American Heart Association, the European Association of Echocardiography, a registered branch of the European Society of Cardiology, the Japanese Society of Echocardiography and the Canadian Society of Echocardiography, Endorsed by the American College of Cardiology Foundation, American Heart Association, European Association of Echocardiography, a registered branch of the European Society of Cardiology, the Japanese Society of Echocardiography, and Canadian Society of Echocardiography. J Am Soc Echocardiogr. 2009;22:975-1014.
36. Khan S, Koerner MM, Pae W, Stephenson ER, Weber H, Brehm C, et al. Successful percutaneous transcatheter aortic valve replacement in multi-organ failure due to aortic bioprosthesis regurgitation in a patient with continuous-flow LVAD. J Heart Lung Transplant. 2013;32:659-63.
37. Parikh KS, Mehrotra AK, Russo MJ, Lang RM, Anderson A, Jeevanandam V, et al. Percutaneous transcatheter aortic valve closure successfully treats left ventricular assist

device-associated aortic insufficiency and improves cardiac hemodynamics. JACC Cardiovasc Interv. 2013;6:84-9.
38. Piacentino V, 3rd, Troupes CD, Ganapathi AM, Blue LJ, Mackensen GB, Swaminathan M, et al. Clinical impact of concomitant tricuspid valve procedures during left ventricular assist device implantation. Ann Thorac Surg. 2011;92:1414-9.
39. Brewer RJ, Cabrera R, El-Atrache M, Zafar A, Hrobowski TN, Nemeh HM, et al. Relationship of tricuspid repair at the time of left ventricular assist device implantation and survival. Intern J Artif Organs. 2014;37:834-8.
40. Miyake Y, Sugioka K, Bussey CD, et al. Left ventricular mobile thrombus associated with ventricular assist device: Diagnosis by transesophageal echocardiography. Circ J. 2004;68:383-4.
41. Scalia GM, McCarthy PM, Savage RM, et al. Clinical utility of echocardiography in the management of implantable ventricular assist devices. J Am Soc Echocardiogr. 2000;13: 754-63.
42. John R, Lee S, Eckman P, et al. Right ventricular failure—a continuing problem in patients with left ventricular assist device support. J Cardiovasc Transl Res. 2010;3:604-11.
43. May-Newman K, Enriquez-Almaguer L, Posuwattanakul P, et al. Biomechanics of the aortic valve in the continuous flow VAD-assisted heart. Asaio J. 2010;56:301-8.
44. Morgan JA, John R, Lee BJ, et al. Is severe right ventricular failure in left ventricular assist device recipients a risk factor for unsuccessful bridging to transplant and post-transplant mortality. Ann Thorac Surg. 2004;77:859-63.
45. Horton SC, Khodaverdian R, Chatelain P, McIntosh ML, Horne BD, Muhlestein JB, et al. Left ventricular assist device malfunction: An approach to diagnosis by echocardiography. J Am Coll Cardiol. 2005;45:1435-40.
46. Weitzel N, Puskas F, Cleveland J, et al. Left ventricular assist device outflow cannula obstruction by the rare environmental fungus Myceliophthora thermophila. Anesth Analg. 2009; 108:73-5.
47. Ammar KA, Umland MM, Kramer C, Sulemanjee N, Jan MF, Khandheria BK, et al. The ABCs of left ventricular assist device echocardiography: A systematic approach. Eur Heart J Cardiovasc Imaging. 2012;13:885-99.
48. Sheinberg R, Brady MB, Mitter N. Intraoperative transesophageal echocardiography and ventricular assist device insertion. Semin Cardiothoracic Vasc Anesth. 2011;15: 14-24.
49. Christiansen S, Klocke A, Autschbach R. Past, present, and future of long-term mechanical cardiac support in adults. J Card Surg. 2008;23:664-76.
50. Ochiai Y, McCarthy PM, Smedira NG, Banbury MK, Navia JL, Feng J, et al. Predictors of severe right ventricular failure after implantable left ventricular assist device insertion: Analysis of 245 patients. Circulation. 2002;106:I198-202.
51. Osaki S, Edwards NM, Johnson MR, et al. A novel use of the implantable ventricular assist device for isolated right heart failure. Interact Cardiovasc Thorac Surg. 2008;7:651-3.
52. Moazami N, Pasque MK, Moon MR, Herren RL, Bailey MS, Lawton JS, et al. Mechanical support for isolated right ventricular failure in patients after cardiotomy. J Heart Lung Transplant. 2004;23:1371-5.
53. Aissaoui N, Guerot E, Combes A, Delouche A, Chastre J, Leprince P, et al. Two-dimensional strain rate and Doppler tissue myocardial velocities: Analysis by echocardiography of hemodynamic and functional changes of the failed left ventricle during different degrees of extracorporeal life support. J Am Soc Echocardiogr. 2012;25:632-40.
54. Firstenberg MS, Orsinelli DA. ECMO and ECHO: The evolving role of quantitative echocardiography in the management of patients requiring extracorporeal membrane oxygenation. J Am Soc Echocardiogr. 2012;25:641-3.

# Coronary Anomalies in Pediatric Age Group: Echocardiographic Imaging

21
CHAPTER

*Munesh Tomar*

## INTRODUCTION

The exact prevalence of congenital coronary anomalies remains uncertain in the general population. Previous studies suggested that these malformations occurred in 0.2–5.6% of a large group of patients studied by coronary angiography.[1,2] The proposed prevalence varied depending on diagnostic criteria, the method used to diagnose the coronary anomaly [e.g. autopsy, echocardiography, coronary angiography, or computed tomographic (CT) angiography], and the populations studied which always targeted the populations, such as athletes or children.[3-5] Since coronary anatomy has substantial variability, *an anomaly should be defined as any coronary pattern with a feature (number of ostia, proximal course, termination, etc.) that is "rarely" encountered in the general population*. With regard to the clinical significance, coronary anomalies cause 10–19% of sports related deaths in athletes and 1.2% of non-sports-related deaths in young individuals.[6-8]

## CLINICAL CONSEQUENCES OF CORONARY ANOMALIES

Symptoms of a coronary abnormality vary from none to a sudden coronary event that may result in death.[9,10] Awareness of subtle as well as obvious symptoms is essential for a timely intervention.

- Related to coronary ischemia
  - Anginal chest pain
  - Sudden death, ventricular fibrillation
  - Cardiomyopathy
  - Syncope
  - Dyspnea
  - Myocardial infarction.
- Unrelated to coronary ischemia
  - Volume overload (e.g. fistula)
  - Aortic root distortion (aneurysms and fistula)
  - Bacterial endocarditis (coronary arteriovenous fistula)
  - Complications in cardiac surgery and angioplasty.

## IDENTIFICATION OF NORMAL CORONARY ORIGIN IN ECHOCARDIOGRAPHY

Even though various coronary anomalies could not be precisely identified by echocardiogram, it is imperative to identify origin of normal coronaries on all echocardiogram and with slight changes in direction of the plane of sound, both right and left coronaries arteries can be imaged from parasternal short-axis view **(Figure 21.1 to 21.3)**.[11,12] Failure to identify normal coronary origin from the mid-portions of the left and right coronary sinuses will give the clues toward a possible anomalous coronary origin. In parasternal short-axis view, left coronary cusp lies between left atrium and pulmonary valve while right coronary cusp lies directly anterior between the septal leaflet of tricuspid valve and pulmonary valve. For better definition of coronary arteries, you need to use a high frequency transducer, increase two-dimensional (2D) gain and come down on compression.

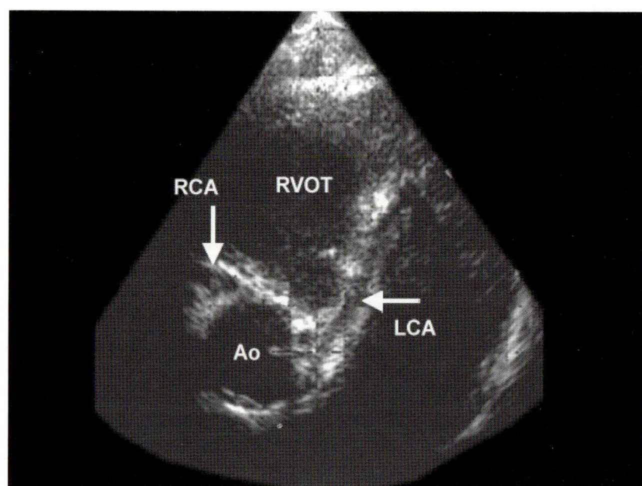


**Figure 21.1:** Parasternal short-axis view at the level of great vessels showing normal origin of coronaries (marked by arrows). *Abbreviations:* Ao, aorta; LCA, left coronary artery; RCA, right coronary artery; RVOT, right ventricular outflow tract.

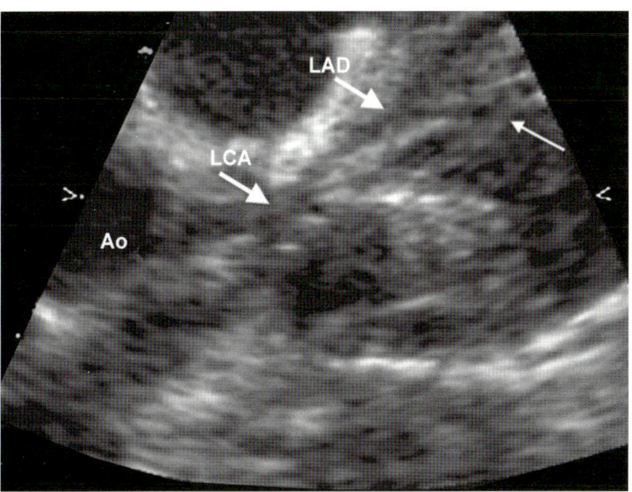


**Figure 21.2A:** Origin of left main coronary artery from left facing sinus and proximal course of left main coronary artery and left anterior descending with its septal branches (thin arrow) is seen (arrow).
*Abbreviations:* Ao, aorta; LAD, left anterior descending artery; LCA, left coronary artery.

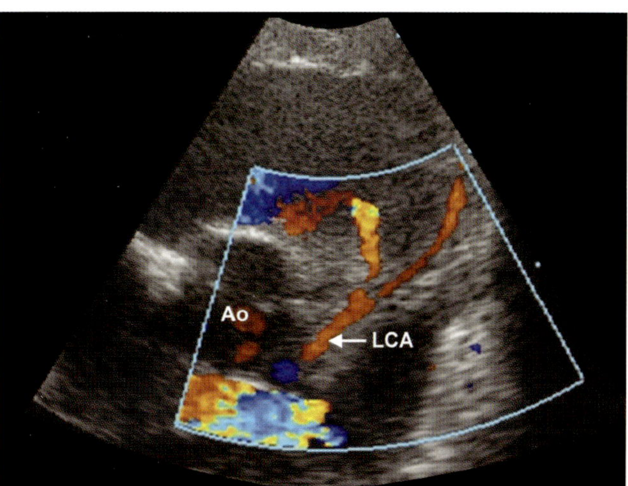


**Figure 21.2B:** On color-flow mapping forward flow in left main and anterior descending is seen (red color).
*Abbreviations:* Ao, aorta; LCA, left coronary artery.

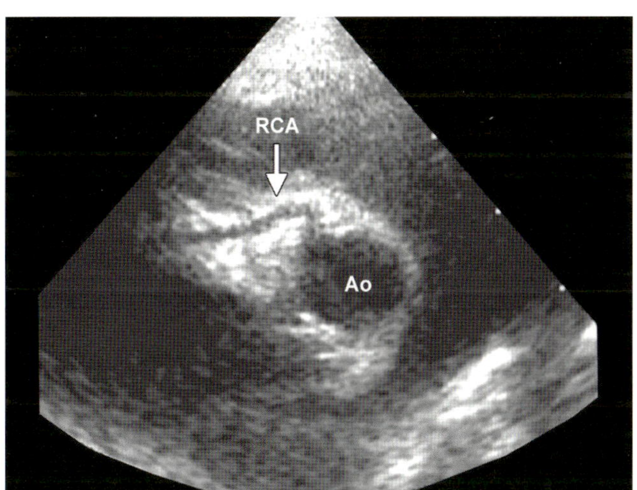


**Figure 21.3A:** The origin of right coronary artery from right sinus (arrow) is seen.
*Abbreviations:* Ao, aorta; RCA, right coronary artery.

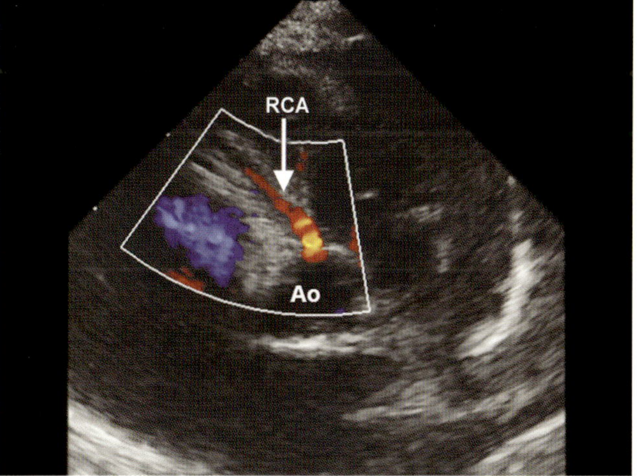


**Figure 21.3B:** On color flow mapping normal flow is seen in right coronary artery (red color).
*Abbreviations:* Ao, aorta; RCA, right coronary artery.

In some patients, it is possible to define origin of both left and right coronary arteries simultaneously. However, it is easier to define both coronaries separately. To visualize right coronary artery, the transducer is angled slightly cranially and rotated slightly clockwise so that tricuspid valve septal leaflet is not seen and you would be able to define origin of right coronary artery from aorta and its course in atrioventricular groove on the anterior surface of right ventricle. With slightly more clockwise rotation of the transducer, entire left main coronary artery from its origin in the posterior left coronary sinus, whole length in left atrioventricular groove, its bifurcation to left anterior descending artery and left circumflex can be profiled. Because coronary arteries are imaged in the direction of the axial resolution of the equipment, they can be easily visualized even in newborn infants.[13] Parasternal long-axis view with anterior tilt can also imagine left coronary artery **(Figure 21.4A and B)**. As the plane of sound is angled between aortic and pulmonary valves, it is possible to define a considerable

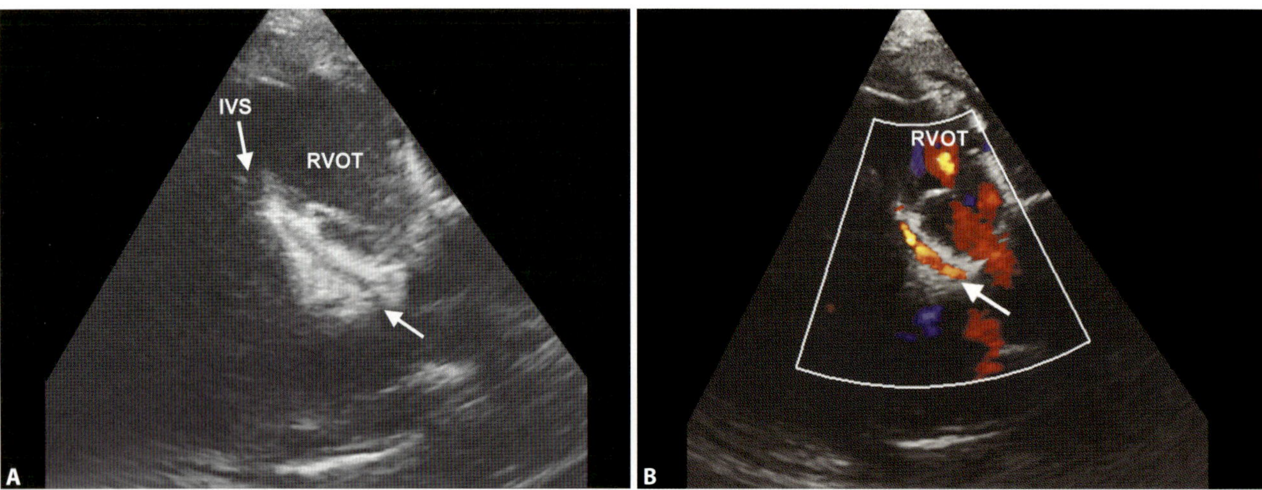


**Figure 21.4A and B:** Parasternal long-axis view with anterior tilt towards right ventricular outflow tract showing left anterior descending artery on: (A) Two-dimensional and (B) Color flow mapping.
*Abbreviations:* IVS, interventricular septum; RVOT, right ventricular outflow tract.

portion of the left coronary artery in left atrioventricular groove, the circumflex artery, and left anterior descending artery coursing down the surface of ventricular septum.[13]

In this chapter, coronary anomalies with concordant atrioventricular and ventriculoatrial connections are being discussed. In later part of this chapter, acquired coronary artery anomaly (Kawasaki disease) has also being discussed.

## CLASSIFICATION OF CORONARY ANOMALIES OBSERVED IN HUMAN HEARTS[14,15]

- Anomalous pulmonary origin of coronaries:
  - Anomalous origin of left coronary artery from pulmonary artery (ALCAPA):
    - Left coronary artery from posterior sinus.
    - From anterior non-facing sinus, main pulmonary artery (MPA), right pulmonary artery.
  - Left anterior descending artery alone from posterior sinus.
  - Left circumflex artery from posterior sinus.
  - Anomalous origin of right coronary artery from pulmonary artery (ARCAPA).
- Anomalous aortic origin of coronaries:
  - Location of coronary ostium within proper aortic sinus of Valsalva but tangential origin (for each artery): high, low, commissural.
  - Anomalous location of coronary ostium outside normal "coronary" aortic sinuses.
    - Noncoronary sinus
    - Ascending aorta, arch, descending aorta, arch branches.
  - Anomalous origin of coronary ostium from opposite, facing "coronary" sinus.
    - Left coronary artery arising from right anterior sinus with anomalous course.
      - Retroaortic or posterior
      - Interarterial
      - Subaortic or septal
      - Prepulmonary or anterior.
    - Right coronary artery arising from left posterior sinus with anomalous course similar to the previous situation.
    - Isolated left anterior descending artery from the right anterior sinus.
    - Isolated left circumflex from right anterior sinus.
    - Separate origin of conal branch from right facing sinus.
    - Single coronary artery (from left or right sinus).
- Anomalies of coronary branching:
  - Absent left main coronary artery, separate left anterior descending artery, left circumflex origin.
  - Left circumflex from right coronary artery.
  - Dual left anterior descending artery, posterior descending artery.
- Coronary arteriovenous fistula—draining to superior vena cava, coronary sinus, right atrium, right ventricle, pulmonary artery, pulmonary vein, left atrium, left ventricle.
- Anomalies of intrinsic coronary arterial anatomy:
  - Ostial stenosis—left main coronary artery, left anterior descending artery, left circumflex artery, right coronary artery.
  - Ostial atresia.
  - Coronary artery aneurysm.
  - Muscle bridge.
  - Hypoplastic coronary.

## Anomalous Pulmonary Origin of Coronary Artery

Anomalous origin of a coronary artery from the pulmonary artery is rare. It is found in 0.01% of 126,596 coronary angiograms performed at the Cleveland Clinic between 1960 and 1988.[14] Four variations of this condition have been described: (i) ALCAPA, (ii) ARCAPA, (iii) origin of an accessory coronary artery from the pulmonary artery, and (iv) origin of the entire coronary circulation from the pulmonary artery.

### *Anomalous Origin of the Left Main Coronary Artery from Pulmonary Artery*

ALCAPA is the most common among these conditions and results in high mortality if not treated on time. Usually left coronary artery arises from lateral or left posterior wall of pulmonary artery from within the left or posterior pulmonary sinus. Rarely, left coronary artery can arise from medial wall of pulmonary artery above the commissure between right and posterior pulmonary sinus.[16]

The heart develops quite normally in fetal life. After birth, as long as the pulmonary arterial pressure remains at or near systemic levels, the left ventricular myocardium supplied by the anomalous artery remains well perfused; the avidity of myocardium for oxygen is such that normal perfusion with blood of mixed venous oxygen content does not present a problem. As pressure in the pulmonary trunk falls postnatally, perfusion of the left ventricle becomes inadequate since the coronary artery pressure falls below the left ventricle end-diastolic pressure. The consequence of the circulatory handicap is a decrease of left ventricular function and further increase of left ventricular end-diastolic pressure with myocardial ischemia.

At the same time, the ischemic myocardium is being perfused increasingly by a developing set of collateral vessels from the right coronary artery, which arises normally. Those with perfectly distributed collateral arteries before the pulmonary artery pressure had fallen escape with ischemic damage of the left ventricular myocardium, which is well perfused, and normal in form and function; this type is often diagnosed in adolescents or adulthood. Surgery is needed at the time of diagnosis. In majority of patients with collateral maldistribution, where there are large interconnections proximal to the branches supplying contracting myocardium that act as a left-to-right arterial shunt, steal from the myocardium to the pulmonary artery, ischemia results in early symptomatology. In such cases symptoms appear within a few days of birth, and death follows within weeks; it is compatible with life only if associated with pulmonary hypertension as associated with large post-tricuspid shunt.

*Echocardiographic evaluation:* Echocardiography has a key role in identification of this major anomaly of coronary arteries in young infants presenting with left ventricular dysfunction. The echocardiographic hallmarks of common type of anomalous origin of left coronary artery from pulmonary artery are listed as follows:

*Two-dimensional echocardiography:* Various views are used to visualize origin of left coronary artery from pulmonary artery, especially parasternal short axis, parasternal long axis, and high parasternal short axis. Sometimes, direct visualization of left coronary artery from pulmonary artery becomes a challenge as left coronary artery falsely appears to connect to aortic sinus due to deficiency in lateral resolution. 2D echocardiographic findings of anomalous origin of left coronary artery from pulmonary artery are as follows:

- Dilated right coronary artery **(Figure 21.5A)** and absence of left coronary artery from left posterior sinus. In infants, the normal ratio of right coronary artery with diameter of aortic root is <0.17 and it increased significantly (>0.21) in infants with anomalous origin of left coronary artery from pulmonary artery.[17]
- Anatomic delineation of the anomalous origin of left coronary artery by 2D echocardiography in parasternal short-axis view at the level of great vessels. As shown in **Figure 21.5B**, the common site of origin of left coronary artery from pulmonary artery. Very rarely, the anomalous left coronary artery may have its origin from the other non-facing anterior sinus of pulmonary artery (**Video 21.1**). Rare instances of origin of left coronary artery from MPA trunk or right pulmonary artery have been reported, often missed on echocardiogram and diagnosed by other means.[18,19] Echocardiographic identification of the origin has a major relevance to surgical strategy, since establishment of dual coronary supply is easily achieved only if the coronary can be mobilized to the aorta.
- Scarring of papillary muscles **(Figure 21.5C and Video 21.2)** as a result of myocardial ischemia, which acts as a very strong clue in infants with severe left ventricle dysfunction to the etiology for the myocardial dysfunction.
- Dilatation of left atrium and left ventricle, left ventricular systolic dysfunction with global hypokinesia and segmental wall-motion abnormality. There will be increased left ventricular mass and volume with low mass/volume ratio.[18,19]

*Color flow mapping:* Color flow mapping has greatly enhanced the ability to detect ALCAPA .

- Turbulent flow in diastole (detection of left to right shunt) in pulmonary artery at the site of connection of left coronary artery. Detection of low velocity flow requires use of low velocity scale of the color Doppler examination and use of low wall filter settings.[18,20-23] The quantity (magnitude) of flow depends upon degree of collaterals from right coronary artery. With normal pulmonary vascular resistance, continuous flow is seen in pulmonary artery at the site of left coronary artery origin.

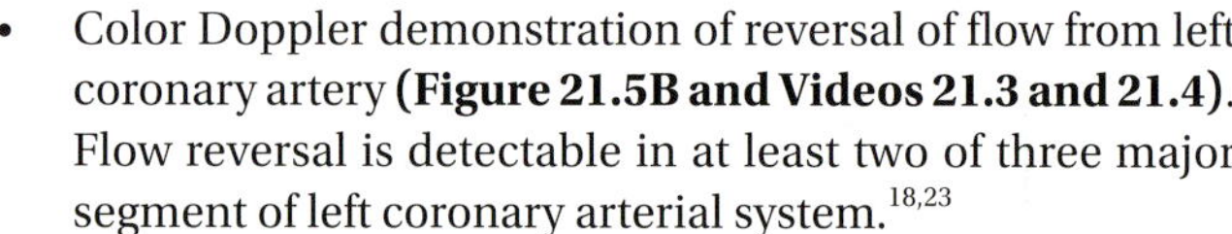

- Color Doppler demonstration of reversal of flow from left coronary artery **(Figure 21.5B and Videos 21.3 and 21.4)**. Flow reversal is detectable in at least two of three major segment of left coronary arterial system.[18,23]
- Ischemic mitral regurgitation **(Figure 21.5D and Video 21.5)**. In all infants and children with unexplained left

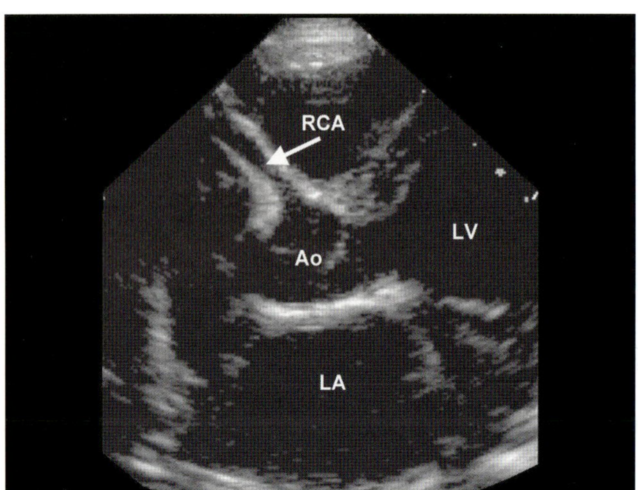


**Figure 21.5A:** Parasternal short-axis view (modified) at the level of great vessels of an infant with anomalous origin of left coronary artery from pulmonary artery showing dilated right coronary artery (arrow).
*Abbreviations:* Ao, aorta; LA, left atrium; LV, left ventricle; RCA, right coronary artery.

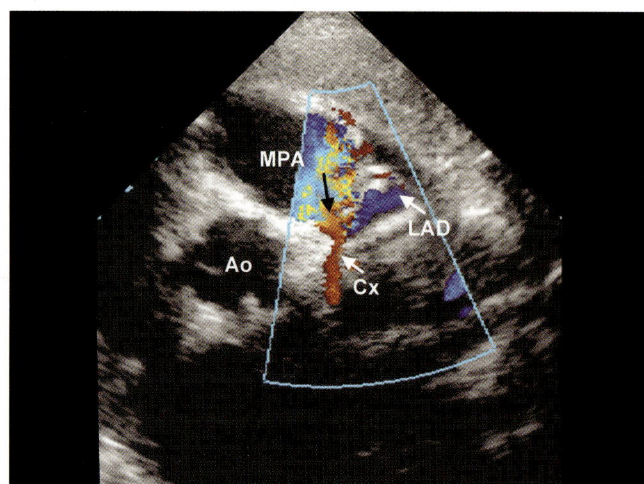


**Figure 21.5B:** Parasternal short-axis view with color-flow mapping at the level of great vessels showing origin of left coronary artery from pulmonary artery. Black arrow points to origin of left coronary artery from pulmonary artery. Flow pattern in left anterior descending and circumflex is reversed (blue flow in left anterior descending and red flow in circumflex) (white arrows).
*Abbreviations:* Ao, aorta; Cx, circumflex artery; LAD, left anterior descending artery; MPA, main pulmonary artery.

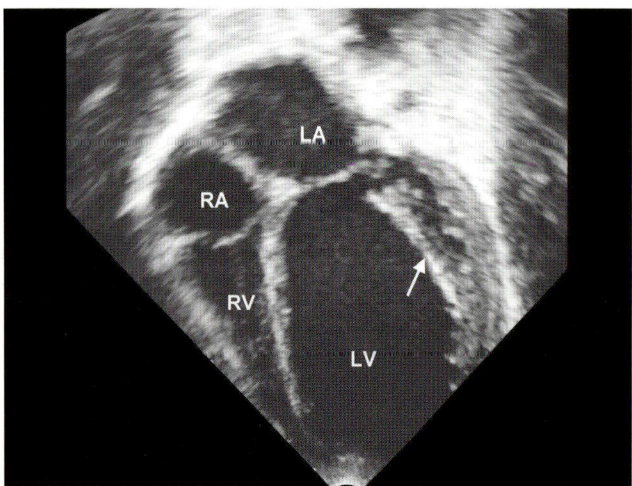


**Figure 21.5C:** Apical 4-chamber view from an infant with anomalous origin of left coronary artery from pulmonary artery showing sclerosed anterior papillary muscle of mitral valve (arrow). Dilated left atrium and left ventricle seen.
*Abbreviations:* LA, left atrium; LV, left ventricle; RA, right atrium; RV, right ventricle.

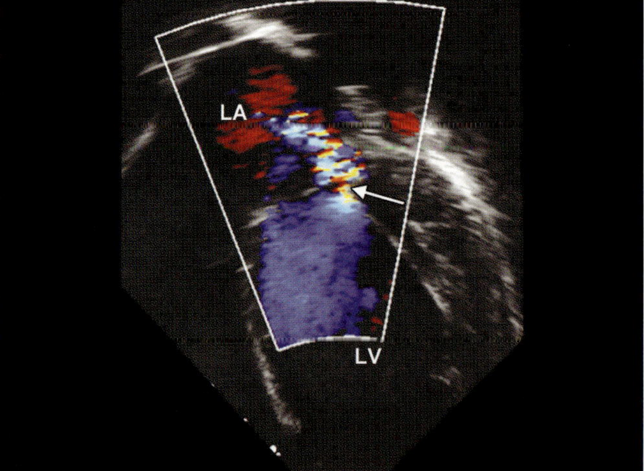


**Figure 21.5D:** Apical 4-chamber view on color flow mapping showing significant mitral regurgitation (arrow). Obvious to note is dilatation of left atrium and left ventricle.
*Abbreviations:* LA, left atrium; LV, left ventricle.

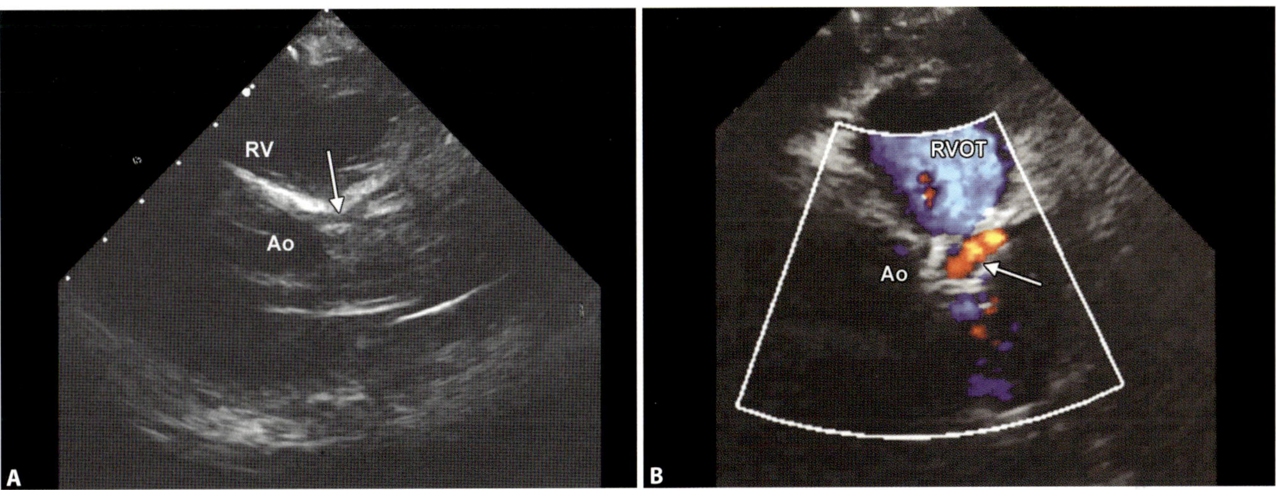


**Figure 21.6A and B:** Same child in **Figure 21.5**, postsurgical translocation of left coronary artery to aorta. (A) On two-dimensional echocardiography, left coronary artery is seen to arise from aorta. (B) On color-flow mapping, normal flow pattern (red color) is seen. *Abbreviations:* Ao, aorta; RV, right ventricle; RVOT, right ventricular outflow tract.

ventricle dilatation and severe mitral regurgitation, anomalous origin of left coronary artery from pulmonary artery should be considered as a possible etiology and actively excluded.

Color Doppler demonstration of myocardial collateral flow in the interventricular septum with flows from posterior interventricular septum to the anterior portions of septum through septal collaterals from right coronary artery to left anterior descending artery, and unlike in other coronary anomalies where various imaging techniques like magnetic resonance imaging (MRI), CT have a major role, anomalous origin of left coronary artery from pulmonary artery is easily identified on echocardiogram.[24]

Echocardiography also has very important role in evaluation of patients postsurgical reimplantation of left coronary to aortic sinus **(Figure 21.6A and B)**.

### *Anomalous Origin of Right Coronary Artery from Pulmonary Artery*

ARCAPA is the second most common of these conditions with an incidence of 0.002%.[14] Typically, these patients are asymptomatic and survive into adulthood; however, sudden cardiac death has been reported.[25] A murmur is the most frequent symptom, followed by chest pain, and congestive heart failure.[25]

The collateral vessels can produce a coronary steal phenomenon due to the relative differences in diastolic pressure between the pulmonary and the systemic arterial beds, and the steal can lead to myocardial ischemia and even sudden death during increased myocardial oxygen demand.[26,27] The severity of ventricular ischemia is determined by the shunt size, presence of collateral circulation, territory at risk, and myocardial oxygen demands. Since right ventricular oxygen demands are lower than the left ventricle demands, ventricular ischemia in ARCAPA is felt to be less common than in ALCAPA.[27] However, conditions that increase right ventricular oxygen demands (i.e. pulmonary artery stenosis) or large territory at risk (i.e. dominant right coronary circulation) may result in increased incidence of ischemic symptoms.[27] Surgical correction with implantation of the aberrant vessel into the aorta is recommended.[28,29]

- Dilated left coronary artery and absence of right coronary artery from right anterior sinus.
- Anatomic delineation of the anomalous origin of right coronary artery from pulmonary artery by 2D echocardiography in parasternal short-axis view at the level of great vessels. Usually, it arises from the right anterior aspect of the MPA immediately above the sinus of Valsalva.
- On color flow mapping, continuous flow into pulmonary artery (detection of left to right shunt) at the site of connection of right coronary artery. The quantity (magnitude) of flow depends upon degree of collaterals from left coronary artery.
- Color Doppler demonstration of reversal of flow in right left coronary artery and adequate intercoronary collateral vessels within the ventricular septum, anterior wall, and inferior wall.
- Chronic volume overload and ischemia would lead to ventricular dilatation and dysfunction. Ventricular

dysfunction, if present, would be limited to right ventricle, septum, and left ventricular inferior wall.

### *Origin of Left Anterior Descending Artery from Pulmonary Artery*

Anomalous origin of left anterior descending artery from pulmonary artery is very rare cause of myocardial ischemia, usually manifesting in adult age.[30] The anomaly differs from ALCAPA in two aspects. First, the area of myocardium supplied by left anterior descending artery is less than that in ALCAPA and, second, the presence of dual coronary arterial supply (right coronary artery and left circumflex) with two aortic sources provides more collaterals to the left anterior descending artery. So, patients with anomalous origin of left anterior descending artery from pulmonary artery have better survival than that with ALCAPA.

*Echocardiographic evaluation*

- Left main coronary artery bifurcation not seen, and it is continued to circumflex.
- Dilated circumflex and right coronary artery.
- Color flow mapping shows normal flow in circumflex, flow reversal in left anterior descending artery. Turbulent flow in diastole in pulmonary artery at the site of connection of left anterior descending artery.
- Prominent collaterals arising from right coronary artery and circumflex both.
- Left ventricular dysfunction with hypokinesia of interventricular septum.
- Sclerosis of anterior papillary muscle of mitral valve with mitral regurgitation.

### *Anomalous Origin of Circumflex Artery from Pulmonary Artery*

Anomalous origin of the circumflex artery from the right pulmonary artery is a very rare pathology.[31-33] These patients can live a normal life till adulthood due to the development of collateral circulation from right coronary artery and left anterior descending artery.[34] Kirklin et al. stated that in the cases who had no problem during infancy, the restrictive character of the coronary ostium originating from the pulmonary artery might also have played a role as well as a rich collateral circulation.[35]

Echocardiography gives clue to the diagnosis of this rare coronary anomaly, but as presentation is in older age group where acoustic windows are not good, CT angiography/MR angiography would be required to confirm the diagnosis.

*Echocardiographic evaluation*

- Left main coronary artery bifurcation not seen, and it is continued to left anterior descending artery.
- Dilated left anterior descending artery and right coronary artery.
- Color-flow mapping shows normal flow in left anterior descending artery, flow reversal in circumflex artery. Turbulent flow in diastole in pulmonary artery at the site of connection of circumflex artery.
- Prominent collaterals arising from and right coronary artery and left anterior descending artery both.
- Left ventricular function usually preserved due to good collaterals from left anterior descending artery and right coronary artery, but some patients present with ventricular dysfunction due to chronic volume overload and ischemia.

## Tangential Origin of Coronary Artery

Normal coronary origin of left coronary artery and right coronary artery is from the mid-portions of the left and right coronary sinuses of aorta; the coronaries are given off perpendicular to the aortic wall **(Figure 21.7)**. In some, coronaries arising in ectopic areas, namely high origin or commissural origin, as well as coronaries arising from the non-coronary sinus, the tangential origin is associated with slit like coronary orifice.[36] Pathologists consistently observe a fibrous ridge at the ostium of tangentially oriented ectopic coronary arteries. Such ridges are often said to have potentially catastrophic consequences. Nevertheless, plaque activation or rupture is seldom documented, even on examination of the histological anatomy. High origin and commissural origin of coronary arteries are also sometimes associated with the same anatomy. In these anomalies, especially high origin of

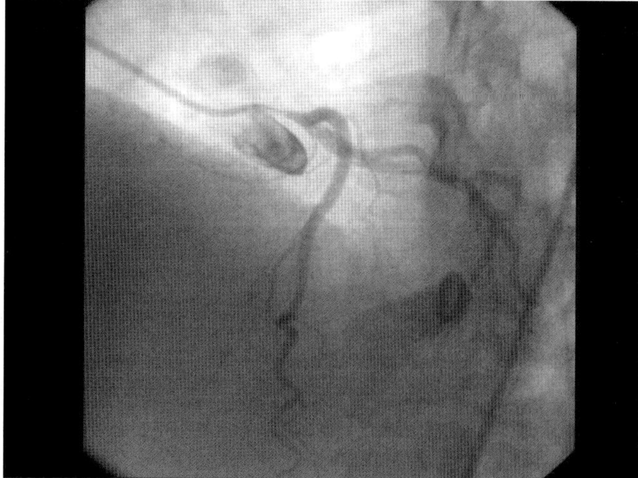

**Figure 21.7:** Selective injection in an adult with large patent ductus arteriosus, severe pulmonary arterial hypertension showing high origin of left coronary artery above left sinus associated with slit-like ostial narrowing.

coronary arteries above the aortic sinuses, abnormal fluid dynamics has been documented for long to cause significantly attenuated blood flows.[37]

### Left Coronary Artery Arising from the Right Coronary Sinus (or Right Coronary Artery)

An aberrant origin of the left main coronary artery or left anterior descending coronary artery from the right sinus of Valsalva is a rare anomaly that has been associated with myocardial ischemia and sudden cardiac death. Depending on the anatomic relationship of the anomalous vessel to the aorta and the pulmonary trunk, the anomaly can be classified into 4 anatomic subtypes by Robert and Shirani:[38]

1. *Anterior or prepulmonic*, left coronary artery courses to the left anterior to the pulmonary artery **(Figure 21.8A)** in 12% of cases and does not associated with cardiac symptoms.
2. *Posterior or retroaortic*, left coronary artery courses dorsal to the ascending aorta and loops behind the aorta to emerge to the left **(Figure 21.8B)**. This subtype occurs in 23% of cases.
3. *Preaortic or interarterial*, left coronary artery courses to the left and posteriorly between the aortic and pulmonary roots **(Figure 21.8C)**. This is the most common subtype and occurs in 53% of cases. This anatomic type is most commonly associated with myocardial ischemia and sudden death in young athlete. The ischemia could be caused by the slit like ostium of left main coronary artery related to its acute proximal bend or compression of left main coronary artery by the aortic rot and pulmonary root, especially when they distend during exercise.
4. *Subpulmonic or septal course*, left coronary artery courses to the left and inferiorly burrowing into the interventricular septum through the crista supraventricularis or outflow septum **(Figure 21.8D)**. This subtype occurs in 12% of cases and does not appear to cause cardiac symptoms.

Parasternal short axis view at the level of great vessels is used to define the origin of coronary arteries. When transthoracic imaging is not adequate as in adults, transesophageal echocardiography may be needed. Basal short-axis view at the level of aorta is used to define the coronary anatomy.

*Echocardiographic evaluation:* 2D echocardiographic features of this anomaly are as follows:

1. Failure to demonstrate the left main coronary artery from its usual site of origin from left sinus.
2. Visualization of ostia and proximal segment of right and left coronary arteries from right sinus of Valsalva.

*Tomographic evaluation:* Contrast-enhanced electron-beam tomography or multislice CT has been shown to permit classification of anomalous coronary arteries.[39] Subtype 3 has been recognized for long to cause sudden cardiac deaths during strenuous physical activity in athletes.[40-43] Anomalous origination of the left coronary artery from the right sinus is consistently related to sudden death (59% of cases), which follows exercise in 81% of events. However, it is recently recognized that even the retroaortic posterior course can lead to serious clinical consequences.[44]

### Right Coronary Artery from the Left Coronary Sinus (or Left Coronary Artery)

This condition is similar to the previous entity. The right coronary artery from left sinus of Valsalva (or from the left coronary artery) can also be cause of myocardial ischemia and sudden death in young athletes. As with above entity, origin of right coronary artery from left sinus (or left coronary artery) has four possible courses **(Figure 21.9 and 21.10)**:

1. Anterior or prepulmonic.
2. Posterior or retroaortic.
3. Interarterial or preaortic (which has been documented consistently with sudden cardiac deaths in athletes).
4. Subarterial or subpulmonic.

Causes of myocardial ischemia would be (a) the slit like orifice, the proximal right coronary artery at its acute bend near the ostium and (b) compression by the aorta and the pulmonary artery as it courses between these two structures to reach the right atrioventricular groove.[45,46] With poor echocardiographic windows, the entity can be visualized by transesophageal echocardiography.[47]

Parasternal short-axis view shows origin of right coronary artery from left and its subsequent course as anterior to pulmonary artery, posterior to aorta or interarterial, and crossing from left to right. With poor echo window, transesophageal echocardiography may be useful. In the interarterial course of coronary arteries, certain surgical strategies are clearly specified.

## Left Circumflex Artery from Right Coronary Artery

One of the common anomalies of coronary artery encountered during coronary angiograms is origin of the left circumflex artery from the right coronary artery. In this common anomaly (incidence of 0.67% in general population), the left circumflex artery arises from right coronary artery and courses posterior to the aortic root to reach the left side.[14] Circumflex from right coronary artery is second most common type of coronary anatomy seen in transposition of great vessels.

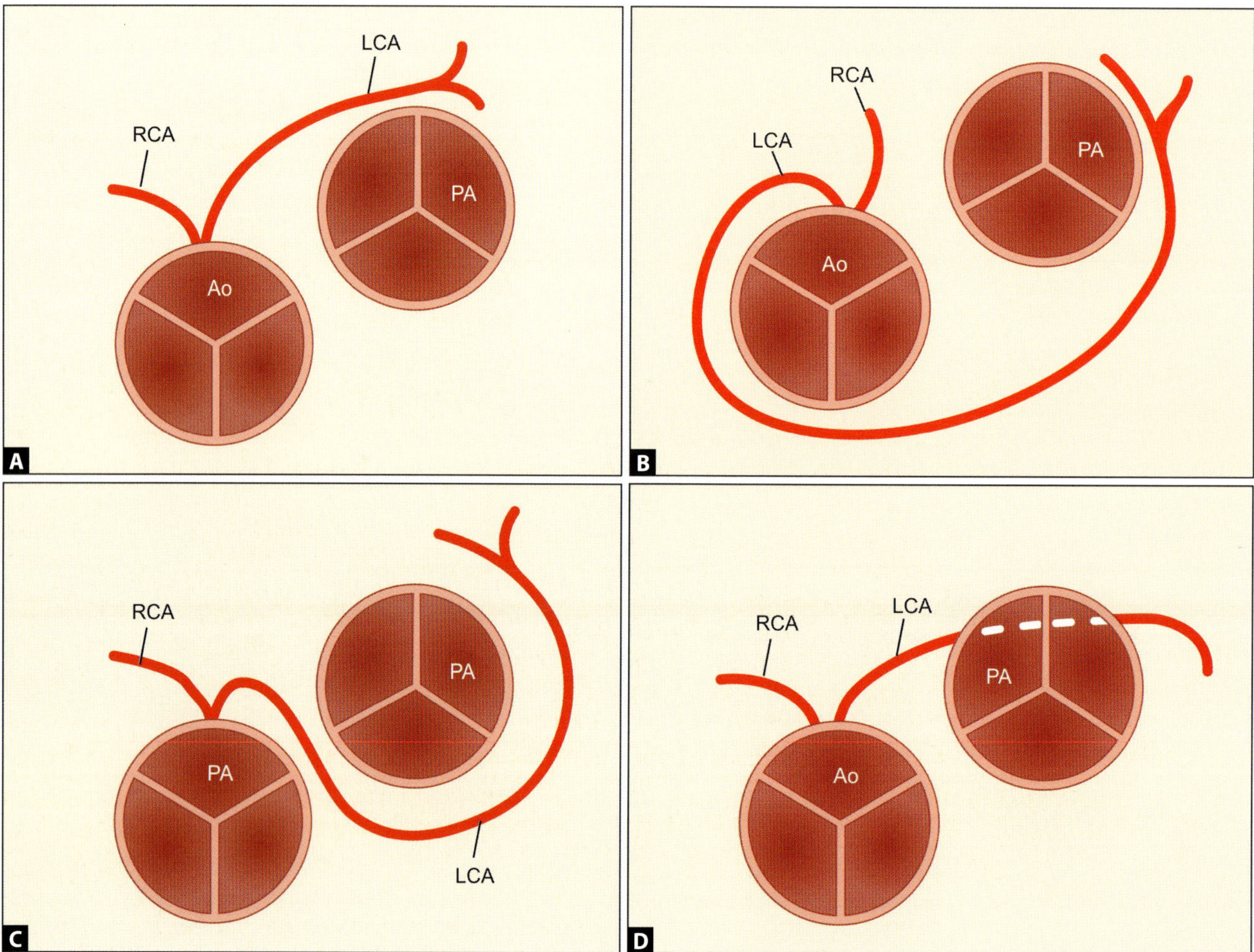


**Figure 21.8A to D:** Line diagram (parasternal short-axis view at the level of great vessels) of origin of left coronary artery from right coronary sinus and its course in relation to great vessels. (A) Anterior or prepulmonic left coronary artery. (B) Posterior or retroaortic course of left coronary artery. (C) Interarterial or preaortic course of left coronary artery. (D) Septal or subpulmonic course of left coronary artery.

*Abbreviations:* Ao, aorta; LCA, left coronary artery; PA, pulmonary artery; RCA, right coronary artery.

### *Echocardiographic Evaluation*

Four-chamber view (subcostal coronal and apical) in posterior plane shows course of left circumflex in posterior atrioventricular groove as it arises from right coronary artery **(Figure 21.11)**. Parasternal short-axis view at the level of great vessels profiles continuation of left main coronary artery to left anterior descending artery and origin of left circumflex from right coronary artery. This abnormal origin of the circumflex artery does not usually lead to any serious complications. However, in certain clinical situations like atrial septal defects undergoing percutaneous device closure, after the placement of the Amplatzer device, effort induced myocardial ischemia resulted from compression of the anomalous artery between the device on one side and the aortic root on the other.[48]

## Left Anterior Descending Artery from Right Coronary Artery

Left anterior descending artery from right coronary artery is a common anomaly of coronary artery and one the most common coronary anomaly seen in tetralogy of Fallot.[49]

In isolation, left anterior descending artery from right coronary artery does not carry any clinical implication but leads to technical difficulty to the surgeon during surgical

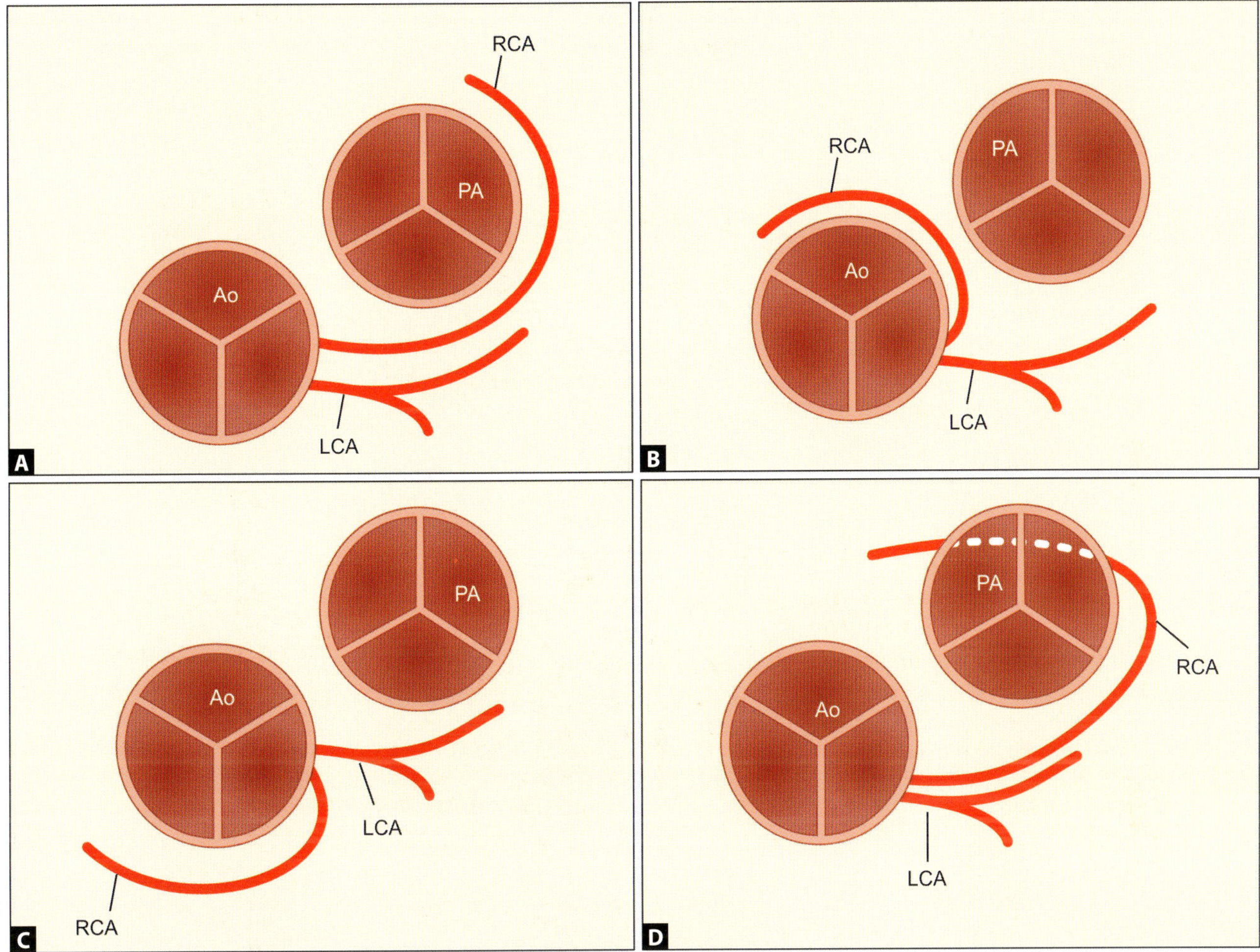


**Figure 21.9A to D:** Line diagram (parasternal short-axis view at the level of great vessels) of origin of right coronary artery from left coronary sinus and its course in relation to great vessels. (A) Anterior or prepulmonic right coronary artery. (B) Interarterial or preaortic course of right coronary artery. (C) Posterior or retroaortic course of left coronary artery. (D) Septal or subpulmonic course of right coronary artery.

*Abbreviations:* Ao, aorta; LCA, left coronary artery; PA, pulmonary artery; RCA, right coronary artery.

correction of tetralogy of Fallot with hypoplastic pulmonary annulus requiring transannular patch. In case of left anterior descending artery from right coronary artery crossing right ventricular outflow tract, right ventricle to pulmonary artery conduit is needed for total correction.

### *Echocardiographic Evaluation*

Parasternal short-axis view at the level of great vessels is best to define this anomaly **(Figure 21.12)**. Coronary from left facing sinus would be continuing to circumflex artery and left anterior descending artery arising from right coronary artery would be crossing right ventricular outflow tract. Subcostal paracoronal view can also be used to define origin of left anterior descending artery from right sinus.

## Coronary Artery Fistula

Coronary artery fistulas are considered a major coronary anomaly by Ogden's classification,[50] and represent an anomaly of termination. Coronary arteriovenous fistulas are present in 1 of 50,000 livebirths (0.002% of the general population) and are visualized in 1 of 500 patients undergoing catheterization (0.2–0.25%). The etiology of these lesions may be congenital or acquired; latter may be broken down into infectious, traumatic, and iatrogenic. Iatrogenic causes may be further

**Figure 21.10A and B:** Spiral computed tomography angiography of a child with tetralogy of Fallot showing **Figure 21.9A** pattern of coronary.
*Abbreviations:* Ao, aorta; LCA, left coronary artery; LMCA, left main coronary artery; PA, pulmonary artery; RCA, right coronary artery.

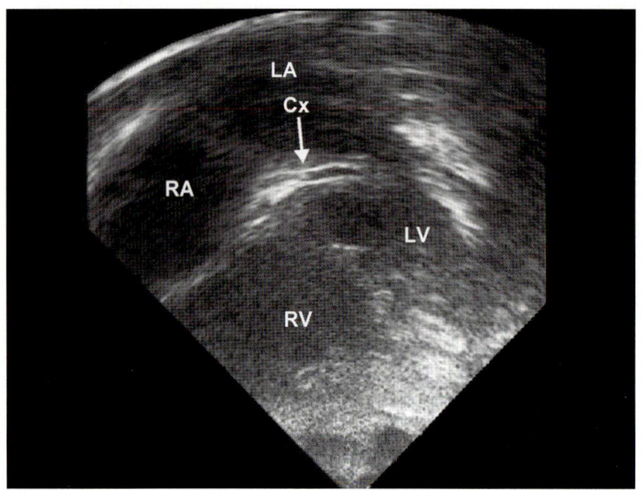


**Figure 21.11:** Apical 4-chamber view from a child with circumflex artery from right coronary artery. Apical 4-chamber view (two-dimensional) showing circumflex artery just anterior to mitral valve and posterior to aorta.
*Abbreviations:* Cx, circumflex artery; LA, left atrium; LV, left ventricle; RA, right atrium; RV, right ventricle.

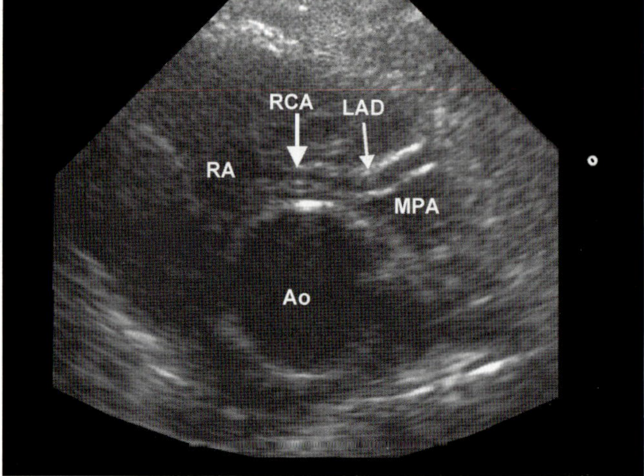


**Figure 21.12:** Parasternal short-axis view at the level of great vessels showing origin of left anterior descending artery from right coronary artery in a child with tetralogy of Fallot (thick arrow). Left anterior descending artery crossing right ventricular outflow tract anteriorly (thin arrow).
*Abbreviations:* Ao, aorta; LAD, left anterior descending artery; MPA, main pulmonary artery; RA, right atrium; RCA, right coronary artery.

subdivided as surgical, postcatheterization, postangioplasty, or postendomyocardial biopsy.

Coronary artery fistula involves right coronary artery in 60% of patients, left anterior descending artery in 25% of patients and left circumflex artery in 15% of patients. Rarely does it involve more than one coronary arteries, diagonal or marginal branches, or a single coronary artery. The common sites of drainage are right ventricle in about 30% of instances, right atrium in about 25% of instances, pulmonary artery in 20% of instances, rarely into left atrium or left ventricle or coronary sinus, or superior vena cava. The termination may be as single orifice or through multiple orifices.

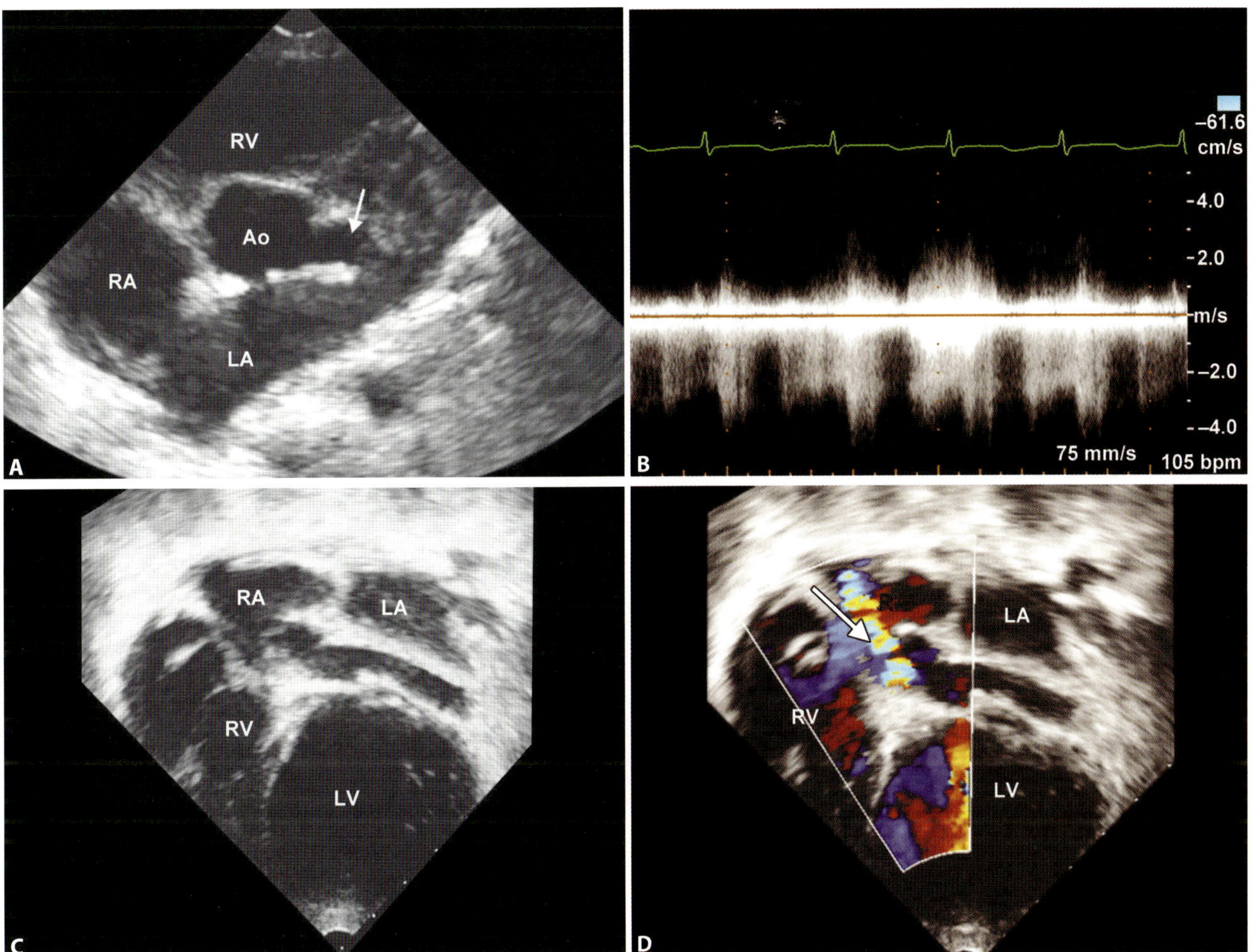


**Figure 21.13A to D:** Echocardiography from a patient with coronary arteriovenous fistula, circumflex to right atrium. (A) Parasternal short- axis view at the level of great vessels showing dilated left coronary artery. (B) Continuous wave Doppler interrogation of communication of coronary arteriovenous fistula showing continuous flow across the communication. (C) Apical 4-chamber view in most posterior plane. Two-dimensional echocardiography showing circumflex artery continues behind the aortic root as a feeding vessel to the fistula draining into the right atrium. (D) Same view with color flow mapping showing turbulent (continuous) flow of coronary arteriovenous fistula to right atrium.
*Abbreviations:* Ao, aorta; LA, left atrium; LV, left ventricle; RA, right atrium; RV, right ventricle.

## *Echocardiographic Evaluation*

Echocardiographic features of coronary arteriovenous fistula are as follows:

- Dilated proximal coronary artery in parasternal short-axis view or transesophageal echocardiography in horizontal plane **(Figure 21.13A)**.
- Continuous color Doppler flows with high velocity rather than diastolic flows seen in normal coronary arteries **(Figure 21.13B)**.
- Course of the fistula to its termination **(Figure 21.13C and D)**.
- Volume overload of cardiac chambers depending on the magnitude of left-to-right shunt through the fistula.
- Rarely, the fistula opens into a large sac (5th cardiac chamber or aneurysm), which opens into one of the cardiac chambers **(Figure 21.14A and B)**.

Thus, echocardiography provides good details of fistula in many patients.

Angiographic classification of surgical relevance is proposed by Sakakibara.[51] Type A (proximal type), proximal coronary segment dilated to the origin of fistula, distal end normal; and type B (distal type), coronary dilated over entire length, terminating as a fistula in the right side of the heart

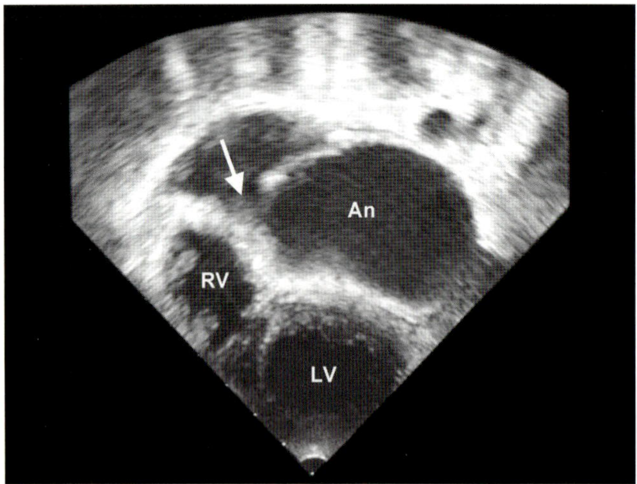


**Figure 21.14A:** Apical 4-chamber view (two-dimensional) with posterior tilt of a child with coronary arteriovenous fistula arising from left circumflex, opening in a large sac [aneurysm (An) or 5th cardiac chamber] and then terminating in right atrium. *Abbreviations:* LV, left ventricle; RV, right ventricle.

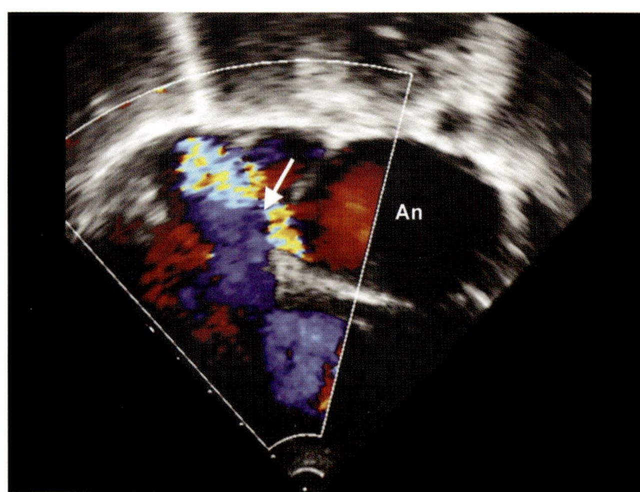


**Figure 21.14B:** On color flow mapping, 5th cardiac chamber opening to right atrium (arrow) is seen. *Abbreviation:* An, aneurysm.

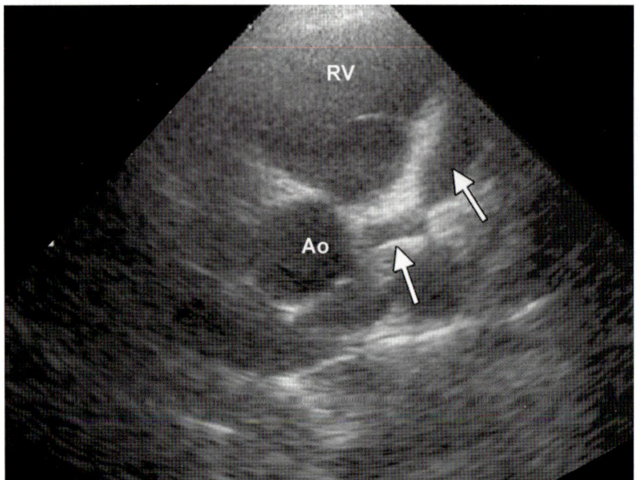


**Figure 21.15A:** Parasternal short-axis view at the level of great vessels from a child with Kawasaki disease showing dilated left main and aneurysmal left anterior descending artery. *Abbreviations:* Ao, aorta; RV, right ventricle.

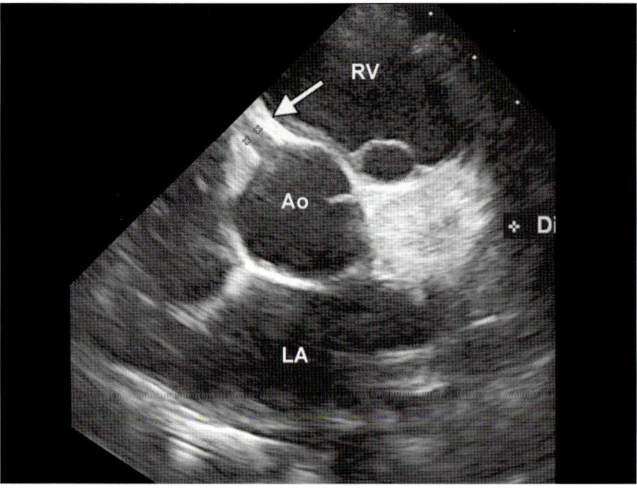


**Figure 21.15B:** Parasternal short-axis view at the level of great vessels with Kawasaki disease showing dilated right coronary artery. *Abbreviations:* Ao, aorta; LA, left atrium; RV, right ventricle.

(end-artery type), proximal to fistula, regular branching of coronary. Surgically, type A is treated by epicardial ligation of the fistula, distal to the fistula origin, maintaining normal branch flow, and no cardiopulmonary bypass is required. Type B requires ligation of the precapillary end by intracameral purse-string sutures at the site of termination, and requires cardiopulmonary bypass. In current era, majority of coronary artery fistulae are managed in cardiac catheterization laboratory by coils or devices. Some fistulae are hemodynamically less significant and may not need any intervention **(Figure 21.15A and B)**.

## Atresia of Left Main Coronary Artery

Atresia of left main coronary artery with lack of luminal continuity from aortic root to left coronary artery is associated with collaterals from the right coronary artery through septal branches.[52]

### *Echocardiographic Evaluation*

- Dilated right coronary artery.
- Left ventricular dysfunction.
- Mitral regurgitation due to sclerosed papillary muscle.
- Collaterals flow. This mimics the septal collaterals of anomalous origin of left coronary artery from pulmonary artery on echocardiography, but there will be no reverse flow pattern seen in left coronary artery and no left-to-right shunt in pulmonary artery.

## Coronary Aneurysms

Aneurysms are defined as dilations of a coronary vessel 1.5 times the adjacent normal coronaries. There exist two forms: saccular and fusiform, fusiform being the most common. Aneurysms may be congenital or could be acquired. Acquired causes are atherosclerotic, Kawasaki's disease, traumatic, iatrogenic (surgical, postangioplasty, postcatheterization, or postendomyocardial biopsy), infectious, and systemic diseases (polyarteritis nodosa, syphilis, Ehlers-Danlos, Marfan's disease, and scleroderma).

## Kawasaki Disease

In clinical practice, Kawasaki disease is the most common problem associated with coronary aneurysms. Moderate coronary involvement with aneurysms is present in 12.8–25% of patients with untreated Kawasaki's disease; the incidence of coronary involvement reduces to one fifth after intravenous gamma globulin therapy.[53,54] The following definitions pertaining to Kawasaki disease are generally accepted in the literature:

- *Segmental stenosis*: A braid-like lesion with multiple tortuosities of the vessel which represents recanalization of an occlusion.
- *Localized stenosis*: A discrete, wedge-like narrowing at the inlet or outlet of an aneurysm. *Ectasia*: 1.5 times larger than normal adjacent coronaries.
- *Dilation/small aneurysm*: Greater than or equal to 3 mm (± irregular lumen).
- *Aneurysms*: 4–8 mm; and *giant aneurysms* greater than 8 mm.

Echocardiography is primary modality for evaluation and serial assessment of coronary artery abnormalities in patients with Kawasaki disease.[55] Cardiac involvement in Kawasaki disease are following:

- *Coronary involvement:* On echocardiography, proximal part of left main, left anterior descending artery, left circumflex, and right coronary artery can be defined from parasternal short-axis view at the level of great vessels as described earlier **(Figure 21.15 and 21.16)**. Apical 4-chamber view with posterior tilt is used to define distal part of right coronary artery in right atrioventricular groove and of left circumflex in left atrioventricular groove. All of the coronary artery branches should be carefully measured from different views. In normal subjects, caliber of the coronary artery shows little variability from origin to 1 cm distally and rages in size from 2 mm in infants to 5 mm in teenagers.[56] On echocardiography, one should look for dilatation of the coronary artery, aneurysm formation (secular/fusiform) and presence of thrombus formation within the aneurysm.
- Ventricular dysfunction.[57]
- Valve regurgitation.
- Pericardial effusion.

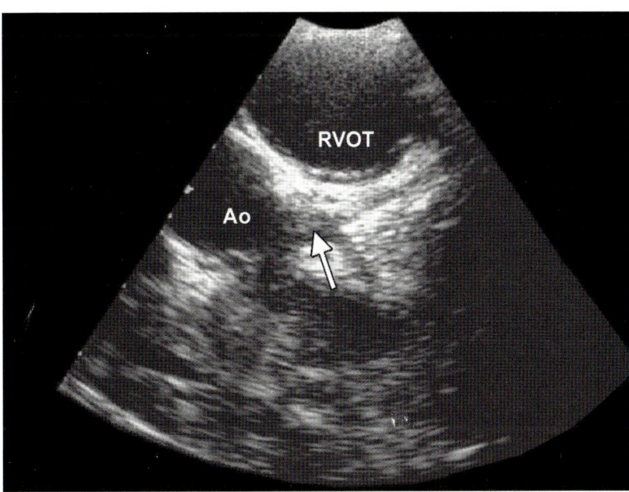


**Figure 21.16:** Parasternal short-axis view at the level of great vessels from a child with Kawasaki disease showing dilated left main coronary artery.
*Abbreviation:* Ao, aorta; RVOT, right ventricular outflow tract.

## DISCLOSURE

After a significant coronary artery abnormality is recognized in a pediatric patient, surgery or appropriate transcatheter intervention should be performed. The risk of fatality from a congenital coronary abnormality far outweighs the small risks of surgical or transcatheter intervention. Angiography, although considered the state-of-the-art method of diagnosis, has significant spatial limitations and is not always diagnostic of aberrant coronary origins from the contralateral aortic sinus. In the hands of an experienced echocardiographer, color-flow Doppler echocardiography is one of the best diagnostic tools for congenital coronary abnormalities. Various coronary anomalies are identifiable with certainty with this imaging modality, but some are suspected by 2D and Doppler echocardiography. For complete evaluation, other cardiac imaging methods like CT, MRI, and conventional angiography may be needed.

## VIDEO LEGENDS

**Video 21.1:** Two dimensional echocardiography in parasternal short axis view at the level of great vessels showing origin of left coronary artery from medial aspect of main pulmonary artery. Caution needs to be exercised as the echocardiography seems to give an impression that the left coronary artery is arising from aorta.

**Video 21.2:** Two dimensional echocardiography in apical four chamber view showing sclerosed dilated left ventricle with severe systolic dysfunction. Mitral valve papillary muscle is also sclerosed.

**Video 21.3:** Color flow mapping in parasternal short axis view showing flow reversal in left coronary artery (blue). Please note, the left coronary artery is seen to be originating from the medial aspect of the main pulmonary artery.

**Video 21.4:** Parasternal short axis view with color flow mapping showing flow reversal in left coronary artery (blue color in left anterior descending artery and red in circumflex artery). Left coronary artery is originating from the left lateral aspect of the main pulmonary artery.

**Video 21.5:** Apical four-chamber view with color flow mapping showing moderate mitral regurgitation.

## REFERENCES


1. Warnes CA, Williams RG, Bashore TM, Child JS, Connolly HM, Dearani JA, et al. ACC/AHA 2008 guidelines for the management of adults with congenital heart disease: a report of the American College of Cardiology/American Heart Association Task Force on Practice Guidelines. J Am Coll Cardiol. 2008;52:143-263.
2. Angelini P. Coronary artery anomalies: an entity in search of an identity. Circulation. 2007;115:1296-305.
3. Zeppilli P, Dello Russo A, Santini C, Palmieri V, Natale L, Giordano A, et al. In vivo detection of coronary artery anomalies in asymptomatic athletes by echocardiographic screening. Chest. 1998;114:89-93.
4. Pelliccia A, Spataro A, Maron BJ. Prospective echocardiographic screening for coronary artery anomalies in 1,360 elite competitive athletes. Am J Cardiol. 1993;72:978-9.
5. Frommelt PC, Frommelt MA, Tweddell JS, et al. Prospective echocardiographic diagnosis and surgical repair of anomalous origin of a coronary artery from the opposite sinus with an interarterial course. J Am Coll Cardiol. 2003;42:148-54.
6. Van Camp SP, Bloor CM, Mueller FO, et al. Nontraumatic sports death in high school and college athletes. Med Sci Sports Exerc. 1995;27:641-7.
7. Maron BJ, Thompson PD, Puffer JC, et al. Cardiovascular preparticipation screening of competitive athletes: a statement for health professionals from the Sudden Death Committee (Clinical Cardiology) and Congenital Cardiac Defects Committee (Cardiovascular Disease in the Young), American Heart Association. Circulation. 1996;94:850-6.
8. Burke AP, Farb A, Virmani R, et al. Sports-related and non-sports-related sudden cardiac death in young adults. Am Heart J. 1991;121:568-75.
9. Alexander RW, Griffith GC. Anomalies of the coronary arteries and their clinical significance. Circulation. 1956;14:800-5.
10. Angelini P, Villason S, Chan AV, et al. Normal and anomalous coronary arteries in humans. In: Angelini P (Ed). Coronary Artery Anomalies: A Comprehensive Approach. Philadelphia: Lippincott Williams & Wilkins; 1999. pp 27-150.
11. Weyman AE, Feigenbaum H, Dillon JC, et al. Noninvasive visualization of the left coronary artery b cross-sectional echocardiography. Circulation. 1976;54:169.
12. Fisher EA, Sepehri B, Lendrum B, et al. Two-dimensional echocardiographic visualization of the left coronary artery in anomalous origin of the left coronary artery from the pulmonary artery: pre- and postoperative studies. Circulation. 1981;63:698-707.
13. The normal echocardiographic examination. In: Snider AR, Serwer GA, Ritter SB (Eds). Echocardiography in Pediatric Heart Disease. Mosby; 1997. pp. 22-75.
14. Yamanaka O, Hobbs RE. Coronary artery anomalies in 126,595 patients undergoing coronary angiography. Cathet Cardiovasc Diagn. 1990;21:28-40.
15. Baltaxe HA, Wixson D. The incidence of congenital anomalies of the coronary arteries in the adult population. Radiology. 1977;122:47-52.
16. Bensky AS, Meyer RA. An unusual coronary artery origin in a patient with anomalous left coronary artery. J Pediatr. 1993; 122:S100.
17. Koike K, Musewe NN, Smallhorn JF, et al. Distinguishing between anomalous origin of the left coronary artery from the pulmonary trunk and dilated cardiomyopathy: role of echocardiographic measurement of the right coronary artery diameter. Br Heart J. 1989;61:192-7.
18. Schmidt KG, Cooper MJ, Silverman NH, et al. Pulmonary artery origin of the left coronary artery: diagnosis by two-dimensional echocardiography, pulsed Doppler ultrasound, and color flow mapping. J Am Coll Cardiol. 1988;11:396.
19. Rein AJ, Colan SD, Parness IA, et al. Regional and global left ventricular function in infants with anomalous origin of the left coronary artery from the pulmonary trunk:preoperative and post operative assessment. Circulation. 1987;75:115-23.
20. Karr SS, Parness IA, Spevak PJ, van der Velde ME, Colan SD, Sanders SP. Diagnosis of anomalous left coronary artery by Doppler color flow mapping:distinction from other causes of dilated cardiomyopathy. J Am Coll Cardiol. 1992;19:1271-5.
21. Fyfe DA, Sade RM, Gillette PC, et al. Pre- and postoperative Doppler echocardiographic evaluation of anomalous left coronary artery arising from the pulmonary artery. Ultrasound Med. 1987;6:101-3.
22. Swensson RE, Murillo-Olivas A, Elias W, Bender R, Daily PO, Sahn DJ. Noninvasive Doppler color flow mapping for detection of the left coronary from the pulmonary artery and evaluation of surgical repair. J Am Coll Cardiol. 1988;11:659-61.
23. Holly DG, Sell JE, Hougen TJ, et al. Pulsed Doppler echocardiographic and color flow imaging detection of retrograde filling of anomalous left coronary artery from the pulmonary artery. J Am Soc Echocardiogr. 1992;5:85-8.

24. Post JC, van Rossum AC, Bronzwaer JGF, et al. Magnetic resonance angiography of anomalous coronary arteries: a new gold standard for delineating the proximal course? Circulation. 1995;92:3163-71.
25. Su JT, Krishnamurthy R, Chung T, et al. Anomalous right coronary artery from the pulmonary artery: noninvasive diagnosis and serial evaluation. J Cardiovasc Magn Reson. 2007;9:57-61.
26. Mintz GS, Iskandrian AS, Bemis CE, et al. Myocardial ischemia in anomalous origin of the right coronary artery from the pulmonary trunk. Proof of a coronary steal. Am J Cardiol. 1983;51:610-2.
27. Williams IA, Gersony WM, Hellenbrand WE. Anomalous right coronary artery arising from the pulmonary artery: a report of 7 cases and a review of the literature. Am Heart J. 2006; 152:1004e9-17.
28. Yao CT, Wang JN, Yeh CN, Huang SC, Yang YR, Wu JM. Isolated anomalous origin of right coronary artery from the main pulmonary artery. J Card Surg. 2005;20:487-9.
29. Li RJ, Yang Y, Li ZA, et al. Right coronary artery arising from the main pulmonary artery: evaluation with 2-dimensional transthoracic echocardiography and multislice computed tomography. Tex Heart Inst J. 2010;37:376-7.
30. Subban V, Jeyaram B, Sankardas MA. Anomalous origin of left anterior descending artery from the pulmonary artery. Heart. 2010;96:170.
31. Ott D, Cooley DA, Pinsky W, et al. Anomalous origin of circumflex coronary artery from right pulmonary artery. J Thorac Cardiovasc Surg. 1978;76:190-4.
32. Garcia CM, Chandler J, Russell R. Anomalous left coronary artery from the right pulmonary artery: first adult case report. Am Heart J. 1992;123:526-8.
33. Doty DB, Chandramouli B, Schieken RE, et al. Anomalous origin of the left coronary artery from the right pulmonary artery. J Thorac Cardiovasc Surg. 1976;71:787-91.
34. Korosoglou G, Ringwald G, Giannitsis E, et al. Anomalous origin of the left circumflex coronary artery from the pulmonary artery: a very rare congenital anomaly in an adult patient diagnosed by cardiovascular magnetic resonance. J Cardiovasc Magn Reson. 2008;10:4.
35. Kirklin JW, Barratt-Boyes BG. Cardiac Surgery, 2nd edition. New York: Churchill Livingstone;1993. pp. 1178-9.
36. Virmani R, Chun PKC, Goldstein RE, et al. Acute takeoffs of the coronary arteries along the aortic wall and congenital coronary ostial valve-like ridges: association with sudden death. J Am Coll Cardiol. 1984;3:766-71.
37. Bellhouse BJ, Bellhouse FH. Fluid mechanics of the aortic coronary flow. Nature. 1968;219:1059-61.
38. Roberts WC, Shirani J. The four subtypes of anomalous origin of the left main coronary artery from the right aortic sinus (or from right coronary artery). Am J Cardiol. 1992;70:119-21.
39. Gerber TC, Kuzo RS, Safford RE. Computed tomographic imaging of anomalous coronary arteries. Circulation. 2002; 106:e67.
40. Ropers D, Gehling G, Pohle K, et al. Anomalous course of the left main or left anterior descending coronary artery originating from the right sinus of Valsalva. Circulation. 2002;105:e42.
41. Basso C, Maron BJ, Corrado D, et al. Clinical profile of congenital coronary artery anomalies with origin from the wrong aortic sinus leading to sudden death in young competitive athletes. J Am Coll Cardiol. 2000;35:1493-501.
42. Kragel AH, Roberts WC. Anomalous origin of either the right or left main coronary artery from the aorta with subsequent coursing between aorta and pulmonary trunk: analysis of 32 necropsy cases. Am J Cardiol. 1988;62:771.
43. Mustafa I, Gula G, Ridley-Smith R, et al. Anomalous origin of the left coronary artery from the anterior aortic sinus: a potential cause of sudden death. Anatomic characterization and surgical treatment. J Thorac Cardiovasc Surg. 1981;82:297.
44. Schwarz ER, Hager PK, Uebis R, et al. Myocardial ischaemia in a case of a solitary coronary ostium in the right aortic sinus with retroaortic course of the left coronary artery: documentation of the underlying pathophysiological mechanisms of ischaemia by intracoronary Doppler and pressure measurements. Heart 1998;80:307-11.
45. Barth CW III, Bray M, Robetrs WC. Sudden death ininfancy associated with origin of both left main and right coronary arteries from a common ostium above the left sinus of Valsalva. Am J Cardiol. 1986;57:365-6.
46. Brandt B III, Martin JB, M arcus ML. Anomalous origin of the right coronary artery from left sinus of Valsalva. N Eng I Med. 1983;309:596-8.
47. Henson KD, Geiser EA, Billett J, Alexander JA, Akins EW, Bopitiya C, et al. Use of transesophageal echocardiography to visualize an anomalous right coronary artery from the left main coronary artery (single coronary artery). Clin Cardiol. 1992;15:462-5.
48. Casolo G, Gensini GF, Santoro G, et al. Anomalous origin of the circumflex artery and patent foramen ovale: a rare cause of myocardial ischaemia after percutaneous closure of the defect. Heart. 2003;89:e23.
49. Jureidini SB, Appleton RS, Nouri S, et al. Detection of coronary artery abnormality in tetralogy of Fallot by two-dimensional echocardiography. J Am Coll Cardiol. 1989;14:960-7.
50. Ogden J.A. Congenital anomalies of the coronary arteries. Am J Cardiol. 1969;70:474-9.
51. Sakakibara S, Yokoyama M, Takao A, et al. Coronary arteriovenous fistula. Am Heart J. 1966;72:307-14.
52. Amabile N, Fraisse A, Quilci J. Hypoplastic coronary artery disease: report of one case. Heart. 2005;91:e12.
53. Akagi T, Rose V, Benson LN, et al. Outcome of coronary artery aneurysms after Kawasaki disease. J Pediatr. 1992;121:689-94.
54. Kato H, Kolke S, Yamamoto M, et al. Coronary aneurysms in infants and young children with acute febrile MCLNS. J Pediatr. 1975;86:892-8.
55. Capannari TE, Daniels SR, Meyer RA, et al. Sensitivity, specificity and predictive value of two-dimensional echocardiography in detecting coronary artery aneurysms in patients with Kawasaki disease. J Am Coll Cardiol. 1986;7:355-60.
56. Arjunan K, Daniels SR, Meyer RA, Schwartz DC, Barron H, Kaplan S. Coronary artery caliber in normal children and patients with Kawasaki disease but without aneurysm :and echocardiographic and angiographic study. J Am Coll Cardiol 1986;8:1119-24.
57. Anderson TM, Meyer RA, Kaplan S. Long-term echocardiographic evaluation of cardiac size and function in patients with Kawasaki disease. Am Heart J. 1985;110:107-15.

# Coronary Arterial Involvement in Connective Tissue Disorders and Other Diseases

22
CHAPTER

*Divya Malhotra, Raj Kumar*

## INTRODUCTION

Cardiac involvement is one of the main complications substantially contributing to morbidity and mortality of patients suffering from systemic autoimmune disease. All the anatomical heart structures can be affected and multiple pathogenic mechanisms have been reported. Inflammatory rheumatic diseases have a long recognized relationship with the cardiovascular system. The treatment of many rheumatic diseases has improved considerably over the past 15 years and increased survival. Patients with multisystem rheumatic diseases may on occasion initially be evaluated by, a cardiologist, a vascular or cardiothoracic surgeon, and early recognition of the immune-mediated basis of the cardiovascular disease reduces morbidity and mortality. The vasculature may represent a primary target organ of the underlying rheumatic disease and can be affected at numerous sites and at all levels.[1] Rheumatic diseases have equally important secondary effects on the cardiovascular system. Chronic systemic inflammation predisposes to endothelial dysfunction and increased arterial stiffness, thereby escalating risk for the development of atherosclerosis. Cardiovascular specialists are increasingly recognizing the significantly increased prevalence of premature myocardial infarction and stroke in patients suffering from rheumatoid arthritis (RA) and systemic lupus erythematous (SLE). Many outstanding clinical challenges remain, and predominant among them are early recognition and diagnosis of patients with rheumatic disease who have the highest risk for cardiovascular complications, alongside improved understanding of the underlying molecular mechanisms, and the development of preventive strategies.

Recognition of the role of inflammation in atherosclerosis has highlighted and stimulated study of the potential relationship between systemic inflammatory diseases and accelerated atherogenesis. This effort has substantially advanced our understanding of both the underlying pathogenic mechanisms and epidemiology. Current priorities include identification of patients most at risk and the development of preventive therapeutic strategies.[1] Evidence supporting an association between inflammatory diseases and accelerated atherogenesis is best developed for RA and SLE. Cardiovascular specialists should consider an underlying inflammatory disease in young patients with otherwise unexplained angina, myocardial infarction, or stroke. Patients with a rheumatic disease who suffer a myocardial infarction have worse outcomes in terms of both heart failure and mortality than does the age-matched general population.

In this chapter, an attempt has been made to highlight the involvement of coronary artery disease (CAD) and other cardiac involvement in patients with connective tissue disorders.

## SYSTEMIC LUPUS ERYTHEMATOUS

SLE is an autoimmune symmetric inflammatory disease. There is female predominance with female-to-male ratio of 9:1. The heart is frequently involved in SLE. Very sensitive methods of cardiovascular investigation have found >50% prevalence of cardiac involvement. In the past cardiac manifestations were severe, often leading to death and they were frequently found in postmortem examinations. Nowadays, cardiac manifestations are often mild and asymptomatic, and they are recognized by echocardiography and other noninvasive tests.

CAD in SLE can be related to arteritis, premature development of atherosclerotic CAD or combination of the two. Premature atherosclerosis in SLE patients has been documented in autopsy, mortality, and population-based observational studies. The prevalence of CAD ranges from 6% to 10%, and in SLE patients, the risk of developing any CAD is 4–8 times higher than in controls. Alarmingly in young women with SLE the risk of myocardial infarction is increased 50-fold.[2]

The role of traditional and nontraditional factors for CAD is still debated. Traditional risk factors, such as age, hypertension, and dyslipidemia are the most common predicators for CAD. Nontraditional risk factors, such as autoimmune inflammation, treatment with immunosuppressive agents, disease duration, high-score activity of disease all contribute to the development of atherosclerotic plaque. Novel risk factors for atherosclerosis have been proposed. They include new inflammatory markers [C-reactive protein (CRP), fibrinogen, interleukin-6 (IL-6)], co-stimulatory molecules (CD40/CD40L), adhesion molecules, such as antiphospholipid (aPL), anticardiolipin (aCL), and anti-β2 glycoprotein I (anti-β2GPI).

In histological studies of human carotid samples, β2GPI was shown to colocalize with T CD4+ lymphocytes in the subendothelial region of atherosclerotic plaques, supporting a possible role of antibodies in the disease progression. aPL accelerates the process of plaques formation, enhancing the macrophages transformation into foam cells by oxidized low-density lipoprotein.

Early endothelial dysfunction studied by abnormal brachial flow mediated vasodilatation, have been reported in patients with SLE. Correlation between aCL IgG antibody levels and increased carotid intimal medial thickness has also been reported. Arterial stiffness is increased in SLE, even in the absence of atherosclerosis. Arterial stiffening is related to disease duration and circulating levels of CRP and interleukin-6.[2]

Presence of autoantibodies complexes, such as antiphospholipid antibodies, anti-SSA/Ro have been implicated in the inflammatory process responsible for pericarditis, endocarditis, and myocarditis.

## Echocardiographic Features

- Pericarditis is the most studied cardiovascular manifestation of SLE. The reported prevalence ranges from 11% to 54%. Deposition of immunoglobulin and C3 demonstrated by direct immunofluorescence support the role of immune complexes in development of pericarditis.[2] Echocardiography represents the standard method to investigate pericardial abnormalities and is able to demonstrate thickening of pericardial layers and quantify amount of pericardial effusion.
- The SLE patients have higher left ventricular (LV) mass index. Arterial stiffness was independently related to LV mass, suggesting that inflammation-related arterial stiffening is the likely mechanism of LV hypertrophy in SLE patients.
- Myocarditis is most characteristic feature of myocardial involvement in SLE. The clinical detection of myocarditis ranges from 3% to 15%.[2] Granular immune complexes and complement deposition in the walls and perivascular tissue are implicated in the pathogenesis of lupus myocarditis. Echocardiography cannot definitely diagnose myocarditis, but global hypokinesis in the absence of other known causes is strongly suggestive. Large echocardiography series have found frequencies of global hypokinesia between 5% and 20% of the patients. However, segmental area of hypokinesis can also be indicative of disease.
- *Valvular disease:* Valvular nodules and have been seen in majority of patients with SLE. This valvular alteration is called verrucous endocarditis (Libman–Sacks endocarditis). Clinically significant valvular heart disease is less common. Varying prevalence of valvular abnormalities has been reported in echocardiographic literature. Significant valvular regurgitation occurs in very few patients. The development of significant regurgitation may be related to high levels of IgG anticardiolipin antibodies. Large transthoracic echocardiography (TTE) studies of unselected patients document an association between higher anticardiolipin titers, valvular nodules and significant regurgitation, particularly involving mitral valve. Libman–Sacks endocarditis on echocardiography presents with sessile lesions on the valves and can be found on any surface of the valve.
- Indices of diastolic dysfunction with abnormal early- to late-diastolic mitral inflow velocity ratio, abnormal tissue Doppler and abnormal mitral flow propagation velocity have also been reported in SLE patients.[3]
- Segmental wall-motion abnormalities secondary to CAD (vasculitis or accelerated atherosclerosis) also has been reported.

### *Case Illustration*

***A 28-year-old lady with known history of SLE, presented to the emergency room with chest pain and shortness of breath for the last 4–5 days. She had no history of hypertension. The electrocardiogram (ECG) revealed diffuse ST segment elevation in anterolateral and inferior leads. Echo done revealed LV hypertrophy with mildly increased myocardial echogenicity (Figure 22.1A). There was minimal circumferential pericardial effusion (Figure 22.1B). Hypokinesia of the apex and mid-anterior wall and mid-septum, LV ejection fraction (LVEF) 35% (Videos 22.1A to C). Tissue Doppler imaging revealed reduced mitral annular systolic and early diastolic velocities (Figure 22.1C). Cardiac-specific troponin and creatine phosphokinase MB, erythrocyte sedimentation rate (ESR) and high sensitivity CRP were elevated. Angiography revealed normal coronaries. Follow-up echocardiography in 4 weeks revealed regression of LV hypertrophy, no pericardial effusion and improvement of LVEF and tissue Doppler parameters (Figure 22.1D to F and Videos 22.2A to C). This is an example of myopericarditis secondary to SLE with regression of LV hypertrophy, and improvement of LVEF over 4 weeks.***

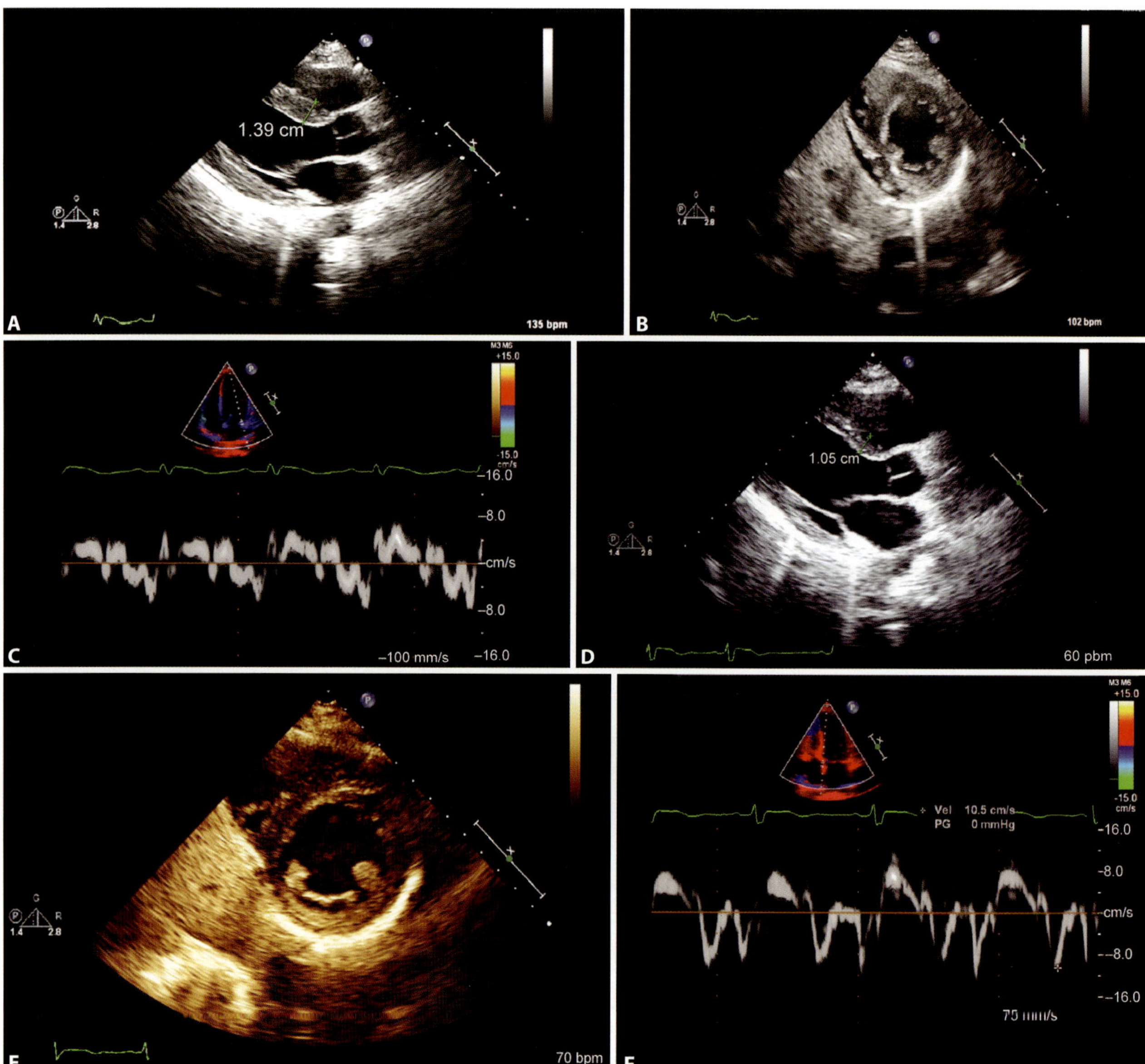


**Figure 22.1A to F:** A patient with systemic lupus erythematous presenting with acute chest pain and breathlessness. (A) Parasternal long-axis view reveals mild concentric left ventricular hypertrophy with mildly increased myocardial echogenicity. (B) Same findings observed in parasternal short-axis view, along with mild pericardial effusion. (C) Reduced mitral annular systolic and early diastolic velocities. (D to F) All these abnormalities disappeared by 4 weeks after the initial presentation.

## RHEUMATOID ARTHRITIS

RA is an autoimmune, symmetric inflammatory polyarthritis with a female-to-male ratio of 3:1. It affects up to 1% of the population in the western world with the onset of symptoms most commonly occurring between 30 years and 50 years of age.

For patients with RA ≥ 50 years of age, a detailed history, physical examination, and ECG to periodically assess for the presence of CAD is recommended. Exercise or pharmacologic-stress testing is suggested for symptomatic patients. Although RA independently raises the risk for atherosclerosis, the precise mechanistic relationship between RA and atherogenesis remains unknown. A recent study of microvascular and macrovascular function in RA has suggested that the classic cardiovascular risk factors may influence endothelial function more than disease-related inflammation. The direct effect of chronic inflammation on vascular endothelium may itself promote atherogenesis, in addition to exacerbating the actions of traditional cardiovascular risk factors. Moreover, the systemic inflammatory environment can contribute to the features of plaque and blood that promote cardiovascular events in patients with RA.

Patients with RA have increased classic risk factors for atherosclerosis. The risk for myocardial infarction in patients with RA is similar to that in those with diabetes mellitus. Women with RA are twice as likely as age-matched controls in the general population to suffer myocardial infarction. Although death rates from both heart attack and stroke are comparable to that in the general population, events occur at an earlier age, with 50% of premature deaths in patients with RA being a direct consequence of cardiovascular disease. The excess mortality becomes apparent 7–10 years after diagnosis and has been associated with persistent disease activity and the presence of rheumatoid factor and anticyclic citrullinated peptide antibodies. Current evidence suggests that patients with RA who suffer a myocardial infarction are less likely to receive acute reperfusion therapy and secondary preventive measures and thus have worse outcomes.

### Echocardiographic Features

- *Pericarditis:* Acute painful pericarditis occurs in less than 10% of patients with RA during their lifetimes. Echocardiography and cardiac magnetic resonance imaging (MRI) is used to identify pericardial effusion and pericardial thickness.
- *Pulmonary hypertension*: It is a rare complication of interstitial lung disease in patients with RA. Echocardiography can reveal right ventricular dysfunction, pulmonary artery dilation and increased pulmonary artery pressures.
- *Aortitis:* It is a rare complication of RA, which, when present, is typically accompanied by rheumatoid vasculitis in other vessels.[4]
- *Disease at the coronary ostia or associated coronary vasculitis*: It can cause myocardial infarction. Dilatation of the ascending aorta is also a common initial finding. Thoracic aortic dissection or rupture have also been reported. An imaging study with transthoracic or transesophageal echocardiography (TEE) is necessary to confirm the diagnosis.

## VASCULITIS

Vasculitides are a heterogeneous group of diseases. The primary systemic vasculitides are classified into large-, medium-, and small-vessel disease. The histologic features of vasculitis include perivascular inflammatory infiltrates, which typically affect the inner layer of the tunica media. Complications include stenosis and occlusions resulting in organ ischemia, thrombosis, aneurysm formation, and hemorrhage.

The immunopathogenesis of the vasculitides is complex, multifactorial, and poorly understood. The endothelium may be subject to complement-mediated injury as a consequence of immune complex deposition in polyarteritis nodosa (PAN) or rheumatoid vasculitis. In the medium- and small-vessel vasculitides, antineutrophilic cytoplasmic antibodies (ANCAs) may activate neutrophils and subsequently damage the endothelium. The proinflammatory cytokines tumor necrosis factor (TNF)-$\alpha$, IL-1, IL-6, and interferon-gamma (IFN-$\gamma$) may activate the endothelium and induce the expression of adhesion molecules, including E-selectin, vascular cell adhesion molecule-1 (VCAM-1), and intercellular adhesion molecule-1 (ICAM-1), thereby facilitating leukocyte adhesion, and recruitment into the vessel wall and surrounding tissue.

Cardiovascular disease in patients with vasculitis, although relatively rare, can be life-threatening. Aortitis, hypertension, coronary arteritis, valvular heart disease, pericarditis, myocarditis, conduction abnormalities, accelerated atherosclerosis, and cardiac failure can all occur. This section focuses on the vasculitides most likely to be encountered by cardiovascular disease specialists.

### Large-vessel Vasculitis

#### *Giant Cell Arteritis*

Giant cell arteritis (GCA) affects large and medium-sized arteries. The disease affects those older than 50 years, with incidence increasing with age. While GCA typically affects the temporal artery, it also affects extracranial branches of the aorta, may involve the subclavian and axillary arteries, thoracic aorta, and on occasion, the femoral and iliac arteries.

Clinical features include fever, weight loss, malaise, headache, temporal-artery thickening with loss of pulsation, scalp tenderness, and jaw claudication. The most feared complication, anterior ischemic optic neuropathy, may be manifested as amaurosis fugax or sudden permanent visual loss.

Histopathologic examination reveals localized fragmentation of the internal elastic lamina closely associated with an inflammatory infiltrate consisting predominantly of IFN-$\gamma$-producing CD4+ T lymphocytes, monocytes/macrophages, and occasional characteristic multinucleated giant cells. Recent studies have revealed that activated CD83+ dendritic cells initiate the arterial wall inflammation and colocalize with activated T cells. Local synthesis of growth factors, such as platelet-derived growth factor leads to concentric proliferation of smooth muscle cells and occlusion of the arterial lumen. On occasion, release of matrix

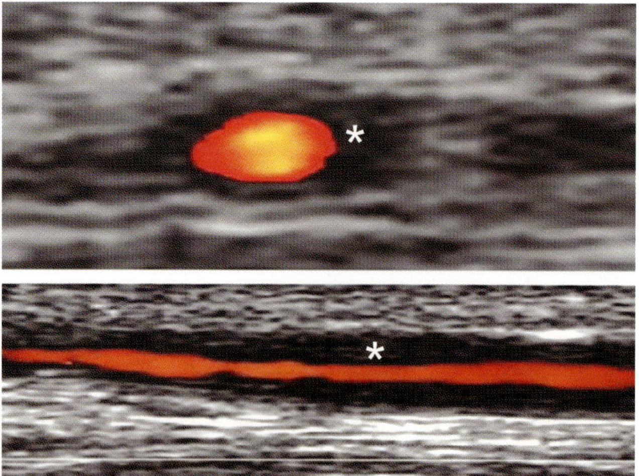


**Figure 22.2:** Temporal artery ultrasound revealing the classic halo sign (*) on short- and long-axis images in a patient with giant cell arteritis.

metalloproteinases and generation of reactive oxygen species result in arterial wall injury and aneurysm formation.

An 18F-fluorodeoxyglucose positron emission tomography (FDG-PET) has confirmed earlier autopsy findings and shown widespread arteritis with increased FDG uptake throughout the aorta and subclavian and iliac arteries in more than 50% of patients.[1]

*Ultrasound and echo features:*[5] Three characteristic ultrasound features of the temporal artery Doppler are as follows **(Figure 22.2)**:

1. A periluminal hypoechogenic halo reflecting arterial wall edema.
2. Segmental arterial stenosis.
3. Arterial luminal occlusion in severe cases.[5]

There have been case reports of such ultrasound findings with thickening of the wall of the aorta with hypoechogenic halo of the aorta on echo or TEE.

Coronary GCA, manifest as tapering lesions in the coronary arteries and myocardial infarction, also has been reported. The frequency of aortic involvement in GCA is not known. It is suggested that all patients with temporal GCA who present with symptoms suggestive of extracranial vascular involvement undergo an imaging study to evaluate the aorta and large vessels. An association has been found between a history of GCA and the development of aortic aneurysm.[6]

## Takayasu Arteritis

Takayasu arteritis (TA) or pulseless disease, a granulomatous panarteritis, affects the aorta and its major branches, typically before the age of 40 years. The disease predominates in women, with a female-to-male ratio of up to 10:1. Initial symptoms typically include nonspecific complaints, such as fever, night sweats, arthralgia, malaise, profound tiredness, and lethargy. The disease may be accompanied by upper extremity claudication, and carotidynia occurs in up to 25% of patients. Examination can reveal diminished pulses, vascular bruits, and hypertension.

In the acute phase, vasa vasoritis is seen in the adventitia and media. There is infiltration by lymphocytes, giant cells, and neovascularization. In the chronic phase, there is fibrosis with destruction of elastic tissue.[7] Arteritic lesions demonstrate adventitial thickening and focal leukocytic infiltration of the media with intimal hyperplasia. The infiltrate is composed of activated dendritic cells, T and B lymphocytes, macrophages, and multinucleated giant cells. Growth factor-driven myofibroblast proliferation leads to intimal hyperplasia and fibrosis and subsequent arterial stenosis or occlusion. Local matrix metalloproteinase synthesis may predispose to aneurysmal dilation.[1]

The aorta may be involved throughout its length, and even though any branches can be diseased, the most commonly affected are the subclavian and common carotid arteries. Stenotic arterial lesions are found in more than 90% of patients, whereas aneurysms are reported in approximately 25%. The pulmonary arteries are involved in up to 50% of patients, and aortic valve regurgitation and coronary arteritis may occur.

Vascular changes lead to the main complications, including hypertension, most often due to renal artery stenosis or, more rarely, stenosis of the suprarenal aorta, aortic insufficiency due to aortic valve involvement, pulmonary hypertension, and aortic or arterial aneurysm.

While computed tomography (CT) scanning and magnetic resonance imaging (MRI) show typical patterns of stenosis or aneurysms of the arteries, angiography remains the standard for diagnosis and evaluation of the extent of disease.

Congestive heart failure is a common finding, much more so than dilated cardiomyopathy, myocarditis, and pericarditis which also have been reported.

*Echocardiographic features:* A detailed echocardiographic evaluation may reveal aortic dilation with aneurysm and segmental stenosis involving any segment of the aorta.

## Case Illustration

***A 26-year-old lady with known history of TA was sent for echocardiography. It revealed focal areas of stenosis and dilatation in the abdominal aorta. Turbulent flow noted in abdominal aorta with increased velocities (Figure 22.3A and B). The aortic arch and Doppler in the descending thoracic aorta revealed normal flow velocities (Figure 22.3C and D).***

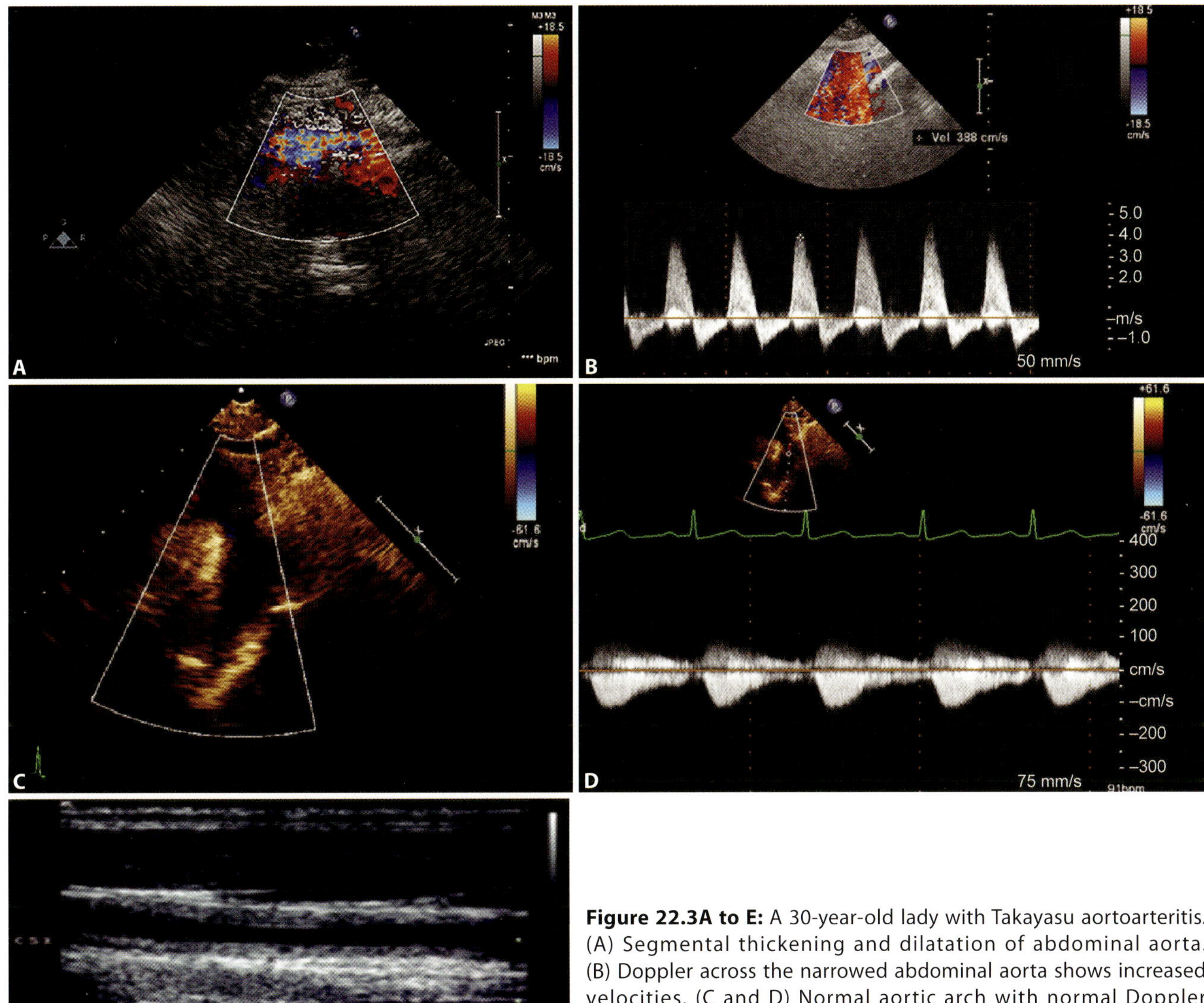


**Figure 22.3A to E:** A 30-year-old lady with Takayasu aortoarteritis. (A) Segmental thickening and dilatation of abdominal aorta. (B) Doppler across the narrowed abdominal aorta shows increased velocities. (C and D) Normal aortic arch with normal Doppler velocities. (E) Left carotid artery ultrasound showing homogeneous circumferential wall thickening, known as the "macaroni sign".

In the Indian population, there is increased predilection for abdominal aorta and renal vessels, while in the Japanese patients, there is increased involvement of the aortic arch and main branches.[7] Case series also have been reported of rapid aortic aneurysm expansion and aortic rupture.

There may be segmental wall-motion abnormality on echocardiogram secondary to coronary arteritis or myocarditis. Aortic regurgitation can be seen secondary to valve thickening or aortic root dilatation. Pulmonary artery dilatation may also be found on echocardiogram. A classic Doppler finding described in TA reveals homogeneous, midechoic, circumferential wall thickening of the carotid artery. This rare ultrasonographic finding (described in the left common carotid artery), was described by Maeda et al.[1] as the "macaroni sign", is considered pathognomonic for TA **(Figure 22.3E)**.

## *Kawasaki Disease*

Kawasaki disease (KD) is an acute self-limiting vasculitis (involving medium and small arteries), predominantly affecting children under the age of 5 years with a peak incidence between 6 months and 24 months.

Characteristic initial features include fever, bilateral conjunctivitis, and mucocutaneous lesions, including red fissured lips and a strawberry tongue. Cervical lymphadenopathy may be prominent, with erythema affecting the palms and soles and a polymorphous exanthema.

The cause of KD is unknown, although infection may trigger the disease and lead to an uncontrolled excessive immunologic response in a genetically susceptibly host. A variety of organisms have been implicated; however, no definitive evidence supports an infectious cause.

Deaths in KD are mostly due to cardiac sequelae. The highest mortality is 15–45 days after onset of fever. At this time, coronary vasculitis concomitant with elevation of the platelet count and a hypercoagulable state occurs. Sudden death from myocardial infarction may occur many years later in individuals who as children had coronary artery aneurysms and stenosis. Many cases of fatal and nonfatal myocardial infarction in young adults have been attributed to "missed" KD in childhood.[8]

In KD, the media of affected vessels reveal edematous dissociation of the smooth muscle cells. Endothelial cell swelling and subendothelial edema are seen, but the internal elastic lamina remains intact. An influx of neutrophils is found in the early stages (7–9 days after onset), with a rapid transition to large mononuclear cells in concert with lymphocytes (predominantly CD8+ T cells) and IgA plasma cells. Destruction of the internal elastic lamina and eventually fibroblastic proliferation occur at this stage. Matrix metalloproteinases are prominent in the remodeling process. Active inflammation is replaced over several weeks to months by progressive fibrosis, with scar formation.

Arterial remodeling or revascularization may occur in KD with coronary arteritis. Progressive stenosis in the disease results from active remodeling with intimal proliferation and neoangiogenesis. The intima is markedly thickened and consists of linearly arranged microvessels, a layer that is rich in smooth muscle cells and fibrous layers. Several growth factors are prominently expressed at the inlet and outlet of aneurysms, where they are activated by high-shear stress.[8]

The key steps leading to coronary arteritis are still being clarified, but endothelial cell activation, CD68+ monocyte/macrophages, CD8+ (cytotoxic) lymphocytes, and oligoclonal IgA plasma cells appear to be involved.[8]

*Echocardiographic features:* Coronary artery aneurysms or ectasia develop in ≈15–25% of untreated children with the disease and may lead to myocardial infarction, sudden death, or ischemic heart disease.

Echocardiography also may be useful in evaluating children with suspected KD, as the left main and right coronary artery (RCA) can be easily visualized. Initial findings in the acute phase are perivascular brightness, ectasia, and lack of tapering of the coronary arteries which may represent coronary arteritis before the formation of aneurysms.

Detailed echoimaging using multiple imaging planes should be utilized to evaluate coronary artery aneurysms. The proximal left anterior descending artery and proximal RCA followed by left main coronary artery are the most common sites for aneurysm formation. The number and location of aneurysms and the presence or absence of intraluminal thrombi also should be assessed.

Depressed LV contractility secondary to associated myocarditis, mild valvular regurgitation (most commonly mitral regurgitation), and pericardial effusion secondary to pericarditis also may be seen in an echocardiogram of a person with acute KD. Cardiac stress testing for reversible ischemia is indicated to assess the existence and functional consequences of coronary artery abnormalities in children with KD and coronary aneurysms. The types of stress tests reported in children with KD include nuclear perfusion scans with exercise, exercise echocardiography, and stress echocardiography with pharmacological agents, such as dobutamine, dipyridamole, or adenosine.[8]

### *Case Illustration*

***An 18-year-old with known history of KD came for follow-up echocardiography. Subcoastal biplane and apical 4-chamber images revealed a large coronary aneurysm with thrombus in the RCA (Figure 22.4A and B). Another large aneurysm with thrombus was seen in the left circumflex coronary artery also (Figure 22.4C and D).***

## *Idiopathic Aortitis*

Idiopathic aortitis is a spectrum of disorders characterized by inflammation of the aortic wall. Various infectious and noninfectious diseases can be complicated by aortitis. Advanced age, presence of connective tissue disorders and diabetes has been implicated as risk factors.

Acute aortic syndromes, including aortic dissection and rupture, can occur in persons with aortitis. Inflammation-associated thrombus formation in the aortic lumen with peripheral embolization also has been reported.

The clinical features are nonspecific and include malaise, lethargy, chest pain, back and abdominal pain, fever, and weight loss, and the diagnosis is often made only at the time of surgery. The ESR and CRP are typically raised, and the extent of the disease can be demonstrated by CT-PET scanning and aortic MR or CT angiography.

*Ultrasound and echocardiography:* Although generally not used as a primary diagnostic modality for aortitis, abdominal ultrasound or TTE or TEE may demonstrate circumferential thickening of the aortic wall. Abdominal ultrasonography is useful for the diagnosis of abdominal aortic aneurysm occurring as a complication of aortitis or in association with chronic periaortitis or inflammatory aneurysm. In addition, echocardiography plays a key role in the assessment of the

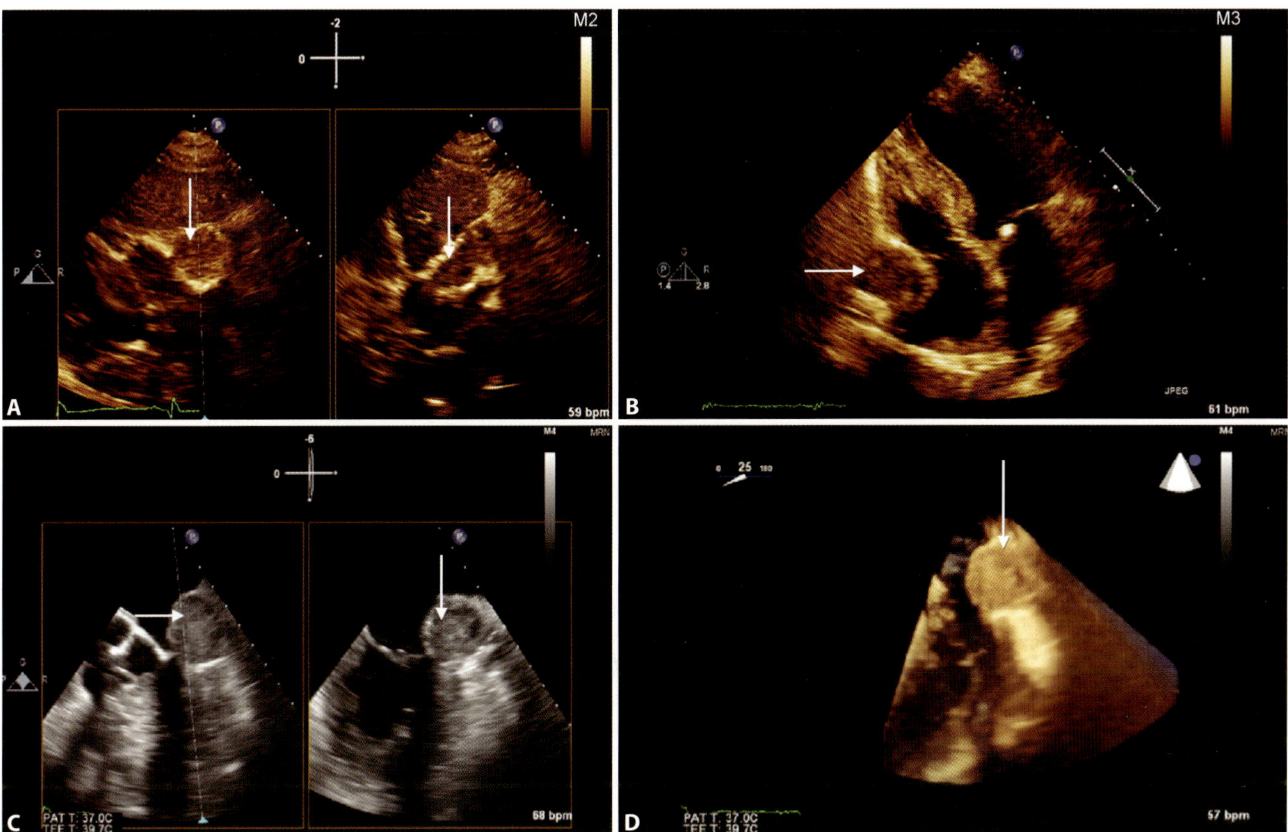

**Figure 22.4A to D:** A patient with Kawasaki disease. (A) Subcoastal biplane image showing a large coronary aneurysm (arrows) with thrombus in the right coronary artery. (B) Apical 4- chamber view showing the same aneurysm (arrow). (C and D) Transesophageal echocardiography showing another large aneurysm (arrows) with thrombus in the left circumflex coronary artery in the left atrioventricular groove abutting the left atrial appendage.

aortic root and aortic valve in the setting of aortitis of the ascending thoracic aorta associated with aortic insufficiency and aneurysm formation.[6]

## Medium-vessel and Small-vessel Vasculitis

These vasculitides include Churg–Strauss syndrome (CSS) or allergic granulomatous polyangiitis, granulomatous polyangiitis (GPA) or Wegener granulomatosis, and microscopic polyangiitis (MPA). Although these diseases have overlapping features, they represent distinct clinical entities. GPA is most frequently associated with a cytoplasmic ANCA (cANCA) staining pattern, whereas MPA is most commonly associated with a perinuclear ANCA (pANCA).

### *Churg–Strauss Syndrome*

CSS is a systemic small-vessel necrotizing vasculitis with a prevalence of 10–14 per million population. An initial prodrome characterized by allergic rhinitis, sinusitis, and asthma is followed by peripheral blood eosinophilia and eosinophilic infiltrative lesions in the lung and myocardium and usually, some years later, by a systemic phase with necrotizing vasculitis affecting the skin, peripheral nerves, gastrointestinal tract, and kidney. ANCA-negative patients are more likely to suffer cardiopulmonary complications, whereas pANCA-positive patients seem to be more at risk for renal and peripheral nerve involvement.

### *Polyarteritis Nodosa*

PAN is a rare disease characterized by a systemic necrotizing vasculitis of medium-sized arteries complicated by aneurysmal nodules. The classic type of PAN is an ANCA-negative vasculitis with the predominant clinical features, including fever, malaise, arthralgia, weight loss, livedo reticularis, cutaneous nodules, and a vasculitic rash. Abdominal, cardiac, and testicular pain may occur, and some patients manifest mononeuritis multiplex. Hematuria, proteinuria, and/or hypertension indicate renal involvement.

### *Granulomatous Polyangiitis (Wegener's Granulomatosis)*

GPA is a necrotizing vasculitis that commonly affects the sinuses, upper airways, lungs, skin, joints, and kidneys. There is predilection to affect upper respiratory passages (sinusitis), lower respiratory passages (pulmonary infiltrates or nodules), and kidney in form of glomerulonephritis. Diagnosis is based on clinical features, biopsy evidence, and typically a positive cANCA. Clinical cardiac involvement is rare, although it has been reported in up to 30% of autopsy cases.

### *Microscopic Polyangiitis*

Microscopic polyangiitis (MPA) is most commonly associated with glomerulonephritis, renal impairment, and pulmonary hemorrhage. Cardiac disease is rarely clinically significant, but pericarditis occurs in 10% of patients, and congestive cardiac failure develops in up to 18%. Subclinical and occasionally symptomatic acute myocardial infarction is seen. Evidences from case reports and small series show that this disease also features symptomatic aortitis and coronary artery microaneurysms.

### *Echocardiographic Features in Medium- and Small-vessel Vasculitis*

Clinically significant cardiac involvement is a rare complication in systemic vasculitides, but it can be life-threatening. As many cardiac manifestations are clinically silent at least during their early stages, heart function should be systematically evaluated by echocardiography. If symptoms appear and the basic investigation is normal, further evaluation using cardiovascular magnetic resonance is of great value, because it is the ideal technique to reveal the presence of myocardial inflammation.

Myocarditis due to vasculitis varies widely from 25% to 70% of cases. It is due to necrotizing vasculitis, presence of granulomas or fibrosis. This can lead to postinflammatory fibrosis and congestive heart failure. In CSS, infiltration by eosinophils is considered as a possible cause and cardiac MRI is of value for early detection of myocardial inflammation, especially in patients with atypical presentation.[9] Arrhythmias (mainly supraventricular), atrioventricular or bundle branch block can also be found due to myocarditis, ischemia or heart failure.

Coronary artery involvement can be detected, due to coronary arteritis that causes thromboses, dissections, stenosis and possible myocardial infarction. Coronary artery involvement can be seen in up to 50% of cases in PAN. Coronary angiography may reveal coronary artery microaneurysms, coronary arteritis, or coronary spasm.

Pericardial involvement in 22% of cases with CSS, 8% in Wegener's, 0–27% in PAN and can lead to constrictive pericarditis.[9] Pericardial involvement may also lead to pericardial effusion and tamponade.

Endocardium involvement is rather unusual, but it can promote valve distortion in some cases.

## THROMBOSIS IN RHEUMATIC DISEASE

Thrombosis is an important pathologic process in many rheumatic diseases and a cause of significant morbidity and mortality. Large-vessel thrombosis, both venous and arterial, can occur in Behçet disease and antiphospholipid syndrome (APS). Thrombosis in situ also occurs in small vessels, principally as the end result of chronic vessel wall hyperplasia or inflammation in diseases, such as systemic sclerosis (SSc), the vasculitides, and pulmonary arterial hypertension. Chronic thromboembolic pulmonary arterial hypertension can complicate SLE and SSc.

Coronary thrombosis and myocardial infarction can complicate primary APS in 0.5–6% of patients, and intracardiac thrombi can also occur. The APS in patients with SLE may enhance their risk for myocardial infarction and stroke. Other cardiovascular complications include pericarditis, myocarditis, and myocardial aneurysm.[1]

## MISCELLANEOUS DISORDERS

Various disorders other than atherosclerotic CAD or coronary arteritis can also reduce or interrupt coronary blood flow and cause myocardial infarction.

- *Congenital coronary artery anomalies:* The coronary anomalies most likely to cause myocardial infarction, ischemia, or ventricular tachycardia are anomalous origin of the left coronary artery from the pulmonary artery (ALCAPA), large coronary arteriovenous fistulas, and those anomalies associated with a coronary artery coursing between the great vessels.

  *ALCAPA:* In this condition, the left main coronary artery arises from the pulmonary artery. The perfusion of the left ventricle begins to suffer as the left main comes off a low pressure system. This leads to a decrease in LV function. At the same time, the ischemic myocardium may be perfused increasingly by developing collateral vessels from the RCA which arises normally.

  Echocardiographic screening studies may show the anomalous origin of the left coronary artery, dilated RCA caused by increased flow, LV enlargement, and depressed ventricular function.

Abnormalities of the origin of the coronary arteries from the aorta traversing between the aorta and the pulmonary trunk may become important in adolescence and young adult life. This is mostly seen when the left coronary artery arises from the right sinus and traverses between the pulmonary artery and aorta. Strong relation to sudden death with severe exertion is known in this condition as the left coronary artery can be compressed between the aorta and pulmonary artery. In contrast, the anomalous origin of RCA from the left sinus is usually not associated with sudden death, because of low perfusion pressure of the right ventricle.

Any child or young person with angina pectoris, myocardial infarction, or cardiac syncope should undergo coronary angiography to rule out coronary anomalies.

- *Coronary aneurysm:* It mostly occurs due to atherosclerotic disease. However, rare causes can be connective tissue disorders (as discussed earlier), trauma, congenital, mycotic, and idiopathic. The primary complication is myocardial ischemia or infarction with rupture being rare and sudden death.
- Intramural CAD due to amyloid heart disease has been reported in 66% patients in one series. They have obstructive intramural coronary amyloidosis, a syndrome of myocardial ischemia consisting of acute myocardial infarction or angina pectoris.
- *Trauma:* Nonpenetrating blunt chest wall injury (steering wheel injury), penetration trauma (laceration from stab wound or bullet) have been reported to cause myocardial infarction.
- *Coronary artery embolism:* A rare cause of myocardial infarction. There have been case reports of coronary artery embolism in patients with atrial fibrillation. In patients with acute endocarditis, there have also been case reports of coronary artery embolism and myocardial infarction.
- Coronary artery thrombosis without underlying atherosclerotic plaque (thrombosis in situ): It is due to leukemia, polycythemia vera, primary thrombocytosis, sickle cell anemia, and thrombocytopenia purpura.
- Encroachment of lumen by disease of arterial wall or adjacent tissues (external narrowing), e.g. sinus of Valsalva aneurysms and epicardial tumor metastases. These conditions can compress the coronary arteries externally and cause myocardial infarction.

## CONCLUSION

Connective tissue disorders are known to result in variety of cardiac disorders, including nonatherosclerotic, and even atherosclerotic CAD. A detailed patient examination, supportive blood tests and echocardiography can be used in initial screening and follow-up of these patients. An increased awareness of the increased risk for silent ischemia, early myocardial infarction, heart failure and sudden death is warranted in this patient population.

## VIDEO LEGENDS

**Video 22.1:** The same patient with systemic lupus erythematosus as in Figure 22.1. There is hypokinesia of mid-anterior septum (A) and left ventricular apex (B and C) with left ventricular ejection fraction around 35%.

**Video 22.2:** The same patient as in Video 22.1, but 4 weeks after the initial presentation. All regional wall-motion abnormalities had disappeared and the left ventricular ejection fraction had normalized by this time (A to C).

## REFERENCES


1. Mason JC. Rheumatic diseases and the cardiovascular system. In: Braunwald Braunwald's Heart Disease: A Textbook of Cardiovascular Medicine, 10th edition. Chapter 84. Philadelphia, PA : Elsevier/Saunders;2015.
2. Tincani A, Rebaioli CB, Taglietti M, et al. Heart involvement in systemic lupus erythematosus, anti-phospholipid syndrome and neonatal lupus. Rheumatology. 2006;45:iv8-13.
3. Kalke S, Balakrishanan C, Mangat G, Mittal G, Kumar N, Joshi VR. Echocardiography in systemic lupus erythematosus. Lupus. 1998;7:540-4.
4. Gravallese EM, Corson JM, Coblyn JS, et al. Rheumatoid aortitis: a rarely recognized but clinically significant entity. Medicine (Baltimore). 1989;68:95-106.
5. Suelves AM, et al. Doppler ultrasound and giant cell arteritis. Clin Ophthalmol. 2010; 4:1383-4.
6. Gornik HL, Creager MA. Aortic diseases, aortitis. Circulation. 2008;117:3039-51.
7. Johnston SL, Lock RJ, Gompels MM. Takayasu arteritis: a review. J Clin Pathol. 2002;55: 481-6.
8. Newburger JW. AHA scientific statement: diagnosis, treatment, and long-term management of Kawasaki disease. Circulation. 2004;110:2747-71.
9. Sophie Mavrogeni. Cardiac involvement in small and medium-sized vasculitides. An article from the e-journal of the ESC Council for Cardiology Practice. 2007; vol. 6, N° 14-04.

# Guiding Medical Intervention by Detection of Subclinical Atherosclerosis in Peripheral Arteries with B-mode Ultrasound

23
CHAPTER

*Ram Bedi*

## INTRODUCTION

This book so far has mainly dealt with ultrasound imaging techniques for diagnosing myocardial ischemia and coronary valvular insufficiency in symptomatic patients. Typically, such patients are examined by highly skilled sonographers, cardiologists, and other imaging experts in suitably equipped facilities that provide secondary or tertiary care. The key question this chapter will try to address is whether ultrasound has a role to play in assessing individuals in a *primary care* setting before symptoms arise. What can be done to detect subclinical atherosclerosis to guide appropriate interventions that might prevent catastrophic complications from occult atherosclerotic vascular disease? Doppler ultrasound-based flow studies have been routinely used in clinical practice for the assessment of carotid stenosis in symptomatic patients to identify those who would benefit from *surgical* intervention. With recent improvements in image quality and built-in automation, perhaps B-mode ultrasound can similarly be employed to assess subclinical atherosclerosis in the asymptomatic population to identify individuals who would benefit from prophylactic *medical* intervention.

## CASE FOR IMAGING

### Problems with Traditional Risk Factor Assessment

Risk stratification strategies based on age, gender, family history, blood pressure, lifestyle choices, and serum markers have served developed healthcare systems well in the past 30–50 years in reducing mortality rates from atherothrombotic events.[1,2] The widespread availability and effectiveness of lipid-lowering agents in particular have contributed immensely in reducing mortality rates from atherosclerotic cardiovascular disease (ASCVD). However, ASCVD risk prediction algorithms are not very well understood or followed in the developing countries.[3] Moreover, exposure to risk factors alone does not necessarily lead to ASCVD events. Data from the Framingham Heart Study with a 26-year follow-up[4] revealed that there was a significant overlap in risk factors between those who suffered a myocardial infarction (MI) and those who did not, as illustrated in **Figure 23.1**. For example, cholesterol levels were the same in 80% of the patients who experienced an MI versus those who did not. In a more recent retrospective study[5] of 232,000 patients admitted to hospitals with coronary artery disease (CAD), low-density lipoprotein (LDL) cholesterol levels were <130 mg/dL in more than 70% of patients and high-density lipoprotein (HDL) cholesterol ≥40 mg/dL in almost half of the patients **(Figure 23.2A to C)**. These studies suggest that the decision for initiating preventative medical intervention, which is based solely on traditional risk factor

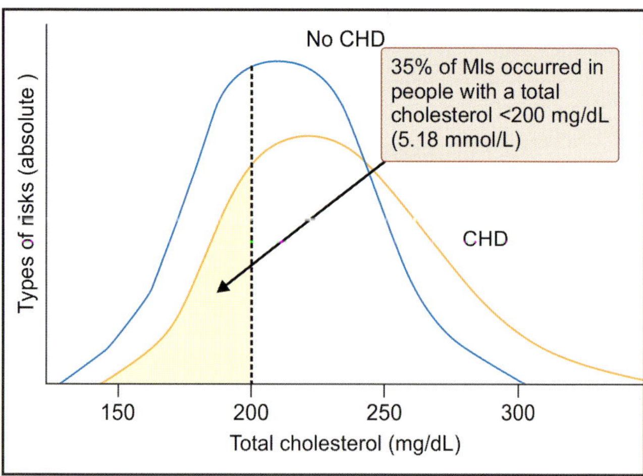


**Figure 23.1:** Incidence of MI in relation to cholesterol levels in the Framingham study.[4]
Data from the Framingham Heart Study with a 26-year follow-up revealed that there was a significant overlap in risk factors between those who suffered an MI and those who did not. Cholesterol levels were the same in 80% of patients who experienced an MI versus those who did not.
*Abbreviations:* CHD, coronary heart disease; MI, myocardial infarction.
Adapted from Castell WP. Lipids, risk factors and ischemic heart disease. Atherosclerosis. 1996;124(Suppl):1-9 (with permission).

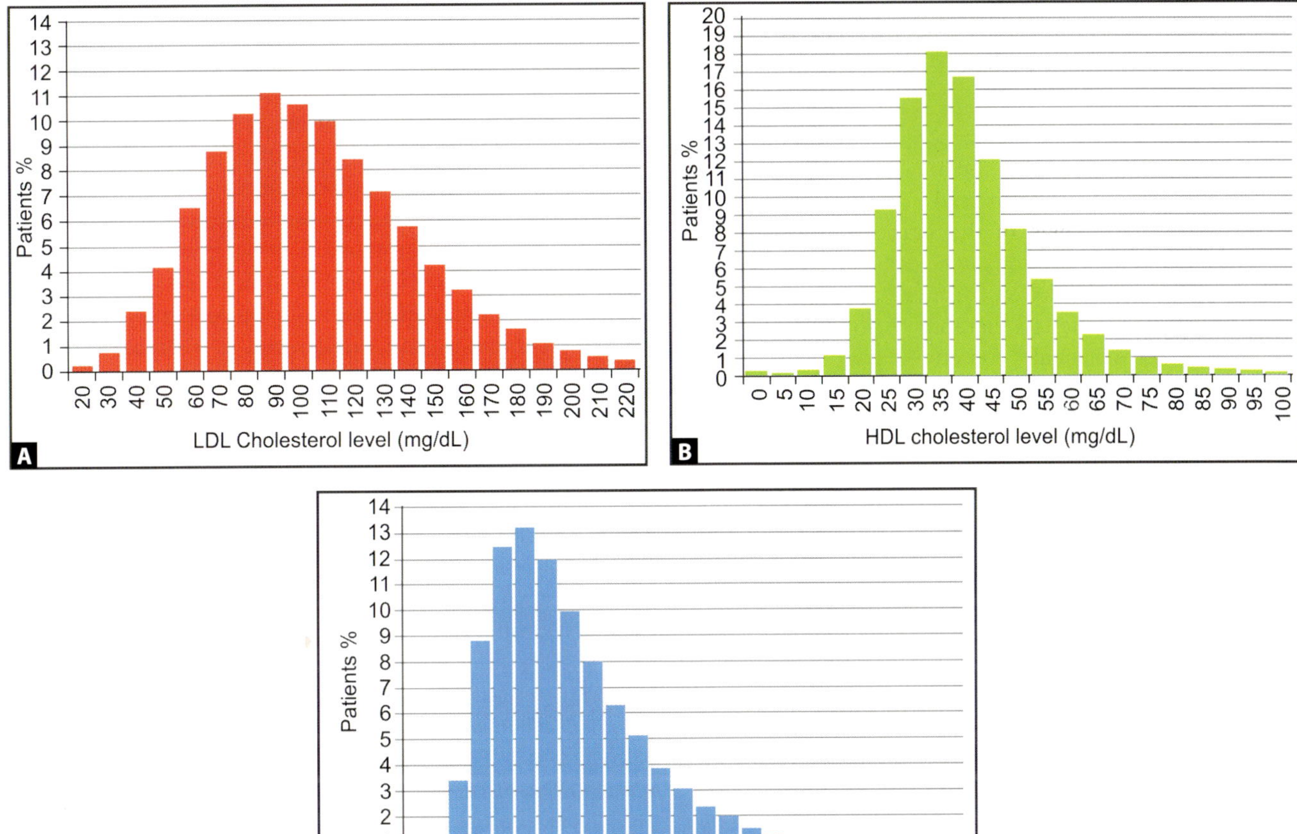


**Figure 23.2A to C:** Distribution of low-density lipoprotein (LDL) cholesterol (A), high-density lipoprotein (HDL) cholesterol (B), and triglycerides (C) in patients hospitalized with coronary artery disease (CAD).[5]

During a 76-month retrospective study of 231,896 cases for CAD hospitalization from 541 hospitals in the US, lipid levels in the first 24 hours of hospitalization were available in 136,905 (59%) cases. A substantial proportion of patients presenting their first or recurrent CAD event were well within the current guideline targets for LDL cholesterol (130 mg/dL or 3.37 mmol/L) and triglyceride levels. These data suggest that the use of imaging tests that identify direct evidence of atherosclerosis may be a better strategy to guide appropriate intervention. Adapted from Sachdeva A, Cannon CP, et al. Lipid levels in patients hospitalized with coronary artery disease: an analysis of 136,905 hospitalizations in Get With The Guidelines. Am Heart J. 2009;157(1):111-7 (with permission).

assessment, needs to be questioned, especially in emerging economies, such as India where mortality rates from ASCVD amongst men and women of working age are significantly higher compared to industrialized countries.[6-9] To reduce societal impact of this epidemic, an alternative strategy might be to initiate prophylactic medical intervention on only those asymptomatic subjects who exhibit direct evidence of early atherosclerotic disease in easily accessible peripheral arterial beds.[10-13] Such a strategy might be particularly applicable where traditional risk factor-based algorithms are not very well established or readily available, as is the case in low- and middle-income countries. At the very least, traditional risk factor assessment needs to be supplemented with a simple imaging study to help better identify those asymptomatic individuals who may benefit from prophylactic medical intervention, if we are to arrest the alarming rise in morbidity and mortality rates from ASCVD worldwide.

## Imaging Coronary and Peripheral Arteries

Atherosclerosis is a systemic process with focal areas of accentuation at various vascular sites. Many clinical, epidemiological, and pathological studies have shown that atherosclerosis develops earlier in the peripheral arterial system[14-16] as compared to the coronary vasculature; studies have also shown that chronic advanced atherosclerosis can exist with minimal or no symptoms.[17] It is reasonable, therefore, to ponder whether detection in one vascular bed can predict presence of atherosclerosis in another. Direct imaging of coronary arteries with ultrasound is not possible because of various anatomical and image resolution constraints. However, peripheral vascular beds, such as the extracranial carotid system and iliofemoral arteries are readily accessible and amenable to good ultrasound imaging quality. A number of imaging studies have attempted to show the correlation between atherosclerosis in the carotids detected with ultrasound and atherosclerosis in coronary arteries detected by coronary angiography or coronary artery calcification (CAC) score or computed tomography angiography (CTA).[18-20] A study by Sosnowski et al.[21] contended that plaque detected with ultrasound in the iliofemoral arteries was an even better predictor of CAD compared to the carotids. Overall, such studies have been largely successful but data are far from conclusive. This is partly because the methods of detection are not exactly alike making comparisons difficult (angiography detects only the level of stenosis, CAC detects only *calcified* plaque and CTA detects highly vascularized and calcified plaque). Furthermore, methodological differences exist in computing the comparative index from ultrasound imaging of peripheral vessels. In some studies, researchers have used intima-media thickness (IMT) in a straight segment of the artery where the measurement is most reproducible (e.g. common carotid artery), some have averaged several IMT measurements taken at different segments of the artery, some have used focally elevated IMT or plaque as the measurement index, and some have used plaque area or plaque volume over an arbitrary segment of the artery. Finally, Institutional Review Board approval for studies involving a coronary angiogram or CTA is typically only granted for symptomatic patients who tend to be older and exhibit more advanced stage of atherosclerosis. This makes it very difficult to apply the results of such comparison studies to the younger asymptomatic population.

An example of discordant observations is illustrated in the study by Cohen et al.[19] in which about a quarter of the subjects had no plaque in their carotids as assessed by ultrasound. Yet, the same subjects exhibited plaque in their coronary arteries as detected by CAC or CTA. Conversely, about half of the subjects found to have no coronary plaque as detected by CAC or CTA exhibited carotid plaque measured by ultrasound imaging. One possible explanation for the latter observation is that plaque in the coronaries had not yet calcified, stenosed or vascularized. Most likely, however, the observed discrepancies suggest that local factors are influencing susceptibility of the vessels to develop atherosclerosis, thus making the comparisons difficult. For these reasons, it is probably best to avoid comparisons altogether. A more pragmatic approach might be to accept that presence of plaque in any arterial bed examined by whatever imaging method is an indication of tissue damage from exposure to risk factors, which suggests higher risk for future ASCVD-related events.

## Intima-media Thickness and Plaque

There is much confounding information in the literature about clinical utility of IMT, carotid plaque, and the use of duplex ultrasound. It should be emphasized that the purpose of duplex ultrasound is to identify individuals who may have hemodynamic flow disturbance and carotid luminal stenosis >50%. In other words, duplex ultrasound is normally indicated for the identification of patients with advanced atherosclerosis who may benefit from surgical intervention. Such an examination is expected to be performed by a highly skilled technician and interpreted by suitably qualified physician. Conversely, a simpler B-mode ultrasound could be performed in an office setting and is adequate for identifying individuals with subclinical atherosclerosis who may benefit from pharmacological intervention.

Lumen-intima and intima-media borders can be traced manually or by computer from a static B-mode ultrasound image of an artery to determine the IMT. The term 'CIMT', frequently encountered in the literature, is often used as an abbreviation for IMT of the common carotid artery. Consider the case of a 49-year-old male illustrated in **Figure 23.3** whose CIMT is perfectly normal (<0.5 mm), yet a significant lesion beneath the near-wall of the adventitial layer of the bulb is very clearly visible. From an ultrasound imaging perspective, there is no difference between IMT and plaque. A plaque is simply a focal elevation in IMT that is interpreted by the reader as a pathological finding. In a paper published by Touboul et al. in 2004, which became known as the Mannheim Consensus,[22] a plaque was defined as a focal structure that (i) encroached into the arterial lumen for at least 0.5 mm, (ii) >50% beyond the surrounding IMT value, or (iii) demonstrated a thickness >1.5 mm as measured from the media–adventitia interface. This definition was subsequently incorporated into North American and European guidelines dealing with ASCVD prevention.[11,12,23,24] For simplicity, it might be reasonable to define a plaque simply as a focal elevation >1.5 mm protruding into the lumen (as in iii above), which is usually hard to miss in modern B-mode ultrasound images. Development of a focal elevation in IMT (so-called plaque) might mean that the local compensatory mechanism to retain natural lumen morphology has failed and natural flow perturbed. As the plaque continues to grow, localized flow velocity increases, which causes a localized Bernoulli pressure depression proportional to the flow velocity squared.[25,26] Interior of the plaque at this location is therefore subjected to the resulting intrastenotic pressure depression, which may lead to intraplaque hemorrhage as illustrated in **Figure 23.4**. This effect is particularly pronounced in patients with arrhythmia who have a higher-systolic blood pressure from the extended R-R interval, resulting in a higher-peak systolic velocity and, therefore, a higher Bernoulli pressure depression that may lead to increased propensity for intraplaque hemorrhage. A more rigorous analysis of flow

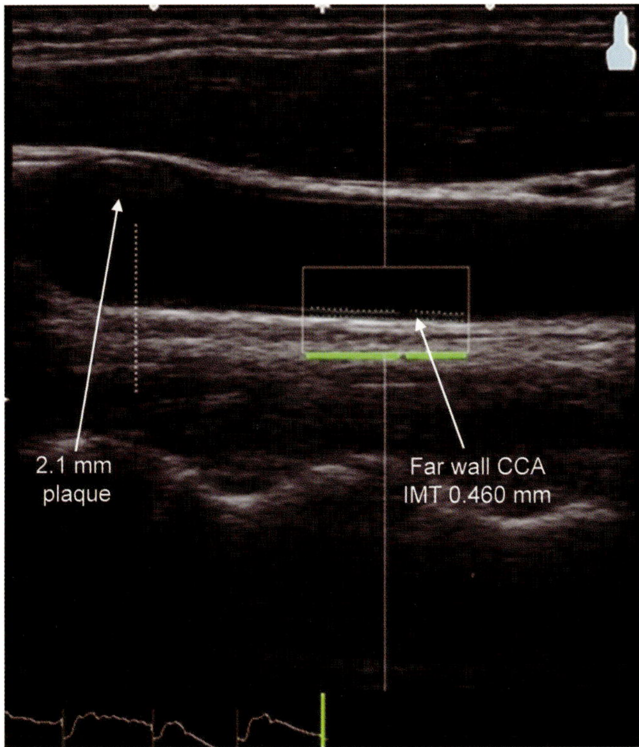


**Figure 23.3:** An ultrasound image to illustrate the difference between "CIMT" and plaque

This B-mode ultrasound image shows the left carotid of a 49-year-old male. The far-wall common carotid intima-media thickness (commonly referred to as "CIMT") is perfectly normal (<0.5 mm). Yet a significant focally elevated IMT protruding into the lumen measuring 2.1 mm beneath the near-wall of the adventitial layer of the bulb is very clearly visible. This focal elevation in IMT is referred to as a plaque in accordance with the Mannheim Consensus Statement.[22]

*Abbreviations:* CCA, common carotid artery, IMT, intima-media thickness.

*Courtesy:* Panasonic Healthcare Co. of North America.

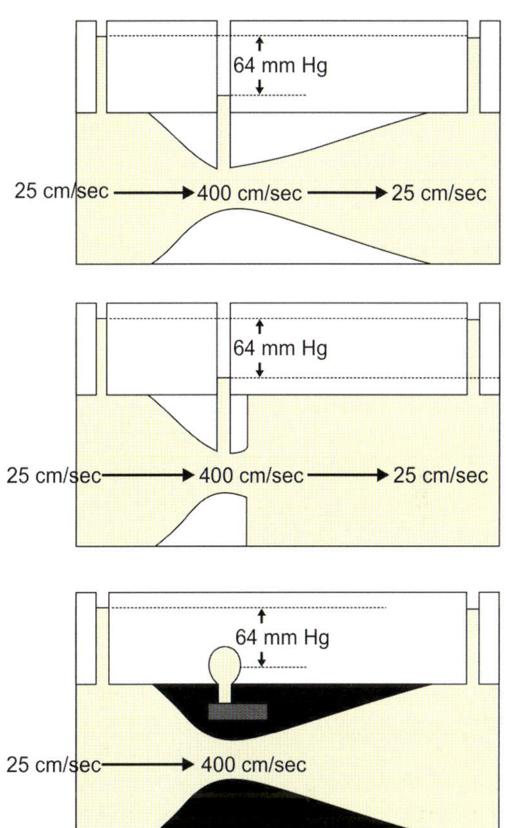


**Figure 23.4:** Potential explanation for how plaques rupture.[25]

Consider a 75% diameter reduction stenosis in a tube. Residual lumen ¼ the diameter of the proximal tube means that area of the stenosis is 1/16th the area of the tube and intrastenotic velocities are 16 times as high as the proximal velocities. The Bernoulli pressure depression is proportional to the velocity squared or to the fourth power of the fractional residual lumen. The Bernoulli effect produces a 'vacuum' on the center manometer port compared with the proximal port. In an artery, the intrastenotic luminal surface of the plaque feels that vacuum compared with the proximal artery.

Adapted from Beach KW, et al. Carotid artery intraplaque hemorrhage and stenotic velocity. Stroke. 1993;24(2):314-9 (with permission).

dynamics that may lead to plaque rupture is provided by Beach et al.[25,26] Plaque findings have been more frequently reported around arterial bifurcations and vessel tortuosity.

## Atherosclerotic Cardiovascular Disease Prevention Guidelines and Imaging

One of the most widely used and cited preventive guidelines is the Adult Treatment Panel III (ATP III) originally published in the USA in 2002.[11] This guideline included a recommendation that persons with clinical forms of noncoronary atherosclerosis should be treated to the same LDL-cholesterol goal (<100 mg/dL) as those with established coronary heart disease (CHD). The investigators went on to state that the extent of carotid atherosclerosis correlated positively with the severity of coronary atherosclerosis and that severity of IMT independently correlated with risk for major coronary events. Therefore, measurement of carotid IMT could be used as an adjunct in CHD risk assessment to identify persons at higher risk than that revealed by major risk factors alone. This guideline in combination with additional observational studies eventually led in 2010 to raising of the CIMT test to Class IIa category by a task force on practice guidelines commissioned by the American College of Cardiology (ACC) and the American Heart Association (AHA).[27] The CIMT test received a stronger recommendation than the followings:

- Genotype testing and advanced lipoprotein analysis, including Lp(a)—Class III
- Hemoglobin A1C— Class IIb

- Resting electrocardiogram (ECG) (in those without hypertension (HTN) and diabetes mellitus) or stress ECG— Class IIb
- C-reactive protein (men ≤50 years and women ≤60 years)—Class IIb
- Lipoprotein-associated phospholipase A2 (Lp-PLA2)—Class IIb
- Resting echocardiography (without HTN) or stress echocardiography—Class III
- Measures of arterial stiffness (pulse wave velocity and augmentation index)—Class III
- Endothelial function with flow-mediated dilatation or peripheral arterial tonometry—Class III.

In a subsequent ACC/AHA guideline published 3 years later by Goff et al.,[28] and commonly referred to as ATP IV, the CIMT test was downgraded from Class IIa to Class III (CAC score was also downgraded from IIa to IIb) without any change in evidence base. This downgrade was based on not new data but a meta-analysis of existing data published by Ruijter et al.[29] in which the investigators completely ignored carotid plaque. In essence, the meta-analysis ignored the most clinically relevant part of the CIMT test (plaque) by focusing solely on IMT of the far-wall of the common carotid—an anatomical site that is less prone to developing plaques. Furthermore, the meta-analysis did not pool individual data. It is interesting to note that the same investigators published completely discordant findings just two months earlier in a meta-analysis of pooled individual level patient data from 36,984 patients.[30] Part of the reason why the conclusions of the updated guideline were so influenced by just one meta-analysis is because this task force adopted the standards of the Institute of Medicine, in which only published randomized controlled trials (RCT) and meta-analyses can be considered (unlike prior guidelines where all available scientific publications were available for consideration). Since no relevant RCT data exist to determine efficacy of any imaging test involving asymptomatic individuals, the task force had no choice but to consider the conclusions from the meta-analysis published by Ruijter et al.[29] Despite the downgrade by the ACC/AHA in ATP IV, the Canadian and European guidelines remain unchanged.[23,24] Incidentally, Class IIa in European Society of Cardiology (ESC) terminology means a test *should be performed* whereas in ACC/AHA terminology Class IIa means a test is *reasonable to perform*.

The question of how effective the published guidelines are in identifying individuals who should be targeted for medical intervention was recently investigated by Bedi et al.[31] In this substudy of 481 asymptomatic individuals only 71 met the criteria for medical intervention under the ATP III guideline. However, an astonishing 82% of the individuals who had carotid plaque did not qualify for treatment, as illustrated in **Figure 23.5**. If the same data were analyzed using the ATP IV guideline, the number of individuals who qualify for medical intervention increased to 217, yet 33% of the cohort with carotid plaque would have remained untreated. Even in the lowest-risk categories, about 15% of the individuals who had

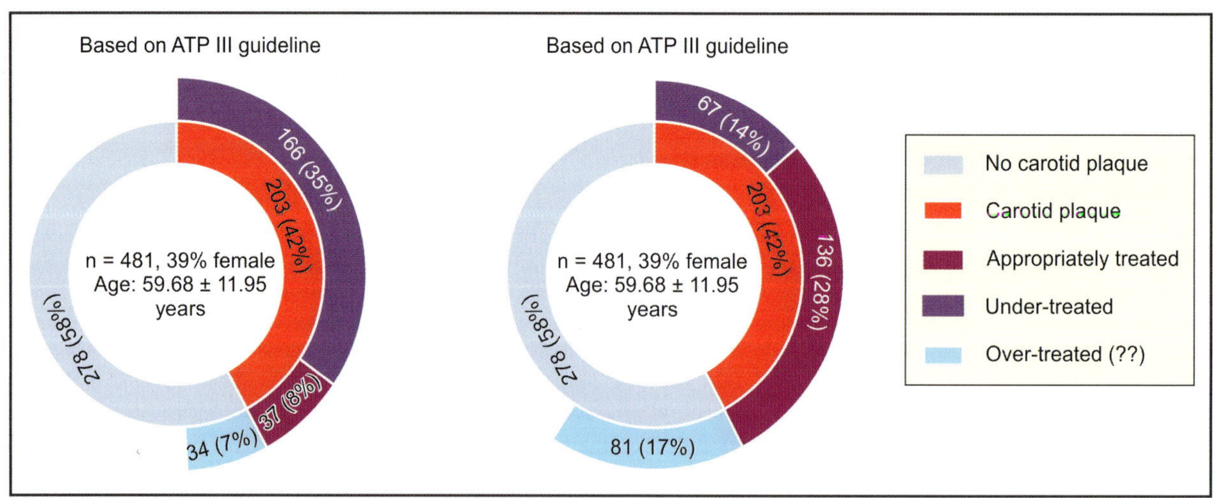


**Figure 23.5:** Plaque findings and eligibility for medical intervention based on atherosclerotic cardiovascular disease (ASCVD) prevention guidelines.[31]

Comprehensive ASCVD risk factor data for 481 self-referred patients analyzed from two clinics in North America showed that 166 (82%) individuals who had carotid plaque would have failed to qualify for medical intervention based on National Cholesterol Education Program Adult Treatment Panel (ATP) III Guideline.[11] Under the recently introduced American College of Cardiology/American Heart Association ATP IV Prevention Guideline,[28] 67 individuals (33%) with carotid plaque would have been ineligible for lipid lowering treatment, yet 81 individuals (29%) who had no carotid plaque qualified for treatment under ATP IV.

Adapted from Bedi R, et al. Detection of subclinical atherosclerosis in peripheral arterial beds with B-mode ultrasound A proposal for guiding the decision for medical intervention and an artifact-corrected volumetric scoring index. Global Heart. 2014;9(4):367-78 (with permission).

carotid plaque failed to qualify for medical intervention under ATP III or ATP IV. The investigators further point out that implementation of ATP IV could potentially be over-treating many individuals who may not necessarily have progressed to developing atherosclerotic disease.

Leaving aside the recommendation of ATP IV, there appears to be good consensus amongst leading academic and clinical organizations around the world that the CIMT test to identify subclinical atherosclerosis is a prudent adjunct to traditional risk factor algorithms when performed correctly. Furthermore, ultrasound imaging provides a safe, portable, low-cost and effective methodology for mass adoption in primary care.

## Should Ultrasound Imaging be the Recommended Test to Detect Subclinical Atherosclerosis?

It can be argued that for primary prevention of any disease, the recommended intervention should be administered to the entire population without requiring any testing. From this perspective, lifestyle modification is an intervention that should be offered to all for the prevention of acute events arising from atherothrombotic complications. However, lifestyle intervention alone is not an effective strategy in reducing ASCVD-related events. Exposure to modifiable risk factors have only a modest specificity and a highly variable relationship to developing atherosclerotic disease. Individuals exposed to atherogenic risk factors do not always go on to develop ASCVD events. The goal of screening the asymptomatic population should be to better identify those individuals who may benefit from pharmacological intervention. In view of this stated goal, the recommended imaging test for the detection of subclinical atherosclerosis is as shown in **Figure 23.6**, which is modified from an editorial comment published by PK Shah.[18] In this article, the investigator proposes two scenarios whereby ultrasound imaging is a gatekeeper to CAC score in one, and CAC score is a gatekeeper to ultrasound in the other. In the end, the investigator prefers CAC score as a gatekeeper, because of its better prognostic value. The reason for discounting ultrasound-imaging-first option was the perceived lack of outcome data and the use of carotid IMT (usually meaning IMT in the far-wall of the common carotid) as a marker to predict ASCVD outcomes; though the investigator goes on to acknowledge that ultrasound-imaging-first option may be preferred, if it is used primarily to detect and quantify plaque. To emphasize this point, it should be noted that the method illustrated in **Figure 23.6** specifically states the identification (and possibly quantification) of plaque in any of the 4 vascular sites examined. Individuals below the age of 50 are spared potential harm from exposure to ionizing radiation because data showing prognostic value of a CAC score in younger populations are scant. The recommended starting age for screening was chosen to be 30 years motivated by a recent study published by Singh et al., involving 776 relatively young asymptomatic (40 ± 14 years) individuals who had undergone aggressive lifestyle management.[3] Even in this population of seemingly well-controlled modifiable risk factors, the prevalence of carotid plaque was 4.3% and 6.1% in 30–39- and 40–49-year-olds, respectively. Data from numerous observational studies supporting the concept of IMT testing are conveniently reviewed and summarized in a consensus statement published by the American Society of Echocardiography (ASE).[12] Outcome data to support the hypothesis that an ultrasound examination should be performed before considering a CAC score is provided by the Carotid and FEmoral ultrasound morphology Screening and CArdio Vascular Events (CAFES-CAVE) study involving >10,000 relatively young asymptomatic adults (mean age 53.2 ± 6.2 years) with a 10-year follow-up.[32] In this observational study, carotid and iliofemoral ultrasound imaging identified 2011 subjects (20.1%) with atherosclerosis and correctly predicted 98.6% of future cardiovascular events during the 10-year observation window. A cardiovascular event was defined as the development of cardiovascular symptoms and/or complications relating to atherosclerosis requiring hospital

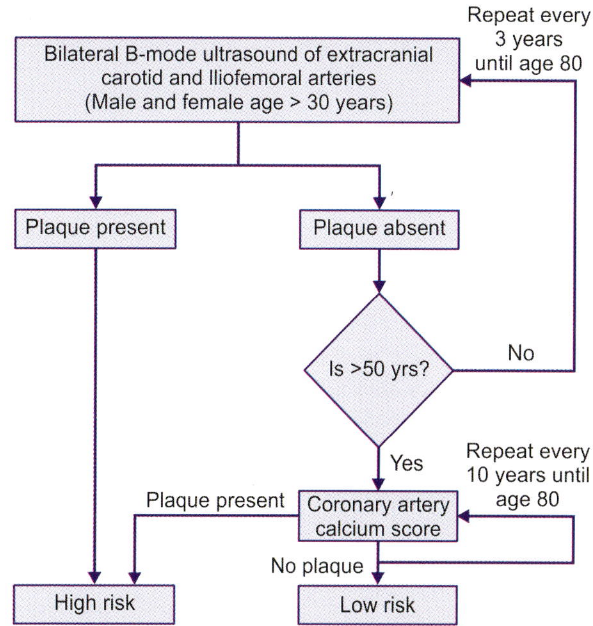


**Figure 23.6:** B-mode ultrasound imaging should be the imaging test to supplement traditional risk factor assessment. Direct evidence of atherosclerosis (tissue damage from risk factors) can readily be assessed with B-mode ultrasound examination of peripheral arteries, especially in the younger population (<50 years). A coronary calcium score can be considered for individuals older than 50, if the ultrasound examination is negative.

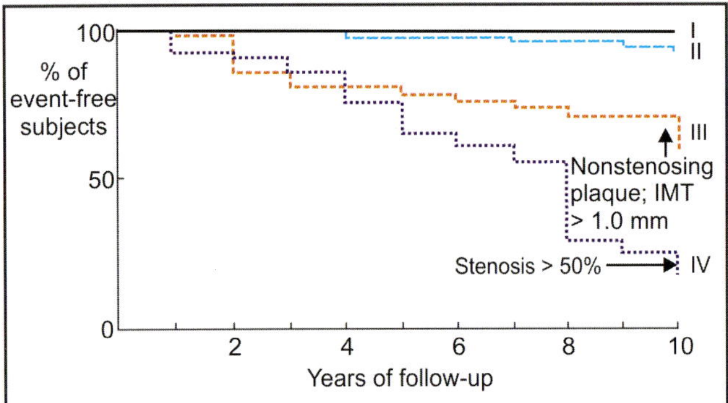


**Figure 23.7:** B-mode ultrasound of peripheral arteries and hard events.[32]

In a large outcome study of 10,000 relatively young asymptomatic subjects (mean age around 53 years) and a 10-year follow-up, carotid and femoral ultrasound identified 2011 subjects (20.1%) with atherosclerosis and predicted 98.6% of future cardiovascular events (MI, stroke, PAD) and deaths. This study of low-risk subjects further concluded that those individuals with a nonstenosing plaque (IMT >1.0 mm) in the carotid or femoral artery had a 10-year CVD event rate of 39% and that 43% of individuals with nonstenosing plaque progressed to a stenosing plaque.

*Abbreviations:* IMT, intima-media thickness; CVD, cardiovascular disease; MI, myocardial infarction; PAD, peripheral arterial disease. Adapted from Belcaro G, et al. Carotid and femoral ultrasound morphology screening and cardiovascular events in low risk subjects: a 10-year follow-up study. Athrosclerosis. 2001;156(2):379-87 (with permission).

admission and treatment for MI, stroke, peripheral arterial disease (PAD) and ultimately death from such events. Arterial wall morphology from ultrasound imaging was categorized into 4 classifications: Class I (normal IMT), Class II (elevated IMT), Class III (nonstenosing plaque), and Class IV (stenosis >50%). Kaplan-Meier plot of event rates for the 4 classes of arterial morphology is reproduced in **Figure 23.7**. This shows that almost 40% of the enrolees who had a nonstenosing plaque (Class III) developed a cardiovascular event within 10 years compared to only 0.13% from Class I (normal IMT). The event rate increased with each classification and 81% of the enrolees found to have stenotic plaque developed events within 10 years. This study further demonstrated that overall 11% of the population experienced disease progression, but none regressed. Progression accelerated with morphology classification; for example, 43% of the enrolees progressed from nonstenotic plaque (Class III) to developing stenotic plaque (Class IV) within 10 years. In view of these compelling data showing natural plaque progression (enrolees who developed symptoms or initiated medical treatment were eliminated from follow-up) and ASCVD event rate data on a relatively young asymptomatic population, the screening method of **Figure 23.6** is recommended. It should be further noted that for screening purposes, there is no need to perform the more complex Doppler examination to determine the level of stenosis. If stenotic disease is suspected (for example by listening for a bruit or other symptoms), that patient should be referred to a specialist for a flow study using Doppler ultrasound. The recommendation shown in **Figure 23.6** is for an examination based on B-mode ultrasound alone to identify plaque and measure IMT (Class I, II and Class III in the CAFES-CAVE Study terminology).

## METHODS

### Clinical Protocol

A protocol for performing bilateral B-mode carotid ultrasound examination for the assessment of subclinical atherosclerosis was published in 2008 by the American Society of Echocardiography, which was endorsed by the Society for Vascular Medicine, often referred to as the ASE Consensus Statement.[12] Basically, the recommended clinical protocol involves identification of focally elevated IMT (plaques) in the extracranial carotid system (including bulb and bifurcation) and measurement of IMT in the far-wall of the common carotid.

Subjects should typically be scanned in the supine position with the neck oriented 45° using a pillow or other similar support. B-mode ultrasound images should be captured with a linear-array transducer that has a center frequency around 7–9 MHz. Presence or absence of plaque should first be determined by acquiring images in the short-axis (transversal) view and then reconfirmed in the long-axis (longitudinal) view. The transducer should be moved in the cranial direction from the proximal common carotid (clavicle) to the highest segment above the carotid bifurcation that is accessible. If a plaque is found, it can be quantified or its presence simply notated on the image. For the second part of the examination, the transducer should be oriented in the long-axis (longitudinal) plane and IMT measured over a 1 cm region of the far-wall of the common carotid approximately 1 cm proximal to the flow divider. The actual IMT measurement can be performed in real time or offline with the aid of software that analyzes contrast of stored B-mode images, depending on the features of the ultrasound instrument. Care should be exercised in positioning and recording the transducer orientation angle, if repeat studies are to be performed. If needed, multiple IMT measurements can be made at predefined transducer orientation angles (anterior/mid/posterior). Cardiac timing should also be recorded so that IMT data are extracted from a known location within the cardiac cycle (typically end-diastole when IMT is maximum).

This protocol can easily be extended to examine the iliofemoral artery in which case the transducer is moved downwards from just below the inguinal ligament to approximately 2 cm below the bifurcation of the common femoral artery (CFA). If the adjacent common femoral vein obscures the image, it can easily be dealt with by a little compression maneuver. Plaques in the femoral artery are frequently found in the bulb and bifurcation in a similar manner as the carotid but the prevalence of plaques in the CFA is typically much higher compared to the common carotid. For illustration purposes, images from a carotid and iliofemoral examination are shown in **Figure 23.8A to E**.

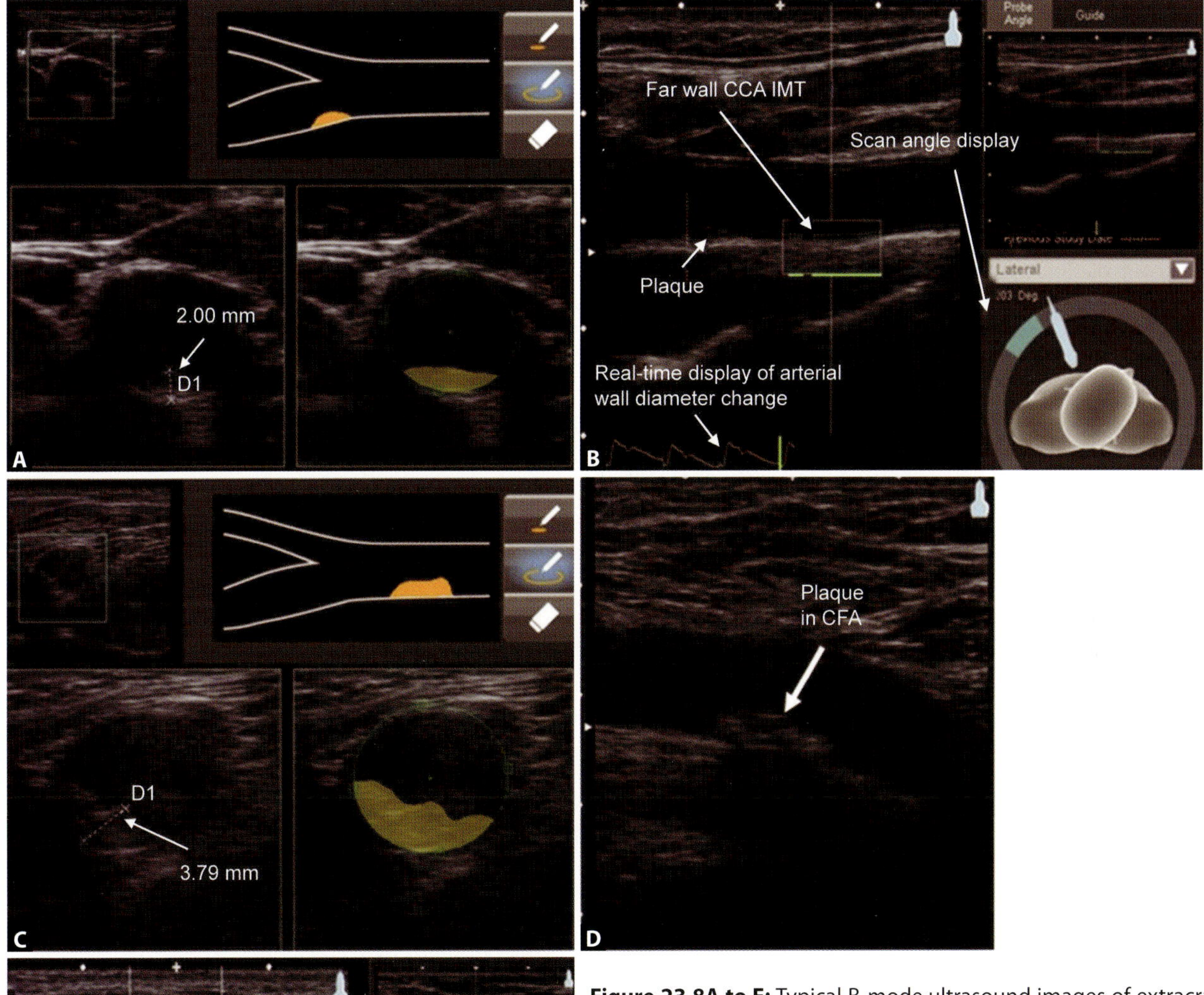


**Figure 23.8A to E:** Typical B-mode ultrasound images of extracranial carotid and iliofemoral artery. The extracranial carotid was scanned in the transversal plane (short-axis view) from the base of the common carotid artery (CCA) up through the bifurcation. An atherosclerotic plaque (focally elevated intima media thickness (IMT) protruding into the lumen by more than1.5 mm) was found in the bulb region, and this was marked up as illustrated in (A). The far-wall IMT of the common carotid approximately 1 cm from the flow divider was then measured and recorded in the longitudinal plane (long-axis view) as illustrated in (B). Similarly, the iliofemoral artery was scanned in the transversal plane from the common femoral artery (CFA) through to its bifurcation. A 3.79 mm plaque in the CFA was found as shown in (C). The same plaque in the longitudinal plane is shown in (D). The IMT of the CFA was measured approximately 1 cm from the flow divider in the longitudinal plane as illustrated in (E).
*Courtesy:* Panasonic Healthcare Co. of North America.

### Common Sources of Error in Intima-media Thickness Measurement

A comprehensive discussion on optimizing IMT measurement technique and reducing errors introduced by suboptimal imaging parameters is provided in the ASE Consensus Statement.[12] A few points are worth expanding upon as follows:

*Cardiac timing:* IMT changes continuously within the cardiac cycle. It decreases during systole owing to the larger arterial diameter and increases during diastole. The maximum IMT is typically at end-diastole. The reported variation in IMT within the cardiac cycle ranges from 4% to 10%.[33-35] This variation decreases with age and with the onset of atherosclerosis. In an unpublished investigation of 30 young and healthy volunteers (mean age 38 ± 6.2 years), intracardiac cycle variation in IMT was observed to be as high as 30% (according to Takenori Fukumoto). It, therefore, becomes paramount that cardiac timing is tracked during any IMT measurement. This can readily be achieved by connecting an external electrocardiogram to the ultrasound console and reading IMT from end-diastolic imaging frames. Some modern ultrasound instruments have such capability integrated into the console itself, see for example the Panasonic CardioHealth® Station.[36]

*Transducer angle:* The IMT can have significant variation circumferentially, especially as the individual ages or if atherosclerosis is present. In order to improve reproducibility of the measurements, IMT measurements at multiple transducer orientation angles are recommended, as outlined in the ASE Consensus Statement.[12] Transducer orientation angle can be determined by placing a protractor called the Meijer carotid artery arc around the patient neck.[37] In younger, healthier patients, circumferential variation in IMT is probably below the resolution of most ultrasound machines, so a single angle measurement may be adequate. Even in such cases, the transducer orientation angle should be recorded with a suitable device, if such capability is not already integrated into the ultrasound console.

*The IMT measurement:* Conventional diagnostic ultrasound imaging machines do not have adequate spatial resolution to illuminate the intimal layer. However, the lumen-intima and media-adventitia borders are seen with relative ease in modern B-mode ultrasound images. The distance between these two borders is called the IMT, which is typically around 0.40–0.70 mm in healthy adults. The axial resolution for a 9 MHz transducer is approximately 0.17 mm, which can contribute a significant amount of error in IMT measurements. Furthermore, some signal integrity is lost when raw ultrasound signal data are processed and converted to pixels displayed on the video screen with varying contrast corresponding to echo strength. This loss in signal integrity combined with limitations of pixel resolution can further compromise overall resolution of IMT measurements. For example, an 8-bit video display screen capable of displaying an ultrasound image to the depth of 8 cm will have a pixel resolution of 0.31 mm, making it difficult to measure IMT precisely. Most manufacturers now provide software tools that automatically identify arterial borders from stored imaging frames by analyzing pixel contrast. Such tools inevitably deploy interpolation to overcome pixel resolution limitations. A better technique is to process the raw ultrasound echo signal separately (before scan conversion) to extract IMT data. A few manufacturers have introduced such systems that process raw radiofrequency data to determine IMT with higher precision.

## FUTURE DIRECTION

### Miniaturization

Though ultrasound imaging has been used in large hospitals and academic centers for over 40 years, it has not realized its enormous potential in the primary care setting. In 2005, the then Chief Executive Officer of Sonosite (a manufacturer of hand-held ultrasound machines) claimed "that by 2010, the handheld ultrasound industry was going to be $1 billion and *half* of that was going to be in doing physical examinations".[38] Similarly, at a launch event for the ultra-portable GE V-scan in 2009, the Chief Executive Officer of the company proclaimed that GE was launching "a stethoscope of the 21st century".[39] In view of such stated grandiose claims, why does the use of ultrasound imaging equipment in the primary care market remain virtually non-existent? Unfortunately, manufacturers appear to be in the erroneous belief that size, weight, and possibly the cost of the equipment are the key barriers to mass adoption. This is evidenced by the plethora of low cost, "hand-held" ultrasound imaging instruments that have become commercially available over the past decade or so. However, these instruments fail to address the fundamental barriers to mass adoption: the need for expertise in acquiring ultrasound images and the need for expertise in interpreting these images. In academic centers and hospitals, highly trained sonographers acquire the data which in turn are interpreted by equally skilled radiologists and cardiologists. This overhead of expertise is perfectly suited for handling the relatively small number of patients who go on to develop ASCVD-related symptoms but is ill-equipped to handle the much larger asymptomatic population who would benefit the most from imaging technology to guide preventative interventions. To help translate ultrasound imaging methods for assessing atherosclerotic disease burden in the asymptomatic population from an academic curiosity to mass deployment requires technological improvements to automate plaque detection and quantification.

## Three-dimensional Ultrasound to Aid Automation

The emerging field of vascular 3-dimensional (3D) ultrasound, though interesting, does not have much clinical utility by itself. Vascular pathological findings are naturally 3D, which can lead to detection uncertainty when using conventional two-dimensional (2D) ultrasound. If an entire volume of interest is interrogated by the ultrasound transducer, a range of computer algorithms can be deployed to manipulate and analyze the volumetric data without introducing operator variability. Therefore, the fundamental role of 3D vascular ultrasound should be to automate plaque detection so as to enable less qualified personnel to administer the examination and interpret the results. Furthermore, volumetric data can be more readily used to quantify pathological findings. The resulting plaque quantification index will most likely become clinically relevant for monitoring response to medical intervention. Some of the considerations for making 3D vascular ultrasound clinically relevant include as follows:

*Transducer:* The best way to gather volumetric ultrasound data and correct for phase aberration error in ultrasound images is by a fully sampled 2D array that can be electronically steered and focused at an arbitrary spatial location. However, such highly complex transducers can be prohibitively expensive. An alternative transducer configuration involves mechanically translating a conventional linear transducer under computer control for volumetric image acquisition. The drawback of this approach is the increase in transducer weight and physical dimensions, which can limit access to anatomy of interest in certain patients. Lastly, volumetric imaging data can be acquired with a conventional linear array provided means are available for tracking free-hand movement of the transducer in multiple dimensions. The positioning information provides knowledge about imaging slice interval and its orientation. Computer algorithms can be developed to align contiguous imaging frames to reduce plaque quantification errors from 3D reconstructed data.

*Image artifact:* Differentiating between pathological findings and image artifacts remains a huge challenge. In arterial ultrasound scanning, the transversal view has been used as the preferred method for identifying focal lesions because it is less susceptible to imaging artifacts. However, image artifacts from refraction and reflection effects may still occur in this imaging plane, such as the acoustical shadowing from the edges of curved surfaces.[40,41] Such anomalies need to be corrected for automatically.

*Tissue interfaces:* Accurately determining the location of lumen-intima, intima-media, and media-adventitia boundaries poses a technical challenge because a certain amount of signal integrity is lost during the scan conversion process. Better algorithms need to be developed that allow analysis of higher fidelity raw radiofrequency data for more precise spatial localization of the arterial wall layers. This process can be fully automated to reduce operator dependency.

## Quantification

Clinical findings need to be presented in a standardized quantitative index that is easy to understand and that is actionable. To date, utility of elevation in IMT in the common carotid as an index of subclinical atherosclerosis has not succeeded as an independent determinant of adverse outcomes.[29] Total plaque area has been proposed as an alternative index,[42] but this method is heavily operator and equipment dependent due predominantly to variability of transducer orientation angle. The error in the measurement may not be so noticeable when examining relatively older patients who have large plaques, but for a younger population with smaller focal lesions, the measurement error might become prohibitively high. Sillesen et al. have recently reported carotid plaque burden as a new measure of subclinical atherosclerosis based on a bilateral examination of the extracranial carotid system with 3D ultrasound.[20] Though this is a step in the right direction, the method as proposed leads to significant quantification errors resulting from inherent image slice misalignment from free-hand movement of the transducer and unknown interslice interval. Improvements to the method were proposed by Bedi et al.[31] whereby free-hand transducer movement was optically tracked in 6-dimensions, and these tracking data were used to correct image alignment and provide known interslice interval for 3D quantification. Furthermore, summation of the intima-media volume (IMV) for 4 peripheral arteries over a standardized 5 cm segment that includes 2 cm distal and 3 cm segment proximal to the flow divider was notated as the FUster-Narula (FUN) Score, as illustrated in **Figure 23.9**. Presence of lesions in the CFA is far more frequent compared to the common carotid, which was the rationale for selecting a standard 3 cm segment proximal to the flow divider. The 2 cm segment distal to the flow-divider encompasses the bulb and approximately 1 cm region into the bifurcation, the segment of the artery that is particularly prone to developing atheroma. The FUN score notation included 4-dots representing each artery examined. A solid dot indicated that a plaque was identified in that artery (any IMT >1.5 mm). The rationale for separately notating plaque findings was to differentiate potentially comparable volumetric FUN scores in those individuals who have systemic elevation in IMT (and thus IMV) but no plaque from those who may have normal IMT but with focal plaque(s).

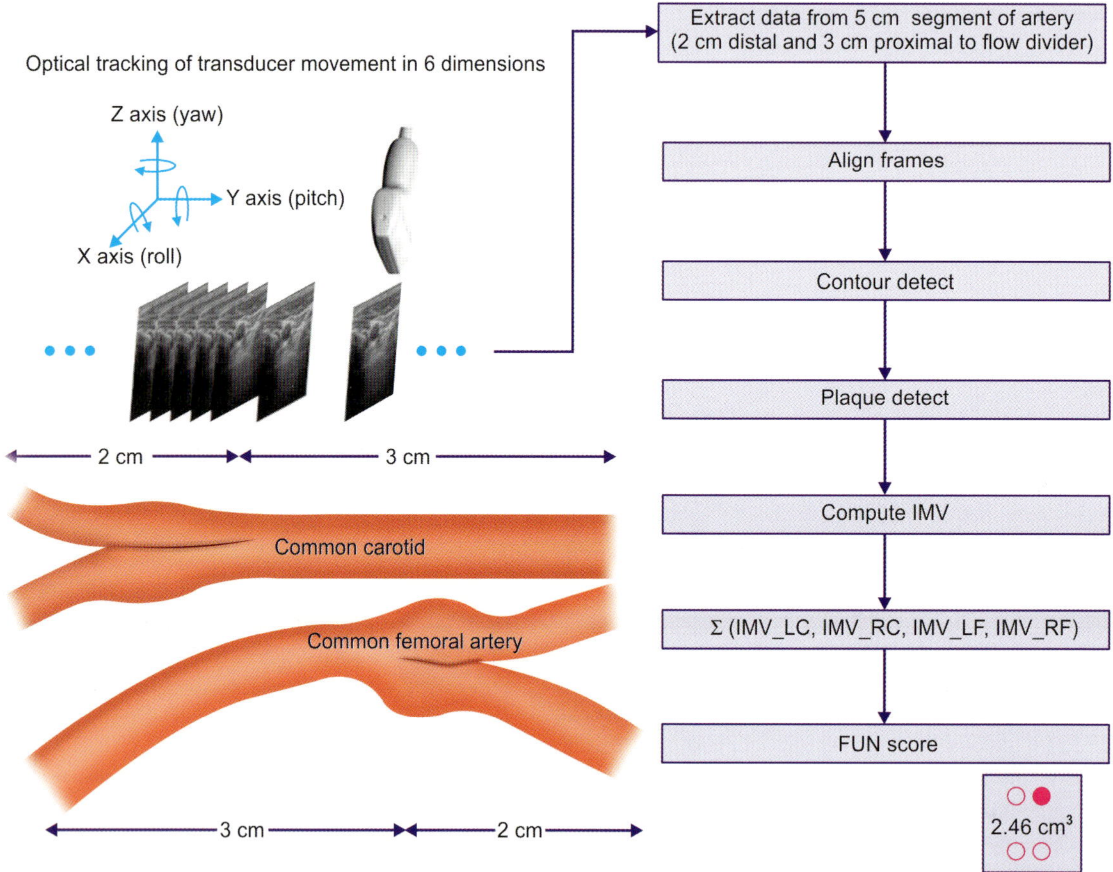


**Figure 23.9:** Quantification of atherosclerotic disease burden—the Fuster-Narula (FUN) score.[31]
The FUN score is a summation of intima-media volume (IMV) in 4 peripheral arteries (bilateral carotids and bilateral iliofemoral arteries) over a 5 cm segment that includes 2 cm distal to the flow-divider and a 3 cm segment proximal to the flow-divider. The presence of lesions in the common femoral artery is far more frequent compared to the common carotid, which is the rationale for selecting a standard 3 cm segment proximal to the flow-divider. The 2 cm segment distal to the flow-divider encompasses the bulb and approximately 1 cm region into the bifurcation, the segment of the artery that is particularly prone to developing atheroma. The FUN score notation includes 4 dots representing each artery examined. A solid dot indicates that a plaque was identified in that artery (any intima media thickness >1.5 mm).
*Abbreviations:* LC, left carotid; LF, left femoral; RC, right carotid; RF, right femoral.
Adapted from Bedi R, et al. Detection of subclinical atherosclerosis in peripheral arterial beds with B mode ultrasound A proposal for guiding the decision for medical intervention and an artifact-corrected volumetric scoring index. Global Heart. 2014;9(4):367-78 (with permission).

## VIGENETTE

Consider the case of a 58-year-old white healthy male who underwent a routine annual physical examination at a primary care clinic in Toronto. This individual was nondiabetic, had no known family history of premature cardiovascular disease, had never smoked nor taken medication to control blood pressure. Below is a summary of his risk profile:

| | | | |
|---|---|---|---|
| Resting blood pressure | = 110/78 | mm Hg | |
| Total cholesterol | = 4.50 | mmol/L | (174 mg/dL) |
| LDL cholesterol | = 3.48 | mmol/L | (136 mg/dL) |
| HDL cholesterol | = 0.97 | mmol/L | (38 mg/dL) |

A bilateral B-mode ultrasound of the extracranial carotid system revealed an elevated IMT in the far-wall of the right CCA of 1.15 mm. More importantly, this individual was also found to have a small non-stenosing plaque in the right carotid bifurcation measuring 1.8 mm. This individual had a 10-year Framingham Risk Score (FRS) of 9%, which is classified as low risk. Because FRS is <10% and LDL cholesterol is <5 mmol/L, this individual does not qualify for lipid lowering therapy according to the Canadian Guideline.[23] However, because he underwent "optional secondary testing", and a plaque was found, this individual qualifies for lipid lowering medication as illustrated in **Figure 23.10**.

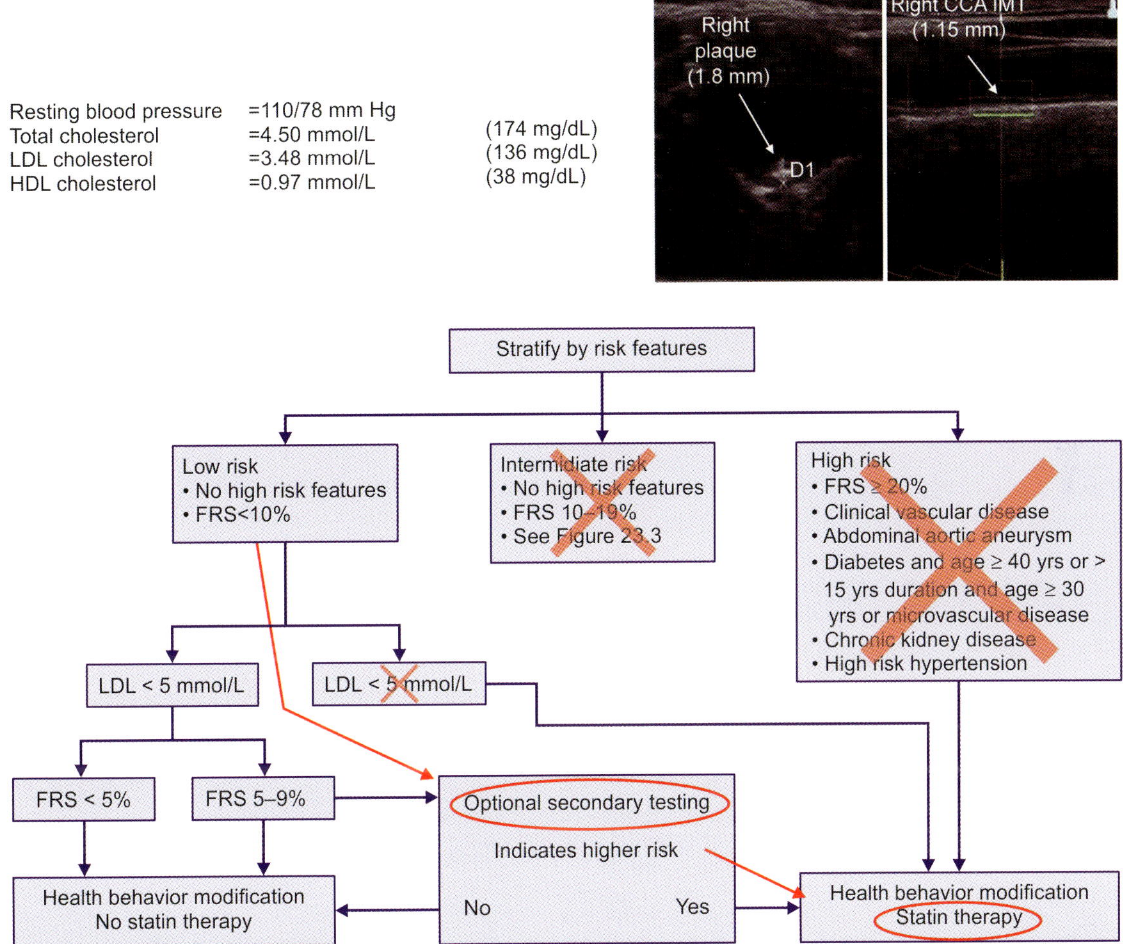


**Figure 23.10:** A Vignette to illustrate application of Canadian Atherosclerotic Cardiovascular Disease Prevention Guideline.[23] This 58 years old asymptomatic white male (nonsmoker) had a Framingham risk score (FRS) of 9% with no prior family history of premature heart disease. Since FRS was <10%, this individual was classified as low risk and because LDL cholesterol was <5 mmol/L, he did not qualify for statin therapy. His doctor ordered a precautionary B-mode ultrasound examination of the carotids as recommended by the Canadian Guideline (optional secondary testing). The results of the ultrasound study revealed a 1.8 mm plaque in the bulb of the right carotid and an elevated carotid intima media thickness (CIMT) of 1.15 mm. According to the Canadian Guideline, *"...Visible arterial wall plaques defined as a CIMT >1.5 mm or in the absence of plaque, CIMT values >75% for age and sex (generally >1.0 mm) are considered as evidence of subclinical atherosclerosis and are generally an indication for statin therapy..."* As a result of the ultrasound study, this individual was offered prophylactic statin therapy.

*Abbreviations:* CCA, common carotid artery; IMT, intima-media thickness; HDL, high-density lipoprotein; LDL, low-density lipoprotein.

Adapted from Anderson TJ, et al. 2012 Update of the Canadian Cardiovascular Society Guidelines for the diagnosis and treatment of dyslipidemia for the prevention of cardiovascular disease in the adult. Can J Cardiol. 2013;29(2):151-67 (with permission).

Similarly, the "adjunct" ultrasound imaging test would allow this individual to be treated to a LDL cholesterol goal of <100 mg/dL according to the criterion of ATP III[11] even though FRS <10%. In the ESC Guideline,[24] B-mode ultrasound examination remains at level IIa (meaning the test should be done). Because the test was done and a plaque was found, this individual would qualify for medical intervention irrespective of the risk profile (HeartScore). If one follows the Pooled Cohort Equations of ATP IV,[28] this individual has a 10-year ASCVD risk of 6.1% which is lower than the treatment threshold of ≥7.5%. As the ATP IV guideline does not recommend ultrasound imaging, this individual would have gone untreated. Having said that, because presence of carotid plaque has already been confirmed, which in ATP IV parlance means presence of "clinical ASCVD", this individual would be a "candidate for high-intensity statin"!

## CONCLUSION

A number of prominent articles in the literature have shown that there is a significant overlap in modifiable risk factors between those individuals who go on to develop ASCVD-related complications and those who do not. Therefore, guiding the decision for medical intervention based solely on traditional risk factor assessment needs to be improved. This need for improvement is particularly acute in developing countries, such as India where a much younger population is afflicted with the devastating consequences of ASCVD-related events. Various noninvasive imaging techniques can be used to improve risk stratification, but the most readily amenable to mass deployment in a primary-care setting is the inclusion of B-mode ultrasound. Diagnostic ultrasound imaging equipment is safe (nonionizing), noninvasive, mobile, and relatively inexpensive. The burden of expertise required to acquire and interpret images can be managed through judicious choice of equipment features and by limiting the technique to easily accessible anatomical windows, such as peripheral arteries (extracranial carotid and/or iliofemoral arteries). Though scientific articles attempting to correlate atherosclerosis in different arterial beds using a variety of imaging techniques (CAC, Angiography, CTA, MRI, ultrasound, etc.) form the basis for vigorous academic debate, from a practical perspective, the prognosis does not change. Pathological studies have already established that atherosclerosis is a diffused phenomenon and that intraplaque hemorrhage is a precursor to atherothrombotic events. Therefore, identification of atheroma in any arterial bed with whatever imaging technique indicates that that individual should be targeted for medical intervention. The method proposed in **Figure 23.6** whereby ultrasound is the "gatekeeper" to guiding the decision for medical intervention in conjunction with traditional risk factor assessment appears to be the logical and practical choice. Furthermore, the anomaly of USA-based ATP IV notwithstanding, most international guidelines for the prevention of ASCVD events support the idea of incorporating B-mode ultrasound imaging of peripheral arteries in routine clinical practice. Automation and overall image improvements over the past decade or so has made this technique clinically viable. Although quantification of atherosclerotic disease burden with further automation and 3D ultrasound remains a subject of vigorous research at present, the simpler 2D ultrasound method is adequate for initial identification of individuals who would benefit from medical intervention. The key message of this chapter is to find a plaque and treat it. Monitoring therapy effectiveness requires accurate quantification with 3D ultrasound which may become routine in the near future.

## REFERENCES

1. World Health Organization. Cardiovascular diseases (CVDs). Fact sheet 317. WHO Media Centre 2011; Available at: *http://www.who.int/mediacentre/factsheets/fs317/en/index.html.* Accessed August 9, 2012.
2. World Health Organization. World Health Report 2003. Geneva: World Health Organization; 2003.
3. Singh S, Nagra A, Maheshwari P, Panwar R, Hecht H, Fukumoto T, et al. Rapid screening for subclinical atherosclerosis by carotid ultrasound examination: The HAPPY (Heart Attack Prevention Program for You) Substudy. Global Heart. 2013; 8:83-9.
4. Castelli WP. Lipids, risk factors, and ischaemic heart disease. Atherosclerosis. 1996;124:S1-9.
5. Sachdeva A, Cannon CP, Deedwania PC, et al. Lipid levels in patients with coronary artery disease: an analysis of 136,905 hospitalizations in Get With The Guidelines. Am Heart J. 2009; 157:111-7.e2.
6. Leeder S, Raymond S, Greenberg H, et al. A Race Against Time: The Challenge of Cardiovascular Disease in Developing Countries. New York, NY: Trustees of Columbia University; 2004.
7. Reddy KS, Yusuf S. Emerging epidemic of cardiovascular disease in developing countries. Circulation. 1998;97:596-601.
8. Yusuf S, Hawken S, Ôunpuu S, et al., for the INTERHEART Study Investigators. Effect of potentially modifiable risk factors associated with myocardial infarction in 52 countries (the INTERHEART study): case-control study. Lancet. 2004;364: 937-52.
9. Goenka SPD, Ajay VS, Reddy KS. Preventing cardiovascular disease in India: translating evidence to action. Curr Sci. 2009; 97:367-77.
10. Greenland P, Abrams J, Aurigemma GP, et al. Prevention Conference V: beyond secondary prevention: identifying the high-risk patient for primary prevention: noninvasive tests of atherosclerotic burden: Writing Group III. Circulation. 2000;101:E16-22.
11. National Cholesterol Education Program (NCEP) Expert Panel on Detection, Evaluation, and Treatment of High Blood Cholesterol in Adults (Adult Treatment Panel III). Third Report of the National Cholesterol Education Program (NCEP) Expert Panel on Detection, Evaluation, and Treatment of High Blood Cholesterol in Adults (Adult Treatment Panel III) final report. Circulation. 2002;106:3143-421.
12. Stein JH, Korcarz CE, Hurst RT, et al. Use of carotid ultrasound to identify subclinical vascular disease and evaluate cardiovascular disease risk: a consensus statement from the American Society of Echocardiography Carotid Intima-Media Thickness Task Force. J Am Soc Echocardiogr. 2008;21:93-111.
13. Roman MJ, Naqvi TZ, Gardin JM, et al. Clinical application of noninvasive vascular ultrasound in cardiovascular risk stratification: a report from the American Society of Echocardiography and the Society of Vascular Medicine and Biology. J Am Soc Echocardiogr. 2006;19:943-54.

14. Mitchell JR, Schwartz CJ. Relationship between arterial disease in different sites: a study of the aorta and coronary, carotid, and iliac arteries. Br Med J. 1962;1:1293-301.
15. Young W, Gofman J, Tandy R, et al. The quantitation of atherosclerosis. III. The extent of correlation of degrees of atherosclerosis with and between the coronary and cerebral vascular beds. Am J Cardiol. 1960;8:300-8.
16. Fernandez-Britto JE, Wong R, Contreras D, et al. Pathomorphometrical characteristics of atherosclerosis in youth: a multinational investigation of WHO/World Heart Federation (1986e1996), using atherometric system. Nutr Metab Cardiovasc Dis. 1999;9:210-9.
17. Berenson GS, Srinivasan SR, Bao W, et al. for the Bogalusa Heart Study. Association between multiple cardiovascular risk factors and atherosclerosis in children and young adults. N Engl J Med. 1998;338:1650-6.
18. Shah PK. Can carotid plaque predict coronary plaque? JACC Cardiovasc Imaging. 2013;6:1168-71.
19. Cohen G, Aboufakher R, Bess R, et al. Relationship between carotid disease on ultrasound and coronary disease on CT angiography. JACC Cardiovasc Imaging 2013;6:1116-7.
20. Sillesen H, Muntendam P, Adourian A, et al. Carotid plaque burden as a measure of subclinical atherosclerosis: comparison with other tests for subclinical arterial disease in the High Risk Plaque BioImage study. JACC Cardiovasc Imaging. 2012;5:681-9.
21. Sosnowski C, Pasierski T, Janeczko-Sosnowska E, et al. Femoral rather than carotid artery ultrasound imaging predicts extent and severity of coronary artery disease. Kardiologika Polska. 2007; 65:760-5.
22. Touboul PJ, Hennerici MG, Meairs S, et al., for the Advisory Board of the 3rd Watching the Risk Symposium 2004, 13th European Stroke Conference. Mannheim intima-media thickness consensus. Cerebrovasc Dis. 2004;18:346-9.
23. Anderson T, Gregoire J, Hegele R, et al. 2012 Update of the Canadian Cardiovascular Society Guidelines for the Diagnosis and Treatment of Dyslipidemia for the Prevention of Cardiovascular Disease in the Adult. Can J Cardiol. 2013;29:151-67.
24. Perk J, De Backer G, Gohlke H, et al. European Guidelines on cardiovascular disease prevention in clinical practice (version 2012): the Fifth Joint Task Force of the European Society of Cardiology and Other Societies on Cardiovascular Disease Prevention in Clinical Practice (constituted by representatives of nine societies and by invited experts). Eur Heart J. 2012;33: 1635-701.
25. Beach KW, Hatsukami T, Detmer PR, Primozich JF, Ferguson MS, Gordon D, et al. Carotid artery intraplaque hemorrhage and stenotic velocity. Stroke. 1993;24:314-9.
26. Lal BK, Beach KW, Sumner DS. Intracranial collateralization determines hemodynamic forces for carotid plaque disruption. J Vasc Surg. 2011;54:1461-71.
27. Greenland P, Alpert JS, Beller GA, et al. 2010 ACCF/AHA Guideline for Assessment of Cardiovascular Risk in Asymptomatic Adults. J Am Coll Cardiol. 2010;56:e50-103.
28. Goff DC Jr, Lloyd-Jones DM, Bennett G, et al. 2013 ACC/AHA guideline on the assessment of cardiovascular risk: a report of the American College of Cardiology/American Heart Association Task Force on Practice Guidelines. J Am Coll Cardiol. 2014;63:2935-59.
29. Den Ruijter HM, Peters SA, Anderson TJ, et al. Common carotid intima-media thickness measurements in cardiovascular risk prediction: a meta-analysis. JAMA. 2012;308:796-803.
30. Lorenz MW, Polak JF, Kavousi M, et al. Carotid intima-thickness progression to predict cardiovascular events in the general population (the PROG-IMT collaborative project): a meta-analysis of individual participant data. Lancet. 2012;379: 2053-62.
31. Bedi R, Nagra A, Fukumoto T, et al. Detection of subclinical athersclerosis in peripheral arterial beds with B-mode ultrasound: a proposal for guiding the decision for medival intervention and an artefact-corrected volumetric scoring index. Global Heart. 2014;9367-78.
32. Belcaro G, Nicolaides AN, Ramaswami G, et al. Carotid and iliofemoral ultrasound morphology screening and cardio-vascular events in low risk subjects: a 10-year follow-up study (the CAFES-CAVE study(1)). Atherosclerosis. 2001;156:379-87.
33. Meinders JM, Kornet L, Hoeks PG. Assessment of spatial inhomogeneities in intima media thickness along an arterial segmnet using its dynamic behavior. Am J Physiol Heart Circ Physiol. 2003;285:H384-91.
34. Cinthio M, Jansson T, Persson HW, et al. New non-invasive method for intimi-media thickness and intima-media compression measurements. IEEE Ultrson Symp. 2005:385-8.
35. Van Bortelm LM. What does intima-media thickness tell us? J Hypertension. 2005;23:37-9.
36. See *http://us.panasonic-healthcare.com/product/cardiohealth-station/*.
37. Bots ML, Evans GW, Riley WA, et al. Caortid intima-media thickness measurements in intervention studies. Stroke. 2003;34:2985-94.
38. Piper Jaffray & Co. 17th Annual Healthcare Conference, January 25-27, New York, USA.
39. *http://usatoday30.usatoday.com/news/health/2009-10-21-pocket-ultrasound_N.htm*
40. Rubin JM, Adler RS, Fowlkes JB, Carson PL. Phase cancellation: a cause of acoustical shadowing at the edges of curved surfaces in B-mode ultrasound. Ultrasound Med Biol. 1991;17:85-95.
41. Steel R, Poepping TL, Thompson RS, et al. Origins of the edge shadowing artefact in medical ultrasound imaging. Ultrasound Med Biol. 2004;30:1153-62.
42. Spence JD, Eliasziw M, DiCicco M, Hackam DG, Galil R, Lohmann T. Carotid plaque area: a tool for targeting and evaluating vascular preventive therapy. Stroke. 2002;33: 2916-22.

# Index

Page numbers followed by *f* refer to figure and *t* refer to table.

## I



## K



## L



## M



## N



## O



## P

## R



## S



## T

## V



## W